What Every Woman Should Know about Cervical Cancer

Nenad Markovic • Olivera Markovic

What Every Woman Should Know about Cervical Cancer

Revised and Updated

Second Edition

Springer

Nenad Markovic, M.D., Ph.D
Global Academy for Women's Health, Inc.
Medical Center Drive
Rockville, MD, USA

Olivera Markovic, M.D., Ph.D
Education
Global Academy for Women's Health, Inc.
Rockville, MD, USA

Additional material to this book can be downloaded from http://extras.springer.com.

ISBN 978-94-017-7559-5 ISBN 978-94-017-7560-1 (eBook)
DOI 10.1007/978-94-017-7560-1

Library of Congress Control Number: 2016950190

Printed on acid-free paper

This Springer imprint is published by Springer Nature
The registered company is Springer Science+Business Media B.V.
The registered company address is: Van Godewijckstraat 30, 3311 GX Dordrecht, The Netherlands

To Our Family

In memory of our wonderful parents
Dr. Trajko & Mila Saljinski and
Prof. Svetomir K. & Olga Markovic,
for raising us to search for truth, their
magnificient devotion to the family
and their love.

Our dear children Svetomir & Mila with love
and hope they will continue our legacy.

Message from the Authors

Every woman should know that among 4000 women she will meet within 1 year, one will certainly have cervical cancer and that she might be this one woman, if she does not participate in regular cervical cancer screening.

During the lifespan while she is at risk (between 20 and 60 years of age), this chance is increasing to 1:10. Having the HPV disease, not the infection only, doubles the chance. At the same time, if detected on time, cervical cancer is completely a preventive disease – after removal of the suspect lesion, the woman is cured.

These statistical assumptions make the cervical cancer screening and removal of suspect lesions one of the most important additions to women's health and well-being.

But knowledge is power, and this power could and should be learned to be executed. Books are only tools that can help readers to improve themselves. The will is the essence of the conduct. The new edition is designed to move the will of women at risk for cervical cancer.

Foreword to the 2016 Edition

In the Afterword of the 2008 Edition, the authors have emphasized the impact different strategies, new tools and subsequent guidelines – promoted by those who think it is their duty to recommend such guidelines – have made to the clinical practice developed to prevent the occurrence, to postpone the development, to facilitate therapy and palliation and to reduce suffering of subjects affected by cervical cancer.

The authors also have responded to the Call to Stop Cervical Cancer promoted by WHO (IARC) in 2008, whose one challenge, "To develop concerted action against cancer of the cervix," is still a very actual one. In 2008, the stance of the authors was to "keep the tradition until the new option proves its superiority."

Since, in between two editions, none of the proposed options proved its superiority to the standard Pap test (as measured by clinical outcomes), the authors have decided to introduce, in this new edition, their experience with MarkPap technology products, which in lieu of growing application of modern IT technology, telemedicine and mobile health seem to be the methodology of choice to move the ailing cervical cancer screening towards new horizons.

The following chapters/articles will present these new ideas:

- MarkPap Test – advantages and weaknesses
- Smart biomarker and digital imaging
- ITTHC and mobile opportunity
- Networking with medical image information
- Screen & Treat, WHO recommendation for one day resolution of cervical lesions, if present
- MEDYKO and one day Screen/Intervention Cycle

Proposal for a New Strategy for LMIC based upon US experience and MarkPap tools provided for specimen self-collection, specimen preparation, staining, reading, and interpretation, together with recommendation for on-site management of women with abnormal specimens.

Between Two Editions

It has been 7 years since the book *What Every Woman Should Know About Cervical Cancer* has been published. The first edition was published as a compendium of information about cervical cancer necessary for women to know and to understand the disease in order to make educated decision and to be equipped with arguments to advocate about their health. The selected format was a monograph with personal experience being added to the medical information.

The expectation that this goal will be achieved was supported by the immense success of the cervical cancer screening campaign in the USA (1945–2005), where the negative trends of increase of cervical cancer prevalence and mortality were reversed into positive trends and both mortality and prevalence have been reduced by 80 % in 60 years of application. This success was undoubtedly related to the successful Pap test – the entire procedure including screening, diagnosis, and removal of lesions that can develop into cervical cancer.

Unfortunately, our book was not followed by proposals for change of health policy around the world and/or with offerings of new tools to enable the application of the new strategy. The cervical cancer market has been driven by the actual needs of local healthcare providers, who have been demanding tools for delivery of acute healthcare services. Cervical cancer prevention with cervical cancer screening, as it happened in the USA, needs large social actions like the cervical cancer campaign led by the American Cancer Society and supported by the US Congress. Without such support, the local healthcare providers are powerless, and women alone cannot help themselves.

This is why the current situation in the world is unacceptable for the twenty-first century.

In 2014, there were 7.33 billion people in the world, 2.5 billion women were at risk for cervical cancer, and only 20 % were protected by any type of cervical cancer screening (frequently substandard procedures); much more resources were spent on diagnosis and treatment for no results than it was invested in prevention for cure. Saving a woman's life is not only her problem, it is a problem for the entire society because women are not only tools for reproduction of population, but they are also competent, although not yet equivalent, partners for improving the society's life by participating in economic and social growth. This aspect will be addressed in more details in the new edition.

The period between 2008 and 2014 has been characterized by fast-growing hopes that cervical cancer could be eradicated (due to HPV immunization and HPV testing) and also the fast balancing of this enthusiasm with the reality check that cancer is something more than a mere viral disease. Anyhow, during this period, HPV testing was improved with methods to assess separate (e.g., oncogenic) strains (16, 18), and testing for HPV was added to cytology screening, to VIA and to colposcopy.

Many competent institutions and professional societies in the USA, usually considered as authority for cervical cancer screening, have responded to this new situation and have changed, adjusted, or improved their guidelines for cervical cancer prevention, particularly, for screening for early lesions indicating possible cervical cancer growth.

Among them, the American Cancer Society (ACS, 2012), American Society for Cytopathology (ASC, 2014), American Society for Colposcopy and Cervical Pathology (ASCCP, 2010), American College for Obstetrics and Gynecology (ACOG, 2009), National Cancer Institute (NCI, 2014), US Preventive Services Task Force (USPSTF, 2012), Centers for Disease Control (CDC, 2012), Centers for Medicare Medicaid Services (CMS, 2014), and the World Health Organization (WHO Guidelines, 2013) have revisited their prior recommendations and came with new guidelines. They are presented in the new edition.

We have reviewed the prior and the updated new guidelines, and we found the following major changes that might have impact on cervical cancer screening practices and, probably, to the prognosis of future cervical cancer in the USA and, maybe, the world.

- Classic Pap smear remains as the basic reference and control test.
- Liquid-based Pap tests (ThinPrep, SurePath) have not produced convincing advantage versus the Pap smear to favor its replacement.
- Testing for HPV is to be reduced to only those strains which are connected to cervical cancer (16, 18).
- It is largely recommended that the period between testing is expanded from annual to between 1 and 3 years – many specific recommendations are given to selected age groups. We prefer annual screening and more sensitive but less harmful tests (perhaps, biomarker-based pathocytological assays).
- Clinical trials should rely more to the robust endpoints than to the surrogate endpoints as currently it will improve the value of the results and their inference.
- We have not found more attention given to modern IT, nor to the improvement of Papanicolaou staining with or without new biomarkers. This lack of attention needs to be addressed, because, as we think, both biomarkers and IT are the core of future cervical cancer screening and preventive medicine applied for cervical and cancer at large.

The most important myth generated after the success of Pap test was declared, and also the major target for those who would like to replace it or to join it partially, is the exacerbation of the cost of Pap test. The myth that Pap test is expensive must be analyzed and then rejected. Below is the first attempt in this direction.

The myth that Pap test is expensive is not true. The test itself – smear preparation, staining, and interpretation – is simple; it may take 1–2 h and the result is ready for reporting. However, the cost is increased because of the following:

- Specimen collection – medical doctor who must examine the subject and perform the pelvic exam
- Expert cytotechnologist and/or pathologist on site to read cytology information and to classify and report the findings
- Colposcopist (gynecologist) on site to validate (confirm) diagnosis
- Needs a medical doctor on site to receive the results and to decide about further procedure and management of women with abnormal specimens

All of this cost is eliminated by using MEDYKO™ (see below in Chap. 6).

These topics are addressed elsewhere in our new edition.

Once we completed these conclusions, the question arises on how to present the actual guidelines. Obviously links or only summaries with references will not have the impact as full guidelines. We decided to present them as originally published by their authors and to get permission for including them here by the publisher. Anyhow, in our new edition, we reserve a full chapter for presentation of the cervical cancer screening guidelines in effect after 2008 until 2015 (Chap. 4).

Tribute to the Readers and the Followers of Our Work

The book *What Every Woman Should Know About Cervical Cancer* is our major publication, but it is not the only one. We were very active in communicating our ideas and achievements via publications, e-mail, or websites (www.bioscicon.com and www.markpap.com) and participating at various scientific and business meetings; promoting ideas in brochures, general public articles in proceedings and daily papers, as well as communicating directly with those who have expressed interest in our ideas, the strategy, and the tools meant to facilitate the application of the strategy.

In the period between 2008 and 2015, we have been very active communicating with scientists, professionals, students, and business and lay people all around the world. In response to many requests, we decided to expand this book with new chapters presenting the true information about different technologies – now in practice for cervical cancer screening – and to give women other options to educate themselves for a better decision on which way to go and what technology to ask for themselves and their families and friends.

Since a book is usually the most comprehensive compendium of answers to all questions, we have added the following new chapters: Chap. 4 “Cervical Cancer

Screening After 2008," Chap. 5 "Global Cervical Cancer Screening," Chap. 6 "New Strategy and Its Global Application," Chap. 7 "New Tools," Sect. 7.1 "MarkPap® Illustrated," Sect. 7.2 "Information Technology Telehealth Center (ITTHC)," Sect. 7.3 "The New Integrative Complex MEDYKO," Sect. 7.4 "Template for Telecytopathology," "Compendium of Guidelines Published Between 2008 and 2014," "Annex with Published Brochures, PPP," and "Media with Video Presentations of the Topics in This Book."

Between the two editions, one important fact has gained more appreciation: the value of outreach. The success of Pap test in America was achieved only when the percentage of screening participants had increased to more than 50 % of women at risk. At this crucial point, the ever-increasing trends of cervical cancer prevalence and mortality in the USA have reversed, and the trend continues to decrease while the outreach stays above 50 %. However, this success was achieved by healthcare providers, US Federal Government, health insurance, and health industry working in concert to provide public and professional education, to develop a national strategy, and to provide tools (infrastructure, equipment, personnel, and supply) to implement mass cervical cancer screening.

This understanding lacks in many developing countries which struggle with cervical cancer-induced problems, and their strategies are failing while the outreach stays low (at average below 20 %).

Fortunately, in case of cervical cancer screening, there are two robust measuring endpoints, the prevalence and mortality which cannot be influenced by many surrogate success/failure endpoints, and the true situation is easily obtainable. The general excuse that the mass cervical cancer is costly and unaffordable in many countries is also not true because of the current availability of modern IT and telemedicine tools and strategies.

Our new edition is dealing with this problem around the world (examples), and we hope, with this new text, to initiate reconsideration of the problem by the policy makers and to inspire them to adjust their policy to new conditions – which are now more favorable for women's protection than ever before.

About the Book and the Authors

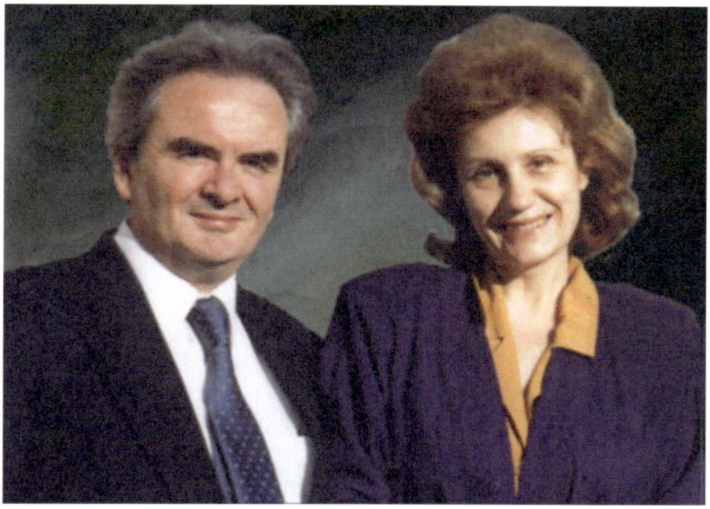

During the 2006 Annual Meeting of the American Association for Cancer Research (AACR) in Washington, D.C., we had the pleasure to meet Dr. Cristina Alves dos Santos, Senior Publishing Editor, Cancer Research at Springer, NL. Discussing our work on cervical cancer screening which was presented at the meeting and how we came to our discovery, Dr. Dos Santos suggested that we consider submitting a manuscript to Springer for publishing.

In the beginning, we thought it would be interesting to write more about us, our work together as a husband-wife team, how we came to these discoveries, and how we proceeded with translational research and brought them from an idea to products.

However, this idea, no matter how attractive it seemed, had to be replaced with the actuality of the momentum – the necessity to provide women with a reference book to help them better navigate among new dilemmas and multiple options that modern medicine was offering.

What happened between the 2006 Annual Meeting of the AACR and our decision to write the book *What Every Woman Should Know About Cervical Cancer*? In 2006, the FDA approved the first HPV vaccine (Gardasil by Merck) and raised everybody's hopes for successful prevention of cervical cancer. It turned the accent from cytological screening to HPV testing and to molecular testing – a logical extension to include detecting viral particles. These molecular biology-related ideas called for a substantial increase of cervical cancer screening cost, and the funds-sensitive health insurance companies sounded alarm. The first signs of the worst solution appeared when Kaiser Permanente, accepting the new technology, recommended extending the periods between two cytological screenings for cervical cancer.

At that time, we were studying the relation between conventional Pap smear and the newly recommended liquid-based technologies in order to position our biomarker-based test to serve women's need best. One of the striking results from this study was the conclusion that the frequency of screening (annually) is probably better related to the success of Pap test (reduction of mortality from cervical cancer for 85 % in the USA) than the testing technology or false readings that have been a widely accepted argument against the Pap test. Recommending to extend the inter-screening periods was an alarming sign signaling to a danger that women could be again insufficiently protected against cervical cancer. More evidence-based information was needed to prevent an unwanted outcome.

We decided to use this opportunity and to write a book with emphasis on health education, a book that will synthesize the new achievements and will present them in the context of basic facts and prior advancements. Dr. dos Santos liked this idea, and when she accepted the proposed synopsis and contents of the book, we started to work. This is how the book *What Every Woman Should Know About Cervical Cancer* was born as a one-stop cervical cancer resource for women. Presenting medical concepts in plain terms with readily available advices, we thought we could help women:

1. To increase the awareness of risks and the availability of methods to prevent cervical cancer
2. To educate them of available cancer control measures: how to detect early curable precancerous disease and stop the cancer before it appears
3. To show them how to seek for appropriate help when cancer is diagnosed

This triad was intended to help women to promote their health, to ask educational questions from doctors, and to participate actively in their disease treatment, when needed.

Having experience with cancer patients and motivated by the current open forums, list-services, and chats on the Internet among women with precancer and cancer, we decided to devote more space in this book for discussions on the emotional, humane side of the problem of how to cope with the disease (Chap. 3). Since many women are interested in complementary medicine, we have chosen to include some carefully selected topics (e.g., relaxation and stress release, eating for optimal health, etc.). Dr. Olivera Markovic, having experience as a university health professor and being acquainted with the needs of health instructors and students, complemented the text to make the book useful for an academic environment. Dr. Nenad Markovic, an experienced oncologist, enriched the book with critical thinking on medical aspects of cervical cancer prevention (including HPV vaccination), control (past, current, and new screening methods), diagnosis (colposcopy, biopsy, histology), and therapy (surgical, radiotherapy, and chemotherapy), with emphasis on controversies and hopes created with the introduction of HPV vaccination. We hope these additions will be of benefit for medical personnel, students, and doctors.

The anticipated story about the authors had to be limited to their joint but abbreviated biography. Drs. Olivera and Nenad Markovic are peers, collaborators, and husband-wife lifetime partners. This was decided when they met in high school as best students in their generations and started and finished medical school on the same day in their hometown, Skopje, Macedonia, former Yugoslavia. They were supported by their wonderful parents. Mr. Svetomir Markovic, Nenad's father, was a renowned educator and professor of mathematics, and his mother Olga devoted her entire life to the family. Dr. Trajko Saljinski, Olivera's father, was DVM and Ph.D. in veterinary microbiology and senior scientific state counsel and director of the State Institute of Microbiology. He inspired her to love science since she was a little girl spending a lot of time with him in the laboratory. Her mother Mila, a talented vocal and instrumental artist and professor, ignited a love for music. Olivera was enrolled since age 6 in the school of music studying piano for 8 years.

After finishing their medical studies, Olivera and Nenad already married planned together their further education and specializations (residency and fellowships). Nenad decided for clinical medicine and specialized internal medicine, hematology, and oncology. Olivera decided for research and teaching and specialized medical biochemistry. At that time, they were immediately hired at the University Medical School in Skopje: Nenad at the University Clinic of Internal Medicine and Olivera at the Institute of Biochemistry, where they began their academic career as assistant professors. Nenad had his residency in internal medicine at the University of Skopje, at the University in Belgrade and later at the University of Lund, GH in Malmo, Sweden. There, working with Prof. Dr. Jan Waldenstrom, he discovered his affection for studying cellular structures and their functional meanings – a step that has influenced his further career. Olivera decided to postpone her specialization becoming a mother of their first child, Svetomir. She then completed the specialization in medical biochemistry at the University in Skopje and at the University in Belgrade. Soon after that, their second child, daughter Mila, was born.

At this time, Olivera was awarded the Fogarty International Research Fellowship at the National Institute of Health, Bethesda, Maryland. The family with two small children and a nanny arrived in Bethesda, Maryland. Olivera started her fellowship at the National Institute of Arthritis Metabolism and Digestive Diseases (NIAMDD) with Dr. N. Raphael Shulman as her mentor. Nenad soon was accepted as a clinical associate at the Leukemia Service, National Cancer Institute, to work with Dr. Edward Henderson.

Olivera started with her research on the maturation and differentiation of megakaryocytic-platelet blood lineage and discovered the importance of the change of the megakaryocytic acid phosphatase isoenzyme spectrum along the lineage maturation. This work was later published in *Blood* together with Dr. Shulman and attracted a lot of scientific interest. Nenad implemented his experience from Malmo and was able to define several image analysis principles that are currently in use in digital image processing. It was an unforgettable time full of hard work, excitement, and scientific achievements. NIH became a second home to Drs. Markovic. At that time, they both started their doctoral dissertations.

After returning to Yugoslavia, they continued their graduate education working with Academic Professor Dr. Stanoje Stefanovic (Nenad) and Academic Professor Dr. Lubisa Rakic (Olivera). They both later defended their doctoral dissertations at the University in Belgrade. Nenad also completed the requirements for subspecialties in hematology and oncology. Olivera has already completed her specialization in medical biochemistry.

Soon, Nenad was awarded the NIH Fogarty International Research Fellowship at the National Cancer Institute, and the whole family moved again to Bethesda. Olivera's mentor, Dr. Shulman, offered her a position as visiting scientist to NIH. At NIH, Nenad and Olivera had the opportunity to work together on molecular imaging and quantitation of biologically active substances, primarily enzymes and their kinetics inside single cells. Together with their American colleagues, they pioneered in the application of image analysis in biomedicine. This was again a productive time full of hard work, discoveries, and publications, but also an amazing time working in the unique atmosphere at NIH meeting new colleagues and friends.

After the second stay at NIH, Olivera and Nenad again returned to the former Yugoslavia to transfer their knowledge and experience in their home country. Nenad continued with his practice, introduced the first leukemia protocols in Yugoslavia, and became head and later director of the University Clinic for Hematology at the University in Skopje.

Olivera developed a new clinical laboratory service at the University Children Hospital and became chief of Clinical Laboratories.

They continued their collaboration with NIH through scientific projects and joint programs involving young people. Nenad became the president of the Association of Yugoslavian Oncologists. At this position, he organized the National Congress with international participation and coordinated efforts of multiple specialists who were involved in providing healthcare in the field of oncology to create a unique policy that was accepted at the Congress. Later, this policy became a Resolution for Management of Malignant Diseases declared by the Federal Assembly of Yugoslavia.

In the follow-up to this Resolution, Drs. Markovic moved to Belgrade and Novi Sad where Nenad started to work on the implementation of this Resolution. With the full support of the Yugoslav Government, Nenad began developing a new cancer institute in Novi Sad, a copy of the NCI in Bethesda. This work was fully supported by the NCI and the US Government who prepared the feasibility study for this development. As a part of the same concept, Olivera developed a new drug and diagnostic test discovery and research laboratory in the University Clinical Center of the University of Belgrade. She was promoted head of the Laboratory for Research and Development at the University Clinical Center in Belgrade.

They both advanced as university professors and continued their joint research, published numerous publications, and participated as presenters, moderators, and organizers on national and international scientific meetings and congresses. To fulfill the Resolution's goals related to education, Nenad created the educational programs for undergraduate and graduate students which were adopted as the regular curriculum for medical studies in the School of Medicine, University of Novi Sad. Professor Dr. Nenad Markovic became the first chair of oncology in the whole of Yugoslavia. Unfortunately, this development was interrupted by the political disintegration of Yugoslavia (1990–1993), and Drs. Markovic returned to the USA where they had established their second residency and where their children were studying.

Between 1983 and 1993, Drs. Markovic were working on both continents being invited as visiting professors at Penn State University, the University of Pennsylvania, and Medical College of Pennsylvania (MCP). During that time, Dr. Nenad Markovic developed the first English medical school at the University in Novi Sad. The medical school was organized according to the curricula of MCP and the requirement of the ECFMG. The affiliation was built between the Belgrade and Novi Sad medical schools and MCP, with joint academic programs and exchange of students and faculties. The contribution provided by Dr. Walter Cohen, the president of MCP, Dean Dr. Alton Sutnick, and the chairman of the Department of Pharmacology Dr. Jay Roberts from the US side was crucial for the success of this affiliation. The school is still active, but the affiliation with MCP stopped by the same reason as the program for developing a national cancer center – political interests were stronger than the public needs for protection from cancer.

In the 1990s, the whole family moved to the USA and continued their scientific and academic careers. Their son, Svetomir, finished medical school and graduate school at MCP and his residency in internal medicine and hematology/oncology at the Mayo Clinic, Rochester, MN. He continues his brilliant career as a physician and researcher, partner, and associate professor at the Mayo Clinic. Their daughter Mila, a talented young lady, graduated from business school and became a business expert in the health insurance industry. She is living with her family in Toronto, Canada. Following the tradition of her mother and grandmothers, Mila is also a devoted parent to our grandson Michael. We are very proud of our children.

Olivera and Nenad continued working together and returned to Washington, D.C., metro area. Nenad joined the Food and Drug Administration, and Olivera continued teaching at universities and colleges in the Metro Area (University of Maryland at College Park, American University, Georgetown University). Besides basic medical science courses (biology, human anatomy and physiology, biochemistry, and pathophysiology), she also enjoyed teaching different health courses (women's health, personal and community health, drug use and abuse, and strategies in stress release). Dr. Olivera Markovic is still an active professor.

In the late 1990s, Drs. Markovic became troubled by the reports of Pap test diagnostic failures, law suits that followed, and laboratory liability and decided to respond to the call for improvement of Pap test technology issued by NIH, NCI Consensus Conference on Cervical Cancer in 1996. They recognized that in their research, they have discovered something that might be helpful to ameliorate this situation, and they decided to explore this option for the benefit of American women in a short term and for the benefit of all women in the long-term planning. This is how they began working systematically on the cervical acid phosphatase (CAP). They found that this isoenzyme molecule is exclusively present in abnormal cervical precancerous and cancerous cells and that normal cervical epithelial cells are entirely negative on Pap specimens. They succeeded to visualize this biomarker of cellular abnormality as an intracellular red insoluble deposit on the bluish Papanicolaou-stained background. Making the abnormal cells more visible with the biomarker, they aimed to alleviate the disadvantage of Pap test related to the high percentage of false-negative results (because of missing abnormal cells). This is how cervical acid phosphatase-Papanicolaou test, the CAP-PAP test, was born and patented in the year 2000. In the meantime, Olivera decided to incorporate with BioSciCon, Inc., the R&D biotech and consulting company, to proceed with this research. Nenad joined later.

The NIH recognized the potentials of the new test and supported BioSciCon with SBIR Phase I and Phase II grants. Again, with the support of NIH, their alma mater, they conducted a translational research on 2000 patients from the general population and women at high risk and showed that the MarkPap® test (trademark for CAP-PAP test) is more accurate, faster, and less expensive. The test was given to a manufacturer to prepare a kit for in vitro diagnostic procedure, and the entire development is now awaiting the FDA approval for marketing in the USA. BioSciCon, Inc., appeared at the NIH success stories page (http://grants1.nih.gov/grants/funding/sbir_successes/155.htm).

The new biomarker also opens a new prospective for telemedicine, MarkPap® Digital (future Tele Pap test). Using an easy-to-use MarkPap Kit, specimens can be processed in a small laboratory or doctor's offices by a low-trained technician or a nurse. Since the abnormal cells are already marked red with the biomarker, the same person could see those cells in the microscope and immediately transmit their images to a laboratory with specialists for final evaluation. The result may be returned within hours. It means that the Pap test could be made available around the world bypassing the need for developing an expensive infrastructure. Drs. Markovic are currently working on the development of MarkPap® Digital.

There is one more important barrier for providing the Pap test globally and save women's lives. Women do not get screened not only because there is no Pap test accessible to them or they cannot afford it. They may have other restraints, like cultural/religious traditions preventing them to visit a gynecologist, or they are simply afraid of a pelvic exam and feel uncomfortable with it. In the USA, there are currently 20 million women who know about Pap test and have this test available, but do not take it. For all of them and the women around the world, our ultimate goal is to develop a self-sampling test, MarkPap® Self (future HomePap). It is the presence of the biomarker that opens this prospective, which has been impossible to accomplish until now. MarkPap® Digital and MarkPap® Self are expected to make the cervical cancer screening available to all women in the world. HPV vaccination and biomarker-based cytological cervical cancer screening, like MarkPap test, open realistic hopes for the eradication of cervical cancer in the twenty-first century.

In order to accomplish this last task in their lifetime efforts, Dr. Olivera Markovic recently incorporated with a nonprofit organization, *Global Academy for Women's Health, Inc.* (www.GAWH@markpap.com). The Academy's mission is the advancement in education and science for women's health. The book *What Every Women Should Know About Cervical Cancer* is the first accomplishment of the Global Academy for Women's Health, Inc.

Drs. Markovic currently reside in Rockville, Maryland, USA, and continue with their research. Until today, they authored more than 200 publications including books, chapters in books, invited lectures, scientific publications and presentations, and patents. Their current activity is devoted to the research and development of their proprietary MarkPap technology, writing and teaching, and hoping that thousands of women around the world will benefit from their hard work and devotion. This will be their legacy.

Drs. Markovic's biographies can be found in several bibliographical records, e.g., *Marquis Who's Who in America*, *Who's Who in the World*, *Who's Who in Science and Engineering*, *Who's Who is Healthcare*, *Who's Who of American Women*, and in *The International Bibliographical Centre, Cambridge, England.*

The New Edition

The new edition covers the period between 2008 and 2015. This period was characterized with substantial changes in concept of cancer prevention, diagnosis, and treatment.

The mass cervical cancer screening for all 2.5 billion women at risk worldwide became the most wanted goal, and the new technology employing electronic devices promised that this goal could be achieved in the near future.

The basic changes and the new ideas are subject of this new edition. Indeed, it is a revised and updated edition, but because of these new issues, it had to be expanded.

The new book contains a prologue and an epilogue, 7 chapters, many sections, and articles. It is now enriched by original text of guidelines and images of new technologies and PowerPoint presentations on how they work. A few videos are added in the Annex to explain some important topics to large audiences.

Although designed as a monograph – a book presenting the personal opinion of their authors – this edition has plenty of information presented in their genuine form, which can be used as reference to the important topics discussed and challenged in the book.

Readers Testimonials

I live on the south of Europe, in Belgrade, Serbia. I am not a medical doctor, but I am witnessing tragic, horrible stories about women suffering from cervical cancer, some of them very close to me. Serbia is a small country in Europe but, unfortunately, leading in mortality and morbidity from cervical cancer. Every year 1400 women get cervical cancer, and 500 lose the battle against this disease. I also found that the situation is the same in the wider region. Now, as the campaign for cervical cancer prevention started, I had a chance to obtain statistical data (not only from Serbia but for the whole region) that during the last 5 years, majority of women had not visited gynecologists' offices and have not had their Pap test done. In general, about two thirds of women do not have a regular gynecological exam. The purpose to investigate women's health situation in my country was the book *What Every Woman Should Know About Cervical Cancer* authored by Drs. Olivera and Nenad Markovic.

Questions started to pile up, e.g., why in the country, with an ancient culture having civilized kingdom in middle ages, whose churches and monasteries are under the UNESCO protection, which had hospitals in the twelfth century with instructions for a proper diet, and why the health education and health culture are on such low level. It is also a paradox that Serbia has excellent widely recognized medical doctors and scientists, but women ask for help when the time between the diagnosis and the end is so short. Dark and cruel Balkan history cannot be the only lasting alibi. In my opinion, the level of health culture is due to insufficient health education. A very thin connection exists between the elite and sophisticated science and the still conservative population, which are not open to each other for a variety of reasons.

Drs. Olivera and Nenad Markovic's book is a big discovery for me. It shows how to connect "difficult theories" of the science and "nontheoretical" mind of the general population. Two brilliant scientists, doctors, and professors have taught us a lesson that should be remembered. In the beginning, I scheduled doctor's appointments for myself and started to remind other women. The acceptance was beyond every expectation.

The unique feature of this book is the fact that it communicates equally successfully with health professionals and with those who are not, systematizing and broadening the professional material and, at the same time, giving to the general audience a proper "curable dose" of facts: carefully chosen and precisely defined subjects that expose problems and provide systematic and clear answers transfer the reader in the zone of sufficient understanding. This book "caught" me and kept me very interested to read everything until the last page. The discovery of a biomarker of cervical abnormality that I named B.M. "Olivera" is spreading in Belgrade because it has a universal value.

I think that what brings an extraordinary value to this book is putting the problem of cervical cancer on the existential level in its psychological and social aspects. With this, the authors have created a universal matrix which unites and organizes all elements for the fight against cervical cancer. I learned from this book, the way to transform endless paralytic energy of fear and despair (that every diagnosis of cancer is a deadly verdict) into a positive energy of fighting against the disease that creates hopes.

The problem is particularly delicate with cervical cancer which provokes multiple frustrations, guilt, and shame that leads to running away from the public scene to isolation and lowliness. The feeling of shame in a conservative environment is stronger than the feeling of fear. The essence of the book is demystification of cervical cancer, putting it together with other diseases which can be prevented, curing and cured IF detected on time.

With demystification of the disease, it comes to the public space where a patient has now a chance to talk about her problems and the disease and to share her worries with others. I have participated in this process so many times trying to give a hand and to help being a careful listener allowing the patient to tell me what she feels comfortable to tell. The attempt to cheer the patient, making her laugh, is sometimes successful, but sometimes it is not. However, real stories about real people with happy ending (particularly about women who the patient is acquainted with), a pleasant company that redirects the attention from the disease, a gentle hug, a small gift, a good book, or a flower would return maybe only for a moment a smile on a patient's face. In all these situations, I have a feeling that this support has an additional value: Those who provide support to cervical cancer patients are emissaries of the core idea of Drs. Markovic's book to bring encouragement and support. The book which these authors have given us is a real friend and companion.

Prof. Dr. Smilja Tartalja

Professor Emeritus
University of Belgrade
Belgrade, Serbia

Sir Francis Bacon said, "Knowledge is power," and when talking about cancer, knowledge brings a power that alleviates fear. After reading *What Every Woman Should Know About Cervical Cancer*, I came away from the book with a much better understanding of cervical cancer and with much less fear of it. As a lay person, who is also a veteran of breast cancer, I often find that it is difficult to read and understand medical books even when they are written for the general public. However, I found *What Every Woman Should Know About Cervical Cancer* to be highly readable. It approached the subject of cervical cancer not only from an individual woman's perspective but also from a global perspective of woman's health. It was very informative about why early detection is so vital and also presented ways to increase early detection of cervical cancer. The book arms women with valuable information in assessing cancer risk and common sense approaches to understanding our physiology. Of particular interest to me was the in-depth discussion of the widely available Pap test and its importance in screening for cancer, including the history of Pap testing from its discovery in the second half of the twentieth century to new technology such as MarkPap technology. Included in this segment is a frank discussion of the limitations of testing procedures including the troubling incidences of false-negative rates and ways to reduce those rates. The book also gives recommendations for women on how to discuss Pap test results with their doctors, something that every woman can benefit from. The book does not stop with just the physical side of health, however. In the final section of the book, there is a wonderful discussion of the mind-body connection and how important a positive, healthy mind-body connection is in promoting healing. I found the chapter on the stages of stress to be very illuminating and relevant not only for cancer patients but for everyone. This is a book I plan to recommend to my friends and relatives. I think it is a book that everyone would benefit from reading.

Educator
Rockville, MD, USA

Ms. Lenore Zahedi

Afterword to 2008 Edition

The manuscript for the book *What Every Woman Should Know About Cervical Cancer* was submitted for publishing on September 30, 2007. The next month, the *2006 Consensus Guidelines for the Management of Women with Abnormal Cervical Cancer Screening Tests* were published in the October issue of the *Journal of Lower Genital Tract Disease* and in the October 2007 issue of the *American Journal of Obstetrics and Gynecology.*

The major difference between these 2006 Guidelines and the previous 2001 Guidelines, recommended by the same consensus conferences, is (1) the introduction of HPV DNA testing in the primary screening for cervical cancer and (2) adjustments made in the management of women with HPV DNA +/– tests. The adjustments were necessary to limit the fast-mounting cost of cervical cancer screening caused by the HPV testing. It is important to note that the authors of this clinical practice guidance document in the preamble stated clearly "these guidelines should never substitute for clinical judgment" giving back the power of decision to doctors and ultimately to patients themselves. This statement is a great support to our book and to our objective to help women understand the value of testing and medical options and to become educated patients who could contribute to the right diagnosis and treatment of their own conditions.

In the follow-up, along with the promotion of HPV testing, many limitations were noted, and the regulatory agencies (FDA, CDC), professional societies (CAP, ASC, ASCP), and even manufacturers of HPV vaccines and HPV tests indicated that the annual cytological testing should be considered as the gold standard not as an unnecessary alternative to the more complicated new testing. The American Cancer Society (ASC) acknowledged the HPV testing, but did not change their 2003 *ACS Guidelines for Early Detection of Cancer*, where Pap test (cytological screening) is the pivotal laboratory instrument to measure women's risk for cervical cancer.

The introduction of HPV DNA testing into the primary screening has brought one big accomplishment; the Pap test is again recognized as the best test for cervical cancer control worldwide. Together with HPV vaccination (cancer prevention), the Pap test is becoming our hope for eradication of cervical cancer in the twenty-first century. This change of perception has set aside the work of WHO, IARC Cervical Cancer Screening Group, PAHO, PATH, JHPIEGO, and other members of the Alliance for Cervical Cancer Prevention who considered Pap test as an unaffordable luxury for cervical cancer screening in low-resource countries and recommended alternative methods such as visual inspection with acetic acid (VIA), DNA HPV testing alone, and/or one-visit screen-and-treat approaches. Now, Pap test (cytological cervical cancer screening) is again the first priority, but the new question is what type of primary screening to be used. All of these options are addressed in our book.

Another major event, already discussed in this book, was the introduction of HPV vaccines (Merck's Gardasil and GlaxoSmithKline's Cervarix). This accomplishment has risen hopes that cervical cancer could be prevented by global vaccination (eliminate the HPV viral strains that can cause cervical cancer by eliminating them from the population), and a lot of money and effort was given to recruit people worldwide to accelerate the access of vaccines to the developing world.

The difference, between the day the manuscript for this book was submitted and the day it is published, was made by an enormous effort given to support those universal noble hopes. Supported by Melinda and Bill Gates Foundation, PATH has launched worldwide marketing to raise awareness of the preventability of cervical cancer deaths among all women in the world (1.7 billion at risk). A *Call to Stop Cervical Cancer*, which has been a logo for this campaign, is now beginning to institutionalize these activities into marketing entities coordinated by PATH. More information is available at http://www.cervicalcanceraction.org.

We have joined the campaign *Call to Stop Cervical Cancer* with a wish to contribute to this noble cause providing women with evidence-based information, which could educate them for making better decision about their own protection from cervical cancer.

Namely, stopping cervical cancer with vaccination, today, is only a wish until more effective vaccines are developed. Current vaccines cover only four HPV strains (out of at least 100) and are intended only for sexually naïve girls. Once infected with HPV, a woman remains infected for life with a weak natural immunity that clears the clinical signs until reinfection or reduction of immunity occurs. The current vaccine cannot add to or change this immunity. New vaccines are necessary. We hope that in the twenty-first century, these technical barriers will be overcome and there will be vaccines for all types of HPV and vaccines or other immunotherapies for noninfected and infected women alike; but, this time has not come yet, and a caution is needed to prevent general public disappointment (with all negative repercussions) when vaccinated women will start getting cervical cancers. To prevent this disappointment, all agencies involved in cervical cancer prevention and control insist on keeping cervical cancer screening programs alive for the next 10, 20, and more years

On the 4th of February, World Cancer Day, the International Agency for Research on Cancer (IARC) has published the *2007 Annual World Cancer Data Update* and *2008 Cancer Challenges*. The first, among General Challenges, is "To prevent those cancers that can be prevented." Two specific priorities are also related with cervical cancer, "To implement what is known to reduce risk" and "To develop concerted action against cancer of the cervix."

The call for "concerted action" was long due. Today, we have available tools for successful cervical cancer control (cytological screening in different versions), and tools for cervical cancer prevention are in the beginning of promising development (HPV vaccination), but we lack a substantial progress in cervical cancer therapy – surgical removal of early lesions that could develop into cancer is still the only therapy providing cure. This is why IARC is highlighting cervical cancer prevention and control.

The *Call to Stop Cervical Cancer* is also dedicated to prevention and control. The programs for development of new vaccines and programs to increase the awareness of vaccine protection are under way and well organized. Cervical cancer control is entangled with some confusion because of different options. The major dilemma is which examining procedure and what type of laboratory technique to recommend for mass cervical cancer screening worldwide. The stance of this book is to keep the tradition until the new option proves its superiority. It means regular annual cervical cancer screening with a biomarker-based cytological test, similar to the conventional Pap test or liquid-based Pap with HPV testing in addition (if necessary).

We see our contribution in this direction with the development of Home Test and MarkPap® Digital, two options available only because of our biomarker previously discussed in this book. We also believe that the medical device industry and the healthcare providers will join our vision to do whatever is possible:

- To make the collection of material and primary screening more affordable and more comfortable for every woman via development of new devices (e.g., Home Test)
- To improve the accuracy of diagnosis by introducing telecytopathology digital screening procedures (based on biomarker-based cytology, digital imaging, and online communication) between field sites where specimen is taken and processed and the remote screening sites where digital images of positive specimens are examined

In addition to the better and new HPV vaccines, we expect these two accomplishments, Home Test and Digital Screening, to become operational new tools for response to the unmet goals summarized in the *Call to Stop Cervical Cancer* in the twenty-first century.

Acknowledgment

Our acknowledgments and gratitude go to the sponsors of this book: BioSciCon, Inc., Rockville, MD, USA, for both editions, and to Joseph E. and Marjorie B. Jones Foundation Washington, D.C., USA, for the first edition.

BioSciCon's mission is the improvement of women's health by saving women's lives and decreasing suffering from cervical cancer via developing new technologies for its prevention and control.

BioSciCon sponsored the formation of the Global Academy for Women's Health, Inc., a nonprofit organization dedicated to the advancement of education and science for promoting women's health around the world. This book is the first objective accomplished by the Global Academy for Women's Health, Inc. The Global Academy for Women's Health, Inc., is now the main sponsor of the second edition.

The Joseph E. and Marjorie B. Jones Foundation is a private, philanthropic institution dedicated to improving the quality of life for all people, particularly those residing in Washington, D.C., metro area, by funding medical research, supporting human services and healthcare initiatives, and furthering the cause of education. The Joseph E. and Marjorie B. Jones Foundation graciously provided a grant to the Global Academy for Women's Health, Inc.

Our sincere thanks to our reviewers: Acad. Prof. Ljubisha Rakic, M.D., Ph.D., Serbian Academy of Sciences and Arts, Belgrade, Serbia; Gary Peck, M.D., Director Cancer Prevention, Cancer Center, Washington Hospital Center, Washington, D.C., USA; and Edward Henderson, M.D. (internist, hematologist-oncologist), retired from NIH, FDA, and VA Administration, Buffalo, NY, USA.

The authors extend their appreciation to the publisher, Springer, the Netherlands: To Mrs. Cristina Alves dos Santos, Ph.D., Senior Publishing Editor, Biomedical Unit, who initiated the creation of this book by inviting us to submit it to Springer, for her support and to Ms. Melania Ruiz, Biomedical Unit, for her contribution during the preparation of the first edition of the book for publishing.

The support of Springer SBM NL Team continues during the second edition. We particularly acknowledge the guidance and help of the senior publishing editor, Ms. Melania Ruiz, and her senior publishing assistant, Ms. Ilse Kooijman.

Throughout the course of writing this book, many friends and colleagues, leaders in their fields, offered their support, enthusiasm, and insight, and we would like to extend our thanks to each of them for their contribution to this book.

We would like to express special gratitude and acknowledgments to a wonderful lady, who made a difference in our lives with her sincere friendship and support. This is Ms. Ann Dobbs, Counselor Emeritus of SCORE, Washington, D.C., Chapter. She was appointed counselor to our company, BioSciCon, Inc., more than 15 years ago. Under her guidance BioSciCon, Inc., became SCORE Client of the Year in 2005. She also played a major role in the incorporation and development of the nonprofit Global Academy for Women's Health, Inc. and became the company's first senior advisor continuing with this role after her retirement from SCORE. Close professional relationship flourished in a sincere lifetime friendship. And not only that, the Global Academy for Women's Health, Inc. is welcoming Ms. Logan Dobbs, Ann's granddaughter, as one of the next-generation leaders to continue our legacy in the years to come.

Professor Annie Dunn, Ph.D., partially edited the manuscript of the first edition, conducted the *Survey on Pap Test*, and contributed with a personal story. We also acknowledge Mr. Jim Grizzell for participating in the electronic *Survey*, Prof. Teresa Bevin for her support and contribution with a story, Dipl. Ing. Cvetko Saljinski for contributing with his artistic talent and knowledge of art photography, and Prof. Harriet Peck for participating in the editing of the manuscript of the first edition.

The authors would like to acknowledge the members of BioSciCon Cervical Cancer Study Group for their participation in the clinical trials on MarkPap test, which provided scientific evidence that was summarized and cited in this book. In particular, we would like to thank Dr. Lewis Townsend, the principal investigator of our Bethesda Clinical Site, who aided in the development of a new application of this test (MarkPap® Self). Our thanks go to Dr. James Sundeen and Dr. William Smith, the principal investigators of our laboratory sites in the state of MD, and to investigators and other members of this study group, Dr. Shelley Parr; Dr. Aruna Kumar; Christopher Kemp, Ph.D.; Dr. Alan Ross; David Hankins, Ph.D.; Ms. Pilar Mollish; Dr. Sasa Kadija; Dr. Vojislav Zizic; Ms. Milena Simic; Ms. Nalini Thavamoney; Dipl. Ing. Marjan Cotic; Dipl. Ing. Cvetko Saljinski; Shriniwas Katti, Ph.D.; Dr. Vladan Posarac; Oleg Panashchenko, Ph.D.; Mr. Peter Ricca; and Mr. Stephen McJonathan. We thank Mr. Alan Key, National Cervical Cancer Coalition, for his support.

After the first edition was published, motivated by the interest of both the general public and professionals, the authors continued with further R&D of MarkPap® technology, which particularly concentrated on developing countries. The reason was that, unfortunately, in spite of all investment and efforts and new approaches (like HPV detection and vaccination, automation), the situation did not improve significantly. The outreach for preventive measures against cervical cancer did not reach more than 10 % in most of these countries. For example, in India, out of 300,000M women at risk, only 20M are being protected.

Realizing that more than price of a certain test and lack of infrastructure at the points-of-care (POC) are responsible for this failure, they concentrated their efforts to further develop infrastructure-independent methodologies.

The first success was the development of the MarkPap Telecytopathology Service for diagnosis at distance. The success was not only with conventional digital technologies (MarkPap® Digital), even more with the possibilities to use cell phone camera for transmission of cytological images (MarkPapMobile, Mobile Pap).

During this period of R&D (2008–2013), the authors acknowledge the support of the Johns Hopkins University, Montgomery County Campus, and its executive director Ms. Elaine Amir to the Global Academy for Women's Health, Inc.

We are indebted to Dr. Oleg Panaschenko who provided his continuous extensive expertise and help as IT architect in the development of the IT Telehealth Centers and Mobile Pap and Mr. Stephen Mc. Jonathan, GT Vision, who provided the digital camera and supported the development of MarkPap® Digital.

Our acknowledgments go to Prof. Smilja Tartalja and Ms. Lenore Zahedi and Dr. Gary Peck and Prof. Harriet Peck for their encouragement and support.

We acknowledge the collaboration with Prof. Ganapathy, President, Apollo Telemedicine Network, India, for helpful discussions on telemedicine and joint attempts to organize the symposium on the new Strategy for Fighting Cervical Cancer in India, based on telemedicine, and Mr. Milan Zatakia, President and CEO of Millennium, for his helpful advises for introducing MarkPap technology in India.

Our special thanks go to Mr. Skipp Boyenga who helped, with his exceptional talent and knowledge, to design and maintain the Global Academy for Women's Health, Inc. website.

The authors would like to thank Mr. Connor Scalzi, a talented artist and video editor for editing our video presentations.

Contents

Introduction 2016

A woman should know that she could change her destiny, if she wishes and if she has the knowledge and tools to do so.

This book is about educating women how to gain knowledge which will empower them to better control their own destiny and the destiny of their children and family at large.

I am a medical doctor practicing internal medicine, hematology, and oncology for more than 40 years, who has spent the recent 20 years in the field of cervical cancer because my wife, Dr. Olivera Markovic, has discovered that female cervical epithelium contains a bioactive protein (biomarker) which may lead and help them to conquer the fear from cervical cancer, and we together decided to devote our lives to bringing this biomarker to benefit all women.

During this period, I've seen thousands of women coming to my office for help because of their concerns, fears, and physical and psychological problems mostly related to cancer. Very early, I learned that the best way to deal with their problems is to hear the patient's complaints, to examine carefully, and to teach them to understand the cause of their concerns and to help them decide the best treatment approach available. I also found how much profound knowledge of the human soul Hippocrates of Kos had (ca. 480–375 BC) who wrote, "In practicing his profession, a doctor can rarely cure, could improve the condition many times, but always must help those who ask for help."

Dr. Olivera Markovic is a medical doctor and a Ph.D. in biochemistry, who was practicing laboratory medicine, but has devoted the last two decades of her professional career to cancer research. She is also a lifetime educator teaching basic medical science, science, and health-related courses. During the recent years, she has taught women's health and related courses at local colleges and universities in the greater Washington, D.C., metro area, where she learned how her students were unprepared for health challenges the adult life is bringing to them and learned how focused education could be both appreciative and successful.

When, because of the biomarker, we both dedicated our lives to women's health, we realized that the best way to accomplish new goals is to combine our research in bringing this biomarker to benefit all women with an appropriate education to help them understand better the beauty and the risks of being a woman in the modern world and the opportunities that all women have to protect themselves from cervical cancer. It is sad and unacceptable that millions of women, mothers, wives, sisters, daughters, and granddaughters, still die from a preventable disease in the twenty-first century.

In the period when we were in dilemma what to do first came the 2006 Experimental Biology Meeting in Washington, D.C., where we met the Springer representative Ms. Christine dos Santos who inspired us to write a book for Springer who will make it available to all women worldwide.

In the meantime, a major change in the strategy for prevention of cervical cancer occurred. Two pharmaceutical giants, Merck and GSK, developed vaccines to immunize women against oncogenic strains of HPV. This achievement has raised hopes for more effective protection from cervical cancer. However, since there is a long way to go to reach those hopes (decades), in the meantime, the newest strategy for cervical cancer prevention placed the emphasis on the motto *no women should be left without cytological screening protection*. Today, cytological screening for cervical cancer (Pap test) is not widely available. Only less than 10 % of 1.7 billion women at risk have the opportunity to use this test in their developed and resourceful countries. The rest, most of them living in low-resource developing countries, does not have this opportunity. The World Health Organization and many governments all over the world are aware of the problems and are struggling to find ways to protect their female population with less expensive screening – but all efforts to replace the standard Pap test have not yet produced convincing results. The alternatives have not been shown to be at least not worse than the cytological testing.

Nevertheless, the news about vaccination has spread among women who are now increasingly asking whether, when, and how to immunize themselves and their daughters against cervical cancer. Because of the inaccessibility of the best cytological test, the cost of vaccination, uncertainty of long-term protection, ineffectiveness in all cancers, and many still unresolved questions but great hopes, the public is alerted, and women are upset which way to go and how. This is a perfect environment for a book like ours to bring a comprehensive insight to the problems as a basic knowledge and reference to websites where women will be able to follow the updated information.

Finally, because of the grave prognosis of cervical cancer, if not detected and treated on time, and the opportunity for cure if detected, and the early detection of cervical cancer or precancerosis, the Pap test became one of the most regulated medical diagnostic tests in the history. In addition to federal regulations (CLIA*88 and amendments), many consensus conferences issued guidelines and guidance for medical procedures designed for early detection of cervical cancer and for products to be used in those procedures. All these documents are in public domain and are available for review on the Internet. As much as this "openness" is important for public education, reading this literature without prior knowledge could be a source of unnecessary misunderstanding, frustration, and pain for readers. Our book will try to provide women with the basic knowledge, so they will read medical information with better understanding and, hopefully, will not regard the current medical strategies as biblical cannons, but as temporary recommendations made by groups of experts based on their best knowledge and understanding. Emphasizing the transition of rules, we would like to open a window that neither bad diagnostic news are always bad as they look nor the good news should always be accepted as a total relief – a certain degree of uncertainty must always be present and second opinion asked. This makes the difference between educated and non-educated patient and could be of importance for women to better protect themselves in their lifelong struggle to avoid cervical cancer or to cure it if the first goal was not achieved.

In the period between the two editions of this book, the clinical trials have become an important medicolegal tool for proving the safety and efficacy of the new medical devices and became the important criterion to measure the compliance of the healthcare service delivery.

Most of those clinical trials were designed as FDA Clinical Trial Phase III in which the new method/device was tested upon a well-establish and validated method versus a standard control method/device with intention to obtain objective data of the new device superiority, equivalence, or inferiority to the standard device. Standard statistical models were established and applied correctly.

The problem, however, rises with the control devices (used as standards).

While Pap test was clearly superior if measured with clinical outcomes (robust endpoints), many of the new devices have shown superiority in some or more laboratory and/or image parameters (surrogate endpoints) and, consequently, were approved for addition or even for alternative to Pap test.

This new policy has introduced more confusion than help, and comparison between screening or therapeutic methods and device supporting those methods became less clear.

This issue, with an attempt to clarify the truth, is discussed in the new edition.

As declared in the beginning, the new edition is the revised and upgraded first edition, which has been extended with several new issues; in particular, the emphasis was given to the New Strategy for Mass Cervical Cancer Screening Worldwide and to tools necessary to enable healthcare providers to implement this new strategy.

For the first time, this book treats the economic factors influencing mass cervical cancer screening and provides solutions on how to fund the crucial outreach of above 50 % of women at risk. This addition is important because it erases some of the myths that are holding wider application of screening methods in low- and middle-income countries; nonetheless, these countries have most needs for health assistance. In lieu of this view, our book could be considered as a contribution to the global efforts to reduce health discrepancies.

Chapter 1
The Female Reproductive System in Health and Disease

1.1 Basic Anatomy of the Female Reproductive System

Introduction to the structure of individual organs of the female reproductive system: Ovaries (egg and ovulation, the corpus luteum). Fallopian tubes. Uterus: The upper part, the body of the uterus (corpus uteri). The lower, narrower part of the uterus is called cervix of the uterus (cervix uteri). Structure of the uterus. Vagina, vulva and perineum. Supportive tissues.

1.1.1 The Ovaries

The ovaries are two small oval, almond-shaped glands ($4 \times 2 \times 1$ cm) located in the pelvic portion of the abdomen on either side of the uterus (Fig. 1.1a, b). They are attached to the uterus and the body wall by ligaments. Ovaries produce eggs, e.g., "ova" and secrete female sexual hormones estrogen and progesterone. The ovaries are covered by a single layer of epithelial cells and beneath this layer ova are produced. The baby girl is born with about 60,000 ova. Each of these ova has the potential to mature, but only about 400 of them mature for fertilization during women lifetime. The process of maturation takes place in a small sack with cells filled with fluid that is called ovarian follicle. As the ovum matures, the cells in the follicular wall start secreting estrogen. When the ovum matured, the follicle ruptures and expels the ovum out of the follicle. This process is called ovulation. The ovum is then swept into the fallopian tube and starts its journey towards the uterus. After the ovum has been expelled, the remaining follicle is transformed into yellowish body called corpus luteum. This structure continues to secret the hormone estrogen, and starts secreting the other female hormone, progesterone. In case the egg is fertilized it continues hormonal secretion for the next 3 months, when the placenta takes over; if fertilization does not take place, corpus luteum degenerates (Fig. 1.1a, b) [68, 80, 87, 158].

N. Markovic, O. Markovic, *What Every Woman Should Know about Cervical Cancer*, DOI 10.1007/978-94-017-7560-1_1

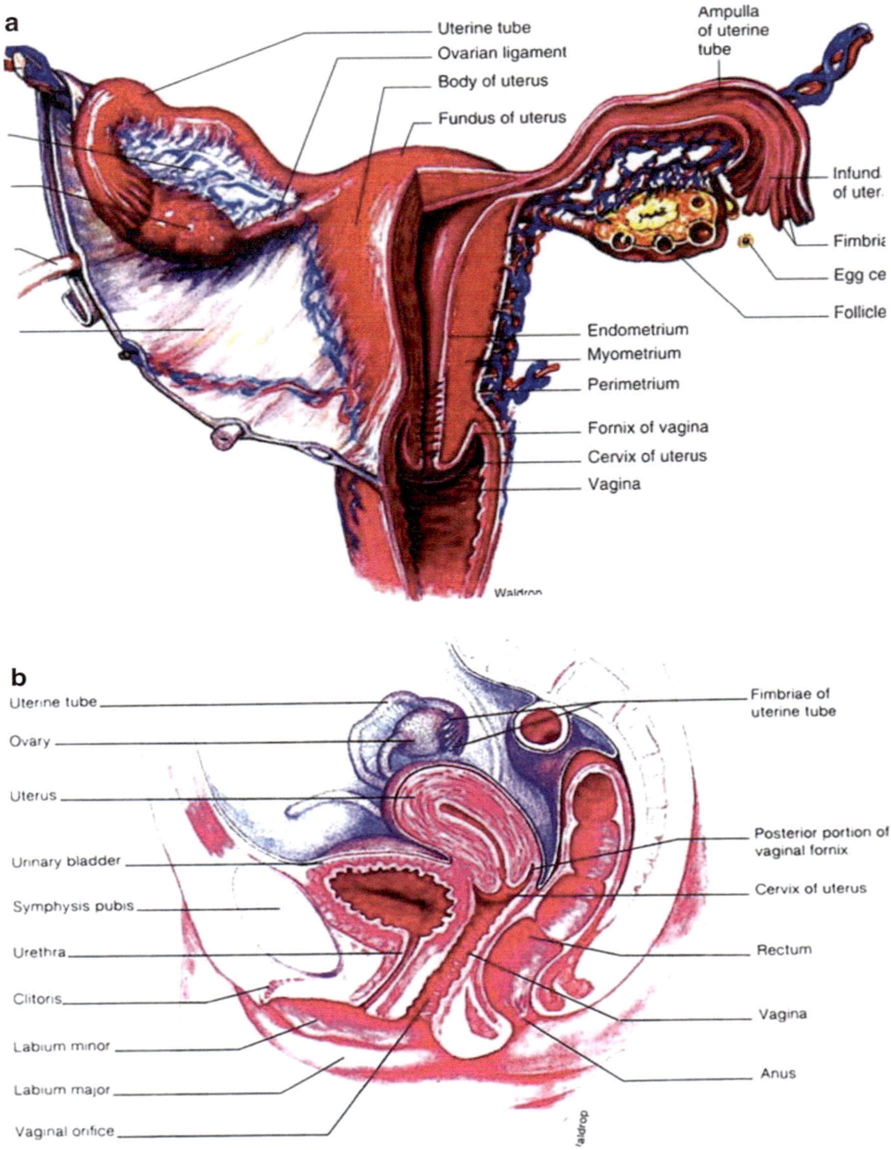

Fig. 1.1 Anatomy of the female genital system: (with permission of the McGraw Hill Companies). (**a**) Front view; (**b**) Profile; (**c**) External view; (**d**) Female reproductive physiology: The cycle of ovulation and menstruation (Prints are from the book *Human Physiology* by Stuart Ira Fox, 6th edition, McGraw Hill Publisher, 1999)

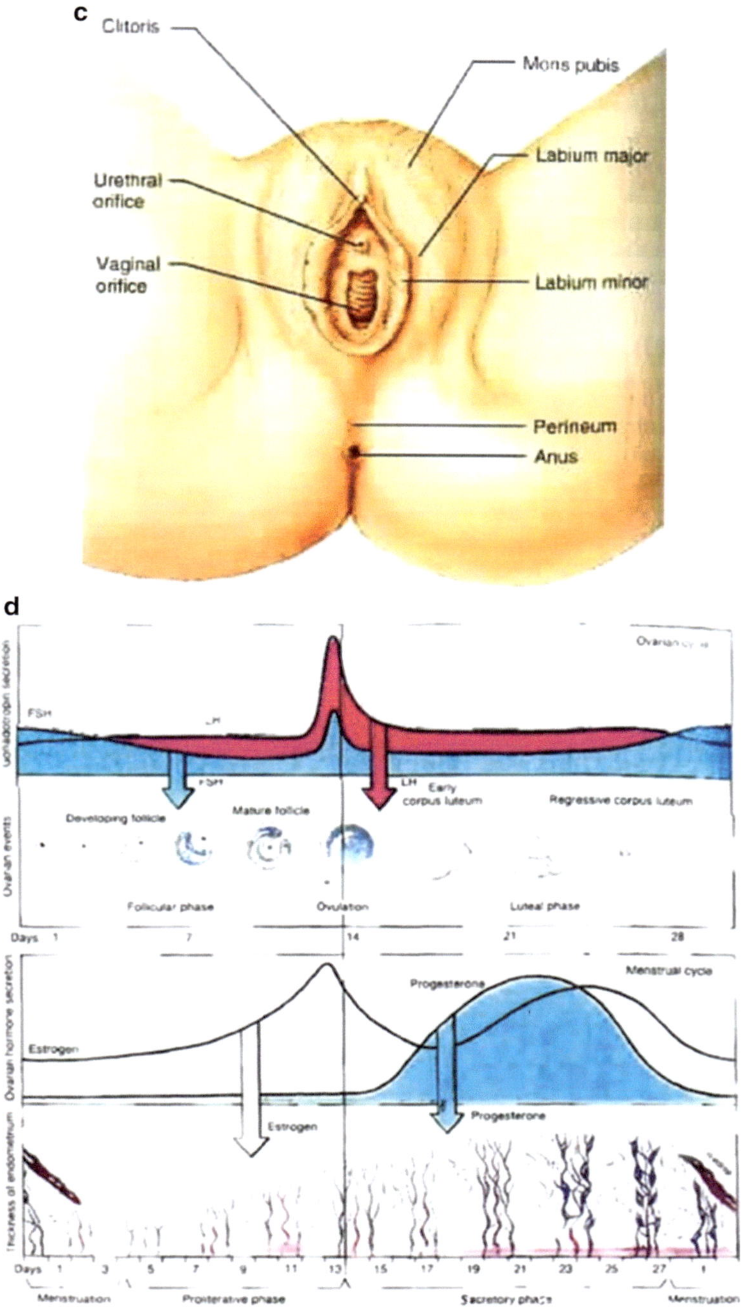

Fig.1.1 (continued)

1.1.2 Fallopian Tubes

Fallopian tubes (the oviducts) are funnel-shaped 12.5 cm long muscular tubes that lie in the pelvic portion of the abdominal cavity, reaching from the ovary to the upper part of the uterus (Fig. 1.1a, b). The ovarian end of the tube contains finger-like projections that sweep the ovum and the tube then carry it to the uterus. The lining of the tube is made of ciliated columnar epithelium and secretory cells. The beating cilia and peristalsis help move the ovum toward the uterus. After sexual intercourse, sperm swim up from the vagina, through uterus into the tubes and this is the place where the ovum meets with sperms and where the fertilization takes place. The secretions are nourishing the egg until it reaches the uterus (Fig. 1.1a, b) [50, 68, 80, 87, 158].

1.1.3 The Uterus

The uterus (the "womb") is a pear-shaped muscular organ (7.5′ 5.0′ 2.5 cm) located in the pelvic cavity behind the bladder and in front of the bowel (Fig. 1.1a, b). The wider upper portion of the uterus is called corpus uteri (the body of the uterus). The lower, narrower part of the uterus is called cervix uteri (neck of the uterus). It is a narrow 2–4 cm long cylindrical part of the uterus. The uterine cavity continues as the cervical canal, which opens into the vagina. The internal ostium (isthmus) of the cervix is where cervix opens into the uterus, the external ostium is where cervix opens into the vagina (Fig. 1.1a, b).

The uterus is composed of three layers. The endometrium (inner layer-lining of the uterus), the myometrium (thick smooth muscular layer) and perimetrium that covers the exterior of the uterus. The lining of the uterus is a specialized epithelium which is involved in menstruation.

The endocervical (inside cervix) lining is with cylindrical epithelium. However, there is a histological transition of the cervical epithelium along the cervical canal. It is called transitional zone between endocervical and endometrial epithelium (towards the internal ostium), and between endocervical and vaginal epithelium (stratified squamous epithelium, towards the external ostium). These transitional zones are usually the place where the abnormalities start. Cervical mucus is produced by the secretory cells of the endocervical glands. Cervical epithelium and the cervix also change during the menstrual cycle.

Supporting tissues, ligaments keep the uterus and the tubes in place. In most women the uterus is oriented forward at a ninety degree angle to the vagina [14, 50, 68, 80, 87, 158].

1.1.4 The Vagina

The vagina is a muscular tube, about 7.5 cm long connecting the uterine cavity with external genitals (Fig. 1.1a, b). The vaginal wall consists of three layers: The inner lining of stratified squamous epithelium, a thin smooth muscular and the outer layer. The lining of the vagina is a wrinkled mucus membrane supplied with numerous blood vessels, where extra blood is pumped when a women is aroused during intercourse. The folds permit enlargement during childbirth. The vagina also is an outlet for blood during the menstruation. A fold called hymen is found at the opening in virgins. Just above each side of the vaginal opening there are two vestibular glands. They secrete mucus at the opening of the vagina [50, 69, 87].

1.1.5 The Vulva and the Perineum

The external parts of the female reproductive system are vulva which consists of several female organs (Fig. 1.1c). This includes: a small pad of fat which protects the pubic bone and twofolds called labia major that protect the inner genitals. Just inside labia major, there are “small lips”, labia minor, which enclose the opening of the vagina. At the upper end is clitoris, a very small sensitive organ with numerous nerve endings, which fills with blood when a woman is sexually aroused. The orifice of the urethra, coming from the bladder, is located above labia minor. In the back, near the anus labia minor merge with the labia major. In front they converge to form a hood-like covering of the clitoris. Before starting sexual activities, virgins have a fold of membrane called the hymen found near the vaginal canal opening. The entire pelvis floor is called perineum (Fig. 1.1c) [50, 68, 80, 158].

1.2 Basic Physiology of the Female Reproductive System

Female hormones, menstrual cycle, pregnancy and menopause.

1.2.1 Female Hormones

It is very important to understand the normal function (physiology) of the female genital system in order to understand the diseased states (pathology).

The main female hormones are estrogen and progesterone. They are produced within the ovaries and will be described in the next section. Estrogen and progesterone, like all hormones, do not function alone but are under influence of other hormones: They are controlled by the hormones in the anterior pituitary gland (follicle-stimulating hormone-FSH and luteinizing hormone-LH) and are regulated by the hypothalamus. Hypothalamus is a part of the brain serving as a body's 'thermostat' and controlling many other important functions in the body. Gonadotropin releasing hormone–GnRH is secreted in the hypothalamus and controls the female hormone balance (activates the FSH an LH) from the anterior pituitary glands. All these hormones decrease and increase in a regular rhythm during the menstrual cycle (Fig. 1.1d) [30, 68, 78, 79].

1.2.2 The Menstrual Cycle

The normal menstrual cycle lasts 28 days at average, ranging between 22 and 40 days, counting the day one from the beginning of the menstrual flow. The changes (different phases) that appear in the uterus corresponding to the phases in the ovaries and the changing levels of ovarian hormones are presented on Fig. 1.1d. Hormones coordinate the ovarian and uterine menstrual cycle preparing the uterine lining (endometrium) for implantation of the fertilized egg and future embryo. The first episode of menstrual bleeding that female experience during puberty is called menarche. Puberty generally begins between 11 and 13 years of age and is completed by 16 years of age.

Uterine Phases In the absence of fertilization, the first phase of the uterine cycle is menstrual flow phase, during which menstrual bleeding occurs because of the shedding of the endometrium that is no longer necessary. Then the thin remaining endometrium begins to regenerate from its base and thickens – this is the proliferative uterine phase. The next uterine phase is the secretory phase, when the endometrium continues to thicken, become more vascularized and develops glands that secrete fluids rich in nutrients to protect the fertilized egg. If fertilization and implantation did not take place, a new menstrual cycle commences (new menstrual flow phase) marking the day one of the next cycle. Each month the body prepares the uterus to accept the fertilized egg and all the effort is "vested" if the fertilization did not take place.

Ovarian Phases Paralleling the uterine cycle is the ovarian cycle. It begins with the follicular phase. Among several follicles that start to grow in this phase, only one continues growing, enlarges and matures (Graafian follicle). The maturing follicle develops an internal fluid-filled cavity and secretes the estrogen. The length of this phase varies between women, even between cycles, but usually lasts 7–14 days and parallels the proliferative uterine phase. At the end of this phase, the follicle ruptures releasing the egg cell – this process is called ovulation and the next ovarian phase is called ovulatory phase. The follicular tissues that remains in the follicle after ovulation is transformed in a yellowish endocrine structure, the corpus luteum, that secrets progesterone and estrogen during the next phase called luteal phase of the ovarian cycle, which parallels the secretory uterine phase. This phase lasts

13–15 days in the absence of fertilization. Degeneration of the corpus luteum at the end of the luteal phase reduces the amount of hormones available to the uterus, the endometrium starts to shed marking again the day one of the next uterine cycle. In the event of pregnancy, the corpus luteum continues to grow and produces hormones, which together with other hormones prevent the loss of endometrium.

Fluctuation of the Ovarian Hormone Levels There are two phases: Estrogen and progesterone phase. Estrogen is secreted in increasing amount by the maturing follicle during the ovarian proliferative phase and is stimulating the uterus to proliferate and thicken (proliferative uterine phase). As it can be seen on Fig. 1.1d, the follicular phase of the ovarian cycle is coordinated with the proliferative phase of the uterine cycle and before the ovulation the uterus is already prepared for the possible embryo. After ovulation, estrogen and progesterone secreted by the corpus luteum stimulate further development of the uterus and growth of the endometrial glands secreting nutrient fluid that can sustain an early embryo before it implant into the uterus. As it can be seen (Fig. 1.1d) the luteal phase of the ovarian cycle corresponds to the secretory phase of the uterine cycle. In the absence of pregnancy, the rapid drop of ovarian hormones and corpus luteum disintegration corresponds to the end of secretory uterine phase and the beginning of menstrual flow phase that is the beginning the next cycle. Cycle after cycle, the maturation and the release of egg cells from the ovary is integrated with changes of the uterus necessary for pregnancy in case the egg is fertilized.

The fluctuations in the levels of other three hormones (FSH, LH, GnRH) controlling the female hormones also occur during the cycle. Early in the menstrual cycle GnRH increases stimulating the release of FSH and LH. LH and FSH secretion increase rapidly just before the ovulation (FSH and LH surge) and then decrease after ovulation.

Cervical Changes During the Menstrual Phases.
The cervical mucosa and the cervix also change during the menstrual phases. The ostium that opens into the vagina progressively widens during the proliferative phase, reaching maximal width before ovulation, and then returns to a smaller diameter again [30, 68, 78, 79].

1.2.3 Pregnancy

The pregnancy begins with the fertilization of the ovum. The sperms deposited into the vagina travel towards the uterus and fallopian tubes, where the fertilization (the union of the sperm and the egg cell) is taking place. This new cell is now called a zygote. The cell starts to divide immediately and it is pushed by the cilia lining the fallopian tube and the peristalsis of the tube. After reaching the uterus the little ball of cells (ovula-blastula) is implanted in the thickened uterine endometrium. After implantation the zygote becomes embryo. The outer layer of the ball sends projections (villa) into the uterine wall what is the beginning of the placenta. This is a new organ that serves for nutrition and excretion of the embryo by means of exchange between the blood of the mother and the blood of the embryo through the capillaries of the placental villa. The umbilical cord is soon developed (between the fetus and placenta) that contains two arteries and one vein carrying the blood to the placenta and from the placenta to the embryo bypassing its lungs. After the third month of pregnancy, the developing embryo is called fetus.

The placenta is also an endocrine organ. Soon after implantation the placenta starts to secrete a hormone human chorionic gonadotropin (hCG). This hormone stimulates corpus luteum to prolong the secretion of estrogen and progesterone for 3 months when placenta is taking over the production of both estrogen and progesterone. Both hormones are essential for the further maintenance of pregnancy. However, the period during 11th/12th week of pregnancy, when corpus luteum disintegrates and the placenta becomes hormonal producer is critical for miscarriage.

During the period of gestation the fetal organ and organ systems are formed and continue to mature. It normally requires 9 months (three trimesters, 266–280 days) from fertilization of the ovum to birth. Usually, the period is divided into three trimesters. The amniotic sac, filled with amniotic fluid surrounds the fetus and protects from mechanical traumas. At birth, the amniotic sac ruptures ("water brake") that mark the beginning of delivery [50, 68, 142].

1.2.4 Menopause

Menopause is the cessation of the menstrual cycle. The period from the onset of irregular cycles to their complete cessation is called perimenopause. Menopause is a normal period in women's lives, which occurs between the ages of 45 and 58. It is caused by decline of the ovarian function, with gradual decrease of estrogen and progesterone leading to considerable changes in the woman body. Ova are not produced anymore and a woman is not anymore capable of becoming pregnant. Although frequently followed by different unpleasant symptoms (e.g., hot flashes, irritability, anxiety, or more severe emotional disturbances), it should be considered as temporary and normal condition. Hormone replacement therapy (HRT) that has been given to women because of the beneficial effects on cardiovascular system and osteoporosis as well as decreased hot flashes, is no longer recommended because of a danger of development of uterine and breast cancers, as well as thrombosis and embolism. HRT, originally given as estrogen only and later combined with progesterone (to lessen the side effects) is still controversial and, if given, must be monitored by the ordering physician. Many women decide not to take HRT and live fulfilling lives using regular exercise and additional calcium to strengthen the bones and the cardiovascular system. Some of them reach maximum in their intellectual and professional lives in this period since, after raising their children, they can devote their time and energy to themselves. It is also important that women should not perceive the menopause as the end, rather the new beginning [78, 79, 142].

1.3 An Overview of the Most Common Women's Diseases

Introduction to most common gynecological diseases other than cervical pre-carcinomatosis and cancer, which are elaborated in Chapter 2. Menstrual disorders, infertility, common vaginal and cervical infections, pelvic inflammatory diseases (PID). Sexually transmitted diseases: Diseases caused by bacteria (gonorrhea), spirochetes (syphilis), chlamydia infections, viral infections (Herpes, human pappiloma virus [HPV], acquired human deficiency syndrome [HIV and AIDS]) and protozoal infections (trichomonas). Benign and malignant tumor of the woman's reproductive system.

Menstrual cycle can be disturbed by many factors. Even stress, psychological pressure of any kind, a change of health status, change of living habits (travels, change of work shifts) may influence the menstruation.

1.3.1 Menstrual Disorders

1.3.1.1 Amenorrhea

Amenorrhea means the absence of menstruation. It can be a primary amenorrhea, when a woman will not begin with menstruation at puberty, or secondary amenorrhea if a woman has had normal menstrual cycles and later stops menstruating. Causes of amenorrhea are connected with many different factors related to pituitary gland hormones, ovarian and uterine causes. The treatment is directed toward the etiology of the disease, e.g., pituitary tumors, ovarian tumors or abnormal ovarian hormone secretion (e.g., polycystic diseases). However, it should not be forgotten that temporary amenorrhea was seen among normal women – athletes and dancers during rigorous exercise, stress and under conditions noted in the previous paragraph. Furthermore, examples of physiological secondary amenorrhea are pregnancy and menopause [50, 110, 111].

1.3.1.2 Dysmenorrhea

Dysmenorrhea denotes painful or difficult menstruation. It may vary from a discomfort on the first days of their period and then subside when the flow is established, About 50 % young women may experience a pain that do not interfere with their normal activities, and about 10 % have cramps that keep them at home. It is rarely associated with nausea, headache, diarrhea that last 1–2 days. Usually, no treatment is necessary. It is called primary dysmenorrhea, without a known physical cause. Dysmenorrhea usually decreases after age 20 and almost disappears after the first childbirth, because of the dilation of the cervical canal. Primary dysmenorrhea usually does not require treatment, however non-steroid anti-inflammatory drugs (commonly called NSAIDs) like Aleve, Advil may be used, if a woman is not sensitive to aspirin or other anti-inflammatory drugs.

Secondary dysmenorrhea is menstrual pain for which an organic cause exists. Causes may be connected with endometriosis, uterine tumor, fibroids, cervical stenosis (narrowing) or pelvic inflammatory disease (PID, see further). Therapy should be directed to remove the cause of dysmenorrhea [128].

1.3.1.3 Abnormal Uterine Bleeding

Abnormal uterine bleeding can appear as excessive menstrual flow on regular menstruation dates or irregular bleeding in between menstruation dates. The first may cause anemia, and the second may be a sign of non-effective ovulation (nonovulatory cycles), hormonal disturbances or more serious disease that needs medical attention. Any, even discrete, bleeding (spotting) after cessation of menstruation may be a sign of a serious disease and a woman should seek doctor's advice [110, 128].

1.3.1.4 Premenstrual Syndrome (PMS)

PMS is a state of irritability, depression and nervousness, mood changes, bloating or sleeplessness that preceded menstruation. Usually one of those symptoms is present. Many women experience a tension, but most of them occupied with everyday duties and responsibilities handle this situation well. It is still a controversial condition, because the precise definition has not been established, the symptoms vary between individuals, cannot be easily monitored and the cause is not known. Hormonal factors (a hormone called prolactin) and serotonin (a chemical messenger in the brain) are some of the factors that may be involved in PMS. There is no laboratory test for this condition.

Concerning treatment, simply reducing caffeine, alcohol, sugar intake (cookies, chocolate) may alleviate symptoms, Avoid salty food to decrease your tendency to bloat. Exercise regularly. Substances called endorphins, natural opiates produced in your brain during exercise may make you feel better. Vitamins (particularly B6 and vitamin E) are also recommended. There are attempt to treat PMS with hormones (progesterone and birth control pills), but regard PMS as a condition, not a disease and handle it as simple as possible [81].

1.3.2 Other Disorders

1.3.2.1 Infertility

A couple is said to be infertile if pregnancy does not result after 1 year after normal sexual activity without contraceptives. About 25 % couples experience infertility at some point of their reproductive lives. The incidence of infertility increases with age. Combination of factors leading to infertility is most frequently common, although about 40 % male partners contribute as a cause.

Infertility may be caused by many different factors such as past infections, endocrine disorders, abnormalities of the structure and the function of individual organs, or psychogenic factors. Each of these disorders can be tested and determined the actual cause of women infertility. It is, however important to test the male partner and exclude status, since male infertility is easier to determine (spermogram). There is an established diagnostic survey with first and second testing cycles. Treatments of infertility have advanced very much, and with the new *in vitro* fertilization methods available, a women who is determined to be a mother, if persistent, will most likely fulfill this eternal role of motherhood [110].

1.3.3 Common Infections in Women

1.3.3.1 Candida (Yeast) Vaginal Infections

Candidiasis is provoked by a fungus *Candida albicans*. Candida may be found as a normal vaginal flora, but in healthy women with acidic vaginal fluid does not cause problems. Candidiasis is transmitted with sexual contact, but it is not considered as a typical sexually transmitted disease. It can appear during diabetes, pregnancy, after prolonged use of broad spectrum antibiotics, or if the immune system is weakened (e.g., by HIV virus, chemotherapy). It is estimated that about 75 % women have vulvovaginal candidiasis during their lifetime. Symptoms are discomfort, itching with white curd-like vaginal discharge. Treatment is local (nystatin) and systematic, when necessary (fluconazole) [110, 142].

1.3.3.2 Vaginitis and Vaginosis

Bacterial vaginitis is inflammation and infection of the vagina. It is a common gynecological problem caused by variety of pathogens. Causes may include candida vaginitis, trichomonas vaginitis and HPV vaginal infection (vaginal warts) and different STDs, which are separately described in this book.

Bacterial vaginosis is considered a polymicrobial disease which is not sexually transmitted. It is an overgrow of normal vaginal bacteria (e.g., Garnerella). Symptoms include malodorous discharge and discomfort, burning or itching in the genital area.

Vaginosis may or may not be combined with vulvitis (inflammation of the vulva) or urethritis (inflammation of the urethra). It is easily healed with local treatment (vaginal creams and gels) or if it is necessary systemic treatment with metronidazole or clindamycin, if necessary [110].

1.3.3.3 Cervicitis

Acute cervicitis is the inflammation of the cervix. It is caused by local infections (streptococcal, staphylococcal, enterococcal), a part of sexually transmitted diseases (e.g., infection by *Naisseria gonorrhoeae* or *Chlamydia trachomatis*) or herpes viruses. Cervicitis may also be a symptom of vaginitis or pelvic inflammatory disease. Signs and symptoms are vaginal discharge (can be purulent and profuse), backache, pain during intercourse, bleeding after intercourse, frequent and painful urination (usually because of the inflammation of the urethra–urethritis), burning or itching in the genital area. There may be slight elevation of the temperature. Diagnosis is made by pelvic exam (red edematous cervix) and bacteriological examination of the swabs taken from the cervix. Your physician may also take Pap test to rule out pre-carcinomatosis or cancer. Treatment consists of limitation of pelvic activity and appropriate antibiotic or antiviral therapy.

Chronic cervicitis is usually minimal, asymptomatic and not clinically apparent. Most frequently an erosion can be found, or cervical ulcer may appear, which are visible during pelvic exam. In this case there are symptoms as vaginal discharge (yellowish, white, thick), postcoital bleeding, backache, urgency and frequency of urination.

In case of chronic cervicitis it is important to exclude dysplasia or malignant process. Pap test should be performed, and biopsy in any suspicious area. The therapy of chronic cervicitis are antibiotics directed specifically towards the pathogen that is found on microbiological analysis (cervical culture) [54].

1.3.3.4 Nabothian Cyst

A Nabothian cyst (the name came from anatomist Naboth) looks like a small fluid–filled lump on the cervix. It appears when the canal of small mucus cervical glands became obstructed and the mucus can not be drained normally. The Nabothian cyst is frequently seen during the pelvic exam and usually does not require any treatment [50, 66].

1.3.3.5 Pelvic Inflammatory Disease (PID)

PID is a polymicrobial infection of the female pelvic organs. It usually involves vagina, cervix, the body of the uterus, uterine tubes or ovaries. This infection may extend from the reproductive organs to the pelvic cavity, and may involve the peritoneum. It can be caused by many microorganisms, but chlamydia and gonococci are usually the initial cause. It can also be caused by endogenous organisms, including anaerobes. PID is most common in young sexually active women with multiple partners. Early symptoms are vaginal and cervical purulent discharge and pelvic pain, with or without chills, fever and/or disturbed menstruation. Untreated PID may lead to sterility.

It is a serious disease and timely antibiotic treatment is very important to stop the spread of PID. With the lack of treatment it is a lifethreatening disease. Hospitalization may be required for intravenous application of antibiotics. General measures, e.g., bed rest and adequate intake of liquids is required. Sometimes even surgery may be needed [65, 110].

1.3.4 Sexually Transmitted Diseases

This chapter will give an overview of the most frequent sexually transmitted diseases. These are diseases that are transmitted by intimate sexual contact between individuals and include the major venereal diseases as Chlamydia infection (non-gonococcal urethritis/vaginitis), gonorrhea, trihomoniasis, genital herpes, genital warts, syphilis and acquired immunodeficiency syndrome (AIDS). Bacteriological examination of a vaginal secretion (either direct microscopic examinations or stained preparations) and bacterial culture reveals the cause of infection. Common symptoms are discomfort, pain, itching, burning and the inflammation of vagina. Urethra is also affected with symptoms of disturbed urination – dysuria (burning, pain, frequent urination and tenesmi). Pelvic exam should be performed to exclude PID [40, 81].

1.3.4.1 Gonorrhea

Gonorrhea is a sexually transmitted disease caused by a bacterium *Neisseria gonnorhoeae*. The organism attaches to the epithelial cells of the vagina and cervix and to the penile epithelium and urethra in male, producing an inflammation. In males it is manifested by painful urination and discharge of pus from the urethra. If not treated may cause serious complications on the reproductive system (sterility) or affect other organs (heart, joints, kidneys). In female early infection may pass unnoticed, later signs of inflammatory process are manifested with vaginal discharge, discomfort, pain, as well as signs of urethritis with disturbed urination (dysuria). Gonorrhea frequently causes PID. The cervix typically does not show signs of dysplasia (pre-cancer). Children can be infected during childbirth. Gonorrhea is easily treatable with antibiotics (penicillin) [65].

1.3.4.2 Chlamydial Infection

This is vaginitis associated with urethritis caused by the bacteria *Chlamydia trachomatis*. Most frequently, it is acquired through sexual contact and is among most frequent sexually transmitted diseases. The symptoms are those of inflammation of the vagina and urethra (discomfort, itching, burning, urgency for urination). Chlamydia induces also inflammation of the cervix (cervicitis) characterized with edematous cervix, discharge and tenderness on the cervical motion. Sometimes, women's disease may pass without symptoms (asymptomatic), but can be dangerous because, if untreated, can cause PID and sterility. The disease is treatable by antibiotics.

Vaginitis and urethritis may be caused by other types of bacteria (see above), and may be a result of trauma or catheterization of the urethra [9, 65].

1.3.4.3 Trichomoniasis

Trichomonas vaginalis is a protozoon found in the vagina and the urethra of males. If the normal acidity of the vagina is disturbed, trichomonas can grow rapidly and result in an inflammation with yellow–green discharge with odor. Trichomonas produces lower genitourinary infection in man mostly with dysuria. It is transmitted by sexual contact, but incidence of non-sexual transmission has been described (infected water in pools and toilets). There is effective treatment of trichomonas infections with metronidazole [128].

1.3.4.4 Herpetic Lesions of the Vulva, Vagina and Cervix

Human herpes viruses cause a venereal disease called genital herpes. Clinically it appears as vesicles (blister-like areas) on vulva, vagina and cervix surrounded by red, edematous areas of inflammation. They progress into superficial ulcers. Symptoms are burning sensations, vaginal pain, vaginal discharge and painful urination. They appear in both women and men. The patient may have fever, malaise and headache. The blister-like areas usually heal after 2 weeks, but virus continues to exist in a latent form, and may reoccur during menstruation, emotional stress or other illnesses. The disease can be passed to the child during childbirth.

A doctor will prescribe therapy against genital herpes, like Acyclovir (Zovirax) that control symptoms, but cannot eradicate the virus [65].

1.3.4.5 Human Papilloma Virus (HPV) Infection: Genital Warts

Human papilloma virus causes genital warts and some strains cause cervical dysplasia that may progress into cervical cancer. Approximately less than 1 % of all women infected with papilloma virus develop cervical cancer. The subject of HPV infection and its connection with cervical cancer is discussed in details in Chap. 2.

Genital warts vary from small separate growth to large cauliflower like clusters (39). Warts are usually not painful, but can cause a painful intercourse and may bleed. Treatment includes topical agents, cryosurgery or other surgical methods. Women with genital warts are at risk to develop cervical cancer and should be controlled rigorously with Pap screening [17, 39–41, 44]. See also Chaps. 2, 3, 4, 5, 6 and 9 of this manuscript.

1.3.4.6 Acquired Immunodeficiency Syndrome (HIV, Aids)

This is an infection caused by the acquired immunodeficiency (HIV) virus, It attacks a special type of white blood cells, T lymphocytes and destroys the immune system. HIV virus is transmitted primarily by sexual contact, but also by sharing needles with an infected person during the administration of illicit drugs. The infection with blood transfusion was also known before rigorous testing has been applied for all blood products. Mother can transmit the virus to her child, too. Accidental transmission has been documented among health workers dealing with infective blood. Normal casual contact with infected person cannot cause infection, neither HIV can be transmitted through toilet seats, food or kissing. Further description of HIV/AIDS clinical symptoms, diagnosis, prevention and treatment are beyond the scope of this book. More information on HIV AIDS can be found in Chaps. 2 and 3 (further readings) [47, 176, 188].

1.3.4.7 Syphilis

Syphilis is caused by the bacteria *treponema pallidum*. It is transmitted only by sexual contact. The disease progress through several stages. During the primary stage, the initial symptoms include a small, hard ulcer (ulcus durum) at the site of the entrance of the infection. The second stage is manifested by many different symptoms: Fever, skin rash, malaise, enlarged lymph nodes, symptoms from renal and central nervous system are present. After this stage the disease may enter in a latent period without symptoms. In about 50 % of cases the third, late stage, appears characterized by inflammatory necrotic tumors and extensive tissue damage that leads to paralysis, insanity, other neurological symptoms and death. Syphilis can be passed on to newborns by sick mother. The disease is treated with antibiotics [65].

1.4 Tumors of the Female Genital System

An overview of benign and malignant genital tumors in women. Benign tumors: Myoma of the uterus, cervical and uterine polyps. Endometriosis. Carcinoma of the endometrium (the lining of the uterus), ovarian cancer, carcinoma of the vulva. Cervical carcinoma is discussed in details in other chapters.

1.4.1 Benign Tumors

1.4.1.1 Myoma (Fibroid, Fibromyoma)

Myomas are the most common benign tumors of female genital tract. These are round, firm, often multiple tumors in the uterine wall that differ in size. Fibroids consist of smooth muscle and connected tissue. Most are small and do not progress into malignant tumors. Fibroids usually do not produce symptoms in non-pregnant women, and may spontaneously disappear after age 50. Otherwise, typical symptoms from fibroids are dismenorrhea (painful periods), heavy bleeding with consecutive anemia, pain, or if become large they compress adjacent organs and blood vessels. In pregnant women fibroids interfere with pregnancy, may cause abortion, premature labor, obstructed labor or hemorrhage.

There are many available methods (ultrasonography, MRI, histerography) to help to diagnose, estimate the size of the tumor and its location. If the fibroid is small it can be easily removed without removing significant part of the uterus; the tumor could be removed with a part of the uterus, or if fibroids are multiple and large, surgical removal of the uterus (hysterectomy) may be recommended [50, 110].

1.4.1.2 Cervical and Uterine Polyps

Cervical and uterine polyps are benign formation in the uterus and cervix. The principal symptom is bleeding/spotting and there may be vaginal discharge. Specifically, cervical polyps could be few millimeters to couple of centimeters in size. Polyps are red pear-shaped. Usually one bigger polyp is present, but may be 2–3 smaller. Polyps can be easily diagnosed with ultrasound and other imaging technologies. Although they rarely progress into malignant tumors, polyps should be removed and submit for histological analysis to differentiate them from neoplastic disease of the endometrium or cervix. The surgical procedure for the removal of a cervical polyp may be performed in the doctor's office [54].

Benign ovarian tumors will be mentioned in the subsection of ovarian tumors.

1.4.1.3 Endometriosis

Endometriosis is an aberrant growth of endometrium outside the uterus. It is caused by abnormal displacement of corresponding stem cells during embryonic development. Endometrial tissue may be at different places (pelvis, ovaries, tubes, bowel). Symptoms depend on the location and the size of the growth. Most frequent it is pain with bleeding. The bleeding may be from the rectum if the implant is in the bowel. Pain starts 2–7 days before the onset of the menstruation and continue during the menstrual phase. Ultrasound examination reveals complex fluid-filled mass that cannot be distinguished from neoplasia. MRI is more specific. The diagnosis of endometriosis must be confirmed by laparoscopy (an instrument is inserted inside the abdomen through a little cut on the abdomen) or laparotomy (operation on the abdomen). Therapy depends of the size, location and a woman's desire to preserve the reproductive function. The therapy is either conservative (hormonal) or surgery to remove the implant. In case of extensive endometrioses with pain, removal of the uterus and ovaries is indicated [110].

1.4.2 *Malignant Tumors Other than Cervical Cancer*

1.4.2.1 Uterine Cancer

The cancer of the body of the uterus is a common cancer of the women's reproductive system. Usually it affects older women 50–70 years of age. Risk factors are intake of estrogen (DES, or HRT) or tamoxifen used for the treatment of breast cancer. Other risk factors are obesity, nuliparity (women who did not have children), diabetes, and hypertension. In the beginning the only clinical symptom is irregular bleeding (for example bleeding/spotting in menopause). However, about 20 % women with incipient uterine cancer may not have symptoms. At a later stage obstruction of the cervix with a tumor may occur. Pap test, which is the best test for cervical cancer screening, may show abnormal endometrial cells, but it is not always positive in endometrial cancer. Direct sampling of the endometrium (endometrial biopsy) is a secure approach for diagnosis. It should be performed in parallel with hysteroscopy, what is entering with the instrument inside the uterus and viewing the inside of the uterus. Vaginal ultrasound can be used to determine the thickness of the endometrium. The uterine carcinoma must be differentiated from a benign uterine hyperplasia that is only thickening of the endometrium. Therapy of the uterine carcinoma depends of the stage of the diseases. Usually it is surgery: Removal of the uterus (histerctomy) with removal of the tubes and ovaries (bilateral salpingo-oophorectomy), and removal of the lymph nodes, if necessary. In some cases, postoperative external radiation and intracavitary radium therapy is needed for uterine carcinoma. There are also some other approaches (e.g., Herceptin treatment) [129].

1.4.2.2 Ovarian Tumors

Ovarian tumors are also common. Most of them are benign. However, malignant ovarian tumors are leading cause of mortality among gynecological malignancies in developed countries where regular Pap test screening protects women from cervical carcinoma. Cervical cancer is still the main killer of women from malignant diseases worldwide.

Ovarian cancer has a proven hereditary connection. Women who have family members with ovarian cancer have up to 40 % chance to have this disease during their lifetime. Frequent ultrasound checking is recommended or, if there are more than one member in the family, oophorectomy is recommended as soon as the childbirth is completed.

The early symptoms of ovarian tumors (both benign and malignant) are very discrete in the beginning; even a women may be asymptomatic. A patient may complain on vague, non-specific symptoms, like gastrointestinal discomfort, pelvic pressure and pain. More advanced malignant disease is characterized with abdominal pain, bleeding and palpable mass, with or without ascites (a liquid in the abdomen). Pelvic ultrasonogram, pelvic examination, and an increase of one biomarker in blood (CA 125) are guidance for early diagnosis of malignant tumor. Treatment is surgery (hysterectomy with bilateral salpingo-oophorectomy, omentectomy and removal of diseased lymph nodes). Post-operative chemotherapy is also recommended [37].

1.4.2.3 Carcinoma of the Vagina and Vulva

Usually appears in women over 50 years old. Human papilloma (HPV) virus type 16, 18 and 31 is found in some, but not all cases. A grading system of different severity of the disease (like for cervical cancer) is established for the vulvar cancer. It is termed vulvar intraepithelial neoplasia (VIN) and it is graded from mild to severe and finally cancer. Symptoms are prolonged irritation, discomfort, bloody discharge and history of warts. Later, tumor mass and growth, or ulceration may be visible. Biopsy is indicated for distinction from non-neoplastic vulvovaginal tumors. Therapy depends on the stage of the diseases from removal of pre-cancerous lesion to radical vulvectomy with inguinal lymphadectomy (removal of the diseased lymph nodes). The prognosis of the disease depends of the stage of the tumor, involvement of lymph nodes and the presence or absence of metastases [110].

Chapter 2
Cervical Cancer

2.1 About Cervical Cancer and Pre-cancerosis in This Book

2.1.1 Introduction

Cervical cancer remains the leading cause of cancer death in women across the globe. In the US, because of Pap test prevention, the number of women who die from cervical cancer has been drastically reduced. This is the best proof that prevention is extremely important to fight cervical cancer.

What is cervical cancer? This is a cancer of the neck of the uterus (see Chap. 1). It is developed gradually starting with abnormal cell changes called pre-cancerosis (dysplasia) that could regress or advance into cancer over the years. Those pre-cancerous changes can be easily detected with Pap test, and the disease prevented before it appears. *Cervical cancer is a preventable disease if detected on time.* Otherwise it is a grave, deadly disease. This is the first and the most important rule. Learn everything concerning cervical cancer prevention. *Be aware of cervical cancer, learn how to:*

(a) *Prevent pre-cancerosis*: learn all about the cancer risks.
(b) *Prevent cervical cancer before it appears*: learn about the importance of regular preventive cervical cancer screening, the Pap test that detects early pre-cancerous changes and prevents the disease before it appears.
(c) *Eliminate/reduce cervical cancer when it appears*: learn about methods of diagnosis and therapy that effectively may help you to conquer this disease.

These are the facts that every woman should know. This is the message that the authors would like to convey to all women.

A strong emphasis in this monograph is given to cervical cancer screening in order to educate women in this proven benefit that dramatically decreased cervical cancer mortality and morbidity in the countries where it is available. Women will learn all that is necessary about screening procedure, pre-cancerous lesions, and

N. Markovic, O. Markovic, *What Every Woman Should Know about Cervical Cancer*, DOI 10.1007/978-94-017-7560-1_2

interpretation of Pap test. Since some women will still be diagnosed with cervical cancer, two sections are dedicated to current concepts for diagnosis, therapy and the prognosis of women when receive therapy.

Instead of fear and avoidance of the Pap test, women can understand the result and ask educated questions. Instead of panicking, those who have cervical cancer will learn how to help themselves by actively participating in their own diagnostic and therapeutic procedures.

2.1.2 *Definition*

Cervical cancer is unstoppable growth of abnormal tissue within the cervix (vaginal portion) of the uteri (womb – where babies are grown). This abnormal growth is hypertrophic (increase of cell size), hyperplastic (increase of cell numbers), anaplastic (atypical cell shape), afunctional (does not function as neighboring tissues), and is aggressive invading surrounding tissues by competing for blood supply and by direct destruction of neighboring cells. Abnormal cells are loosely attached to each other, and easily shed into vaginal fluid (where they can be detected by Pap test) or into lymph ducts (enlargement of local lymph nodes – local metastases) and further into blood and other places (distant metastases) where they appear as local tumors.

Cervical cancer is specific among other cancers with slow growth (1–3 and more years from the first detectable growth to the detectable disease). However, there is a number of conditions causing cervicovaginal tissue to respond with inflammation (acute, subacute and chronic) which may create cervical lesions identifiable indirectly by Pap test as cervical dysplasia categories ASC-US through HSIL and diagnosed by colposcopy-biopsy and histology as CIN (1–3) or cervical dysplasia (mild, moderate and severe). Most of these lesions resolve spontaneously with removal of the causal factor or by improvement of the host immune response. Few of them may persist and, if untreated, may proceed into cervical cancer; consequently, the name pre-cancerosis is given to indicate to this probability (Table 2.1).

The table shows that a single Pap test result had very unstable predictive rates (both positive and negative). This is perfectly in the context of a screening test, it should be an alarm to initiate further diagnosis and therapy if necessary, not any

Table 2.1 Natural history of cervical epithelial lesions (Adapted according to Malinowski [112])

Pap test result	No report of change within 2 years[a]	Regression to normal within 24 months (%)	Progression to HSIL within 24 months (%)	Progression to invasive carcinoma within 24 months (%)
ASC-US	24.4	68.2	7.1	0.3
LSIL	31.6	47.4	20.8	0.2
HSIL	40.2	35.0	23.4 (persistence)	1.4

[a]New estimates

type of diagnostic method that can predict therapeutic outcome – as many are trying to pursue. Therefore, regular screening (e.g., repeat Pap annually) would be the most reliable protective measure.

Because there is no way to predict which lesions will resolve, progress or transform into cancer, the recommendation is to remove them as soon as histological diagnosis is made. Timely removal of lesions has reduced the incidence (frequency of occurrence) of cervical cancer both in the population participating in Pap test screening and in general population at large.

Recently, many researchers are reporting different biomarkers having correlation with disease prognosis (early assessment of disease future progress). Unfortunately, these prognostic factors can only provide an estimate of probability – this is not helpful for a single patient who needs more certainty to rely upon. Therefore, we still recommend early removal of the pre-cancerous lesion as the best alternative for the safety and well-being of involved patients.

2.1.3 Interpretation

2.1.3.1 How to Approach These Issues from a Lay Person Perspective

If you open any medical textbook or health education book for college students, you will see four important sections: prevention, control, diagnosis and treatment. It is true for almost all diseases and conditions of altered health, but it is not completely true for cervical cancer. Why? The answer is simple: There is no effective therapy for cervical cancer; prevention is curative. How is this possible?

Let me use an analogy to explain what I mean. Just imagine driving a new, big car on a straight, empty highway over Plains. On a sunny day, with nobody in my horizon, I may get a temptation to press the gas pedal and increase the speed over the allowable limit of 65 miles per hour. If I actually do so, this will be as I have got a HPV infection. I may reduce the speed, and nothing will happen. However, I could be spotted by a policeman. This would be the Pap test. He may only warn me (this will resemble ASC-US) or he may give me a ticket to pay directly resembling (LSIL), or may send me to a judge for speeding only (ASC-H) or for negligent driving (HSIL). Before appearing in Court, I am in the control; I can always reduce the speed, do not allow next temptations, and I will be OK. The judge may order monetary penalty (e.g., conservatory treatment), may give me points and order a new driving course (surgical removal of the lesion), and if I accept all of this and continue driving, nothing will happen to me. However, instead of meeting the policeman, I could have hit some one and could have inflicted injury on myself and the other person. This situation resembles carcinoma in situ – I may get out of it, but the outcome is not always clear. Rarely, I could have killed someone or got permanent injury – this would be cancer. In any case, I would have to pay dearly, and to be very happy if I would be able to get out with limited, although permanent, consequences. Of course, the road patrol could miss my speedy driving and I could hit somebody (this would be false negative), or the road patrol could stop me as a part of a routine check up and, after short examination, let me go further (that would be false positive). Obviously, the false negative would be many times more dangerous than false positive. The Pap test is to reduce those false negatives to minimum.

I hope this analogy will provide basic understanding that cervical cancer is a slow progressive disease that has two different phases. One is from the first epithelial cell becoming malignant (ability for unstoppable growth of abnormal cells that compete with normal tissues) through development of invasive carcinoma (at average 3 years). Other phase is independent – it includes many conditions that may bring to development of cancer but which are not cancer by themselves. All these conditions, known as pre-cancerosis, could be detected with the Pap test. Consequently, Pap test is an alarm warning us to take care of ourselves and to protect us from cervical cancer – this alarm is saving lives of about 50,000 American women per year who are diagnosed with CIN 1–3, and to many more women who have been happy to see their Pap test reversed from positive to negative.

If this is clear, than you will understand why, in this book, the authors will try to keep separate the Pap test as a screening (preventive measure) from the diagnosis of cervical cancer (medical diagnostic procedure). Consequently, the cytological screening is presented as one entity with the diagnostic procedures (colposcopy, biopsy with histology, and with ancillary HPV infection testing) as another entity. However, if a woman is Pap positive, all of these tests are only parts of a single procedure dedicated for fast, true diagnosis and timely therapy intended to cure.

2.1.3.2 Caution

When we began writing this book, we did not believe the time would come to caution our readers on the "free use" of names with different interpretation. However, working on this book we contacted colleagues around the world in order to collect as true information as possible. This is when we were stricken with a revelation that the name Pap test does not mean the same in different countries. How has it happened? We have developed a system for telecytopathology, a diagnostic telemedicine for microscopic specimens. Having been in contact with researchers in many countries, we asked them to send us microscopic images of selected examples of their Pap test specimens. Surprisingly, when images were compared, we found substantial difference in staining procedures (India – predominately red, Japan – predominance of blue, England – slightly different terminology) and the interpretation was not always consistent with our impression of the same images.

In the meantime the new global strategy for cervical cancer prevention has evolved: HPV vaccination plus cervical cancer screening (Pap test preferably, but other options could be considered) [91]. This is causing concerns and calls for alert. In the US, Pap test has been successful only because it has been standardized (CLIA*88) – specimen collection, specimen processing, staining and interpretation are strictly regulated [48]. Cytotechnologists, performing specimen reading and interpretation, are subject to regular proficiency testing and keeping the standard of interpretation is *conditio sine qua* non their job. We are not aware of any other country where such regulations are in effect. This makes comparison between results of screening from different sources difficult and not sufficiently reliable. (After 60 years of Pap test introduction, it is clear that a worldwide standardization of cytological cervical cancer screening is not possible while the standard Papanicolaou staining is used – new techniques are necessary and, we believe, this is the place for biomarkers to help cytological screening).

We think this caution had to be included here to prepare readers of this book to question, not the quality, but the reliability of laboratory results (was the standard Pap test used, was it an alternative, what control is used) that will be decisive for doctors' recommendation and actions, which will affect lives of our readers.

Another, not less important, caution is against misuses of cytological and histological terminology for interpretation of cytological results. This situation could appear when somebody uses histological diagnosis carcinoma in situ (CIS), adenocarcinoma in situ (AIS), or cervical intraepithelial neoplasia (CIN 1–3) for reporting Pap test results or any other cytological result of cervical cancer screening. Even cytopathology atlases are not free from lacking clarity on this subject. Using histology for interpretation of cytological specimens does not mean "better diagnosis" but a lack of sufficient sensitivity for clinical decision making needs, which may cause doctors to delay or skip the next diagnostic procedures (colposcopy – biopsy – histology) and to recommend appropriate surgery on time. Unfortunately, this confusion between cytological and histological diagnosis is more frequent than it is believed and is present even in credible literature. This is why we decided to alert our readers on this unwanted possibility.

2.2 Epidemiology of Cervical Cancer

Epidemiology is the study of factors affecting the health and illness of populations, and serves as the foundation and logic of interventions made in the interest of public health and preventive medicine. It is highly regarded in evidence-based medicine for identifying risk factors for disease and determining optimal treatment approaches to clinical practice [179]. Randomized clinical trials (RCT) are tools highly recommended to provide scientific evidence in epidemiologic research, and for achieving a critical mass of information for guidance of diagnosis and therapy.

Epidemiology of cervical cancer is determined by two parameters, incidence or incidence risk of invasive cervical cancer (number of new cases per a population of 100,000 women at risk per year) and mortality (number of deaths per a population of 100,000 women per year). In this book we will not use the incidence rate because, in this parameter, the denominator is person-years which is a statistical tool for correction of a dropout rate, but is not accurate as the risk and could complicate reading and interpretation [8, 94].

Today, cervical cancer is a preventable disease if detected on time, and if proper measures are taken to remove the lesions that, if untreated, could develop into cervical cancer [175]. This is exactly the theory behind the Pap test. So, the experience accumulated over the years of Pap test application and changes in the natural progression of cervical cancer must be taken into consideration. We recommend that the percent of Pap positive (abnormal) results and the percent of histologically diagnosed severe dysplasia (CIN 2/3 and CIS) be added to the first line of epidemiological parameters for the assessment of cervical cancer epidemiology. Both indicate two clinical outcomes: Positive Pap test requires further diagnosis, and positive histology requires surgical intervention.

In this chapter, we will discuss epidemiology of cervical cancer using objective measuring parameters for the assessment of the epidemiological condition: cervical cancer incidence, mortality, percent of positive (abnormal) Pap tests, and percent of histological diagnosis of severe dysplasia/pre-cancerosis or cancer (CIN 2/3, CIS or AIS).

Until the middle of the twentieth century, cervical cancer was generally considered as a chronic neoplastic (malignant) disease affecting all women (endemic globally) with ultimate fatal outcome. The average incidence risk was about 30 and the average mortality was about 15.

During the second part of the twentieth century these numbers have changed due to the new strategy for prevention and control of cervical cancer. In the 1950s, the American Cancer Society (ASC) promoted a new test for cervical cancer screening (Pap test) as a method "for early detection of cervical lesions that, if not removed on time, could progress to cervical cancer." This approach enabled doctors to diagnose and remove pre-cancerous lesions, thus to reduce the probability of their transformation into cancer. This cancer control measure became very effective and in countries where Pap test was made available, major reduction of mortality was registered (70–90 %). Pap test has been acknowledged as the "best cancer prevention measure available." In 2002, worldwide statistics showed that cervical cancer, once the major killer of women among malignant disease, has moved to the fourth place (after breast, lung and stomach), while in the US it has moved to the sixth place [106].

NOTE: The cited results are estimates based upon well documented reports, mostly from developed countries.

In the past 20 years the epidemiology of cervical cancer has changed dramatically. Basic and epidemiologic research have provided evidence for a connection between certain strains of human papilloma virus (HPV) and both, cervical cancer and high-grade pre-cancerous lesions. According to Franco [69], virtually all cervical carcinoma specimens contain HPV DNA. The authors of this book have seen many koilocytic (HPV infected cells specific morphology) features in malignant cells on smears taken from women with advanced cervical cancer (Figs. 2.1d, 2.3c and 2.4a). Saslow [69] argues that HPV and other cervical cancer risk factors "must be understood in the context of mediation or acquisition of HPV infection," a statement what we consider too strong, but they also continue with, "influencing the events of the natural history of cervical neoplasia that occur following the establishment of a persistent HPV infection," which is more acceptable. As a medical doctor, I was trying, so far unsuccessfully, to find solid evidence that HPV virus (oncogenic strains) could cause cervical cancer in a healthy woman. Why was I doing it? Because there are so many women infected with HPV (40 % of all population in the

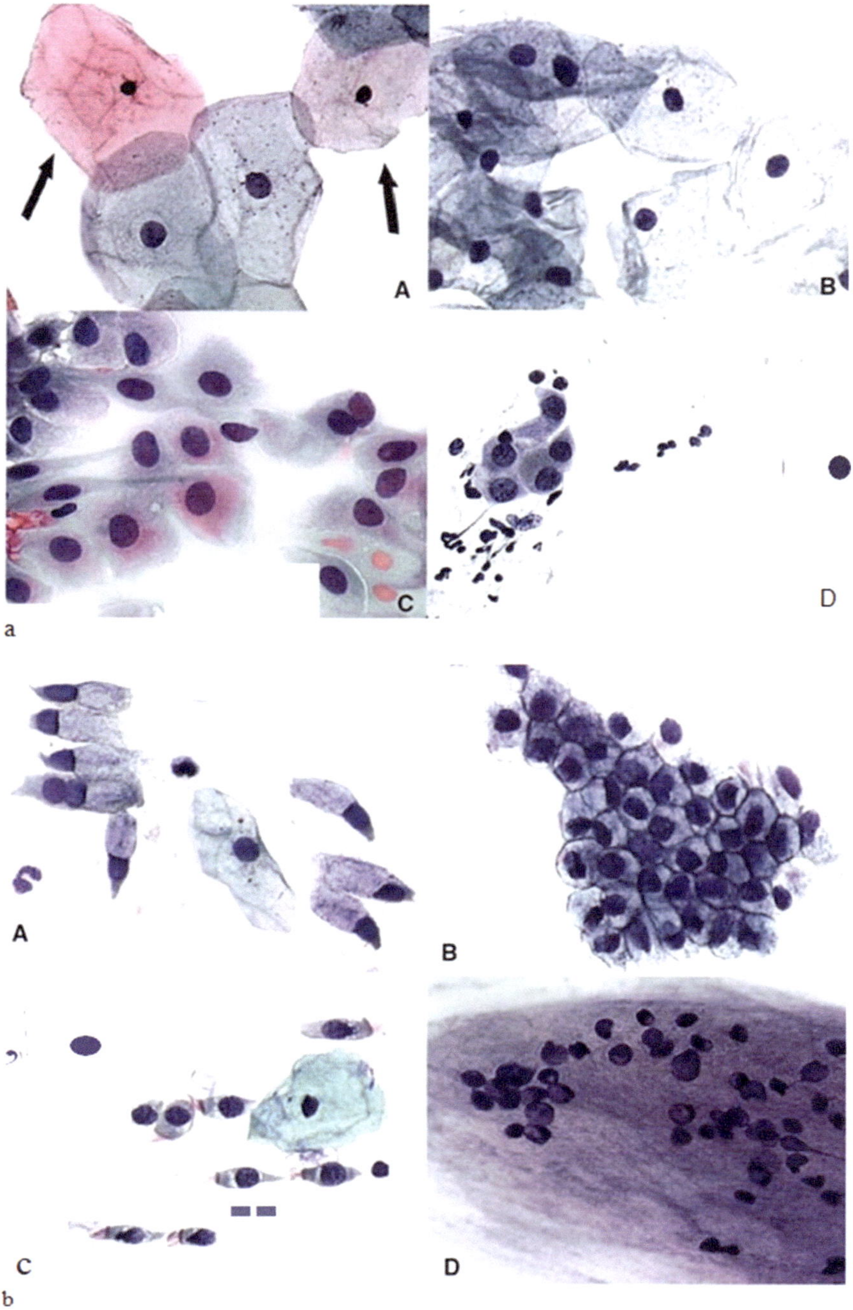

Fig. 2.1 Cytology (with permission by IARC, WHO) (**a**). Normal squamous cells. Normal images obtained from Pap specimens: (A) Superficial squamous cells, (B) intrermediate squamous cells, (C) parabasal squamous cells, (D) metaplastic cells; (**b**). Normal endocervical cells, Normal images obtained from Pap specimens: (A) and (C) Ciliated glandular cells, (B) secretory glandular cells, (D) naked nuclei; (c). Exocervical smear, slightly inflammatory, an intermediate cell with an enlarged nucleolus and homogenouschromatin; d). A group of immature, atypical cells with

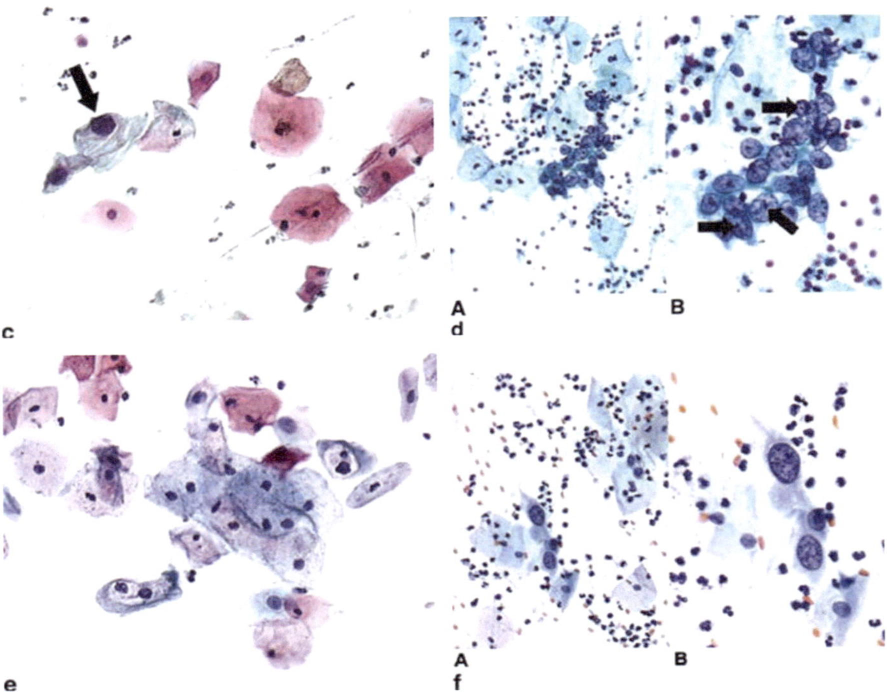

Fig. 2.1 (continued) prominent nucleoli; (e). Basophilic squamous cells with perinuclear cavity and moderate nuclear enlargement – typical koilocytes; (f). Parabasal cells with an enlarged and irregular nucleus among normal superficial and intermediate cells and endocervical cells, mucus, inflammation (Images are reproduced from the Cytopathology of the uterine cervix – Digital Atlas. Edited by L. Frappart, B. Fontaniere, and R. Sankaranayanan. 2004. http://screening.iarc.fr/pic/…)

US) and only 10,000 annually develop cervical cancer. Why is this difference? As solid evidence, I expect to see a study in which a group of women volunteers agree to be infected with oncogenic strains of HPV, and then allow investigators to observe the gradual increase of cervical dysplasia (e.g., disease progress at 3 months from normal to ASCUS, then LSIL, HSIL and CIS) before a doctor will cure this virus-induced disease. The other group could be immunized before infection – the effect of immunization would be immediately established. Unfortunately, such evidence does not exist in available literature. On the other hand, in the Chinese province of Shandong, between 24-year periods (1970–74, and 1990–94) mortality of cervical cancer was reduced from 21.11/100,000 to 4.40/100.000, due (according to the authors) to the effective reduction of syphilis [42]. Does syphilis cause cervical cancer? No, but the chronic inflammation, and syphilis is such an inflammation, can cause it. And this is probably true for other chronic inflammations affecting epithelial tissues everywhere in the body (e.g., lips, oral, anal regions)

Having said that, we would try to present data from published literature with intention to emphasize the problem as a worldwide disease that does not recognize borders and is equal for women of every race, ethnicity, education, religion or social status. The difference comes later, when Pap test or diagnostic and therapeutic methods are needed but are not available to every woman equally.

Examples will be given to illustrate the importance of the preventive screening and to convey the message to all women. At the end of the twentieth century, worldwide, because Pap test was not available to all women, only 6.5 % women got screening, there were 500,000 new cases of cervical cancers per year and 250,000 women died from this preventable disease. Cervical cancer was the leading cause of death from malignant diseases in developing countries. More women die from cervical cancer than from childbirth.

In the beginning of the twenty-first century, this situation began to improve. The understanding that cervical cancer is preventable disease if detected on time become almost universal knowledge, and WHO (IARC, Cervical Cancer Screening Group), followed with many governments, started serious campaigns to include their female population in cancer screening programs [91]. A typical example is China. Several years ago, they did not have regular Pap test screening. In 2006, China reported over 70 million tests, and the estimate is that the number of tests will grow by a rate of ten million tests per year until the majority of the 300 million women at risk will be protected. Similar, but less spectacular, trends are present in other countries (e.g., Vietnam, India). New emerging biomarker-based technologies are not only providing a better and more accurate Pap test, but are expected to make it available to all women in the world and save lives. These efforts resulted in changing the natural history of cervical cancer and, according to one recent statistics, in a combination of developed and developing countries (but performing cervical cancer screening campaigns) the mortality of cervical cancer has moved from first to fourth position of all cancers [106]. Without those efforts, still in too many countries, the situation has not been changed.

A special section in this book (2.3.6 HPV and cervical cancer) is provided to understand the importance of HPV testing and novel HPV vaccines. It is clarified that the HPV vaccination will not decrease the need for cervical cancer screening; the cytological screening (Pap test and alternatives) will continue in the years to come (CDC, CMS, WHO) [41].

Cervical cancer, which is worldwide the second major killer of women from malignant diseases (after breast cancer) [148] is closely related to sexual habits and to certain strains of human papilloma virus infection that can cause sexually transmitted diseases (STD), genital warts and anal-genital cancers. Probably, due to the increasing women's sexual freedom and to the contagiousness of transmission, cervical cancer is now affecting approximately 500,000 women per annum, but if this trend is not interrupted, the incidence is expected to increase to 1,000,000 per year by 2050 [Dr. Boyle, Director IARC, 2005].

The incidence of cervical cancer is also increasing in the population of HIV/AIDS patients who have reduced immuno-competence allowing other risk factors, including HPV, to promote the cervical cancer occurrence. World Health Organization (WHO) is reporting worldwide programs for reduction of HIV/AIDS infection as STD (sexually transmitted diseases). Those programs include intensive education on sexual habits, thus, they also include prevention of cervical cancer [176].

In this text, we will discuss mortality, incidence of cervical cancer, incidence of CIN and incidence of Pap test positive results, both in the US (where excellent statistics are available) and worldwide (according to scanty reports and WHO summaries).

Mortality from cervical cancer is different around the world, ranging from 2.3 for white American women to 93.9 for Haitian women. This difference is related to the availability of Pap test. WHO is largely using data available in the Globocan Statistical Database (IARC) and to NCI SEER database [8, 92, 135] (Table 2.2).

Based on the same source of data, we identified three points to consider as essential for improving this unacceptable discrepancy:

- Reducing the cost of Pap test to make it affordable for worldwide application. The cost to be reduced includes all crucial elements of the test: the specimen collection, processing, interpretation and quality control. However, the cost reduc-

Table 2.2 Cervical cancer epidemiology according to published studies [21]

Country & source		Group	Mortality	Incidence	Test/year	Pap +
USA [135]		Average	2.9	8.7	50 million annually 2000–2004	3.5 million, or 7 % of 50 million tests per year
		Latino	3.3	13.3		
		White	2.3	8.5		
		American-Indian	4.5	11.5		[144] insufficient Pap
China [68]	1970–74		21.11		In 2005, 72 million tests	Reduction of syphilis Shandong Province
	1990–92		4.40	12.3		
India [23]			8.5	17.1		No Pap test available
Central America [67]		40.28	16.84	2001		
South America [67]		30.92	17.03			
Brazil [12, 27]		Statistical package Globocan 2000	11.8	31.3	New 24,445	
Haiti [12]			93.9	24.28	New 2428	Highest
Puerto Rico [12]			10.3	4.3	New 262	Pap test available
Mexico [12]			16.8	40.5	New 16,448	
Europe EU25 [13, 35]			3.74	10.43	2004	
Russia [13]			5.2			
Poland [8]			7.8	14.4		
Australia [42, 173]			2.66	7.72		
Melanesia [42]			23.78	43.81		

tion should not reduce the quality of testing and follow-up diagnosis and treatment. New methods are sought.

- Health Service should organize cervical cancer screening to be accessible and affordable for the majority of population at risk.
- Transform health care campaigns into a health care service available to every woman by making the funding for cervical cancer screening and the follow-up diagnosis and treatment a permanent asset.

In the medical literature, cervical cancer epidemiology is largely associated with studies related to the comparison of invasive cervical cancer incidence and its relation to the number of so called risk factors. Studying the probability of their relationships causality may be established. If this causality will be established with external risk factors, there has been a hope that medical or behavioral/educational interventions could reduce those risks, consequently the incidence of cervical cancer. This brings the fourth point to consider:

- Include education for reduction of risk factors as an essential part of the campaigns. Setup outreach goals and milestones to reach these goals.

We also believe that, in the case of cervical cancer, the prevention is more powerful than many would like to believe. Table 2.3 presents our vision on how different cancer prevention measures could change the natural history of cancer in the US.

This table shows that the hopes for eradication of cervical cancer [178] in the twenty-first century may not be groundless. However, instead of giving the crucial role to the HPV testing or HPV vaccination, we believe that a concentrated action of all factors cited in this table could be the only means to achieve such a noble goal.

Worldwide the situation will change to the extent local governments will be able make modern preventive achievements available to their female population. The following literature examples are only the tip of an iceberg of world scientific literature related to cervical cancer prevention and risk factors.

Interestingly, in 2007, the World Health Organization agencies have been very active in recommending guidance and guidelines for developing countries on how to organize their preventive actions against the "epidemic" of cervical cancer. One of those agencies, the Department for Vaccine Research and Biologicals has issued technical information on HPV and HPV vaccines, targeting policy-makers and

Table 2.3 Cervical cancer mortality and factors influencing IT (estimate)

Time	Cervical cancer prevention in the US	Mortality deaths per 100,000	Comments
<1941	Natural history	30	W/O Prevention
1945–75	Any cancer screening	12	Pre-pap test
1955–2005	Pap test	3	After 50 years
?	Biomarkers	2	Estimate
1945–2007	Education for risks	1	Estimate
>2006	HPV vaccines	<1	After 20 years
?	New therapies	0?	Hope

health professionals worldwide [177]. The essence of this document is that cervical cancer is caused by HPV infection and development of cervical cancer is 100 % related to HPV virus. This contradicts reports from another agency, the International Agency for Cancer Research, which maintains that the role of HPV in cervical cancer carcinogenesis is probably serious, but not 100 %.

When we read published material, we found that in many different WHO reports published by WHO Press, there is a sentence stating, "This report reflects the opinion of the authors, and does not represent the position of WHO." We would like our readers to be aware of this clear distinction between the authors of the recommendations and the publisher or the sponsoring organization.

According to Brinton [29] there is a strong association between cervical cancer occurrence and religions, and the behavior of marital and sexual partners. It is not clear how these factors interact with HPV infection which is the major infective etiological agent. Also, Herpes Simplex virus infection may increase the risk. More speculative factors include cigarette smoking, oral contraceptive usage and certain nutritional deficiencies. Numbers of studies implicate male partners as the risk factor.

In 2004, an NCI study group reported that because the oncogenic HPV infections (HPV type 16, 18, 31, 45, 52) are common but usually clear within 1–2 years, it is of utmost importance to determine the role of cofactors, which may promote development of cervical cancer instead of the HPV disease spontaneous healing [160]. They examined 235 cases of squamous cervical carcinoma and 486 controls. Among HPV exposed women having a Pap test, black race and yeast infections were significantly associated with increased cancer risk. Current smoking was associated with a twofold increase in risk. Increased risk tendency was found in women with lower education, low-income and history of unspecified genital infections. Oral contraceptive use was not related and multi-parity was only weakly related.

Similar studies were conducted worldwide, most of them to show connection between HPV and cervical cancer, but also to indicate cofactors and other risk factors. Most of them confirmed coincidence but not causality.

A study from Colombia and Spain included 436 histologically confirmed squamous cell carcinoma and 387 age-stratified controls [27]. An association between HPV DNA and cervical cancer was confirmed in 70 %, suggesting that the rest of cases were associated with other STD and risk factors. Among other factors, this study identified oral contraceptives, early age of the first intercourse and early age of the first childbirth as independently correlated. Low education and the number of sex partners were surrogates for HPV infection.

A study from Denmark included 59 women with invasive cervical carcinoma, 596 women with CIS (carcinoma in situ, or CIN 2/3) and 614 controls. The study showed that cervical carcinoma and CIS shared risk factors strongly associated with sexual behavior and STD factors, and with adolescent HPV infection (warts). In addition, a cohort study including 11,088 showed 199 cases with LSIL/HSIL Pap test, and 131 with ASCUS. HSIL cases were closely associated with HPV high-risk infection, up to 80 %, which was a 33-fold increase in comparison with HPV negative cases in the same study [98].

A study from Brazil (Sao Paolo area with the highest cervical cancer rates in the country) included 199 histologically confirmed invasive cervical cancer cases and compared with 225 age-frequency-matched controls. The study showed HPV DNA in 84 % cancer cases compared with 17 % in negative cases [62]. The study also emphasized the role of additional risk factors such as prior Pap smears reducing the risk, while number of sexual partners, the early age at first intercourse, parity and duration of contraceptive use; all were associated with increased risks.

In a predominantly monogamous population in Bangkok, Thailand, 190 women with squamous and 42 women with adenomatous cervical carcinoma were compared with 291 cervix-free disease women for association between HPV DNA and neoplasia. The study found high correlation with HPV-16 and HPV-18 types. However, other risk factors were also involved, husbands visit to prostitutes, early age of first intercourse, parity and use of oral contraceptives [168].

Many similar studies (like 14, 16) between 1990 and 2006 confirmed an association between oncogenic HPV types and the occurrence of cervical neoplasia; no direct evidence was presented, but much circumstantial evidence what, according to the epidemiological criteria, could sustain a conclusion that this association is more causal than coincidental.

An interesting study in the US was reported in the February 2007 issue of JAMA. Dunn et al. reported that prevalence of HPV infection is greater than expected in American females aged 14–59 years (26.8 % with 95%CI between 23.3 and 30.9 %) but the relative percent of high-risk types (HPV16 and HPV18) was relatively low (3.4 %) questioning the effectiveness of mass HPV vaccination with Gardasil (Merck) or Cervarix (GSK) [60].

A recent meta-analysis of eight case–control studies of cervical cancer conducted in three countries revealed that cervical adenocarcinoma is associated with the HPV infection almost the same way as the squamous cell carcinoma [38]. This study suggests that anti viral measures will affect both types of cervical carcinoma. This also indicates that HPV infection is neither cell type specific nor behaves as a monoclonal disease (cancer). It is possible that HPV virus infects growing cancer cells and remains in this association further.

An interesting study was conducted in the US between years 2003 and 2004. The National Health and Nutrition Examination Survey was conducted and the results are published by CDC on their MMWR [44]. According to this study, the prevalence of HPV infection (not HPV disease) is largest in sexually active young women (40 % between ages 15–19, and 50 % between 20 and 24) as it could be detected by HC 2 test. Other age groups show gradual decrease of HPV infection. Cervical cancer is not a problem for women at age between 14 and 24 – it comes much later. We read this study in favor of HPV being a cofactor not a causative agent for cervical cancer.

Some strange risk factors were also reported incidentally. One of them was the wood-burning in the kitchen of Honduras [174]. Their value is to be established by scientific criteria.

However, none of those factors have shown such a powerful influence on the incidence of invasive cervical cancer as was established for the regular Pap test checkups in developed countries. In the US, for example, between years 1955 and 2005, the incidence risk of invasive cervical cancer and of cervical cancer mortality has been reduced fourfold; this reduction has been largely credited to the Pap test. If this is true, and all evidence is supporting this assessment of Pap test, then NOT having Pap test regularly should be considered as a substantial risk factor and should be put on the List of risk factors for cervical cancer.

Having given such credit to the Pap test, we would like to emphasize now that Pap test is only a tool to detect early cervical lesions that, if untreated, could develop into cervical cancer. It is the management of women with abnormal Pap test that eliminates suspect lesions and reduces other risk factors that could alter prognostically unwanted trends and prevent the occurrence of the disease.

As Pap test is a guidance for elimination of suspect cervical lesions, the HPV testing could be considered as guidance for elimination of high-risk HPV strains. Because the antiviral therapy against HPV is still not available (surgery can only reduce the viral load), the most promising means to protect women is the HPV vaccination. Whether elimination of high-risk strains would reduce the incidence of Pap test positive results, the incidence of CIN/CIS growths, or the incidence of cervical cancer, remains to be seen within the next 20–30 years when more robust data will be available. In the meantime, we are living with hopes created by statistical analyses and the optimistic estimates of the future without cervical cancer.

In 2007, cervical cancer screening in the US is facing specific problems:

- The screening role of Pap test is losing grounds to a new diagnostic role. This (new?) role includes test prognostic elements such as diagnosis of HPV types involved and other DNA PCR markers (e.g., chlamydia and neisseria). The new role adds to the cost, improves specificity but reduces sensitivity and fewer women are being seen by specialist to make decision of their further treatment (reduction of frequency to compensate for the increase of the cost).
- Growing impression that HPV vaccination will prevent all cervical cancers and that Pap test is not needed anymore; a trend causing prolongation of the period between two controls (over 2 years) is increasing the probability for higher incidence of cervical cancer.
- Transforming the specimen collecting solution from a cervical sample only into a general female genital health sample for multiple assays is diffusing the concentration of the health care providers to the main purpose of cervical specimen – the cervical cancer screening. Pap test is not easy to properly conduct, and not comfortable for women, therefore, using this specimen collection for other purposes is ethically unacceptable – but this is up to the American Medical Association to evaluate.

We think that the role of the absenteeism from regular Pap test screening as a risk factor has not been emphasized sufficiently. Consequently, the value of regular testing has been challenged by many "business" oriented scientists who recommended adding "diagnostic" and "prognostic" values to the screening test. Naturally, a conventional Pap test cannot answer to such "high-quality" requirements, and the label of "not good enough" has been added to the best cancer screening test. It is important for every woman to know that no other test has shown such a consistency of providing benefit to women in the fight against cervical cancer as the conventional Pap test.

Epidemiology of cervical cancer is still an evolving story. Incidence and mortality are excellent but not sufficient measures for assessment, and new parameters indicating outcomes of preventive and cancer control measures should be included (e.g., positive/negative Pap test and HPV induced disease). New biomarker-based tests will probably add to more aggressive early surgery eliminating lesions that could progress into invasive cancer, and a revision of risk factors could improve our understanding that not-taking preventive measures (behavior that can be changed by education) is increasing substantially the risk for missing cervical cancer occurrence and/or progress.

2.3 Prevention and Control of Cervical Cancer

Prevention of cervical cancer is a term intended to include better understanding of cervical carcinogenesis, factors triggering malignant transformation and growth, and knowledge on how to eliminate, avoid or reduce those factors with an ultimate goal to reduce (if not eliminate) cervical cancer occurrence.

> As all other cancers, cervical cancer is an autonomous disease characterized by unstoppable growth of abnormal (malignant) cells which destroy surrounding tissues forming local tumors (lump, swelling), move via lymph pathways to surrounding lymph nodes (regional spread), or via blood to distant places where they continue their abnormal growth with all collateral consequences (distant metastases).

Cervical cancer starts to grow when a single cell with potential to replicate itself (from the basal or para-basal epithelial layers – see Fig. 2.3) begins to produce cells with malignant characteristics such as the following:

- Resistance to normal growth control signals including oxygen supply
- Unstoppable replication with destruction of the surrounding tissue and creating genuine blood supply (cancer invasion)
- Loosing intercellular connections with ability for and easy separation of cells with the same destructive abilities which use lymph and blood flow to migrate in distant sites of the body (cancer metastases)

> We do not know what is a primary trigger of this transformation (spontaneous mutation, radiation, drugs, viruses, all of them or none of them), but we know that the body has immune-defense mechanism to identify and destroy those abnormal cells. Consequently, there must be two events to concur: origination (birth) of a malignant tissue and the insufficiency of the defense mechanism to control this growth.

All we can do is to try to control these two events by controlling the so called risk factors which, we know, could promote cancer growth or alter the defense mechanism. This section will discuss the known risk factors that may increase or decrease the probability for a woman to get cervical cancer. Our current knowledge about risk factors for cervical cancer is coming out of epidemiological studies, which could only establish an association between events. However, if the results of these studies are repeatedly seen in study-by-study, our confidence is increasing that this association may contain some causality. Unfortunately, real causality may be proven only by experiments, and for cervical cancer such experiments are still to be performed because of many ethical issues involved.

2.3.1 Risk Factors and Education to Reduce Their Influence

> *All women should be aware of the risks and how to avoid them whenever possible.*
>
> Risk factors for cervical cancer are closely related to women's behavior (particularly sexual life style) and, therefore, medical interventions must be combined with educational efforts to make the protection more permanent. It is a big task, but we need to plant awareness of the importance for these interrelations if any success is to be expected.
>
> This chapter will cover the known risk factors and will outline education on how to avoid them in order to decrease one's chance to develop pre-cancerous changes and cervical cancer. All women should know about the risks and how to use this knowledge for self-protection against cervical cancer.

Let us talk about the risk factors that health education literature is mostly recommending. According to the American Cancer Society (ACS) most recent web page (June 20, 2007) [4] the following list includes most of the known risk factors:

- Human papilloma virus infection
- Certain types of sexual behavior such as
  - Having sex at an early age
  - Having many sexual partners
  - Having partner who has many sex partners
  - Having sex with uncircumcised man
- Smoking
- Human immunodeficiency virus (HIV) infection
- Chlamydia infection
- Diet
- Oral contraceptives (birth control pills)
- Multiple pregnancies
- Low socioeconomic status
- Diethylstibestrol (DES)
- Family history of cervical cancer
- Other Sexually transmitted diseases (STD).

We would add three more factors that belong to the general risks for cancer:

- Exposure to radiation, any type
- Exposure to drugs that may affect nuclear genetic material
- Prolonged stress.

Finally, we would like to propose a new risk factor:

- The Absenteeism from Pap test screening within the recent 3 years.

We have summarized those risk factors on Table 2.4 below.

This table is adding a new group of risk factors "the Participation in cancer screening" and reveals that both nonparticipation and false results lead to the lack of medical protection, and recommend education and medical help as necessary interventions for reducing risk factors in this group.

Let me now address few thoughts to each of these factors and you will find which one could be relevant for your specific situation. You will find more information in the referenced literature.

Table 2.4 List of risk factors, interrelations and recommended interventions

Group	Risk factor		Interrelation	Intervention
Behavior	Sexual behavior	Early age	With HPV	Education[a]
		Many sex partners		
		Partner with many sex partners		
		Sex with uncircumcised man		
	Smoking	Statistics only		
	Diet	Vitamin E, raw food, fruit & vitamin C, folic acid, vegetables, selenium, macrobiotic diet, meat		
Participation in cancer screening	Absenteeism from regular screening	No Pap test within 3 years	Lack of protection	
	Insufficient health care protection	False negative Pap		Medical help[b]
		Inaccurate Pap		
		Alternative Pap		
STD[c]	HPV	Persistent	Other factors	Medical help
	HIV	AIDS	Immunocompetence	
	Chlamydia	Chronic infection	HPV?	
	Syphilis			
	Chronic cervicitis	Any genesis		
Social	Oral contraceptives	Long term use, HRT	HPV?	Education
	Multiple pregnancies	Statistics, not direct proof	STD?	Education, Medical help
	Low SE status	Multiple factors	STD	Free education

(continued)

Table 2.4 (continued)

Group	Risk factor		Interrelation	Intervention
Genetic	Family history	Complex of geno- and phenotypic predisposing factors	Any other risk factor	Medical help
Exposures	DES – diethyl-stilbestrol	Mutagenesis	Clear cell carcinoma	Cancer control
	Radiation	Carcinogenesis	Direct effect	Environmental
	Mutagenic drugs			Medical help
	Chemotherapy	Immuno-competence	STD	Medical help

[a]Education as a part of cancer prevention activities
[b]Medical help as defined in cancer control, diagnosis and treatment
[c]Sexually transmitted diseases includes HPV

2.3.1.1 Human Papilloma Virus (Genital Warts)

This risk factor will be discussed more in the Sect. 2.3.6 (HPV and cervical cancer) of this book.

Genital warts (condylomata acuminata, veneral, anal and anogenital warts) is a highly contagious sexually transmitted skin disease (estimated prevalence among sexually active population in the US is 10–20 %), caused by some types of HPV (6, 11), with lower pathogenicity (1–2 % of the population at risk), and with good prognosis (90 % resolve spontaneously), but could continue transmitting the infection.

Warts grow as clusters from size of 1–5 mm to large masses protruding around the genital area. They affect male and female partners. Diagnosis is by biopsy – papillomatosis with typical cells – koilocytes and parakeratosis. It could be missed for early cervical cancer – visual appearance and acid test, as well as HC-2 test, which are positive.

Here, I would like to emphasize several important facts.

- Medical diagnosis of HPV infection is neither diagnosis of cervical cancer nor the verdict that cervical cancer will occur. It is only a sign that one risk factor is present, nothing more. And this HPV high-risk strain should persist for more than 2 years in order to be considered as a disease of high risk for cervical cancer.
- A group of about 30–40 HPVs are typically transmitted through sexual contact and infect ano-genital region. (Recent reports focus on oro-pharyngeal region). Most of HPV types cause benign papilloma (warts). A persistent infection with any type of the subset of 13 so-called "high-risk" HPV (16, 18, 31, 33, 35, 39, 45, 51, 56, 58, 59 and 69) can lead to development of cervical dyskaryosis or a pre-cancerous lesion. Once the lesion is present it can produce a positive Pap test. Such a lesion may resolve by itself (most likely) or, if untreated, progress into cancer (least likely).

- HPV disease is STD (sexually transmitted disease) caused by an opportunistic pathogen (virus is usually present without causing disease in healthy women or men). The virus is present in the genital fluids and is transmitted with direct contact. The virus is highly contagious, but of low virulence and requires an altered body defense system to begin the disease. The probability that an infected woman will develop cervical cancer is about 1 pro mille (~0.001).
- HPV oncogenes, E5 and E7, which are considered to be virusrelated genes promoting cervical cancer are also genes promoting the growth of warts (benign papilloma), and warts are more frequent outcome than cancer.
- However, detecting HPV infection indicates to a sexually active woman and to a certain type of sexual behavior such as having sex at an early age, having many sexual partners, having partner who has many sex partners, having sex with HPV infected man, and to a probability of exposure to many other risk factors. This is the secondary, but important meaning of HPV testing; the one that is most controversial from the social aspects.

2.3.1.2 Human Immunodeficiency Virus (HIV) Infection – AIDS

HIV is the virus causing AIDS (autoimmune deficiency syndrome) that is a viral disease characterized by increased sensitivity to infection including opportunistic pathogens such as HPV. AIDS patients are more prone to developing cervical dysplasia, and they should be more vigorously examined with Pap test because they are also at high risk for any cancer including cervical cancer.

Both CDC (Centers for Disease Control and Prevention) and AHCRQ (Agency for Healthcare and Research) recommend that women with HIV be screened more frequently than healthy women (at least 1–2 times annually).

2.3.1.3 Smoking

Smoking is recently recommended for consideration as a risk factor for cervical cancer. Indirect, epidemiological evidence is offered to support this recommendation. One study in Sweden [145] included 375 Pap positive women with 363 Pap negative. The authors called them as women "with" and "without" the earliest stages of cervical cancer. Among smokers, those who tested positive for HPV-16 were 14.4 times more likely to get cervical cancer than those who did not have the infection. Among smokers, those who had high HPV-16 viral load were 27 times more likely to develop cervical cancer than those who did not have the infection. Among nonsmokers, those who tested positive for HPV-16 were only six times more likely to get cervical cancer than nonsmokers without the infection [56].

Until more convincing evidence is offered, we would consider smoking as a cofactor to other behavioral and STD risk factors for cervical cancer with some additive effect.

2.3.1.4 Chlamydia Infection (Lymphogranuloma Venerum)

Chlamydia trachomatis infection is another low symptomatic STD that, until recently, has been considered as a cofactor (with HPV) for causing a more persistent inflammation of uterine cervix and probably cervical cancer. More research in this area has been conducted since 2001 [189]. Most of the studies reported epidemiological connection between chlamydia infection, HPV and cervical cancer, but the results were not conclusive. More basic research tried to establish whether chlamydia infection could affect cancerogenesis, but also no conclusion was made. An excellent review of literature data on chlamydia infection and cervical cancer is available on the Internet [9].

Nevertheless, chlamydia infection is formally accepted as a risk factor for cervical cancer (ACS Guidelines) and measures for detection and clearing of this infection are recommended within the preventive measures for cervical cancer.

Interestingly, both chlamydia and HPV infections indicate to a type of sexual behavior that supports persistent inflammation – a verified causative factor in cancerogenesis. We think that better sexual education, telling women the truth, not frightening them, and combined with treatment of genital inflammation, will bring more success than mass screening for HPV or chlamydia that has been recommended.

2.3.1.5 Diet and Cervical Cancer

Food has always been associated with cancer as a factor that may reduce or increase the risks for getting this disease. It is easy to connect the lack of food (malnourishment) with impaired immunity and cancer development because of breaks in the body defense system. It is more difficult to connect overeating (obesity) with cancer, but many have found metabolic defects that could affect cancer development [6].

Cervical cancer has been closely associated with consumption of vitamin E, raw foods, fruit and vitamin C, folic acid, vegetables, selenium, macrobiotic diet, and meat [95].

Antioxidants are substances that may protect cells from damage caused by unstable molecules known as free radicals. These radicals are produced by radiation, chemotherapeutic drugs (e.g., adriamycin), aging, ischemia and similar, but they may produce DNA/RNA damage that can initiate cancer progress. Cells have their own natural mechanisms for protection against free radicals, but sometimes, this mechanism could be overwhelmed, or insufficient to cope with the size of the tissue injury and number of newly formed radicals. In such situation, disease occurs and progress. Antioxidants are available in most raw foods, and as vitamins in supplemental therapy [132].

Vitamin E is an antioxidant and could protect cells from damage caused by unstable molecules known as free radicals [93]. Free radical damage may lead to cancer. Antioxidants interact and stabilize free radicals and may prevent some of the damage free radicals otherwise might cause. Examples of antioxidants include beta-carotene, lycopene, vitamins C, E, A, and other substances. However, clinical trials have been inconclusive [139]. Nevertheless, antioxidants are recommended as food supplements for prevention of cervical and other cancers.

Raw food (not cooked vegetables, fruits, seeds) has superior nutritional value than cooked food. Many vitamins such as vitamin C, vitamin B and vitamin E are destroyed when food is cooked; vital enzymes are destroyed and essential fatty acid become unstable in high temperatures. The recommendation to prefer raw over cooked food has come after a report by the United States Academy of Science which surveyed over 10,000 research papers and found dangerous compounds in food coloring, preservative compounds and tap water. No special emphasis was given to cervical cancer.

Vitamin C reduces production of nitrosamines, a cancer causing chemicals that are formed in the body during digestion of nitrates and nitrites. High content of these chemicals could be found in tinned, smoked and cured meets and fish, sausages, bacon, pickled foods and smoked cheeses. Tap water may contain nitrates and nitrites in areas were fertilization is widely used. One study found that women with abnormal Pap test had lower amount of vitamin C [95], but there was no conclusive evidence connecting cervical cancer and vitamin C. Tobacco-specific nitrosamines are best studied in lung cancer, but cervical cancer is not included [156].

Women with cervical dysplasia, particularly those who used the pill, have lower levels of **folic acid** than those who did not. In one study on oral contraceptives, cervical dysplasia gradually decreased in the group supplemented with folic acid tablets, but remained unchanged in the group given placebo [191]. Again, drugs were involved, and folic acid served as a food supplement depleted by oral estrogens – not a direct connection between the vitamin and cancer.

At least two large studies addressed the issue of **vegetables** reducing the risk of cervical cancer [145, 192]. In the prospective study [145] lower levels of folic acid, beta carotene, and vitamin C were found in patients with cervical cancer, and in the other [193] both dark-green and yellow-orange vegetable consumption and multivitamin supplementation were each strongly related to reduced risk.

Both studies stressed the importance of a diet balanced with vitamins particularly those having antioxidant effect. However, direct relation between vegetable food and cancer has not been convincingly established.

Selenium attracted attention in the second part of the last century because of its ability to work with vitamin E as an antioxidant and to boost the production of immune antibodies. Selenium is found in garlic, brewers yeast, mushroom, sesame seeds, brazil, cashew nuts, asparagus seaweed, cabbage and cruciferous vegetables – it all were found to inhibit growth of cancers; however, no convincing data related to cervical cancer have been reported. However, at least one study clearly did not support the relationship between serum selenium and invasive cervical cancer at typical serum selenium levels in the US [141, 169].

Macrobiotic diet has been investigated after reports that the Oriental diet, low in fat and high in carbohydrates and fiber has helped some people to enter remission of cancer. Nothing more than anecdotal data are reported, but the change of lifestyle – typical for this diet – could be responsible more than the diet itself [95].

There are many studies connecting eating **meat** (both red meet and poultry) with all forms of cancers. They all stress the importance of vegetarian diets because vegetarians have, at average, less cancers than omnivores. One study from Hawaii found positive correlation between frequency of uterine cancer and the consumption of animal fat and animal protein [101].

2.3.1.6 Oral Contraceptives and Cervical Cancer

Female genital system is under hormonal control. Both estrogen and progesterone cause structural changes of genital epithelium during the menstrual cycle and pregnancy. Hormones also influence cervical epithelium. Cervix grows in size (hypertrophy) and in number of cells (hyperplasia). In the next phase, superficial epithelial cells separate from the tissue and shed into vaginal fluids (exfoliation).

These are well known phenomena related to human reproduction in women.

The question is whether estrogen and progesterone given as contraceptive pills or HRT (hormone replacement therapy) may incite cancer development as an adverse event. Many studies have addressed this issue. There is substantial evidence that long term hormonal use (5 years and above) could increase the risk for breast and endometrial (uterine) cancers – this is the basis for the recent recommendation to gynecologists to stop prescribing hormonal therapy for alleviation of peri-menopausal syndrome. With regard to cervical cancer, there are many studies indicating that oral contraceptives pose risk for cervical cancer [136]. However, recent reviews of those studies have questioned their value because most of them have not included HPV infection as the confounding variable. The issue remains controversial [127].

We believe in basic principles: the rule of probability and the chance of spontaneous mutation. Additional estrogen certainly incites basal cells to further reproduction, chance of spontaneous mutation increases, but the probability of cancer development in healthy women is so low that the benefit overweighs the risks. However, in presence of persistent HPV infection (with high-risk viral strains), or immuno-incompetence (chemotherapy or HIV), the pill or HRT may have a cooperative effect and increase the chance for cervical cancer.

2.3.1.7 Multiple Pregnancies

Multiple pregnancies are always cited as a risk factor for cervical cancer, but we have not seen a randomized clinical trial to confirm, with statistical proof, that the real connection exists. Multiple pregnancies are usually connected with multiple cervical injuries, cervico-vaginal infections including HPV, therefore, a theoretical justification is present, but nothing more conclusive has been reported.

2.3.1.8 Low Socioeconomic Status

This is probably the most relevant single risk factor for development of cervical cancer, but because of the multiple factors involved under the same term, it is almost impossible to select proper preventive recommendation. Socioeconomic status is directed by the family income and it is responsible for lifestyle, individual behavior and environmental influences. I usually use analogy while teaching students: "Empty wallet cannot cause cervical cancer, but causes many other unwanted conditions, which may contribute to the development of this disease."

However, many governments are trying to reduce this social status influence using taxpayers' money via promoting cervical cancer prevention programs or campaigns. Due to the modern communications and worldwide media coverage, the knowledge that cervical cancer is a preventable disease has been spread widely – the policy-makers who want to be reelected could not risk to be seen as someone who is neglecting the health benefit of a half of his constituency. Making Pap test widely available to all women is a typical governmental response to this challenge.

In countries that cannot afford the Pap test, other cervical cancer screening techniques were tried, but none has reached the protection rate of the Pap test. After the introduction of HVP vaccines, some countries are trying to approve it for their citizens, and to mandate Pap test as to control the success of vaccination (Serbia, Macedonia). In India, the strategy is to develop 2d generation HPV vaccine out of herbs and make vaccination affordable (currently Merck is charging $500.00 for three vaccines). In China, the government has ordered all hospitals to perform Pap test for small compensation – in 2 years China has reached a number of 72 million Pap test annually, and expects further growth of ten million tests per year. China and India have approximately 300–400 million women at risk for cervical cancer which need annual protection. International charity organizations such a the Melinda & Gates Foundation are pouring money into developing countries to improve sexual education, HPV prevention, and to subsidize the cost of vaccination. We only hope that those efforts will continue for the next 10–20 years when the effects will be seen as a reduction of cervical cancer mortality for at least 50 % from the current rate per country.

In the US, mostly because of the cost and lack of health insurance, almost 20 million women do not participate in cervical cancer screening – it is not known how many of them belong to the group of 40 million uninsured citizens of this country.

Lower economic status dictates the level of education, type of jobs available, selection of marital partners, and many known types of behavior in the adult life of women. Obviously, all of these aspects and many others have been examined in different behavioral and medical studies as risk factors for cervical cancer. Again, not a single factor was selected as being dominant over the others.

2.3.1.9 DES – Diethylstilbestrol

In the middle of the twentieth century, a synthetic hormone diethylstilbestrol (DES) was one of the best drugs used to protect pregnancies against miscarriages, and millions of women used it in large amounts [43]. It was necessary tens of years to pass before it become obvious that DES induces many adverse events on newborn girls – many were born with enlarged vulva, some had menstrual bleeding at birth, but many developed an early childhood leukemia (up to the age of 10) and some developed vaginal carcinoma (clear cell carcinoma) and other malignant diseases later in their lives including cervical cancer – all of this significantly more frequent than in their peers born by mothers who did not receive DES during pregnancy [190]. This is one risk factor which is causing cancers, but its causality is not proven for cervical cancer alone.

2.3.1.10 Family History of Cervical Cancer

Although family history is important for some cancers, cervical cancer has not been yet connected with this risk factor or a specific gene change. Simply, cervical cancer does not appear to run in families. In a review, Zelmanowicz and Hildesheim [190] evaluated 19 studies (most from Scandinavia) and found a twofold increase of probability that cervical cancer will occur in a family where it was already present. However, data were not convincing.

2.3.1.11 Other Sexually Transmitted Diseases

This group is not included in the ACS list of risk factors for cervical cancers, but some of them are included into other lists and we will mention them here.

- Herpes Virus. A STD that presently has no cure. However, treatment is available and successful [64].
- Hepatitis. All three types of hepatitis, HA, HB and HC could be passed through sexual contact. Although there is no cure for the disease, there is a vaccine for HB (HBV) which can prevent this type of disease.
- HIV/AIDS. It is clearly connected with increased risk for cervical cancer. The mechanism is via reduction of host immuno-competence. Most information is available at the CDC web site [47].
- Syphilis. It is historic STD for which has cure today.
- Trichomoniasis. Probably most common parasite affecting female genitalia. Not connected with cervical cancer.

2.3.1.12 General Cancer Related Risk Factors

- Exposure to radiation, any type
- Exposure to drugs that may affect nuclear genetic material
- Prolonged stress.

These three factors have been known for years as risk factors for different cancers. We will not discuss them here, but will refer our reader to any oncology textbook, or any Internet reference under "cancer risk factors."

2.3.1.13 Absenteeism from Pap Test Screening. False Negative Pap Test

All previous risk factors are something that women do and can stop doing in order to reduce the risk for cervical cancer. We would like to propose a new risk factor which is opposite; it is something what women do not do, but should do. This is the regular Pap test screening (at least once in 3 years). We are suggesting calling this new risk factor the "Absenteeism" from Pap test within 3 years.

The value of asking about the "Absenteeism" and recording it as a risk factor will be seen in the near future when, upon many predictions, the number of Pap tests will be reduced and replaced with non-cytological alternatives such HPV testing, molecular DNA/ RNA biomarker testing, VIA or "See & Treat." In the US, introduction of liquid-based Pap technologies increased the cost of regular screening; consequently, a new compromise was made between adopting the new techniques for specimen collection and prolonging the interval between screenings. With HPV vaccination and emerging assays for new molecular biomarkers, the cost will be further increased and, we are afraid, the periods between screenings will be further elongated. It could result in an unacceptable return of cervical cancer. To prevent such an outcome, we think that recording and reporting the Absenteeism will show that this new risk factor could be of essential importance.

The same value of "absenteeism" has the "false negative Pap test," but we cannot record or measure the rate of false negatives. According to the current practice, the false positive results cannot be confirmed before the progress of disease is established.

Historically, false negative Pap test results have been the major moving force for improvements of the clinical practice of cervical cancer screening in the US. A woman should know that false negative Pap test results do exist, that their rate could be as high and 20 %, and that she could contribute to their reduction by asking doctors about the false result rates in the laboratory to which she will be sending the Pap test specimen for processing and evaluation.

In summary, the awareness about risk factors and the available measures to reduce the risks cannot prevent every woman from getting cervical cancer, but will certainly dramatically reduce the probability of an educated woman to get cervical cancer below the average rated for her peers.

2.3.2 Cancer Control: Cervical Cancer/Pre-cancerosis Screening

Every woman should know that the risk factors can be controlled only to a certain extent and that cervical cancer could occur silently in healthy women living without any apparent risk factor. Therefore, an active search for early signs of cervical lesions that could develop into cervical cancer must be practiced by a woman who wants full protection against this grave disease (please see Table 2.3). Protecting asymptomatic women from this silent danger is the purpose of the cervical cancer screening, a health care procedure designed to help healthy women to not miss early sings of cervical cancer. Because cervical cancer has been the major killer of women worldwide from malignant disease, every country or region has devised their own program for protection of their female population. The purpose of these programs is to examine healthy women having no symptoms of genital disease for early signs of cervical lesions that, if not treated on time, could develop into cervical cancer, and to remove those lesions if detected.

There are many programs for cervical cancer screening but one of them, Pap test, has become so successful that, today, we can easily classify all cancer screening programs into two categories: the Pap test-based and Non-Pap test-based. The common denominator for all these programs is the emphasis on:

- Outreach – bring as many healthy women into the program as possible
- Screening technology – use methods for detection of cervical lesions that can provide least omissions (false negative results)
- Timely intervention – apply diagnostic and therapeutic modalities that could provide cure of the lesion and full protection against cervical cancer occurrence or progress.

2.3.2.1 Pap Test or Cytology-Based Cervical Cancer Screening

Overview

Currently, the term Pap test encompasses a series of well defined medical procedures and use of medical devices intended to examine healthy women in order to detect cervical dysplasia (pre-cancerosis – lesions that could develop into cervical cancer if not treated) and cervical cancer (if present without clinical symptoms) – and to provide doctors with the decision making key information on how to manage women with cervical specimens showing cells with abnormalities (indicating to cervical cancer or pre-cancerosis). It is a screening method intended to detect each and every woman who might have such a lesion and to inform her doctor about the alarming signal requiring a full diagnostic workup for cervical cancer. Screening test must be highly sensitive not to miss any woman, but the diagnostic workup must be highly specific to prevent any fast conclusion and unnecessary treatment. This is how the Pap test was envisioned.

The cervical cancer screening using Pap test requires three profiles of professionals to act in concert: (1) Primary physician (family medicine, women's health, or gynecologist) to examine woman and to acquire specimen, (2) Cytotechnologist to process this specimen and read it with assistance of cytopathologists for interpretation of the clinical condition, and (3) Gynecologist for completing diagnosis and recommending or applying treatment when necessary. Currently, women with cervical cell abnormalities are treated as recommended in the 2001 ASCCP Guidelines [183]. Lack of coordination within this system, or an insufficiently developed infrastructure because of the cost, is probably the major cause why failures occur and why women are not completely protected worldwide.

All current Pap test-based health care screening practices belong to in vitro diagnostics and have three common elements: (1) specimen collection with a medical device to scrap cervical epithelium, (2) specimen processing using Papanicolaou stains, and (3) specimen interpretation using cytopathology criteria for reading images of specimens stained with Papanicolaou stains. Currently in use are cytologic criteria compiled in the 2001 Bethesda System Terminology [162].

According to different use of these elements, we would sub-classify the Pap test-based screening technologies into: (1) Pap smear (classic, conventional Pap test), (2) Liquid-based Pap (LBP), and (3) Biomarker-improved Pap test. HPV testing, which is currently advertised as a possible alternative for Pap test is only a "biomarker" improved Pap and will be discussed later together with other biomarkers. However, the issue of HPV vaccination is of specific interest as a new preventive measure (immunization) and is discussed separately.

History

About 60 years ago screening for cervical cancer was not known. Women were getting this cancer, it was developing in their bodies as a silent danger and, when first clinical symptoms (e.g., contact bleeding, lumbar pain, abnormal bleeding, and increased vaginal discharge) appeared, the sufferers would have visited doctors only to find out that the disease had advanced to a stage when the prognosis was ominous. Cervical cancer was known as the main killer of women dying from malignant diseases. This situation is still almost the same in many countries around the world, but it is not in the developed countries where mortality has been reduced for more than 80 % (see section on Epidemiology above and Fig. 2.2).

Cancer, and the cervical cancer is not different, is a disease that does not recognize borders, a disease that affects women without preference or prejudice for race, ethnicity, socioeconomic status, religion or education. Like all cancers it is more frequent in older age groups. So, what is the matter? What makes this difference between developed and developing countries? Why do women in developed countries have better prognosis in comparison with those who live in developing countries?

There is a solid base of evidence that this difference is due to the regular participation of women in a cervical cancer screening program – popularly known as the

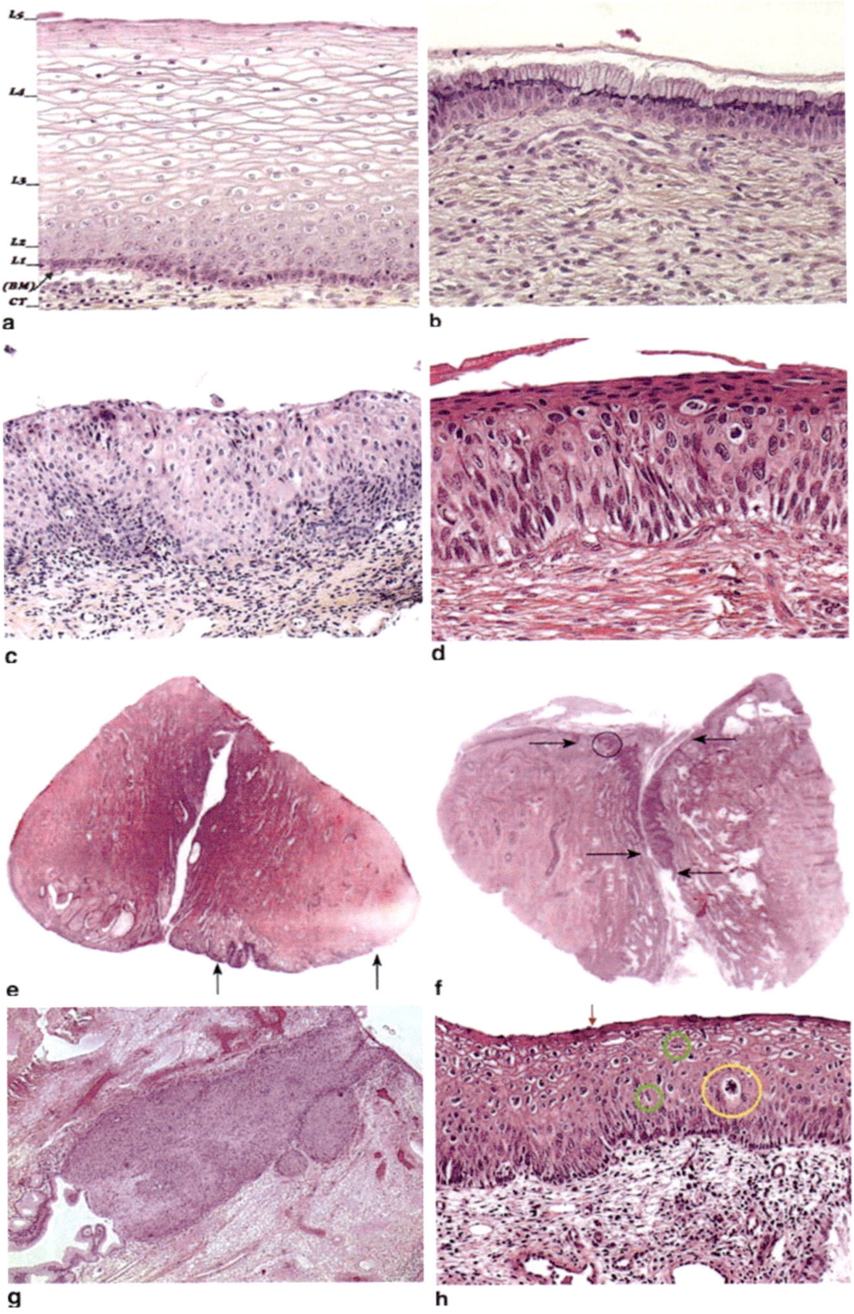

Fig. 2.2 Histology, CIN (With permission by IARC, WHO) (**a**). Normal ectocervix: L1 = basal cells – one layer, L2 = parabasal cells – 2 layers, L3 = intermediate cells – 8 layers, L4 = superficial cells – 5–6 layers, BM = basal membrane, CT = connective tissue; (**b**). Normal endocervix: A layer of columnar cells secreting mucus (above) and of layer of reserve cells above the connective tissue;

Regular Pap Test [136, 139]. This evidence clearly supports the conclusion that women participating in regular screening (at least once in 3 years) have significantly less chances to be diagnosed with cervical cancer (either CIS or advanced) than those who do not participate, participate irregularly, or have been falsely diagnosed as negative. The emphasis is on regular screening and on the accuracy of the Pap test (less false negative results).

There are few events in the history of medical devices that have made a larger impact on the natural course of a malignant disease, and on our thoughts of the value of preventive screening, than the application of the Pap test for cervical cancer screening in the second part of the twentieth century.

The name Pap test was created in honor of Dr. George Papanicolaou, an American-Greek pathologist from New York, who, when studying the oestrus in mice, recognized that specimens collected by excoriation from the cervix (using scrapping device) are more consistent and provide better cytological information than specimens collected from vaginal fluids (exfoliated cells). In the middle of the past Century he convinced a gynecologist (Dr. Thorn from Rockefeller Medical Center in New York) to check whether specimens obtained from women would show the same quality. Indeed, this small change in specimen collection made a whole world of difference. It was a basic change for collection of gynecological specimens from exfoliative cells (spontaneously shed) to excoriated cells (scrapped from the superficial layers of epithelium). After receiving human specimens, Dr. Papanicolaou was not satisfied with standard staining techniques (hematoxylin-eosin for histology or Wright-Giemsa for hematology) and he experimented with different stains to improve cytoplasmic transparency and visibility of nuclear chromatin structures. He introduced hematoxylin, eosinalcohol (EA) and orange G (OG) stains. The experiments were successful and he recognized that this test could become essential for detecting early cervical lesions. These stains remained the core of the Papanicolaou staining until today. The new staining technique was met with a considerable resistance by other pathologists, and Dr. Papanicolaou had to develop an entire new set of criteria for reading and interpretation of slides stained according to his recommendation. This was recognized as Papanicolaou staining [102].

The results were published between 1943 and 1950 and attracted attention of the American Cancer Society (ACS), a non-profit organization with a mission to pro-

Fig. 2.2 (continued) (**c**). koilocytosis, disorganization of the lower layers of the epithelium, cellular criteria of dysplasia and HPV infection: binucleated cells, abnormal mitotic figures, koilocytes; (**d**). Disorganization at all layers of the cervical epithelium, but above an intact basal membrane; (**e**). Thin slice of a cone. Disorganized epithelium in a region between two arrows. Free margins on all sides. Operation leads to cure; (**f**). Thin slice of a cone including cervical canal. Squamous cervical carcinoma in situ – no invasion visible. Operation leads to cure; (**g**). Adenocarcinoma in situ. Proliferation of a abnormal glandular cells into uterine wall, but without spreading – invasion of connective tissues; (**h**). HPV disease: Flat condyloma, HPV infects superficial layers and induce koilocytic appearance of cells in the superficial layers and induce koilocytic appearance of cells in the superficial and intermediate layers (Images are reproduced from the Histopathology of the uterine cervix – Digital Atlas. Edited by L. Frappart, B. Fontaniere, and R. Sankaranayanan. 2004. http://screening.iarc.fr/pic/…)

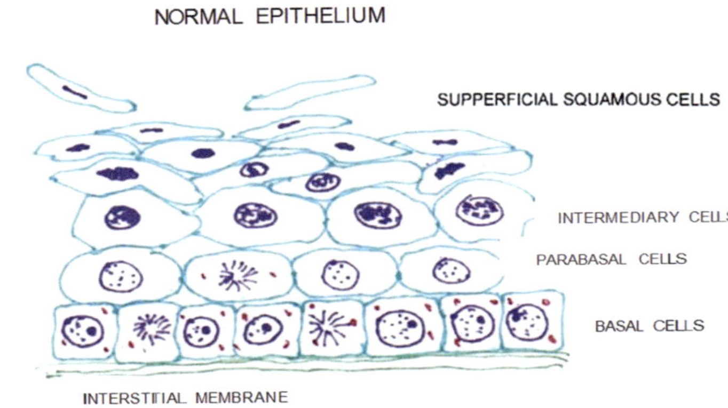

a

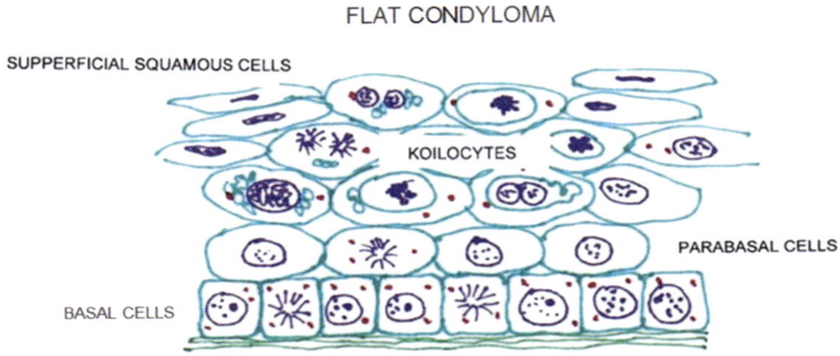

b

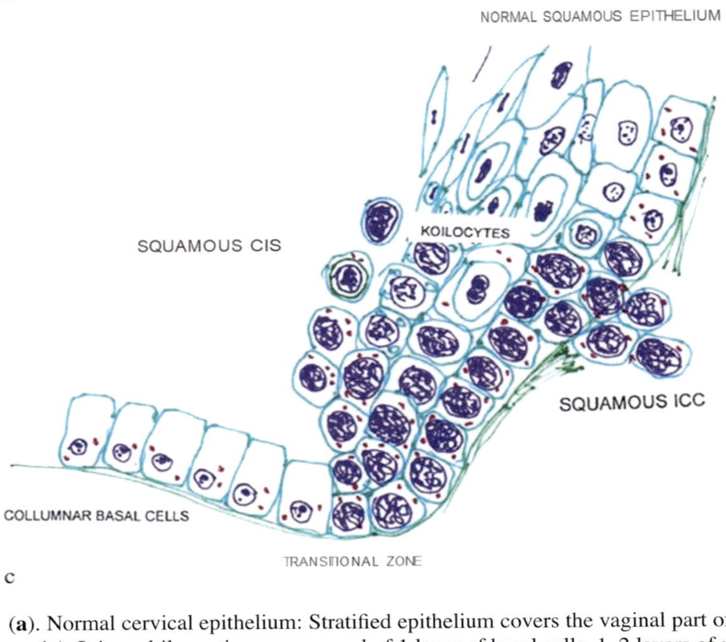

c

Fig. 2.3 (**a**). Normal cervical epithelium: Stratified epithelium covers the vaginal part of the cervix (ectocervix). It is multilayer tissue composed of 1 layer of basal cells, 1–2 layers of parabasal cells, 6–8 layers of intermediate cells, and 6–8 layers of superficial cells. From inside, it is bordered by the interstitial membrane, and from the outside is covered with the mucus (containing mote new ideas for cancer prevention and treatment [5]. The method for obtaining specimens, staining smears according the new technique and stains, and reading and interpreting cytological specimens became known as the Pap test (Dr. Pap was Dr. Papanicolaou's nick name in the hospital). Pap test has never been patented (stains are not patentable, and their use is a subjective assessment that, also, is not patentable). To secure consistency among results obtained in different laboratories, Dr. Papanicolaou started a School of Cytotechnology where he trained laboratory technicians to prepare cervical specimens, stain with his procedure and read them. This was an efficient approach, which became crucial for the wide acceptance of this test. However, being a pathologist himself, Dr. Papanicolaou kept the final decision about the medical condition on the slide for the pathologist or the laboratory supervisor. Cytotechnologists are trained to recognize what is normal, what is artifact, and are required to suggest what is abnormal and the degree of abnormality – final diagnosis is left to pathologists. This is one of the weaknesses of the manual Pap test as it is practiced today.

In the early 1950s ACS launched a campaign to screen all women (above age 18) for cervical cancer, and the results soon became evident. Today, a qualified cytotechnologist must have BS degree, 2-year School of Cytotechnology, and regular Proficiency Testing Certificate provided by an accredited Laboratory Personnel Proficiency Testing Agency (such as CAP, ASCP or MIME in the US). The schools still operate and the cytotechnologists' skills are mandatory in the US and regulated by the Clinical Laboratory Improvement Amendments (CLIA) under the enforcement authority of CDC and FDA [48] (Fig. 2.3).

This requirement does not exist outside of the US, and the quality of screening provided by less qualified personnel is dubious; thus, it is subject to much larger errors of interpretation. Training cytotechnologists and maintaining their proficiency is a requirement unmet in other countries. This is why Pap test is difficult to implement in developing countries, and this is why we believe a biomarker technology combined with digital imaging (e.g., MarkPap – see below) has a real prospect in the global cervical cancer screening.

Pap test related measurement of cervical cancer mortality rates (number of deaths per 100,000 population at risk) began in 1955. In that year, the US mortality

Fig. 2.3 (continued) exfoliated cells) and open into the vaginal cavity. CAP (*red dots*) is always absent in cells on Pap specimens from healthy women. (**b**). Flat condyloma: HPV disease is characterized with growth of cells with characteristic cytology: destruction of cytoplasm collected in perinculear hallo and/ or micro vacuoles, and with nuclear irregularities (bi-nucleous, change of nuclear size and shape). They grow in form of tumor (condyloma) but, unless is combined with cancer, do not destroy surrounding tissue. Cervical acid phosphatase (*CAP*) is present in basal, parabasal and abnormal (dysplastic) cells. (**c**). Cervical cancer: Squamous cell cervical cancer usually starts in the transformational (transitional) zone, and spreads around destroying the surrounding epithelium above the membrane (carcinoma in situ), and later, breaking the membrane, invades the deeper tissues. If operated on time, it may be cured (margins free of tumor cells). It may, or may not get HPV infection. Further promotion of tumor growth depends on the infection. All abnormal cells included in this abnormal growth (cancer, precancer, koilocytes) are CAP positive and could be detected on PAP smears rate from cervical cancer was 12/100,000. Between 1955 and 1996 these numbers declined at a standard rate of 4 % each year. Between 1955 and 2002 the mortality from cervical cancer in the US was reduced to 3/100,000. This is a reduction of over 75 %. Similar results were obtained in other countries where this test was made available to public and was promoted by governments and professional societies. Some countries, like Island, had reduced their mortality rates for 90 % (IARC Cervical cancer screening statistic reports) [92]. Nevertheless, the classic Pap test (Pap smear) in addition to its advantages also has some obstacles. The test has an unacceptable high negative rate, and in several US court cases (women had developed cervical cancer and died while the test was found to be false negative) the court ruled against laboratories. In 1996, in Bethesda, an NIH Consensus Conference on Cervical Cancer developed Guidance for Pap test and clinical actions after the test [14]. It was largely accepted that the standard Pap test has approximately 20 % false negatives, one-half because of sampling error, one-half because of errors in staining and interpretation. Later, a College of American Pathologists (CAP) Advocacy Group established that a 5 % false negative rate is inherent to the Papanicolaou staining, it cannot be escaped, and the target for "ideal" specimen processing would be to have false negative rates as close to 5 % as possible [36].

As a consequence, the Bethesda System Terminology was recommended to reduce the error of reading and interpretation [140, 162] and a Working Group combined of professionals from all societies involved in women's health recommended new criteria for approval of medical devices intended for gynecological cytology [114]. Soon, Cytyc Corp. proposed a proprietary specimen collecting solution (and a cell transferring device) intended to eliminate the sampling error by collecting the whole specimen and making it available for examination [18]. The classic Pap smear got an alternative – the liquid based Pap (LBP). The new technology was well accepted by pathologists (cleaner specimens – easier recognition of abnormal cells), women (in case of insufficient smearing the second specimen has already been available), and industry (the specimen collecting solution became a medium for additional testing such as HPV, chlamydia, neisseria), but it has never reduced the need for regular testing or reduced the sampling error. However, LBP has spread rapidly and in 2006, almost 80 % of all Pap tests in the US are performed on the specimens collected in solution. One of the supporting factors to this spreading is the increased profit the laboratories are making using this expensive test (reimbursement is approximately $50–60 per test) in comparison with the well controlled conventional Pap smear (only $15).

What is the Purpose of Pap Test?

Stopping cervical cancer before it appears.

What Women Should Know About Pap Test?

Cytological screening with Pap test is the most powerful way to prevent cervical cancer. This is a microscopic examination of cells obtained from scraping the cervix and swabbing the cervical canal.

Every woman must know about the Pap test. How it is done (pelvic exam, smear, LBP), what are the risks, disadvantages, false-negatives and false positive rates. What is pre-cancerous lesion (dysplasia)? Classification system for Papanicolaou smear: Negative (NIL), Negative with inflammation or reactive changes (RCC), Atypical Squamous Cells with Undetermined Significance ASC-US, or with possible high grade (ASC-H), Low Grade Squamous Intraepithelial Lesion (LSIL) or High Grade Squamous Intraepithelial Lesion (HSIL). In Chap. 3 of this book we include the original 2001 Bethesda System terminology, where explanations for those terms could be found [183]. She should also know what the recommendations are for clinical actions according to these diagnostic categories. These recommendations have been published by the American Society for Colposcopy and Cervical Pathology in 2001 and the new Guidelines are expected in 2007 [162]. Such knowledge will help her to be well-prepared to receive any Pap result and to take the best possible measures as soon as possible.

This section is designed to help women understanding better the cervical cancer screening and to learn what they could expect of this preventive measure.

What to do if Pap test is positive? What is necessary for diagnosis of cervical cancer (colposcopy, biopsy, histology)? What is colposcopy (viewing of the cervix with 10–20× magnification). What is biopsy (colposcopy directed punch that is taking a small piece of tissue for histological analysis). Remember, the Pap test is a screening method that is referring women for further investigations. Histology (examination of the tissue removed by biopsy) provides the final diagnosis. What is the meaning of histological diagnosis CIN 0 (no dysplasia), C 1 (mild dysplasia), CIN 2 (moderate dysplasia), CIN 3 (severe dysplasia) and CIS (carcinoma in situ). What is AIS (adenocarcinoma in situ). A woman who understands those terms will be better equipped to cope with the problems.

How to gain this knowledge? What are the most important questions you should ask your doctor? What the doctor may not tell you about abnormal cervical smear?

Questions and Answers About Your Pap Test

Pap test is a medical cancer prevention procedure intended for healthy women and conducted by:

1. Medical doctors for obtaining cervical samples from healthy women
2. Pathologists to process those samples, stain them with Papanicolaou stains on microscopic slides, and interpret the cytological microscopic images according to the Bethesda System terminology for assessment of the condition of health from the specimen
3. Medical doctors again to follow-up with clinical actions according to the Pap test results.

The goal of this test is to detect early signs of lesions that, if untreated, could develop into cervical, endometrial or vaginal cancer, and to remove those lesions with intention to cure the condition [5].

Since 1950, American Cancer Society adopted the new achievements (sampling, staining and reading cervical specimens) as a single Pap test, and promoted it for cervical cancer screening of all women at risk (age 18 and above) in the US. The test was adopted by health professionals, particularly gynecologists and pathologists, by professional organizations, health insurance and governments. Consequently, within 50 years, almost 80 % of American women at risk participated in Pap test, 50 million tests were performed annually, and the mortality from cervical cancer was reduced for 75 %. The Pap test was soon acknowledged as the best preventive anticancer test available and began to spread in other countries – almost exclusively in the developed world because of the need for infrastructure and the cost to build this infrastructure [92].

Let us now discuss about cervical cancer in the US, how Pap test is performed and what every women should know about the test.

Frequency

How often should a woman at risk go for cervical cancer screening?

Our recommendation is at least once in 2 years.

Why so frequently when American Cancer Society, the National Cancer Institute (NCI), and other authorities on this matter recommend once in two or three years? Our answer is very simple. The guidelines are prepared referencing results from clinical trials. We have read reports from the same trials, and we have seen that "the most participants fit within the recommended range." However, there was still a disease progression that occurred earlier (2.5 %) and later (2.5 %). Obviously, it is less harmful if the disease occurs later than earlier. This is particularly important if false negative results have not been eliminated. More frequent screening will eliminate this danger and women should be safer.

There are many recommendations for how frequently a woman should go for cervical cancer screening. Almost all are coming from respectable and influential sources like American Cancer Society, Centers for Disease Control and Prevention, but many are coming from health insurance, health management organization or industry.

The National Comprehensive Cancer Network (NCCN) has recently published a comprehensive NCCN Clinical Practice Guideline in Oncology aimed for 2008. They are recommending the screening interval adjusted according to the method of screening, results and woman's age. Here are their guidelines for 2008:

- After initiation of screening (3 years after the onset of vagina intercourse), cervical screening should be performed annually with conventional cytology smears (Pap test) OR every 2 years using liquid-based cytology; at of after age 30, women who had three consecutive, technically satisfactory negative cytology results may be screened every 2–3 years (unless they have a history of in utero DES exposure, are HPV+, or are immunocompromized).

- Human papillomavirus (HPV) DNA testing for primary screening has recently been approved by the FDA for women over 30 years of age. It is reasonable to consider that for women age 30 and over, as an alternative to cervical cytology testing alone, cervical screening may be performed every 3 years using conventional or liquid-based cytology combined with a test for DNA for highrisk HPV types.
- Until more data are available, women who test positive for HPV DNA should continue screening at the discretion of their health care provider.
- Frequency of combined cytology and HPV DNA testing should NOT be more often than every 3 years, if both tests are negative.
- Counseling and education related to HPV infection is a critical need.
- Women who received HPV vaccination should continue cervical cancer screening according to the guidelines [184].

This citation is an example how the healthcare market is influencing the frequency of testing. Neither LBP not HPV DNA has been proven to influence the prognosis as to extend periods between screenings for 1 year for each of them. However, the cost of Pap smear (conventional is about $15.00, for LBP is about $60.00 and for HPV DNA an additional $40.00–60.00. On the US market (50 million tests per year), the difference is between having Pap smear only and having (LBP + HPV) is substantial, but this difference is reasonably reduced if divided by three. The extension of periods between screenings could have been a compromise, and women should be aware of this when asking for the next Pap test.

What Type of Screening?

A woman should always ask for pelvic exam and specimen collection. Although the specimen collection could be, sometimes, performed by a specially trained health professional, we would recommend that a medical doctor be the person to perform the pelvic exam and to collect the specimen. Medical study provides physicians with a certain background knowledge that simply cannot be replaced by others with alternative training.

Recently, with the advancement of home-based technologies, there are some signs that home Pap test will soon be taken under consideration. As a matter of fact, the self-collection of cervico-vaginal specimens at home has been an old concept, but because of cellular destruction in fluids the technique was not practical for use; however, the resistance of MarkPap biomarker in the same environment makes the substantial difference [119]. The chemical/physicochemical characteristics of this biomarker provide hopes that such a home test is probable. If one day the Home Pap becomes a reality, we would recommend more frequent home testing (at intervals of 3–6 months) and consulting doctors at the first sign of test abnormality or, at least, to see the doctor once in 3 years [22].

Another type of primary screening is currently getting attention outside the US. This is HPV Testing alone. The idea is based upon expectations that modern

DNA/RNA techniques may make HPV testing inexpensive (approximately $1.00 per test) and amenable for frequent testing at home. If persistent (two and more years) HPV infection is detected, then cytological screening will be indicated. This is a reverse approach to the current Pap test, but it could be attractive if any logic other than business could be proven. In spite of many discussions in favor of frequent HPV testing, we would be very cautious to ever recommend HPV testing alone. Without a parallel cytological screening, the probability to miss the disease is too high. There are cervical cancers without HPV disease – although rarely. However, HPV frequency in healthy population is too high to be used for cancer screening (abundance of false positive results), and the cost will be unbearable for developing countries.

What Type of Specimen Collection?

Prior to the last 10 years of the twentieth century, there was only one option – Pap smear. In 1996, the National Cancer Institute in Bethesda, Maryland, organized a consensus conference on cervical cancer [138]. One of the important issues at this conference was how to improve cervical cancer screening in order to reduce the high percent of false negative results and the liability of laboratories for cancer caused death of women who had negative Pap test [162].

It was reported that one half of all false negative results occurred because of poor sampling (insufficient specimen) and the rest was caused by inadequate specimen processing (staining) or interpretation (diagnostic error). This conference adopted a consensus statement with recommendation of a new Bethesda System terminology to improve cytological interpretation (reduces diagnostic error).

In the follow-up, several companies came out with their products aimed to improve specimen processing. Some (e.g., ThermoShandon Varistain Automatic Slide Stainer) added Papanicolaou staining software to their automatic slide stainers. It was easy. A new program was added to the computer to move a rack with slides from staining station to station and to keep slides in staining and clearing stations for precise periods of time. Papanicolaou staining was not changed; just the consistency of processing was significantly improved [170]. Automatic staining improved significantly the consistency of Pap test smear processing.

A major change came from those who recommended replacing specimen smearing with its collection into a preservative solution. Two attractive marketing ideas underlined those offerings. First, the specimen will be collected in its entirety, and the laboratories will be able to examine the whole specimen – or, a woman will not be called for another specimen if the first was inadequate. Second, transferring specimens from solution onto microscopic slides is a procedure requiring filtering from debris, mucus, and inflammatory cells. Consequently, the images became better and pathologists prefer them to the conventional smears. This is the technology known as ThinPrep Pap Test (Cytyc, MA) and SurePath Liquid Pap (TriPath Imaging, NC) [53, 172].

Unfortunately, the first goal was not met. Laboratories do not examine the whole specimen collected in solution – just the first slide prepared by transferring cells from suspension onto microscopic slides. Instead of examining all available cells, the leftover was used for ancillary methods such as HPV testing. The next consensus conference (2001 Bethesda System) acknowledged this failure to examine the entire specimen and accepted the technology as sufficiently good for the purpose [162].

Recently, new specimen collection technologies are trying to enter the Pap test market. One of them is Diamics Cervical Analysis System (C-Map) which is using a proprietary specimen collector to make a "touch prep" of woman's cervix on microscopic slides [58]. Once the specimen is transferred onto microscopic slides, the authors will use several (six at this time) antibodies and rapid immunocytochemical protocols for identification of proteins (antigens) known to be present in transforming cells. This is an interesting system, but still lacking clinical confirmation of the hypothesis. We think the concept of transferring cervical cells with a balloon is similar to swab technology and does not include scrapping, and that the concept of using antibodies to keratins will not resolve the problem of identifying cells transforming into malignant. Maybe, an array of antibodies and FISH technology will make this test more usable for the purpose.

There are many non-approved devices for self-collection of vaginal fluids such as swabs, Q-tip-like devices, catheter-like devices, etc., but we will not comment on them here. None of them will be discussed with the doctor before the FDA approval.

LBP technologies are using special broom-like devices for specimen collection – these are plastic brooms shaped to enter the cervical canal and to collect material from the surface. They are elastic and the pressure the specimen provider must exercise, to bring sufficient number of endocervical and transformation zone cells, is difficult to control – this may cause additional confounding inconsistency of collecting material and help increase the probability for sampling errors.

Based on the comments presented here, our recommendation would be to keep the conventional Pap smear specimen collection technique unless there is a need for HPV testing when the manufacturer's recommendation for sampling should be respected.

Why Waiting for Pap Test Result Is so Long?

There is nothing secret with the laboratory processing of the Pap test specimen. It is a laboratory test composed of two parts – specimen preparation and staining, and microscopic examination. It is actually completed within a couple of active hours. The delay is between phases – collection of specimen, specimen processing and reading with interpretation. Result? Two to three weeks period is usually needed between the day of specimen sampling and the day of receiving the laboratory result.

The usual explanation is work overload. Let us see if this is true. In the US there are 50 million Pap tests performed annually – approximately 200,000 specimens daily are collected by approximately 100,000 providers or two specimens daily on average. The bottleneck is not in doctor's offices. There are about 4000 cytopathology laboratories accredited to perform Pap test – this equals 12,500 tests per laboratory, or 48 tests daily. A laboratory usually employs a general laboratory technician (cytoprep) for specimen processing, a cytotechnologist for slide reading and interpretation, a pathologist for quality control and final cytological diagnosis, and an administrative person for receiving specimens and reporting results. Specimen processing time is one hour per sample, a number that must be divided with the capacity of automatic instruments. Usually, no more than one hour is needed for processing 60 slides. There is no bottleneck here.

Average screening time is 6 min per slide. One cytotechnologist could comfortably examine 50 slides per day. The pathologist (supervisor, quality control) examine at average 25–30 % of slides. Again, this is a job to be completed within one day.

At worst, in the US, there is an infrastructure able to provide Pap test results within 3 days after sampling. Why then waiting of 2–4 weeks? Obviously, laboratories are not giving priority to preventive medicine testing such as Pap test because they are usually overwhelmed with routine work dealing with curative medicine – everybody knows that the patient in trouble should not wait. STAT orders are frequent, and many interruptions in the standard procedure are done because of emergencies. But, Pap test is not an emergency.

Pap test is done to healthy women – no emergency is involved, this test can wait (?). But, what about women who wait? How do they feel? These and similar questions are still to be answered. Maybe separate laboratory units (the old Papanicolaou's idea) should be dedicated only to Pap test? This is a probability to be considered when planning major cervical cancer screening programs in any country, not only the USA.

Another reason for the delay of sending "Pap negative letter" to healthy women is inherent in the regulations imposed on laboratories for performing Pap test. According to CLIA*88 "(f) Test results must be released to authorized persons and, if applicable, the individual for using the test and the laboratory that initially requested the test. An authorized person means an individual authorized under the State law to order tests or receive test results, or both" [71]. Laboratories are informing doctors about the result, and they are informing patients according to their priorities.

We think, whatever is the real reason, the period of more than a couple of days for informing a healthy woman that her cancer screening test is negative, should be considered as unacceptably long, and a better way must be sought. One of the solutions is using a biomarker-based test combined with digital imaging and telemedicine and provide results within hours. (see under MarkPap technology).

What to Expect from the Pap Test Result?

As with many other tests, this test could be reported as: Unsatisfactory, satisfactory and negative, satisfactory and positive, and with the degree of positivity (abnormality) determined in one of 2001 Bethesda System categories [162]. What should women know about each of these reports?

1. Unsatisfactory

   This report means that something has happened with the specimen and the doctor was not able to make the diagnosis. Usually, this could be a call for repeat. However, if the processing was done properly, the problem is with sampling and a healthy woman should consider going for a new test. Repeating sampling for Pap specimen is safe after 3 months. Three months between sampling is a period considered necessary for full reparation of the scrapped cervix. What women will feel in the meantime, it depends how the doctor will explain the recall.
2. Satisfactory and negative

   Having received this result, a healthy woman should be assured that no silent danger has occurred and that she should continue to live the same live as before testing. However, since this result has a false negative rate of up to 20 %, the woman should be aware of the necessity to avoid risk factors and to stay alert and to consult her doctor as soon as any of the alarming symptoms appear before her next scheduled appointment.
3. Satisfactory and positive

   This result should alarm a woman that she should see the doctor and ask for explanation and advice. Usually, the doctor's office will call for an appointment automatically. How to manage women with cervical epithelial abnormality largely depends upon the cytological diagnosis of this abnormality [162].

In 2001, the American Association for Colposcopy and Cervical Pathology (ASCCP) issued Guidelines for Management of Women with Cervical Epithelial Abnormalities and has adjusted this guidance thereafter [183]. The most recent recommendations largely rely on HPV testing, giving the presence of HPV high risk viruses, particularly the repeated presence (persistent infection) a role of a negative prognostic sign that should be used increasing the cytological category. Therefore, a woman with low grade Pap test positivity but with HPV high-risk positivity should be advised to continue with diagnostic procedures earlier than it would have been recommended if only cytology was used. Naturally, this recommendation raises fear of cancer and concern among affected women. This approach will also increase the rate of false positive alarms manifold.

4. Degree of positivity

   Papanicolaou and the immediate followers used the term dysplasia (Gr. *dys* – disordered, *plassein* – to form) to indicate that some abnormal tissue is forming within the normal. The name cervical dysplasia was used to describe all forms of cervical cell abnormalities found at Pap test examination, and the grading: No Dysplasia, Mild, Moderate and Severe Dysplasia were added to quantify the extent of this abnormal tissue/cells presence.

   Later, this taxonomy was changed several times before the 2001.

Bethesda System [89, 162] was accepted as the universal terminology for describing microscopic images of abnormal (positive) Pap smears. For details, please see Table 2.5 (2001 Bethesda System).

Although this System is intended for doctors only, we think that some general information should be provided for all women to know.

Table 2.5 The Bethesda System (Cited IARC Screening Group, http://screening.iarc.fr/atlasclassifbethesda.php)

SPECIMEN TYPE	
Indicate	
□	conventional smear (Pap smear)
□	vs. liquid-based preparation
□	vs. other
SPECIMEN ADEQUACY	
□	Satisfactory for evaluation (describe presence or absence of endocervical/ transformation zone component and any other quality indicators, e.g., partially obscuring blood, inflammation, etc.)
□	Unsatisfactory for evaluation …(specify reason)
□	Specimen rejected/not processed (specify reason)
□	Specimen processed and examined, but unsatisfactory for evaluation of epithelial abnormality because of (specify reason)
GENERAL CATEGORIZATION (optional)	
□	Negative for Intraepithelial Lesion or Malignancy
□	Other: See Interpretation/result (e.g., endometrial cells in a woman >= 40 years of age)
□	Epithelial Cell Abnormality: See Interpretation/result (specify "squamous" or "glandular" as appropriate)
INTERPRETATION/RESULT	
NEGATIVE FOR INTRAEPITHELIAL LESION OR MALIGNANCY	
(when there is no cellular evidence of neoplasia, state this in the General Categorization above and/or in the Interpretation/Result section of the report, whether or not there are organisms or other non-neoplastic findings)	
ORGANISMS:	
Trichomonas vaginalis	
Fungal organisms morphologically consistent with Candida sop	
Shift in flora suggestive of bacterial vaginosis	
Bacteria morphologically consistent with Actinomyces spp	
Cellular changes consistent with Herpes simplex virus	
OTHER NON NEOPLASTIC FINDINGS (Optional to report; list not inclusive):	
Reactive cellular changes associated with	
inflammation (includes typical repair)	
radiation	
intrauterine contraceptive device (IUD)	
Glandular cells status post hysterectomy	
Atrophy	
OTHER	
Endometrial cells (in a woman >= 40 years of age) (Specify if "negative for squamous intraepithelial lesion")	
EPITHELIAL CELL ABNORMALITIES	
SQUAMOUS CELL	
Atypical squamous cells	
of undetermined significance (ASC-US)	
cannot exclude HSIL (ASC-H)	

(continued)

Table 2.5 (continued)

Low grade squamous intraepithelial lesion (LSIL)
(encompassing: HPV/mild dysplasia/CIN 1)
High grade squamous intraepithelial lesion (HSIL)
(encompassing: moderate and severe dysplasia, CIS, CIN 2 and CIN 3)
with features suspicious for invasion (if invasion is suspected)
Squamous cell carcinoma
GLANDULAR CELL
Atypical
endocervical cells (not otherwise specified (NOS) or specify in comments),
endometrial cells (NOS or specify in comments),
glandular cells (NOS or specify in comments)
Atypical
endocervical cells, favor neoplastic
glandular cells, favor neoplastic
Endocervical adenocarcinoma in situ
Adenocarcinoma:
endocervical
endometrial
extrauterine
not otherwise specified (NOS)
OTHER MALIGNANT NEOPLASMS: (specify)
ANCILLARY TESTING
Provide a brief description of the test method(s) and report the result so that it is easily understood by the clinician.
AUTOMATED REVIEW
If case examined by automated device, specify device and result.
EDUCATIONAL NOTES AND SUGGESTIONS (optional)
Suggestions should be concise and consistent with clinical follow-up guidelines published by professional organizations (references to relevant publications may be included).

- The 2001 Bethesda System is a taxonomy of microscopic images that could be seen from Pap test specimens at certain pathologic conditions, but it is not a classification of cervical or genital diseases that can cause those images to appear.
- There are three main categories in this taxonomy: Specimen Adequacy, General Categorization, and Interpretation/Result. In this book we are using the General Categorization (Negative, Positive – Epithelial cell Abnormalities and Other).
- Pap positive results (Epithelial Cell Abnormalities) are divided into subcategories according to the cell type (squamous cell – frequent, glandular cell – rare), and according to the assumed lesion they are classified into undetermined [ASC-US], low risk intraepithelial [LSIL], and high risk intraepithelial lesion [HSIL] or cancer [CIS]. As it is written, this taxonomy calls for further examination (colposcopy/biopsy/histology) in order to determine the diagnosis of the disease and refer to therapy.

- Pap test positive results, unless it is a frank cancer, should only be used as a call for further diagnostic examinations in order to determine the diagnosis and to use it for planning therapy.

5. Ancillary methods – HPV testing.

HPV testing has introduced in cervical cancer screening a factor that is not by itself an early sign of a lesion that, if untreated, could develop into cervical cancer; therefore this factor is neither cancer nor pre-cancerosis. Rather, detecting HPV infection speaks about a presence of a virus that may contribute to development of such a lesion. Consequently, the attention should be directed towards the infection. There are two ways to treat this infection:

1. Reducing viral load (search for a benign growth – wart – causing shedding of cells with viral particles) and removing this piece of sick tissue, and
2. Increasing the non-specific immune competence of the host.

Removing a lump tissue with HPV infected cells is not removing cervical cancer or pre-cancerosis. This is the crucial difference where neither the Guidelines are clear nor every pathologist or gynecologist agrees upon. Many studies have reported successful elimination of such lesions as removal of CIS (carcinoma in situ) which is not the true, but it stays reported and entered into statistical summaries reporting success/failures of HPV testing and cytological only testing. Currently, the leading recommendation is that both HPV and cytology should be used for decision about what to do next [183].

We recommend reliance on cytology because HPV testing (as it is performed today) could introduce more false positive alarms and cost women unnecessary stress, emotional, physical and financial damages. It means, we recommend (1) intensive treatment of virus infection to be followed by (2) cytological examination within 3–6 months.

6. What to do?

Pap smear is a screening method designed to eliminate from further investigation all Pap negative women (above 90 %) and to reduce the number of those referred to colposcopy to only those who might have a hidden disease. Is it only an alternative method to delay colposcopy? No, we don't think so. We are not recommending any delay of colposcopy, if it is necessary. However, colposcopy in the US is usually combined with biopsy (many times blind biopsy – just to be on the safe side?) and the colposcopy, which otherwise is quite safe, becomes a procedure with risks of bleeding, infection and consequences of frequent scarring if used indiscriminately.

Therefore, when Pap test report is "satisfactory and positive," the woman should be aware that even the medical guidelines recommended to establish standard of healthcare have their own limitations and, before those guidelines are applied to her case, she should ask her doctor to advise her what to do next, not mechanically complying with guidelines, but after serious consideration of her particular case. In many cases, such a modest request may be extremely helpful to women in resolving the problem easier.

What if Disease Is Present?

For many women and medical advisors, a positive Pap test is a signal of imminent or pending cervical cancer. This is simply not true. Pap test is a screening method to detect early signs of a lesion that could develop into cervical cancer, and HPV infection is only a sign that this infection could contribute to cancer development if remains persistent. The emphasis here is on the word "could." This is a conditional; therefore, a woman should first ask, "what should I do NOT to allow cancer to develop?"

We have been amazed to learn that many women received answers such as "wait and check" to this quite legitimate question. This answer creates stress and fear. Fear from cancer and stress of "not doing anything to prevent it." A better approach is to explain everything, but is questionable as to how many women would like to know and will be able to understand the logic of medical prognosis and the uncertainties included in this. Probably very few! Another option is for the doctor to take the role of decision maker and the responsibility that goes with this. Many women would like this, but many doctors would not. This book is intended, among other issues, to help women understand dilemmas when clinical decision is to be made and to motivate them to become an active participant (not only a passive receiver) of the necessary medical help.

At the end of this section we would like to emphasize again that Pap test is only a screening procedure and if positive, another, more profound examination is needed to detect the lesion than could develop into cervical cancer and to remove this lesion on time. For details, please see sections on Diagnosis and Therapy later in this book.

Problem. Why Some Women Do not Take a Simple Pap Test and Get a Deadly Disease?

For the most of the world Pap test is not available. Where it is available, not all women use this opportunity to protect themselves. Why? This question has been addressed many times before, and the following suggestions have been made:

1. The high cost of Pap test
2. Women are uneducated or not sufficiently educated about cervical cancer prevention (why should I go, I feel fine)
3. The Pap test is not available (no infrastructure and professionals to do the Pap test)
4. Women do not have access to a doctor (live in remote places)
5. Women are prevented from seeing gynecologist (cultural, religious issues)
6. Women are afraid of Pap test
7. Uncomfortable with Pap test
8. Do not trust the test (false-negatives).

All of these answers (#1–#8) have been reported in many surveys, and women have repeated them in our currently ongoing survey [20]. In comparison with others, we have found more women being well aware of Pap test (above 90 %), but who willingly do not participate (25 %) because one or more of the reasons cited above. Only 5 % of participants in our survey said that they do not know and they do not want to know about Pap test – because of the same reasons. (Please see the Pap test Acceptance Survey in the Chap. 3 of this book).

We hope, this book will eliminate at least one reason, the lack of reference (resource where to ask for additional knowledge). This book is intended for every woman's library.

Solution to the Problem. Could Something More be Done in Cervical Cancer Prevention to Reduce the Impact of the Reasons why Women do not Participate in Cervical Cancer Screening?

The answer is YES. Novel approaches to improve the Pap test with discovery of related biomarkers will bring solution to most of these problems and will bring the answer YES to almost all of these questions.

- Is it possible that the Pap test can be less expensive and affordable for women? YES
- Could the Pap test accuracy be improved? YES
- Can cervical cancer screening be made available to all women in the world? YES
- Could hundreds of thousands unnecessary deaths be prevented: This is somebody's daughter, wife, mother or sister who is dying because she cannot have a Pap test? YES
- Would it be possible to have Home Pap test in the near future? It means to take a sample in the privacy of your home (self-sampling using a simple kit) and to send it to the doctor? YES
- Could a woman in a remote province (where there are no professionals to perform and read Pap test) get the result in couple of hours? Is telemedicine a solution for mass cervical cancer screening? YES
- The next section on Biomarkers, will shed more light on our optimism.

2.3.2.2 MarkPap Technology for Cervical Cancer Screening. What Is this?

MarkPap is a trademark for Cervical Acid Phosphatase – Papanicolaou Test, a biomarker-based Pap test. The scientific information on this test and detailed technology is presented in Chap. 7 "MarkPap® Illustrated" see also Ref. 212, 116 and 122.

Why Should Women Know About this Emerging Technology?

MarkPap technology is developing to meet the unmet needs of women who participate and who do not participate in regular cervical cancer screening based on Pap test (cytological screening). Once the technology is approved for marketing, we hope, it will become the substance matter for all YES answers given in the previous section above.

Let us now try to explain our confidence why this technology will provide tools to make the cervical screening more accurate, faster, less costly, and accessible to almost every woman.

- The core of this technology is the biomarker of cervical cell abnormality, which labels only abnormal cells and has never been positive in normal squamous cells presented on Pap smears or monolayers of LBP specimens (Fig. 2.4). A single biomarker positive squamous cell found during microscopic examination of a gynecological specimen indicates that this cell has been separated from a lesion or any abnormal growth occurring in the tissue from which the specimen was separated (cervix). In the Chap. 7.1, please see the series of pictures and legend explaining how this biomarker makes a difference for locating abnormal cells and for determination of cytological condition on the slide (Chap. 7.1).

This biomarker's advantage for locating rare abnormal cells is expected to reduce false negative rates for manual cervical cancer screening much below the Pap test false negative rates, and to almost eliminate the false negative results when digital imaging scanners are used for screening [220].

- The presence of this biomarker is visualized as a red granular pigment precipitated inside the cytoplasm of abnormal cells. If cellular background is stained with a modified Papanicolaou staining technique (MarkPap® Test), and the cellular components are colored in blue, the red biomarker label contrasts distinctly and is very much amenable for digital imaging (Fig. 2.4).

This advantage will be used for developing tools for automatic (robotic) cervical cancer screening instruments, and for their use for mass cervical cancer screening

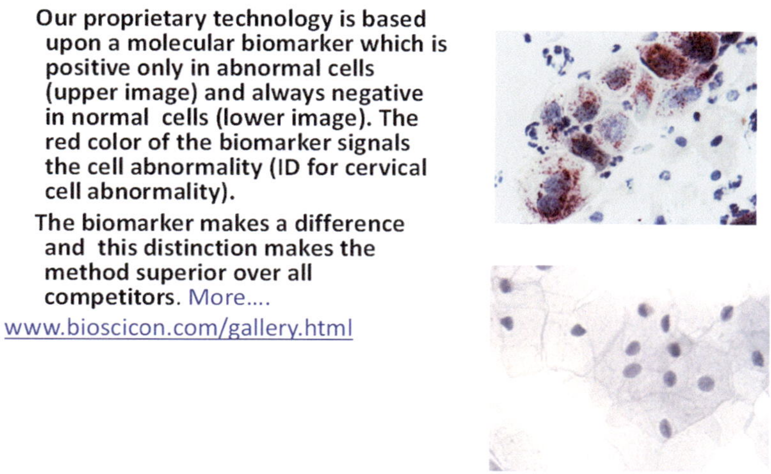

Fig. 2.4 MarkPap® Platform technology illustrated

because they provide speed, accuracy and low cost non-comparable with manual technologies. The first instrument of that category has already been conceived.

This is the MarkPap® Digital which is a combination of the biomarker-based cytology, digital imaging and a Web-based IT communication protocol for telecytopathology (Chap. 7)

- The label of biomarker's presence is a pigment precipitated inside cytoplasm. As a chemical substance it is indestructible in vaginal discharge regardless of the cause of this discharge. Finding a single biomarker positive cell or a piece of such cell in vaginal fluids has almost the same meaning as finding the biomarker labeled squamous cell on cervical smears.

This advantage will have tremendous impact on future cervical cancer screening because it is enabling development of collecting vaginal specimens that might be collected by women themselves (MarkPap® Self) or may become a basis for future development of Home Pap which will use chemical reaction to identify presence/absence of abnormal cells in the self-collected specimen [Chap. 7].

- Last, but not least important advantage is the ability of this test to identify women with HPV disease – this is a condition in which an HPV infected woman begins to respond to the infection with a disease which could be manifested as abnormal growth – warts or, many times rarely, cervical cancer. This advantage is a real chance for MarkPap based cytology to become a prescreening test for HPV disease. (Chap. 7)
- The important advantage of the MarkPap technology (manual version), which has been developed to improve the classic Pap test, is that it uses:

  1. The same Pap test infrastructure (doctors for specimen collection, cytopathology laboratories for specimen processing, staining, reading and interpretation)
  2. The same technology (screening and clinical actions contingent to the cytological results)
  3. The only difference between Pap test and MarkPap test is the biomarker, which itself is providing visual means for more accurate detection of abnormal cells

MarkPap Test is a better Pap test because it is more accurate, faster, and less expensive and, we think, it should be considered to replace the Pap test based on Papanicolaou staining when the time comes.

Because of those obvious advantages, the MarkPap technology is considered disruptive to the global cervical cancer market and many market competitors, already on the market, who have control over it, have started putting road blocks to delay, if not completely to prevent, the arrival of this biomarker-based cytology with digital imaging and Web-based communication technology.

2.3.3 Non Cytology-Based Cervical Cancer Screening

Most of the world outside the US does not have facilities to build an infrastructure necessary to carryout the Pap test as it is required in the US. Although cervical cancer is still the major killer of women from malignant diseases, the fight against this killer is still not well organized; it is more campaign than services, more enthusiastic efforts than an established organization, and it has been inspired more by the public opinion (media influenced) and political needs than by scientific analyses of the needs in each country and the awareness that the prevention of cervical cancer is equal to cure [55]. As a result, no significant change of mortality has occurred in many countries undergoing cervical cancer prevention campaigns (Table 2.2). A significant impact to developing countries is coming from the industry fighting for new markets and having recognized that 1.7 billion women are not protected against a preventable disease. This is a huge market with defined needs where they can offer their products. Typical example is the HPV testing as offered for replacement for the "expensive" Pap test.

Most of developing countries are currently in search for the best technology that will allow their health care services to provide cervical cancer screening contingent on their abilities. They have been widely supported by the World Health Organization, its agency the International Agency for Research on Cancer (IARC), international non-profit world health dedicated organizations as the Alliance for Cervical Cancer Prevention (ACCP) including five international organizations and charity institutions including the Melinda & Bill Gates Foundation. Considerable funds have been recently dedicated to HPV vaccination because of the feeling that developing countries cannot afford to pay for a still not proven prevention, while they should be able to provide funding for cervical cancer screening as a well documented and proven protective measure.

In April 2007, ACCP published "10 Key Findings and Recommendations for Effective Cervical Cancer Screening and Treatment Programs" [1]. The recommendations provided by the Alliance are outlined here:

1. Every woman has the right to cervical cancer screening at least once in her lifetime. In low-resource settings, the optimal age for screening to achieve the greatest public health impact is between 30 and 40 years of age.
2. Although cytology-based screening programs using Pap smears have been shown to be effective in the US and other developed countries, it is difficult to sustain high quality cytology programs. Therefore, in situations where healthcare resources are scarce, those resources should be directed towards cost-effective strategies that are more affordable and for which quality can be assured.
3. Studies have shown that the most efficient and effective strategy for secondary prevention of cervical cancer in low resource settings is to screen using either HPV DNA testing or VIA (visual inspection), then treat pre-cancerous lesions

using cryotherapy (freezing). This is optimally achieved in a single visit (currently possible with VIA plus cryotherapy) and can be carried out by competent physicians, including nurses and midwives.
4. The use of HPV DNA testing followed by cryotherapy results in greater reduction of cervical cancer precursors that the use of other screening and treatment approaches.
5. Cryotherapy, when conducted by competent providers, is safe and results in cure rates of 85 % or greater.
6. Studies suggest that cryotherapy is protective against the future development of cervical disease among women with current HPV infection. Because of this, and due to the low morbidity of cryotherapy, the occasional treatment of screen-positive women without confirmed cervical disease is acceptable.
7. Unless there is a suspicion of invasive cervical cancer, the routine use of an intermediate diagnostic step (such as colposcopy) between screening and treatment is generally not efficient and may result in reduced programmatic success and increased cost.
8. Women, their partners, communities, and civic organizations must be engaged in planning and implementing services, in partnering with the health sector.
9. For maximum impact, programs require effective training, supervision, and continuous quality improvement mechanisms.
10. Additional work is needed to develop rapid, user friendly, low cost HPV tests and to improve cryotherapy equipment.

The impact of these recommendation could be very big, therefore, they deserve a special attention in this book.

Here are our comments:

1. The ACCP acknowledges that the cytology based cervical cancer screening is the best preventive measure, but it is not for women in low-resource countries because of the cost to develop the infrastructure (high quality cytology programs). The fact is that the cytology screening programs (Pap smear, LBP) have already been implemented in most "low-resource countries" but, at this moment, the technology is only affordable to this part of the society who could pay for the test. Governments are subsidizing the cost (China), or offer alternative such as VIA to those who cannot pay the cost (India). We think, it would have been better if ACCP had recommended the Pap test – like screening for all women, and would have called for development of new efficient technologies to help all women worldwide.
2. The main study cited in the Recommendations is one study from India published in the International Journal of Cancer [154]. Conclusions in this study have relied mostly on the statistical analysis of success/failure rate among groups. Unfortunately, the success was measured as incidence and mortality in comparison with a questionable denominator (person-years) instead of number per 100,000 population at risk. Another statistical analysis used the right denominator and the results were different – no significant difference was found between groups. This additional analysis clouds the ACCP Recommendations and calls

for caution when somebody is trying to apply them. Consequently, similar caution should be applied to all other "study reports" cited in this ACCP document.

3. Particularly not convincing are studies recommending HPV DNA testing plus cryotherapy for reduction of cervical cancer precursors. The goal of cervical cancer screening is to reduce the cervical cancer incidence and mortality, not the precursors – whatever they may be. What would be the reason for reducing HPV infection or warts, but having increased the incidence of invasive cervical cancer? ACCP report does not provide answer to such questions.
4. Cryotherapy of cervical lesions is not like cryotherapy of skin moles. This is many times more than difficult to eliminate a mole without damaging the normal tissue, it does not eliminate cervical cancer, may produce collateral damage, needs follow-up controls, and doing it in one day settings is not recommendable for the safety of patients.
5. Colposcopy with biopsy and histology is not an "intermediary" procedure, it is highly efficient diagnostic intervention that can be curable for carcinoma in situ and could not be replaced by the ACCP recommended options.

On the other side, according to the recent reports, the cytologic cervical cancer screening is spreading exponentially among the members of the United Nations. China reported 70 million tests in 2006; India has already tens of million tests preformed per year. Mexico, Brazil, Japan, Vietnam, South Africa, all report results from their Pap tests. At this moment, we would like to caution the readers of this book against a possibility for misjudgment because of the inconsistence of the meaning of the Pap test in different countries. Recently, we asked colleagues from several countries to send us their Pap test images. The surprise was great. From India we got images taken from specimens stained more reddish than the standard Pap test should be; from Japan, the images were more dark blue. Our cytotechnologists, who are trained in the US, were not able to confirm the diagnoses made in India and Japan. We think, it is time to consider worldwide standardization of cytological screening and we think that telemedicine with telecytopathology and standard specimens (slides) will be the best answer to this emerging problem.

Some countries are still looking otherwise and are testing other approaches. Among more attempts, three strategies gained recognition: See & Treat, One day, One dollar primary screening.

"See & Treat" strategy is coming with the recommendation of IARC (WHO's International Agency for Research on Cancer) and is based upon a 7-year Indian study in which providers used VIA technology. VIA, which comes from the Visual Inspection and Acid (vinegar), combined with touch cryoablation of white patches on cervical lesions as identified after exposure to vinegar. This technique is recommended to become a standard of care, at least in India. We think, it will change their current practice for better because it will bring more women to examination (providers are nurses or specially trained technicians) and they will be able to select women with cervical cancer and to refer them to doctors. Otherwise, treating each "white patch" with cryoablation could be dangerous because cervical cancer will not be cured, warts will not be eliminated, new lesions could be provoked and there will not be histological verification. However, under assumption that 90 % of women will be negative, at least for India this prevention could be a certificate of cervical health at this moment. Another problem, more serious for us, comes from the tendency to claim this technique as replacement of regular scheduling for cervical cancer screening, and this is unacceptable [155].

A similar approach, "Screen-and-treat colposcopy" has been recommended for cervical cancer detection in high risk populations [113]. In a rural region of Southern Mexico 8281 women considered to be at high risk were evaluated. 4881 had vaginal symptoms before colposcopy. 5646 underwent colposcopy. Abnormal result (HPV, CIN 1–3) was diagnosed in 1073, but only 9 (1 %) had carcinoma. 238 were treated on site. Women gladly accepted the "one day" diagnosis and treatment.

An expensive alternative to VIA is TruScan. A Sydney, AU, based company Polartechnics Ltd and CSIRO developed device with pen-like probe to collect visual information directly from the cervix and is combined with the computer with mathematical algorithms to analyze data and detect cervical cancer. An interesting device, which has not utilization in the routine cervical cancer screening [82].

"One Day" strategy is led by recognition that in many developing countries it is difficult to bring women for examination once, but almost impossible to bring them for follow-up. Therefore, the theory behind "Screen & Treat" is applicable here. Instead of VIA (or VILA – visual inspection helped by Lugol), any other technology could be used for inspection and verification of the lesion the same day when the doctor will intervene. Again, this is a statistical approach. Ninety percent will be negative, 6 % of the rest will have no visible lesions, and only 4 % will receive treatment, about 1–2 % will be followed – result is statistically defendable but not medically [155].

In 2007, Suba et al. recommended a combined-modality of "Screen & Treat" strategy. The new strategy will include Pap test cytologic screening of all VIA positive cervices and immediate decision to apply conization (LEEP) for excision of the sick tissue rather than cryoablation as currently preferred treatment [164]. The reason behind this suggestion is that cryoablation usually leads lesions with abnormal cytology (invasive cancer could not be eliminated) and does not treat cancers. The authors suggest, this approach for developing countries where the "single-visit" programs are the preferred strategy.

"One-Dollar Pap test" is an attempt to replace Pap test with biomarkers. The most advanced is the concept to use low-cost technology for identification of HPV oncogenic strains in cervical specimens by highly virus specific DNA/RNA-related techniques. It follows the mindset that the presence of oncogenic strains should be considered as the cytological signs of early lesions that could develop into cervical cancer. This is not true because detection of viral infection is neither detection of viral disease (body's response to infection) nor pre-cancerosis or cervical cancer. However, this approach is getting attention of big companies, and soon new methods could be approved for detection of viral particles but be advertised for prevention of cervical cancer. It would be fair to consider those technologies as pre-screening for cytological examination but, we are not aware of such intentions yet.

In other words, if Pap test is not available, the whole world is looking for alternatives. Neither of them is equal to the Pap test. This is why we are recommending those alternatives that preserve the most of the Pap test by using modern technology such as automation, digital imaging, telecytopathology, web-based communication to reduce the cost and increase the speed and accuracy of cervical cancer screening. At this moment, the only approach promising to meet all those requirements is the MarkPap technology [122].

2.3.3.1 Instead of Conclusion

Since the goal of cervical cancer screening is to detect early signs of lesions that could become malignant in healthy women (the lesions are to be seen and verified by colposcopy), there is a limit to the acceptable cost for this preventive measure. This limit is defined as the cost of diagnostic colposcopy when applied to healthy women. Because colposcopy requires quality instruments and experienced examiners, this is not VIA as recommended by IARC for developing countries, bit it is still not an unreachable goal; particularly in countries with socialized healthcare systems.

Consequently, we believe, the future is in the cytological biomarkers identifying needs for colposcopy, the markers similar to MarkPap test described in this book.

2.3.4 Management of Women When the Pap Test Result Returns

What should a woman do when the Pap test result comes back? She should immediately call her doctor and ask for an urgent appointment. When she meets the doctor she should receive advice according to the Guidelines for management of women with Pap positive test. What those Guidelines are all about?

American Society for Colposcopy and Cervical Pathology (ASCCP) has taken a leading role to guide medical doctors what to do with their patients when their Pap test results return as positive. In 2001, the Society has issued Consensus Guidelines for Management of Women with Cervical Cell Abnormalities [183] and these guidelines are regularly updated with new recommendations. ACS, the US Preventive Services Task and the American College of Obstetricians and Gynecologists have added their contribution [41]. The new consensus Guidelines are expected in October 2007. (Information by Kathleen Poole, Executive Director, ASCCP). Both cytology and histology guidelines will also be reprinted in the October 2007 issue of the *Journal of Lower Genital Tract Disease*. Algorithms for the guidelines will be published in the *Journal of Lower Genital Tract Disease*. As with the 2001 Guidelines, ASCCP will post free links to the AJOG published guidelines and the algorithms on its website. The algorithms will be available online on October 1, 2007 [15].

Whatever the Pap test result is, the woman should ask her doctor what are her specific options within the limits of the clinical actions those Guidelines are recommending. The Guidelines are neither a law nor are applicable to every woman. Individual variances should always be considered.

The Guidelines are a medical document. To help our readers to grasp easily and understand better what is recommended there, we have compiled these guidelines and have summarized them into a table (Table 2.6), which is supposed to be a simplified version customized for general public. If new Guidelines are issued before this book is in print, we will update this table.

There are two major components in the table: The 2001 Bethesda System Terminology and the ASCCP Guidelines. The Pap test and the cytological abnormalities found on Pap test are discussed in the previous section (2.3.2).

The 2001 Bethesda System terminology is a consensus taxonomy trying to systematize cytological results describing normal or pathological clinical conditions which were identified on cervical specimens obtained from healthy women, or women with hidden disease during cervical cancer screening procedure. A woman with symptoms or Pap test positive result requires gynecological diagnosis, not a screening test. How to reach this diagnosis has been left to doctors to decide.

However, because approximately 50 million Pap tests are performed yearly in the US, and about 3.5 million are found Pap positive, the members of ASCCP have thought they can contribute to the standard of healthcare in the US by recommending criteria for management of women with positive Pap test results hoping to improve the prognosis of women in the follow-up to screening. In 2001, the ASCCP 2001 Guidelines were published as another consensus document, but with recommendations as to what doctors should do after receiving the Pap test result. In these Guidelines, the ASCCP is recommending clinical action options to doctors who are making decisions what to do in the follow-up of women with positive Pap test.

Those intentions were good and widely accepted. Our table summarizes those recommendations [183]. For detailed information we recommend reading the new ASCCP Guidelines that will be published in October 2007 (see above) [15].

The term consensus means an agreement – a document agreed upon by a group of experts. Why is the consensus necessary? Because opinions are different; therefore, the consensus is a collection of opinions on which everybody (or at least the majority) has agreed. It also means that there are many other issues, not mentioned in this document, on which the experts did not agree. One of those issues is the personalized medicine approach. It seems, there is no agreement how to approach an individual healthy woman who suddenly received information that she might have a hidden cancer. The lack of consensus on this matter is making women frustrated, feared, and antagonistic towards the test. This chapter was intended to bridge this gap and to help women understand better what the Pap test is all about, and how to handle different information which they may receive from their doctors.

Let me try to explain the whole procedure presented on this table step-by-step.

Table 2.6 Pap test screening results and management of women with abnormal Pap test

<table>
<tr><th colspan="3">2001 Bethesda System Pap test</th><th colspan="3">2001 ASCCP Guidelines for management of women with cytological abnormalities</th></tr>
<tr><td rowspan="8">Negative</td><td colspan="2">NIL</td><td colspan="3">Repeat annually or less frequent</td></tr>
<tr><td colspan="2">Infection</td><td colspan="3">Treat infection</td></tr>
<tr><td rowspan="6">BCC –
RCC
Benign</td><td>Repair – inflam</td><td rowspan="6" colspan="3">Repeat testing after 6 months – wait and watch</td></tr>
<tr><td>Radiation</td></tr>
<tr><td>IUD</td></tr>
<tr><td>GC</td></tr>
<tr><td>Atrophy</td></tr>
<tr><td>EC post 40 years</td></tr>
<tr><td rowspan="15">Positive</td><td colspan="2" rowspan="2">ASC-US</td><td>HPV No</td><td colspan="2">Repeat at 12 months</td></tr>
<tr><td>HPV HR</td><td colspan="2">Colposcopy and control 4–6 months</td></tr>
<tr><td colspan="2">ASC-H</td><td colspan="3">Colposcopy and further</td></tr>
<tr><td colspan="2" rowspan="2">LSIL</td><td rowspan="2">Colposcopy</td><td>0</td><td>Repeat cytology</td></tr>
<tr><td>+</td><td>Biopsy</td></tr>
<tr><td colspan="2">HSIL</td><td colspan="3">Colposcopy with endocervical sampling, or diagnostic excision</td></tr>
<tr><td colspan="2">SCC</td><td colspan="3">Surgery</td></tr>
<tr><td colspan="2">AGC-NOS</td><td rowspan="3" colspan="3">Colposcopy with endocervical and/or endometrial sampling with control at 4–6 months. Diagnostic excision if persistent</td></tr>
<tr><td colspan="2">AGC-H</td></tr>
<tr><td colspan="2">AIS</td></tr>
<tr><td colspan="2">Adenocarcinoma</td><td rowspan="4" colspan="3">Surgery</td></tr>
<tr><td rowspan="3"></td><td>Endocervical</td></tr>
<tr><td>Endometrial</td></tr>
<tr><td>Extra uterine</td></tr>
</table>

NIL Negative for intraepithelial lesion or malignancy, ***BCC*** Benign cellular changes (normal repair after inflammation or injury, radiation induced changers, intrauterine device [IUD] induced changes, hormonally induced changes including atrophy after hormonal reduction), EC – endocervical cells from cervical channel, ***ASC-US*** atypical squamous cells of undetermined significance (first degree of abnormality, mostly subject to spontaneous resolution), ***ASC-H*** atypical squamous cells but high degree of abnormality could not be eliminated (the screener has found one or more cells which look abnormal but their number, distribution, shape and chromatin density do not allow classification into HSIL group), ***LSIL*** low grade squamous intraepithelial lesion (cellular changes similar to those caused by HPV disease – koilocytosis; could resolve spontaneously with improvement of immuno-competence or HPV load reduction), ***HSIL*** high grade squamous intraepithelial lesion is a sign of a more serious cervical lesion, which is not likely to resolve by itself and will need further examination and intervention, ***AIS*** adenocarcinoma in situ (cancer started in glandular cervical channel cells, but still refrained within the epithelium – between the base membrane with basal cell layer and the superficial layer), ***AGS NOS*** atypical glandular cells (analog to ASC-US) but with involvement of cells from the cervical channel, ***AGS-H*** analog to ASC-H but with glandular cells, ***SCG*** squamous cell carcinoma (cervical cancer either in situ – local, or invasive, but the diagnosis needs biopsy and histology)

2.3.4.1 Pap Test Negative

If the result is "Pap test negative" it is a relief for a woman whose specimen was examined. However, the category "Pap test negative" includes three subcategories: Infection-inflammation, Benign/reactive cervical cells (BCC/RCC), and Endometrial cells after 40 years of age. What is the meaning of these subcategories?

- *Infection/inflammation* term is reserved for conditions when infection by bacteria, fungi or parasites is present, the body responded with inflammation (presence of many inflammatory cells such as polymorphonuclears [PMN], monocytes [histiocytes], lymphocytes), but cervical squamous cells show normal cytology. We have seen severe acute gonococcal infections, but the parenchymal cells of the cervix were not affected. Naturally, a woman with such result must be treated for the infection.
- *Benign cervical cells*, this term is reserved for atypical cells which usually occur in conditions that are considered as repair from previous inflammation, radiation, women carrying IUD (intrauterine devices), older women with atrophic epithelium or women at any age if their epithelium shows predominance of squamous cells with increased amount of keratin. Cytokeratin is a callous, horny intracellular protein which presence is usually reactive (in response to external factors), but could be an additional sign of pre-cancerosis (keratin plus diskaryosis), too.

  NOTE: Search for epithelial cells with keratin in blood has become a popular test for diagnosis of cancer (cervical also) in blood. We do not recommend this test because it is non-specific, and has nothing to do with early diagnosis of cervical cancer – it could be of interest only for those women who do not go to gynecologists from non-defendable reasons such as behavioral eccentricity. Cytological diagnoses BCC (benign cellular changes) or RCC (reactive cellular changes) are categorized as Pap negative, but should be considered as an abnormal condition which deserves control of its progress.
- Between menarche and menopausal women cervical specimens must have endocervical cells (collected by cytobrush from cervical canal) and, sometimes, may have endometrial cells (spontaneously separated during menstruation). Atypical endocervical or endometrial cells on Pap test may be associated with the presence of a wide variety of processes, including polyps, chronic endometritis, hyperplasia, and carcinoma. Again, this is not a result that should be considered as negative and be forgotten. It should be considered a result that indicates to an abnormal condition, which is not cancer, but which should be followed.

The best description of cytopathological images of these "benign" conditions could be found in the Comprehensive Cytopathology of M. Bibbo [19]. We do not expect our readers to read a medical reference textbook, but it is important to note that, even in this book, the criteria between cytological categories are not clear, there is overlapping, and prediction on lesion histology is included in the pure cytological description of images. In other words, the temptation to explain the origin of atypical cells found on smears is overwhelming, and the real intention of a screening test, to identify a possible lesion that has to be further examined, has been obscured. In this book, and only for the purpose of more critical reading, we are trying to make distinctions between subcategories of Bethesda System terminology clearer and better divided.

This entire group of Pap negative tests but with abnormal cytological results has been barely considered in the 2001 ASCP Guidelines.

In addition, every woman should know that Pap test has been found to be of medium sensitivity (only 51 %) and much better specificity (above 90 %), and that false negative readings have been noted at average in 20 % of Pap test results. This group is also not included in the 2001 ASCP Guidelines [183].

Having said that, we do not wish to frighten women with negative Pap test results. We only wish to remind all women on the limitation of such consensus statements and the relativity of the guidelines for clinical actions they recommend, and to inspire women to ask doctors for more explanation, and to become active participants in the protection of their own health.

2.3.4.2 Positive Pap Test

If a woman receives information that her specimen was found Pap positive, she should ask what the sub-classification of this category is because this will determine how her doctor will proceed.

There are ten sub-categories in the Pap positive group (Table 2.6). The 2001 ASCCP Guidelines recommend a different approach for each of them. New partial guidelines (after 2001) have been even more specific with the "necessary" procedures. Every gynecologist has been regularly updated with those instructions and every woman can find them on the ASCCP Home Web Site on the Internet [14].

How to manage a woman with Pap positive test is really a compromise that doctor has to make between the cytological result and the special circumstances that may exist in each case. We have summarized those recommendations on (Table 2.6) in a simple table and understandable manner. This is probably the best procedure that a doctor should advise.

However, whatever Pap test positive result is, every woman should be aware of three things:

- The result might be wrong
- The result indicates a condition that could resolve by itself
- The result needs confirmation by diagnostic tests (pelvic exam, colposcopy, etc.)

Recently, HPV testing has received more attention as an additional test to cytological Pap test. The ASCCP Guidelines have also incorporated or are incorporating HPV testing to different sub-categories of Pap positive results. Why? The reason behind such an approach is the fact that persistent HPV disease (not infection only) is a risk factor for cervical cancer. Another reason is the availability of cervical cells collected in Pap test specimen collection solution. After the Pap test is completed, the residual cells could be used as free specimen for HPV viral particle determination assays such as HC 2 (Digene), or any of DNA/RNA viral probe assay available as biomarker test – analyte-specific reagent – for research only. Having material available, every additional test would add value to the diagnostic value of Pap test (don't forget that the Pap test is only a screening test – diagnosis is the next issue), and any test that could indicate to the presence of an additional risk factor should be helpful. This fact was acknowledged in FDA approval of HPV testing as the ancillary test which could be used in the management of women with positive cytology (ASCUS). The same caution is also expressed by the authors of the Bethesda System who carefully discern the use of HPV testing from diagnosis of the clinical condition [163].

We are not against HPV testing, but we would like women to be aware that Pap test is screening test (not diagnostic), HPV infection is not HPV disease, and HPV disease is only a risk factor not cervical cancer. However, the presence of HPV positive test for "oncogenic" strains of the virus is a signal that additional attention must be taken, and that this woman is at increased risk requiring more frequent Pap tests and/or additional diagnostic testing. Part of this philosophy is included in the Table 2.6. The danger of false alarms using HPV testing has been recognized long time ago. In 1999, the Papanicolaou Society Annual Meeting indicated to this unwanted effect [128].

2.3.4.3 What to Do?

The ASCCP Guidelines are recommendations for diagnostic and treatment procedures. Because they are discussed in details in the next Sects. (2.4 and 2.5) we will not talk about this part of the table here.

In general, after receiving Pap test result every woman should be alerted to talk with her doctor and ask for advice. She should ask if the recommended action is based on the cytological result only, on HPV test only, or is it based on the cytological result upgraded for HPV result. Fortunately, all those combinations have one outcome: colposcopy. This is a visual examination of the cervix in search for visible lesions and is safe and painless. However, increased cytological category sometimes requires biopsy. Biopsy, which could be painful and may have complications such as bleeding and/or infection, should be avoided if not necessary. Doctors like to discuss liability with educated patients, and this opportunity should be utilized on mutual benefit.

We believe that this book will serve as a guide for women to ask proper questions and receive the best answers. We also would like to convey that women should not be afraid of Pap test (as many of them are now), but they should learn by using this book how to help themselves find the best option what to do after receiving the Pap test result.

2.3.4.4 Points to Consider

Women in the US are faced with a problem they cannot solve, but can help solving. The name of this problem is the Frequency of Pap Test Screening.

Originally, Pap test was recommended for annual screening. The same recommendation is still valid for the countries where this test is to be introduced for the first time. There is solid evidence that in these countries the mortality of cervical cancer might be reduced to 50 % within 3 years – but only among women who will be participating in the annual program.

Currently, there are 100 million American women at risk for cervical cancer. According to the National Health Interview Survey (NHIS) in 1980, the estimated number of Pap tests performed in the US per year was 50 million. This estimate suggests that each woman had a chance to see the doctor once in 2 years. But, in reality, 20 million American women do not participate; therefore, this period between two screening periods for preventive program participants has already been extended to 3 years. Recent analysis by the same NHIS has projected reduction of annual Pap test for 43 % from current 50 million test because of the impact the HPV testing and HPV vaccination could have on the frequency of Pap test screening [63].

A reduction of 43 % is a total of 22 million tests per year. Although this will not be written in the new Guidelines, the reality is suggesting that an extension of the period between two tests to five years will be considered "safe." We think, this extension, even as a theoretical chance, could cause an unnecessary risk for American women and the reoccurrence of cervical cancer within such less protected population will became a predictable outcome.

Our message in this book is that every woman should take her share of the responsibility for her own health. Insistence on cytological screening per year or once in 2 years has been proven as safe for participants. This should not be changed unless, after 10 or 20 years, sufficient evidence will accrue that HPV vaccination has prevented the occurrence of cervical cancer (not the HPV infection as the current scientific reports declare). Until this time, the best cancer preventive measure should be kept available at the frequency of testing that has been confirmed in 50 years of experience.

2.3.5 *Biomarkers and Cervical Cancer*

Since the liquid-based-Pap test (LBP) was introduced, this new specimen collection technique has not met the goal for which it was introduced for (reducing the sampling error) but has fought for new applications in order to stay on the multibillion market of cancer screening.

When HPV was recognized as being intimately connected with cervical cancer and the first HPV testing was performed in the Pap test specimen collecting solution, the interest of molecular biologists turned towards LBP specimens as a source of human nuclear material for their genetic experiments. Indeed, it was true, LBP cervical specimens could be used as material resource for molecular biology methods (e.g., DNA/RNA, PCR, immuno-hybridization), which, in turn, could be applied for studying cells in transformation from normal to dysplastic and malignant. Many hopes were entrusted into studying HPV viral particles in transforming cells, changes in proteins, enzymes, signals, and pathways caused by HPV and/or cancer.

Many connections were found in laboratory experiments (cell cultures), some correlations between molecular markers and histology were identified, but no significant correlation with cytology was identified; consequently, no Pap specimen-related biomarker assay usable for a routine clinical application has been developed yet [133].

In the meantime, consensus conferences on cervical cancer have declared that:

- Pap test is not perfect (cit: nobody has ever said so)
- Pap test sensitivity is low (approximately 50 %) for a screening test – reported in a meta-analysis published by AHRQ (Agency for Healthcare Research Quality), but accepted widely
- Pap test specificity is better but not sufficient (many false positive results with costly unnecessary biopsies ending with a blind biopsy because the lesion was not seen on colposcopy indicated by the positive Pap)
- The prognosis of the disease progress was poor (cit: screening test is not for this purpose)
- The therapy cannot be ordered according to the Pap test results – only further diagnostic procedures (cit: this was known from the very beginning) [115].

These conclusions show an increasing tendency to add values to the conventional Pap test, but these new values are expected to come from increasing its potentials for clinical diagnosis and for prognosis of the disease. It is an area where biomarkers can demonstrate their advantages. However, it should not be done for the cost of loosing the main purpose of the Pap test – no woman with epithelial cell abnormality should be missed. At this moment, biomarkers based on molecular methods without cytology cannot meet this requirement.

We think, the efforts should be directed towards development of molecular biomarkers within cytologically identifiable cells on Pap specimens. MarkPap technology is an example of such an approach (see below).

2.3.5.1 Biomarkers as Analyte-Specific Reagents (ASR)

This is how the story of molecular biomarkers began.

Biomarker assays are modern tools intended to improve diagnosis and therapy of cancers. Cervical cancer in particular has been a subject of many efforts to discover reagents targeting specific molecules or processes involved in cancerogenesis or promotion of cancer (cancer biomarkers), which have been intended to improve an early assessment of disease prognosis and to guide therapeutic measures. Table 2.7 summarizes several biomarkers associated with cervical cancer.

A popular example of such in-house developed biomarkers is the ProEx C Analyte Specific Reagent promoted by TriPath Imaging in 2005 [18]. At this moment, I would like to attract your attention onto the phrase Analyte Specific Reagent (ASR). This phrase is reserved for all assays developed to detect or to demonstrate activity of biologically active molecules, which could be used for research only. Biomarkers are the same active molecules, but applied in clinical medicine as

Table 2.7 Biomarkers (Analyte-specific reagents for research use only) with clinical or potential clinical usefulness

Biomarker	Method	Reported	Date	Comment
Genes: APC, DAPK, MGMT, GSTP1	Quantitative hypermethylation specific PCR	Reesink-Peters N, et al. [152]	2004	Call for more genes and more specific
Cervical Aid Phosphatase on cervical smears or monolayers	Nanotechnology, cellular microarray, signal amplification by chemistry	Markovic N, Markovic O [118]	2006	Trademark: MarkPap® available at www.bioscicon.com
Telomerase – nuclear enzyme in cytoplasm	Protein released in cell when chromosomes become genetically unstable	Medical Laboratory Observer [11] Lang LH [104]	1999	Nonspecific
HTERT, IGFBP-3, transferrin receptor, beta-catenin, HPV E6 and E7	Molecular diagnostics	Shoji Takahashi [166]	2006	Concept based upon literature search
Panel of molecular biomarkers	Different techniques	Malinowski DP [112]	2007	Uncontrolled signal transduction, cell cycle deregulation, activation of DNA replication, altered extra-cellular matrix interactions.
Serum markers	Proteomics and glycomics in HPV and cervical cancer	Greenwell P [76]	2007	Only a project, no data. Fishing expedition – no idea
E7 protein	HPV – optical imaging of nanogold particles, E7 antibody, confocal microscopy – contrast enhancing	Kumar S [103]	2006	Promotes reentry in S-phase of differentiated keratinocytes
Biomarker in serum	Oncogene protein epitope identified as Y(355) LGTRR(360)	Yoon SK, et al. [186]	2004	Non specific– found in hepatocellular carcinoma (virus)
MCM7	E2F-induced cellular DNS replication factor – staining	Brake T, et al. [28]	2003	Only HSIL and SCC, nothing earlier
Biomarker	Method	Reported	Date	Comment
MCM proteins	Immunocytochemistry in tissue microarray	Oberman et al. [144]	2005	
		Cortez et al. [51]	2005	

(continued)

Table 2.7 (continued)

Biomarker	Method	Reported	Date	Comment
SCC-ag in serum	Serum protein (?)	Bischoff R, et al. [24] – project	2003	Only for recurrence
CIN	Surrogate endpoint marker	Ruffin MT, et al. [153]	1995	Cytological biomarker
Search for biomarkers	NCI, NIH – collects tissue specimens for DNA and RNA analyses	McFarlane KL [59] Contract solicitation	2002	Project – fishing for new biomarkers
VEGF	Angiogenesis	Obermair A [143]	1999	VEGF in CIN (1–3)
Pap smear[a]	Biomarker for colposcopy	FDA approved Weinstein [108]		In use
MarkPap® smear	Proposed as a new biomarker for colposcopy	Not approved by FDA, Markovic [115]	2003	In process of approval

[a]Pap smear is the only cervical cancer biomarker recognized by FDA for colposcopy [108]

a marker for specific clinical action. Biomarkers need FDA approval, otherwise should be considered as ASR. Some confusion in terminology is still present, and we hope our readers will have the privilege of having more clear insight into this emerging field.

In an excellent review of molecular diagnostics application in cervical cancer prevention, Malinowski (2007) concluded that the multiple biomarker panels have potentials to develop clinically useful molecular diagnostics [112]. His article is a well-documented admission that, in spite all of efforts, molecular diagnostics has not reached the level to replace the Pap test, and it should not be considered for anything more than as an adjuvant methodology for certain prognostic aspects.

In his conclusion he writes something important for our book. "The molecular diagnostic is likely to develop into," he said, "a cell-based assay where the detection of over expressed proteins in a cytology specimen can be correlated with current morphology-based classification of disease and confirmed with biopsy sample. As this correlation becomes established and the molecular diagnostics assay gain validity and clinical acceptance, the reliance on cell-based association will be diminished. This will ultimately lead to the migration of molecular diagnostics test to a no slide assay format. The use of morphology-based classification for cervical carcinoma and the malignant precursors that are currently detected using the Pap smear will eventually be eliminated and replaced with more quantifiable and robust molecular diagnostics assays."

This long statement is important – he thinks that those new methods will replace Pap test, but he does not specify whether it would be the Pap test as a cervical cancer screening device, or the Pap test liquid sample where genetic and other type of testing could be performed.

For those who believe the Pap test should stay the best cancer screening test, this discussion is only another attempt to open the huge cervical cancer market to molecular biology industry without real justification.

Interestingly, in this review, the author is exclusively concentrated on molecular diagnostic assays, genomic analysis, multi-gene diagnostic expression signatures, combination of biomarkers and immunocytochemistry, but is not mentioning a very simple MarkPap assay, which encompasses all the requirements for a specific biomarker for cervical cells abnormality and has produced images amenable for digital image analysis at distance and telecytopathology. Consequently, we will address the omitted technology at the end of this section.

For the purpose of better understanding the scope of cervical cancer biomarkers, for this book only, we will try to summarize the information provided in Table 2.7 above and referenced in the literature. Generally, there are four groups of biomarkers and/or ASR considered of importance for cervical cancer:

1. Cytological (Pap smear, CAP, CIN)
2. Molecular and HPV related (genetic and DNA/RNA related such as cyclin E, Ki-67, and p16) [2]
3. Serum (still not proven)
4. Biomarkers, still in research phase, coming from different sources such as microarray analysis of cervical carcinoma cell lines, signal transduction and mitogen activated protein kinase pathways in keratinocytes (superficial cervical cells infected with HPV and showing signs or reentering into cell cycle), proliferation expression signatures (CDC, MCM, TOP2a), extra-cellular matrix proteins (cathepsin, metalloproteinases, integrin) and others, none of which has proven clinical use yet [11, 112]
5. Potential biomarkers, like the role of angiogenesis (vascular endothelial growth factor) in development of preinvasive lesions [143].

However, most of these biomarkers are not recognized as having clinical value. Therefore, only a few are included into the FDA list of approved biomarkers [112] and/or used in the clinical TNM (tumor/nodus/metastasis) classification for tumor staging. Only Pap smear is in this list.

2.3.5.2 Cytological Biomarkers

We will continue discussion only on cytological and HPV related biomarkers. Cytological are clearly defined:

- **Pap smear** is a biomarker for colposcopy, meaning that the Pap test negative result excludes, and Pap test positive result indicates to a need for colposcopy. Years of experience have proven the value of Pap smears for this purpose [33].
- **CIN** is histological diagnosis made on thin slices of biopsy-collected cervical tissue. CIN 0–1 indicate to no intervention, CIN 2–3 + indicate to surgery.
- **CAP** is indicating the presence of cervical dysplasia and HPV disease. CAP negative result is indicative of healthy cervico-vaginal epithelium, CAP positive results call for colposcopy and HPV testing after and when needed [84].

All **HPV**-related biomarkers are considered to provide prognostic factors to improve cytological screening. Indeed, they provide information of the presence of HPV infection, HPV disease, type of the HPV strains involved, evolution of cervical disease (cancer or else), but they should not be used separately; therefore, their value as cervical cancer markers is diminished. In studies followed the most cited ALTS trial, the authors carefully discern the role of HPV testing and propose it to be used for management strategy, not for diagnosis [127]. With the advent of HPV vaccination, these makers, together with anti-HPV (strain specific) antibody in serum may provide convincing evidence of the value for controlling the specific immunity – this time is still in front of us.

Because Pap smear and CIN are well known and described elsewhere in this book, we will concentrate now on cervical acid phosphatase (CAP) which will be elaborated in Chap. 7.

2.3.5.3 MarkPap Test a Biomarker or a Surrogate End-Point for Colposcopy

The reader is advised, at this moment, to refer to Chapter 7, Sec-1, where the new version of MarkPap Test is presented in details together with IT technology adjacent.

Readers are advised to Chap. 7.1 (New Tools, MarkPap Platform Technology Illustrated) where the upgraded and expanded description of the removed text from this page was completely presented.

The following sub-chapters should be found:

1. **MarkPap Test**
2. **MarkPap Reagent Kit with Accessories**
3. **MarkPap Specimen Self Collection Kit™**
4. **MarkPap Telecytopatholgy Services ™**
5. **MarkPap Digital TelePap**
6. **MarkPap Mobile, Mobile-Pap.**

2.3.5.4 PAP Smear as a Biomarker for Colposcopy Versus MarkPap Test

Finally, we would like to discuss a not so well known fact that Pap smear has been accepted by FDA as a biomarker for colposcopy [108]. It has not been incorporated into cervical cancer grading or staging diagnostic procedures, but is considered to be a biomarker because it is a guide for clinical action. All Pap smear positive women (ASCUS+) should go to colposcopy for further diagnosis; all Pap test negative women should come for the next scheduled screening test.

To be clinically acceptable, a biomarker assay should be sensitive, specific, cost-effective, fast, and robust against inter-operator and inter-institutional variability. It must demonstrate clinical value beyond that of other types of information that are already available at the time of diagnosis [114]. Biomarker candidates must undergo clinical validation before receiving US FDA approval. This has happened for Pap smear.

All other biomarkers are designated analyte-specific reagents (ASR) for research purpose only. MarkPap assay includes Pap smear (PAP) plus detection of an analyte specific reagent (CAP). MarkPap equals CAP+PAP. Having Pap smear is already an FDA approved biomarker for colposcopy. It needs additional clinical evaluation for CAP.

MarkPap was initially recommended as a biomarker (surrogate end-point) for colposcopy [16, 115] (Fig. 2.5).

2.3.6 Human Papilloma Virus and Cervical Cancer

(A cervical cancer risk factor and how to avoid or reduce it).

Human papilloma virus (HPV) is considered to be the most significant risk factor for cervical cancer not because the virus can produce cancer directly (e.g., by altering the affected normal cell genomic structure and bringing the viral ability for self replication), but because it can act in concert with other risk factors and cause crucial events to occur (genetic mutation, failure of the repair system and failure of immune control) that will lead an "abnormal" cell to progress into cancer and/or to promote a HPV infected cancer growth [35].

HPV denotes a family of more than 100 types of viruses. Certain types cause warts (papilloma) and most of them do not cause cancer. High risk subtypes (strains) linked to cervical cancer are 16, 18, 31, 33, 35, 45. Digene's Hybrid Capture 2 test is a diagnostic test for detection of genital HPV infection (a single test detects more "highrisk" viruses) [85]. There are new tests designed to detect viral particles, or nuclear proteins (DNA fragments) of affected cells – this is considered to be of help for assessing prognosis of the lesion from which cells are separated. None of these new methods examines cells, therefore, for both screening and diagnostic purposes, virus-detecting or virus-effect-detecting methods must be combined with cytological methods (e.g., Pap test for screening, or histology for CIN diagnosis) to determine the status of health on the cervical specimens [107].

When the first antiHPV (high-risk strains) vaccine has been approved (Merck, Gardasil in 2006), the hopes have been risen that this could be the first anti cervical cancer vaccine and that every woman should be protected from this grave disease. The second vaccine (GSK – Cervarix for HPV types 16, 18) is getting approvals around the world (European Union approval published in September 2007), but we still do not know whether our hopes for prevention of cervical cancer occurrence will be realized and when in the foreseen future [73].

2.3.6.1 HPV Disease

Fortunately for women, HPV virus is indeed contagious, sexually transmitted, but not very virulent causing warts in 1 of 64 infected women, and cervical cancer in 1 of 2000 infected women. Occurrence of the disease is related to the immune defense

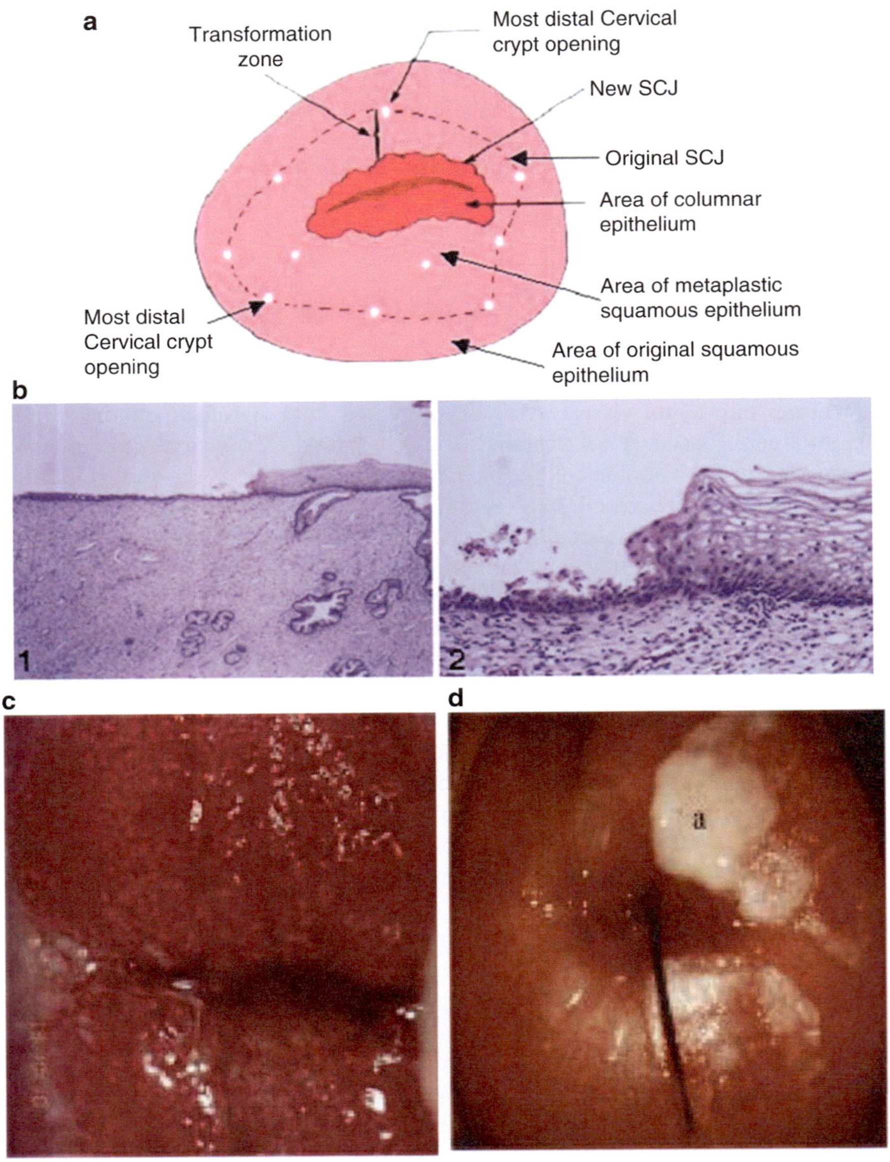

Fig. 2.5 Cervical cancer images – colposcopy. (**a**). Colposcopy = scheme: IARC, Colposcopy book. Images used by permission from IARC (Source: Colposcopy and Treatment of Cervical Intraepithelial Neoplasia. A Beginner's Manual. Eds. J.W. Sellors and R. Sankaranayanan. English edition. IARC, 2007. ISBN 92 832 0412 3). (**b**). Transformational Zone – histology (IARC, Atlas of histology). (**c**). Cervicitis: IARC, Colposcopy book, #sfig9.2. Chronic cervicitis. Reddish appearance and bleeding on touch. Scattered acetowhite small areas. (**d**). Leukoplakia: IARC, Colposcopy book, #sfig7.4. Large acetowhite plaques of hyperkeratosis, (e). CIN 1 lesion

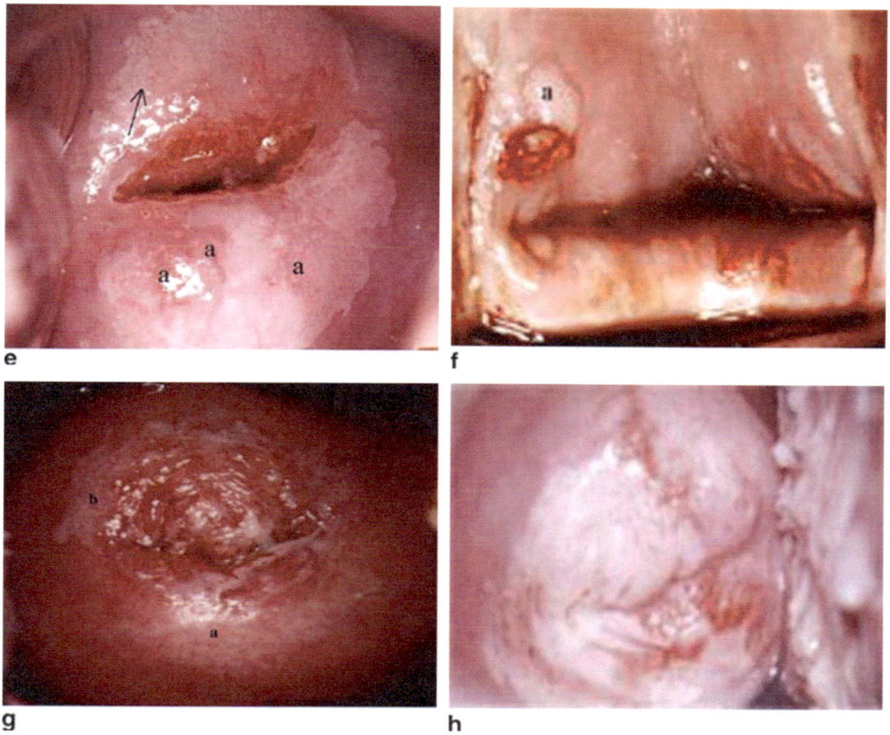

Fig 2.5 (continued) macroscopic appearance: IARC, Colposcopy book, #sfig7.16. Circumorificial acetowhite lesion with fine mosaic. Histology indicated CIN 1. (f). Exophytic condyloma: IARC, Colposcopy book, #sfig7.7. Wart, HPV infected tissue, tumor-like growth. (g). CIN 2 lesion macroscopic appearance: IARC, Colposcopy book, #sfig7.20. Acetowhite lesions with coarse punctuation and mosaics. Histology confirmed CIN 2. (h). CIN 3 lesion macroscopic appearance: IARC, Colposcopy book, #sfig7.27. A dense, acetowhite, opaque, complex circumferential lesion. Histology CIN 3 [88]

of each infected women, and the spontaneous resolution of the infection is the most frequent outcome. If an infection continues – persistent or chronic, one should always search for additional risk factors that may contribute to HPV disease. Only persistent infection (above 1 year) was connected to cervical cancer. The low virulence of this virus may also shorten the period of protection after HPV vaccination – this would be a non-desirable, but possible situation with all consequences related to a late development of HPV disease (warts, cancer) in previously immunized girls.

On the other side, it is well documented that invasive cervical cancers are "contaminated" with HPV and, what is particularly intriguing, with only certain types in vast majority of cases. In 2007, Smith et al. published a meta-analysis of HPV virus type distribution among 7094 cases of invasive cervical cancer (ICC) and 14,595 cases of HSIL reported worldwide. They found an overall prevalence between 86 % and 94 % of HPV16 and HPV18 as the most common types. Some differences were found between ICC and HSIL cases suggesting a possible type-specific influence on the disease progression [161]. Again, this study confirms a strong association between HPV and cervical cancer and justifies vaccination as a preventive measure to reduce HPV, but for a single woman, it does not establish a true causal relation; rather a relation of a co-factor in cancer promotion and progress.

(a) ***HPV Disease Epidemiology.***

HPV is the common wart virus spread over the globe. It is the cause of the various kinds of warts (genital warts, plantar warts, flat warts) as well of cervical dysplasia, vaginal dysplasia, and cervical cancer. HPV has been implicated as a cause of infertility, miscarriages, vaginosis, vulvar vestibulitis syndrome, prostate disease in men, and laryngeal papillomatosis (both genders). Genital HPV is highly contagious sexually transmitted infection which does not cause a symptomatic disease in men, but in women cause development of either benign proliferation of infected tissue (genital warts) or cervical cancer.

HPV affects both women and men. It is easily transmitted. Centers for Disease Control and Prevention (CDC) estimates that 20 million people in the United States already had HPV in 2005. Approximately six million new cases of genital HPV (more than 30 genital HPV types) appear each year; most of them (74 %) in 15–24 year age group [124]. However, the HPV disease rates are much better. Again, according to CDC, in 2005, only 357,000 women were registered because of genital warts, but more than four million had vaginal infection and 424,000 vaginal trichomoniasis, or 106,000 vaginal herpes [40]. Invasive cervical cancer was found in 10,000 women and CIS (carcinoma in situ) in about 40,000 (this information was not confirmed by CDC) [41, 88]. These numbers confirm high contagiousness, low virulence and uncertain natural immunity.

HPV is not always transmitted sexually. However, the types that cause anoperineal and genital warts (also called condyloma acuminata, venereal warts, genital warts, vaginal warts and penile warts) and cervical dysplasia are most commonly sexually transmitted, like low risk HPV types 6, 11, 42, 43, and 44. For this reason, HPV is classified as an STD (sexually transmitted disease) that can be transmitted through sexual intercourse, oral sex, anal sex, or any skin-toskin contact.

HPV is contagious even when warts and dysplasia are not present. Some HPV types have a greater association than others with cervical dysplasia and cancer like high risk HPV types 16, 18, 31, 33, 35, 39, 45, 51, 52, 56, 58, 59, and 68. All HPV types are contagious [74, 83, 85]. Some women develop genital warts, cervical/vaginal dysplasia, or both, while others become carriers with no signs or symptoms, or they become immune to certain HPV types. Men generally develop genital warts, become carriers, or develop immunity.

HPV infection and HPV disease rates should not be mixed with rates for cervical cancer. However, in countries where cervical cancer rates are very high, like in Mexico, where a woman dies from cervical cancer every 2 h, there is a solid ground for alarming against HPV infection [70]

(b) ***HPV Disease Pathogenesis.***

It is believed that HPV virus enters the body after slight trauma to the epithelium and needs superficial, highly differentiated cells for replication. Basal cells could be infected but are unable to produce virus because they do not contain basic material for viral replication. However, the viral DNA is often integrated in host chromosome in malignant HPV associated lesions. There is no solid evidence to support any theory how a HPV infected cell could be transformed into malignant. The evidence of a relation between HPV and cervical cancer is mostly epidemiological – correlation. There is a theory that virus, integrated in cell chromosomes is responsible for transformation during cell replication, but no hard evidence was provided [97, 185]. Based on indirect information, we would rather consider that cervical cancer starts in a basal cell (mutation), begins to grow and, when passing HPV infected tissue (condyloma) gets HPV virus and continue to grow together thereafter. Figure 2.3c presents an imaginary of this situation.

(c) ***HPV Disease Clinical Symptoms.***

HPV disease in women is almost an asymptomatic disorder if not for small discomfort during intercourse and/or increased vaginal discharge. The only visible signs are warts, small, soft, red or white papillomatous tissue growth on vaginal lips, inside vagina, on cervix or in the vulvar region. Sometimes they accumulate forming larger tissue formations – condyloma acuminata.

(d) ***HPV Disease Diagnosis.***

History, pelvic exam and Pap smears with HC 2 HPV test are the first line of diagnostic procedures to be considered if any suspicion of HPV infection appears.

It is impossible to determine how long someone has had an HPV infection. Incubation period ranges from 1 to 3–6 months. Neither men nor women are routinely tested for HPV. Women, participating in regular cervical cancer screening (Pap test) are indirectly tested for HPV disease. This is a condition when cervico-vaginal epithelium responds to HPV infection by producing abnormal tissue growth (papilloma, condyloma, or cancer). Typical "HPV induced cytological characteristics" are a combination of nuclear images seen in cervical dysplasia (bi-nucleosis, karyorrhexis, karyopycnosis, karyolysis) and "koilocytic characteristics" such as cytoplasmic vacuolization and/or perinuclear hallo. If cells do not show cytological abnormalities described above, the HPV infection goes undetected unless a Digene Hybrid Capture HPV DNA Test is performed. (see Figs. 2.1e, 2.2e, and 2.3c for cytological details).

Other testing methods (specific blood tests) may show that there has been HPV infection in the past, but they cannot determine if HPV is currently present. HPV is usually diagnosed because the cervical or vaginal cells obtained by Pap smear or biopsy have the "characteristic appearance of HPV-infected cells" under microscope. We prefer MarkPap test because it can detect HPV infected cells separated from intraepithelial condyloma even before "koilocytic" shapes become obvious, and is free of contamination with virus that may come from inactive cells (dormant phase) [21]. Figures 2.1e, 2.3b and 2.4c presents several HPV infected cells with and without "koilocytic" appearance.

There are more than 100 types of HPV detectable by current laboratory technology. Most of them are detected by tests conducted in addition to the Pap test (like reflex testing or ancillary methods to improve the assessment of prognosis). According to Zuna et al. [193], when cytology diagnoses were compared with HPV test results, HPV DNA was present in all HSIL (23 different types) and in 94 % invasive carcinoma (13 types). P16 biomarker was the most frequent in all categories.

HPV types 16 and 18 are involved in 70 % of cervical cancer cases, and together with HPV types 6 and 11 are involved in 90 % genital warts cases. Gardasil may not fully protect everyone and does not prevent all types of cervical cancer, so it is important to continue regular cervical cancer screenings [41, 124].

(e) ***HPV Therapy.***

There is no therapy for HPV virus. However, there is therapy for warts – medical creams (imiquimod, podofilox), cryotherapy and surgical excision including LEEP. Additional therapy is available for diseases that present significant risk factors for cervical cancer, such as HIV/AIDS, metabolic and hormonal disorders, etc. [97].

(f) ***HPV Prognosis.***

The infection subsides spontaneously (following improvement of subject's own immune defense – immuno-competence), and doctors rarely need to intervene.

In healthy women, HPV can cause genital warts and cervical dysplasia (precancerosis). Warts are usually diagnosed at the pelvic exam, dysplasia at the cervical cancer screening (Pap test). Positive cytology is a sign of abnormal growth and requires further diagnostic procedures or expectation to observe the disease progress. Improving the host immune defense during this time could frequently resolve the problem. Intervention is necessary to "reduce the viral load." It is usually done by removal of warts. At this moment there is no specific antivirus therapy (like Ribavirin for herpes virus infection).

The prognosis *quo ad vitam* is excellent because measures are available for prevention of HPV disease development and removal of HPV induced lesions. However, prognosis *quo ad sanationem* (cure) is uncertain.

2.3.6.2 HPV Prevention and Vaccines

There are three levels of prevention to consider here:

1. Prevention of HPV infection
2. Prevention of HPV disease
3. Prevention of cervical cancer that could develop if HPV disease is persistent.

Each level requires a separate set of measures.

Prevention of HPV infection requires safe sex. In the US this term implicates sexual abstinence and use of condoms [119]. Asking for safe sex is a behavioral intervention including education, providing participants with tools to apply the education, and monitoring for compliance. Although it is easy to say, this is very difficult to implement.

Prevention of HPV disease requires an individual to concentrate on maintenance and/or permanent improvement of her immuno-competence. To convince patients to improve their self-defense against STD infection such as HPV is easy because diet, exercise, and/or well-being are components of everyday life and girls and women are susceptible to advices that will help. HPV vaccination belongs in this category. Please see the next section for more discussion on this issue.

Prevention of cervical cancer in women with HPV is a combination of the above mentioned measures, and the application of therapeutical measures to reduce the viral load (medical creams and surgery) is helpful. These measures should be combined with measures directed to reduction of all other cancer risks, if and when present. This is why regular cervical cancer screening with cytological tests such as Pap test are not expendable and women should know that, when going to see their doctors for regular gynecological exam, they should ask for Pap test.

HPV Vaccines

In the US, only 10,000 women get cervical cancer annually (0.05 % of HPV infected) and about 4000 (0.02 %) die from cancer. Obviously these rates do not justify the assumption that HPV vaccination will prevent cervical cancer. However, because most of cervical cancer cases show presence of high-risk HPV strains, it is widely accepted that prevention of infection with those strains could reduce the probability for cervical cancer occurrence – elimination/reduction of a significant risk factor [41, 70].

HPV vaccination is a procedure of teaching the body's immune system, using harmless viral particles, to recognize the harmful HPV virus (with infected cells) and to destroy it in the next contact; thus, to prevent or to alleviate the HPV disease that could lead to development of cervical cancer.

In June 2006, the FDA approved the vaccine Gardasil, which is highly effective in preventing persistent infections with HPV types 6, 11, 16 and 18, which are involved in about 70 % of cervical cancers and about 90 % of cervical warts [124]. The vaccine is based on technology developed by NCI scientists whose work laid the foundation for the production of HPV "virus-like particle" or VLP (virus-like particle) vaccines. Using genetic engineering techniques to manipulate the genetic material of the virus, scientists created a vaccine consisting of non-infectious VLP formed by a single protein – the L1 protein – from the outer surface of HPV. The L1 protein triggers a robust antibody response that neutralizes HPV infection. Gardasil is comprised of a mixture of HPV type 6,11,16, and 18 VLPs. Studies to date have shown that this vaccine provides protection against HPV 16 infection for at least 4 years. The vaccine is approved for use in females 9–26 years of age, but is most effective if given before the onset of sexual activity [130]. There are also reports of adverse events including three deaths that question the safety of vaccination [96]. However, this report did not cause an alarm because, in comparison with millions of vaccines already distributed, this "is a neglectable number." We think, for those who died, their deaths are not neglectable. Every woman should know that adverse events after HPV vaccine happen and even death cannot be eliminated as one of the risks. In May 2007, a comprehensive report based on scientific studies was published in LA Times [123] cast doubts to the previous optimism about the success of HPV vaccines.

The real problem is that, as of present, HPV vaccines may protect only against several specific strains of HPV; they do not protect from cervical cancer – although, we all would like to have them having this anticancer protection. This is the main cause of the dispute. HPV disease is of minor significance – highly contagious by sexual activity, none to mild clinical symptoms, frequently with self-resolution. Notably, nobody will ever consider vaccination to prevent this type of disease. However, cervical cancer is a grave disease and any preventive vaccination is highly preferable. Currently, there is confusion even among health professionals how to measure the effectiveness of these vaccines. A recent report from the FUTURE II (Females United to Unilaterally Reduce Endo/Ectocervical Disease) Study Group published in the New England Journal of Medicine (NEJM) has used a composite endpoint to measure the effectiveness of vaccination. The problem is that this composite endpoint included cancer and non-cancer diagnoses (HSIL, CIN 2/3, AIS and invasive cervical cancer) instead of viral antibody that would be the most appropriate [100]. The composite endpoints are usually used when the study is small and cannot prove the point – in this case the endpoint would be cervical cancer. Since it is a very rare disease, to have a group of vaccinated and a group of non-vaccinated women with at least several cases of cervical cancer per group, and to search for statistical significance, it would need probably tens of thousands subject/specimens and many years of study. Therefore, this was a compromise. However, every woman should know that such compromises are allowable in science, but not in medicine when the truth is necessary for decision what to do with the patient.

There are more than 100 types of HPV. Of the 15 types that are considered to be cancer causing, or oncogenic, HPV types 16 and 18 – which were first identified and molecularly cloned by the researchers at the German Cancer Research Center – are responsible for about 70 % of cervical cancers worldwide. In most women infected with HPV, however, the infection will clear by itself and cervical cancer will not develop; therefore, HPV infection is necessary but not sufficient for development of the disease. Indeed, in the US the prevalence of HPV infection is as large as 40 % of sexually active women (40 million), 2–3 million are getting this infection each year, but only 10,000 develop cervical cancer. The probability of a woman in US to develop cervical cancer after being diagnosed HPV positive is 1 in 2000 cases. Does it justify mandatory vaccination? Surely does not at this time. However, it is good to have the vaccine available, and it is good that Merck, GSK and other vaccine makers increase their production with new strains, but the decision to take or not the vaccine and when, must be left to individual decision.

We wish every woman should understand how much it is important to make difference between public advertising of the "vaccine for cervical cancer" and the real benefit she or her daughter could have from vaccination, and how much is important for her to be able to make an educated decision.

Tomorrow

Scientists are striving to better understand why HPV infection clears in most women, but persists in others and leads to cervical cancer in only some women with persistent infections. Efforts to characterize the molecular pathways in cervical cancer cells, and to better understand how the interplay between these cells and their environment (in particular the effects of hormones and immune system factors) may affect cancer development and progression, should provide critical insights. We believe, another tool, biomarkers, could be of substantial benefit on this road [120].

At the time this book will be published, many currently present dilemmas may be solved. Here, we would try to identify some of these questions that are asked by women and their caregivers in Summer 2007.

Dilemma about HPV vaccine is to take (who, when, why) or not to take it? Who should be vaccinated? Most recent recommendations from the regulatory agencies FDA, CMS, CDC will be presented [41]. In September 2007, the National Coalition for Cervical Cancer, a non-profit organization of women with cervical cancer, held 2007. National Conference in Washington, DC. The conclusion of this conference represents the newest initiative for prevention of cervical cancer including HPV vaccination and cytological screening [45]. On September 18, 2007, Women in Government, a non-profit organization from Washington, DC, issued New State Policy Recommendations encouraging insurance providers to adequately cover FDA-approved cervical cancer/HPV vaccines, Pap tests, and HPV tests [77]. On the other side, Judicial Watch uncovered three deaths related to HPV vaccine out of 1637 adverse events reported within recent 4 years. Neither adverse events nor deaths sounded an alarm against vaccination because of rarity of these events [19].

We hope, the more grounded answers will be soon provided to common questions such as: How much and how long am I protected with HPV vaccination? Should I continue with regular Pap test? Does HPV vaccine mean that Pap test should be cancelled, or replaced by HPV vaccines? The answer is NO, and it will be explained.

In summary, only a woman with cervix can get cervical cancer, but it does not mean that a woman with cervix must get cervical cancer. The same analogy goes for HPV (at least at the 2007 level of understanding): a woman having HPV infection could get cervical cancer, but it does not mean she must get this cancer. In both examples the probability is very low (below 1 %).

In 2015, some of these questions have been addressed, but not complete answers are available. For details see Sect. 4.1.6.

In summary, HPV infection is well documented, but the pathogeneses is still more inclined to the tumor growth, than tumor-genesis. This inclination is raising hopes that HPV immunization may be extended to cervical cancer treatment – elimination of active virus may suppress further growth of the invasive tumor. However, it needs more work to be done.

At present, HPV screening has been accepted as obligatory addition to cytological Pap test and vice versa. Some attempts to replace Pap test with HPV alone have been shown with insufficient evidence, and the cytological screening is still number one in prevention and diagnosis of cervical cancer.

The attempts to make cervical cancer screening mandatory worldwide have failed and the outreach is still below 10 % worldwide. This failure to increase the outreach is due mostly to the need for infrastructure – not only the cost of the test, by the entire procedure from healthy subject recruitment, testing and removal, of suspect lesions. American experience, to reverse the cervical cancer prevalence and mortality trends in individual countries seem unreachable is some new ideas are not involved. This second edition is addressing this problem with two major novelties: MeDyKO (a composite biomarker) and Telemedicine with mobile phone camera component in combination with worldwide networking (see New strategy, Chap. 6 and New Tools Chap. 7).

There is also a moderation of the initial enthusiasm to vaccinate young girls and even boys – the occurrence of side effects (some of them serious) although very rare, have raised the threshold of caution and individual responsibility of parents have been alerted rather than the government liability for mandatory vaccination – as it was in prior period.

More technical improvements were provided by the health industry – mostly for detecting high risk ("oncogenic") HPV strains 16, 18. The new automatic HPV particles reader is Cobas, manufactured by Roche, which got FDA approval for primary screening for virus infection. This machine could be very useful for adding to better prognosis of advanced lesions, LSIL and above, particularly CIN 2/3+. In the context of using HPV vaccination for treatment of advanced cervical cancer, such a specific diagnosis (only "oncogenic" strains) could be essential for disease follow-up.

Anyhow, the interrelation between HPV disease and cervical cancer is well established and this relationship lead to the description of a new composite biomarker (MeDyKo, see Chap. 7.2) which integrates instant information on cervical cancer potential development, presence and prognosis. More work on this composite biomarker is warranted and offers new hopes for further advancement I the fight against cervical cancer.

2.4 Diagnosis and Treatment of Cervical Cancer

Overview

Cervical cancer is a malignant disease – a qualitatively different condition from the risk factors or any of the abnormal conditions identified in Pap test as pre-cancerosis.

There are biomarkers, frequently found in cervical cancer cells, but they are typically identifying DNA/RNA or mitotic abnormalities, or HPV infection particles, but not the malignancy itself. Not any single biomarker, no matter how specific it is for demonstration of abnormal changes in cellular genomic or proteomic structure, qualifies for being considered as cancer. Cervical cancer as an autonomic disease could develop at any moment, in any precancerosis, and any level of "disease progress." This truth defines our approach to cervical cancer.

Prevention and Control is an approach dealing with everything we know that may precede or may trigger, support or promote cervical cancer occurrence, growth and invasion. This approach includes procedures to avoid exposure to risk factors, to reduce this exposure, to detect early signs of lesions that could develop into cervical cancer and to remove them (this is how the Pap test was described).

Diagnosis and Treatment is another approach dealing with:

- Cancer diagnosis – histological diagnosis: squamous cell carcinoma adenocarcinoma, clear cell carcinoma, sarcoma
- Staging – assessment of cancer spread locally, regionally and through the entire body (TNM classification – T (local spread – size of tumor; N – regional lymph nodes; M – distant spread, metastases)
- Planning appropriate therapy based upon histological diagnosis, staging and the relevant individual characteristics of the patient
- Assessment of the prognosis under different plans for therapy and decision which plan to use.

There are a number of medical procedures in use for making objective and correct diagnosis, planning appropriate therapy and making reliable prognosis. Some which are frequently used will be discussed in this book. Internet is great source of information for cervical cancer diagnosis and treatment. The best American hospitals have recognized the impact Internet can provide and have used its web pages for informing general population of their own experience, and CNN is publicizing their views and recommendation to public [46].

2.4.1 Diagnostic Methods

Diagnosis is a process in which a physician is using medical skills and tools to confirm, modify or reject an initial hypothesis about what is wrong with the patient and to come to the conclusion how to help her best.

Diagnosis of cervical cancer begins after Pap test result has returned as positive, if the patient has history of cervical cancer, or complains of symptoms that could raise a suspicion of cervical cancer. When faced with a suspicion that the patient might have cancer, the first objective of the doctor is to examine her thoroughly and to confirm this diagnosis or reject the suspicion. Today, doctors have available all tools necessary to make proper diagnosis with very little chance of mistake.

We shall now discuss some of these tools called diagnostic methods.

2.4.1.1 Anamnesis – History

This is an extremely important part of the medical diagnostic procedure. This is really an interview of patient's complaints, but also, a guided inquiry of risk factors, patient's habits and concerns, and other information that may influence making an exact diagnosis and application of the most promising plan for therapy. This interview begins with the first information the patient provides at the nursing station, continues with answering specific questions on the medical questionnaire, discussing with the nurse, and finally, summarizing this information with the doctor before the physical exam.

An overt cervical cancer will present itself with easily recognizable signs and symptoms: pelvic pain, bleeding between periods, difficulties with urination, losing weight, fatigue, and depression. No woman or man who cares about his woman should ever allow her to come in such situation.

Cervical cancer screening and the Pap test is a preventive medical procedure (cancer control) designed for healthy, asymptomatic women who might have precancerosis or early signs of lesions that could develop into cervical cancer. Women coming to Pap test are typically without complaints and symptoms and in good health including sexual health. Diagnosis is the next procedure, designed for patients, women who failed on the screening test and women who could be considered as having a serious disease.

2.4.1.2 Pelvic Exam

Pelvic exam is a complete physical exam of woman's pelvic organs by a health professional. The exam is intended to determine the position, shape, size and sensitivity of the vagina, cervix, uterus, fallopian tubes, ovaries and the surrounding organs, urine bladder and bowel; also, to collect cervico-vaginal fluid and to inspect this discharge for any presence of infection, abnormal spotting or bleeding and tumors.

The procedure is safe and painless unless disease exists. Details about the procedure could be found elsewhere [187].

Invasive cervical cancer is detectable by pelvic exam. An experienced physician can detect a presence of an abnormal mass, detect its location, size, relation with other pelvic organs, detect sensitivity/ pain, and examine the condition of the surrounding organs and tissues.

This is an excellent, safest, and most informative technique that should not be avoided or replaced with instrumental examinations.

2.4.1.3 Colposcopy

Colposcopy is a diagnostic medical procedure intended to allow doctors to examine visually with colposcope (Gr. kolpos – vagina; *skopein* – to view, examine) – an instrument equipped with directional lights and magnifying glasses – the female organs vulva, vagina and cervix.

During this procedure, a speculum (L. *speculum* – mirror) is placed into vagina, colposcope brought to approximately 15 cm, and a doctor inspects the superficial areas of those organs looking through the magnifying glasses. Usually, it is important for the doctor to brush off some vaginal fluid for better viewing. If cervix is not within the best viewing distance, the doctor may use an instrument (forceps) to pinch cervix and bring it closer. To improve the probability for correct visual diagnosis, doctors usually use vinegar swab (acetic acid 5 %) to present the abnormal parts of epithelium as white patches over red background. These patches are considered to be cervical lesions causing abnormal cells to appear in Pap test [88, 141].

In the US, colposcopy is a gold standard for validation of Pap test. However, it would be only a half of diagnosis unless a piece of the affected tissue is removed immediately and sent for histological diagnosis. This procedure is called cervical biopsy and is described below.

2.4.1.4 Biopsy

Biopsy is a diagnostic procedure designed to collect a piece of the sick-looking tissue from the body and to give it to pathology laboratory for processing and histological analysis. Biopsy could be done on normal tissue to serve as control or by mistake. Normal tissue biopsy should be avoided because of small, but still present, risks for bleeding and infection. Multiple biopsies may produce scars with disfigurement of the cervix.

In cervical pathology, biopsy is performed during colposcopy and the doctor is targeting white patches. The material is taken with a special cervical biopsy forceps with cutting edges at the tip. The sampled tissue should be diagnostic of the condition causing this epithelial abnormality. All epithelial abnormalities are determined using histological analysis and terminology.

There are Pap test providers who, because they cannot be sure in their findings on colposcopy (usually the borderline images between normal and abnormal epithelium) conduct cervical biopsy more frequently than necessary – just to be on the safe side. Sometimes, performing biopsy with colposcopy could be a request from the clinical trial in which the doctor is participating. However, if biopsy is diagnostically unnecessary, we are recommending an Informed Consent to be taken from the patient before this procedure is performed. This simple procedure will protect the patient's rights and the doctor's compliance with medical ethics and the DHHS OHRP (Office of Human Research Protection) requirements.

2.4.1.5 Histology

Histology (Gr. *histos* – web, tissue) is the study of tissue (a mass or layer of cells forming the basic structural material of an animal of plant) separated from the source by biopsy and processed in pathology laboratory for a pathologist to examine the tissue and make histological diagnosis. This procedure is separate for normal (microscopic anatomy) and for sick tissue (microscopic pathology) [89, 180].

Histological diagnosis of cervical tissue obtained by biopsy is determined in terms of CIN (Cervical Intraepithelial Neoplasia) categories [93]. There are four grades of CIN: CIN 0 or no CIN, CIN 1 of mild dysplasia, CIN 2 or moderate dysplasia, and CIN 3 or severe dysplasia. The CIN 3 is usually alternated with CIS (carcinoma in situ diagnosis), which is the first degree of cervical cancer [84] (see Fig. 2.2 for details).

How is this done?

The specimen, a piece of tissue pinched from the cervix, is processed in a pathology laboratory. It is usually embedded into paraffin to preserve the structure, sliced in thin slices and stained with histological stains hematoxylin-eosin to present the tissue composition for microscopic examination.

A pathologist is examining the stained tissue specimen with microscope and is looking for histological features concerned with differentiation, maturation and stratification of cells and nuclear abnormalities. The proportion of thickness of epithelium showing mature and differentiated cells is used for grading CIN. More severe degrees of CIN (CIN 2–3) have a greater proportion of undifferentiated cells with only tiny layer of mature, differentiated cells on the surface. If the basal membrane is disrupted, and the undifferentiated cells invade the subepithelial tissue, the diagnosis of invasive cervical cancer is made (ICC) [84].

Nuclear abnormalities include, but are not limited to nuclear enlargement, nuclear-cytoplasmic ratio, and increased intensity of nuclear staining (hyperchromasia). Mitotic figures are rare in normal tissue; their frequency is increased in immature tissue. These features are used for grading CIN. The type of cells involved is crucial for diagnosis of CIS (carcinoma in situ – cervical cancer confined within the epithelium at one place), condyloma (Gr. *kondyloma* – knob) HPV induced growth of abnormal cells (but not cancer) or other growth of morbid excrescence (e.g., polyp).

HPV virus is known to produce a specific type of cells (koilocytes), which typically have nuclear alterations (morphologically indistinguishable from images typical for cervical dysplasia) and a cavity within the cytoplasm containing cellular debris. It happens because HPV virus (oncogenic strains) affects cell nuclei and initiates apoptosis (programmed cell death); nuclear abnormalities and cellular cavities are cytological presentation of these events. The virus usually affects cells from more superficial layers; consequently, cytological images will include cells with parakeratosis, abnormal nuclei and keratin (protein present in superficial layers). Some authors believe that HPV virus can cause reverse differentiation (dedifferentiation) of superficial cells and initiate new cycle of mitotic replication, but we think this is not likely, and that virus is affecting the cells from a neighboring layer (intermediary) which nuclei still have this ability although abated (Fig. 2.3).

The virus could be integrated in the host genome early and can cause disruption of normal maturation (can be identified by expression of E6/E7 oncoproteins) and the loss of growth control. If infection is persistent, koilocytes grow into papillomatous benign tumors (warts) or, rarely, into cervical cancer.

Histological classification must be definite for diagnosis of cancer. Clinical actions are determined by CIN classification. See Fig. 2.2 and Table 2.8 and the text below.

2.4.1.6 Ancillary Methods

The term ancillary method is applied for non-standard laboratory techniques that could, under certain conditions, improve the diagnostic accuracy of the standard diagnostic practice. The Bethesda System recognizes cytological staining with Papanicolaou stains as the only standard method for cervical cancer screening. The Gynecological Histopathology recommends hematoxylin/eosin staining for tissue slices. All other methods are considered as ancillary [162].

The 2001 Bethesda System has included all non-cytological testing into the ancillary category, which includes HPV testing by any of available molecular biology techniques using nucleic acid probes (e.g., Hybrid Capture 2 test) that is a nucleic acid hybridization signal amplification system, Southern blotting utilizing direct hybridization with complementary DNA probes, or target nucleic acid amplification (notably the polymerase chain reaction) for HPV detection, genotyping, and viral load detection [57].

Microscopic methods for detection of organisms such as trichomonas vaginalis, fungi (candida), actinomyces, shift of flora suggestive of bacterial vaginosis, or cellular changes consistent with herpes simplex infection, belong in the same category [165].

In this book, we present an emerging new biomarker-based method for detection of cervical acid phosphatase as a biomarker of cellular abnormality. This method is very simple although, because of the techniques used, it is defined as "*nanotechnology-based cellular micro-array method for measurement of molecular signals amplified by chemical reactions*" [21]. In 2007, this method is available in the US *For Investigational Use Only*, before it is approved by FDA.

2.4.1.7 Diagnostic Interventions

Excisional biopsy is the first and the most important diagnostic procedure to determine the prognosis of surgical therapy. This procedure is combined of surgical removal of cervical lesion with a significant part of normal-looking tissue around this lesion (sides and depth), and histological analysis to determine whether the borderline regions are free of tumor, or tumor had invaded surrounding and/or deeper tissues. If the borderline regions are free of tumor (CIS), this diagnostic procedure becomes therapeutic, and the removal of the lesion is equal to cure. This is why the excisional biopsy must be done by specialist and properly followed by competent histology. There are two most frequently used methods for this diagnostic removal of tumor: Loop Excision, and Cone Biopsy (Conization).

Table 2.8 Diagnostic procedure after positive Pap test

Diagnosis and therapy of cervical cancer			
A. THIS IS HOW IT BEGINS			
Pre Pap	Anamnesis, Pelvic exam, Speculoscopy[a]		Vaginal fluids, if necessary
Pap screening	Pap smear of Liquid-based specimen		
Pap negative	Repeat procedure after at last one year		
B. DIAGNOSTIC PROCEDURES AFTER POSITIVE PAP TEST			
Pap positive	Colposcopy	Negative	Reevaluate cytology
		Positive	Biopsy – Histology
ASC-US+ AGC+	Histology	CIN 0	Reevaluate colposcopy and cytology
		CIN 1	Test for HPV type
		CIN 2	Diagnostic excisional biopsy
		CIN 3	Therapeutic excision
		CIS	Staging & Surgery (see below)
C. DIAGNOSIS & THERAPY OF CERVICAL CANCER			
Diagnosis: Cervical cancer	Staging Methods	Chest X-ray, CT scan (CAT), Lymphangiogram, Pretreatment surgical staging, Ultrasound exam, MRI (magnetic resonance imaging)	
Stages	Definition	Therapeutical options in 2007	
0	CIS	Intraepithelial (CIS)	LEEP, Laser surgery, Conization, Cryosurgery
1	1A	Invasive, microscopical size	Hysterectomy, Conization, Radical hysterectomy
	1B	Invasive, visible size	Radiation therapy (int + ext), Radical hysterectomy, Chemotherapy
2	2A	Cervix + vagina – not other tissues	Combination of internal and external radiation, radical hysterectomy with lymph node removal, chemotherapy
	2B	Upper vagina and uterus	Internal and external radiotherapy with chemotherapy
3	3A	Whole vagina, pelvis wall	Internal and external radiotherapy with chemotherapy
	3B	Block ureters, lymph nodes	
4	4A	Bladder, rectum, regional LN	Internal and external radiotherapy with chemotherapy
	4B	Pelvis, abdomen and distant MS	Palliative radiotherapy and or surgery, chemotherapy, clinical trials
D. THIS IS HOW IT MAY END: HEALTHY 0.9, PAP POSITIVE 0.1, COLPOSCOPY POSITIVE 0.02, CIS 0.001, SCC 0.0001, DEATH 0.00002			

[a]Speculoscopy – visual examination without colposcope. *CT* computed tomography, *LEEP* loop electrosurgical excision procedure, *MS* metastasis, *LN* lymph node

Table 2.9 TNM classification of malignant tumors (Based upon UICC Guidelines)

Introduction	
TNM (Tumor-Nodus-Metastasis) Classification of malignant tumors has been developed and is maintained by the International Association Against Cancer (UICC). This globally accepted classification is also used by the International Federation of Gynecology and Obstetrics (FIGO), and is applicable for cervical cancer staging.	
Mandatory Parameters ("T", "N", and "M")	
T (a, is, (0), 1–4):	size or direct extent of the primary tumor
N (0–3):	spread to regional lymph nodes
M (0/1):	distant metastasis
Other Parameters	
G (1–4):	the grade of the cancer cells (low – well differentiated; high – poorly differentiated)
R (0/1/2):	the completeness of the surgery (resection, boundaries free of cancer cells)
L (0/1):	invasion into lymphatic vessels
V (0/1):	invasion into veins
C (1–4):	a modifier of the validity of the last mentioned parameter.
Prefix Modifiers	
c:	stage given by clinical examination of a patient. The c-prefix is implicit in the absence of p-prefix
p:	stage given by pathologic examination of surgical specimen
y:	stage assessed after neoadjuvant therapy

Loop Excision

Loop excision (known as LEEP and LLETZ) uses a fine wire loop with electrical energy flowing through it to remove the abnormal area of the cervix (lesion). This wire loop serves as a surgical knife but is less damaging to cervical tissue. The tissue removed is sent to the laboratory for examination. Loop excision is commonly done under local anesthesia and causes little discomfort. However, loop excision is a surgical procedure, it is designed to follow, not to precede the pinch biopsy, and should be used with caution when indicated. Overuse of LEEP may cause unnecessary discomfort and damage to the patient [93].

Cone Biopsy

Cone biopsy (or Conization) removes a cone-shaped or cylindershaped piece of the cervix. It is usually done in the operating room and can be done with a laser or with conventional surgical instruments (cold-cone). The tissue removed is also sent to the laboratory for examination. Cone biopsy has a higher rate for complications including interfering with childbirth. Many surgeons are avoiding it and prefer LEEP.

Two other procedures used for excision of cervical tissue, cryotherapy and laser treatment, destroy the tissue, the sample is not available for histological diagnosis, and should be used only for therapy (see below) of cervical dysplasia or pre-verified CIS.

For some time now, the WHO is recommending to developing countries to implement the "Screen & Treat" strategy. This is one time cervical screening procedure, combined with cryoablation of any visible lesion. Since cryoablation is destroying tissue, wide implementation of this policy could cause an increase of invasive cervical cancer occurrence. This is a medical intervention without histological verification, and should be avoided – cytology after cryoablation is abnormal, and cryoablation does not cure cancers – invasive cervical cancer could emerge unnoticed.

2.4.2 *Staging System*

Once the diagnosis of cervical cancer is made, the patient is referred to a specialist who will organize the next diagnostic steps and will plan therapy.

Approximately 40 years ago, the International Union Against Cancer (UICC) has developed a system of procedures necessary for oncologists to take before planning therapy for any single patient. The name of this clinical diagnostic tool is TNM Classification of Malignant Tumors [171]. It is so important that we have copied an overview of this tool from the Internet in order to give our readers at least a simple information what could be necessary for them to undertake if diagnosis is cervical cancer. Please review the Tables 2.10 and 2.11. They contain basic information what doctor is expected to know about his patient before beginning to plan therapy.

According to the TNM Classification, each cancer should be determined by its local growth (T – size in three dimensions), involvement of local lymph nodes (N – even one lymph node positive is sign for radical operation or wider zone radiation), and distant metastases (M – a single distant metastasis indicates to chemotherapy – no local treatment alone could be successful).

This classification was accepted by the American Joint Committee on Cancer (AJCC) and of the International Federation of Gynecology and Obstetrics (FIGO).

The extent of cervical cancer must be described in term of this classification. It requires many additional tests necessary to demonstrate local growth of tumor, involvement of regional lymph nodes and presence/absence of distant metastases.

Twenty years ago this task would have been very difficult and subject to many errors in diagnostic procedures. Fortunately, with the advance of medical imaging, the entire story has changed and the total staging is possible with extraordinary accuracy.

Table 2.10 TNM classification (UICC)

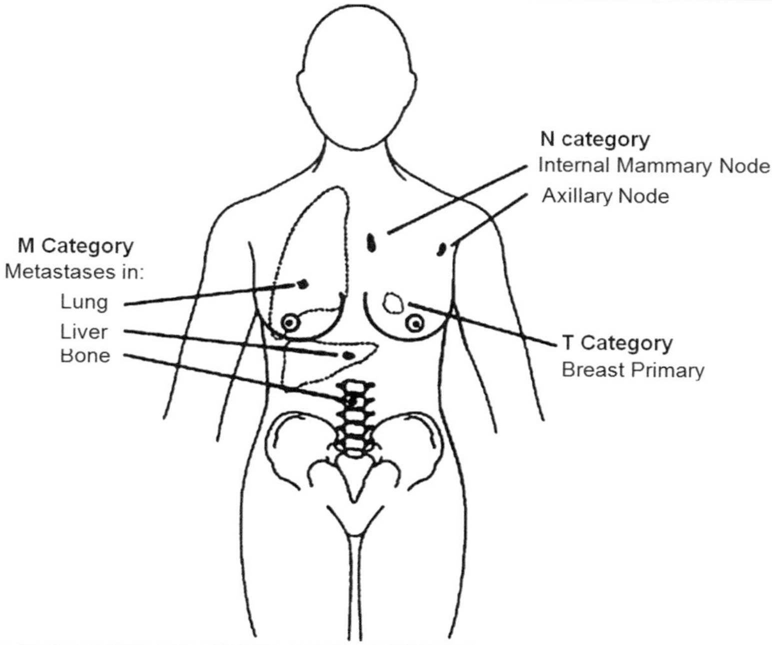

Table 2.11 History of invasive cervical cancer incidence and survival after treatment for US seer estimates in 2004 [63]

Stage	Percent	Survival 5 years	Lifetime risk 2004	Prevalence 2004
T1N0M0	51	92.0 %		
T1N1M0	34	55.7		
T1N1M1	9	16.5		
Unstaged	5	60.1		
All	99 % of 13,050 new	71.05	1:142 for born in 2004	250,726 total 251/100,000

For therapy options available to each stage, see in Table 2.8 above

2.4.2.1 Medical Imaging Used for Staging Cervical Cancer

Invasive cervical cancer is assessable for manual exam, but the precise size of local tumor growth could be measured only with medical imaging instruments. These instruments (X-ray, ultrasound, CAT, and MRI) are also used for detection of enlarged lymph nodes or other affected organs [171].

Ultrasound (abdominal and vaginal), Computerized Axial Tomography (CAT) and Magnetic Resonance Imaging (MRI) are medical imaging techniques widely in use to determine the location and the size of a cervical cancer and the involvement of regional lymph nodes or/and other organs in contact with cervix.

Chest X-ray examination is used for detection of distant metastases. Lymphangiography is used to search for lymph node metastases in deep pelvic, para-aortic and inguinal areas. Bone radiography is used for detection of distant bone metastasis, if any. PET Imaging (positron emission tomography, PET Scan) is a newest technology available for detection of distant metastasis or vital tumor mass in pelvis.

Any other medical imaging or diagnostic technology should be used in search for distant metastasis if any suspicion exists that they are present in the body, but not detected with the routine diagnostic methods cited above.

2.4.3 Planning Therapy

We cannot overemphasize the fact that the cervical cancer therapy, whatever it will be, must be planned individually for each patient upfront; the patient should always be informed about different options regarding survival, late consequences, pain and fatigue, adverse events, and plans how to minimize those risks or alleviate them. Informed Consent would be the best way to protect patients and physicians from disappointment and possible conflicts that may arise during the failing treatment.

Once the staging is completed, the therapy could be planned according to the previous experience of the success/failure of different therapeutic approaches applied on the certain type of tumor and TNM stage [90]. The Table 2.8, *Diagnostic procedures after positive Pap test and Therapy for cervical cancer* according to the diagnosis, is an example of such planning. Unfortunately, in the case of cervical cancer, therapeutic options are very limited once the cancer entered the invasive phase. This can be seen on the next table, where radical surgery is indicated from stage 1A, radiation and chemotherapy from stage 1B. Lower stages have better prognosis with 5-year survival of about 90 % (stage 1). Higher stages have poor prognosis and 5-year survival rate could be as low as 16 % (Table 2.9). This is unacceptable, and every effort should be given to prevent disease progression to the level of invasive cervical cancer. This book is dedicated to help women to be aware of the disease and the current possibility to prevent, diagnose and treat it, and to ask their doctors for regular examinations and removal of pre-cancerous lesion and risk factors on time before cervical cancer occur.

An important parameter for estimating the probability of success is the reported data of studies designed to assess survival of patients if treated with a certain type of therapy. Although this is only an estimate, medical doctors rely on this information once they have completed histological and staging diagnostic procedure. The following table is an overview of such data available for every woman to see and to compare her situation (diagnosis), the recommended therapy and the expected results (Table 2.11).

This table speaks for itself. Modern diagnosis and therapy are so effective, that more than one half of patients are captured at the early phase (T1N0M0) and the 5-year survival rate is above 90 %, which is almost as good as it could be. Obviously, the nature of cervical cancer has not changed over time because those who are diagnosed later (T1L1M1) have a very low 5-year survival rate (16.5 %) in spite of the best therapy available.

The table also shows that among late diagnosed patients (approximately 1200 new cases) almost 900 died within 5 years. If diagnosis was made early, 1100 of them would have survived. This is a striking difference in comparison with 6655 new cases early diagnosed of which, in the 5-year period, only 665 died while 6000 survived.

If a newborn baby girl has a chance to get cervical cancer 1:142 during her lifetime, this chance should be tremendously improved if she will participate in cervical cancer screening – the chance estimate is approaching zero, or 1:∞. Similar calculations make a basis for an optimistic prognosis that cervical cancer could become the first cancer brought under control in the twenty-first century.

2.4.4 *Cervical Cancer Treatment*

Overview

Modern gynecological oncology has simplified the options for therapy of cervical cancer. First, the decision must be made whether this cancer is curable by surgery, or it has spread beyond the local reach of gynecological surgery. The Staging TNM System has been developed to help doctors make this decision (Table 2.9). Unfortunately, successful options are limited, once cancer has grown beyond (Tables 2.8 and 2.11).

Once the staging is completed, the doctor will have to consider three major therapeutic options, surgery, radiotherapy and chemotherapy. Each of these three options has its own advantages and limitations. Patients are also interested in alternative medicine, and doctors should be able to help them with advice as how to use the benefit without causing damage of different alternative methods.

Conventional therapy is surgery, radiotherapy and chemotherapy. Surgery is extremely effective when used to eliminate local cancer (CIS and Stage 1A). For upper stages, indications for surgery, radiology and chemotherapy are distinct, but doctors usually decide for combinations [32]. Although we cannot speak for every doctor, we believe that the decision for combination is given in good faith and wishing the best to their patients – doctors are aware of the limitations of each and every therapy available.

In addition, in the US, there are specialized institutions such as Cancer Treatment Centers of America, where patients are offered Complementary and Alternative Medicines under medical doctors' control [33]. They offer:

- Nutrition Therapy (e.g., nutritional assessment, diet, supplementation [beta-carotene, selenium, vitamin C, eicosapentaenoic acid, vitamin E] and education)
- Pain Management (e.g., drug support and no drug management using behavioral techniques, radiation, surgery, neurological and neurosurgical interventions, traditional nursing and psychosocial interventions)

- Naturopathic Medicine which is intended to lessen the side effects of chemotherapy, radiation and surgery. It uses natural (e.g., Chinese medicine, psychological medicine, homeopathic medicine)
- Mind Body Medicine (e.g., stress management, relaxation and imagery training, spiritual meditation, support groups, counseling, humor therapy, psychoeducational groups)
- Physical Therapy (such as manual [Swedish massage, reflexology, lymphoedema massage] and occupational therapy)
- Spiritual Support (e.g., personal exploration of spiritual issues, symbolic language, socialization, suffering, healing, death/dying issues, grief/loss, God/church, guilt/forgiveness and prayer support)
- Image Enhancement (cosmetic image enhancement, and plastic and reconstructive surgery) – mostly for those on chemotherapy.

Interestingly, outside US, this type of support is expected from primary caregivers, medical doctors and nurses. They may have special training, but this training is usually incorporated in medical studies, residency or graduate study for those who would devote their lives to work in end-stage disease facilities.

In this book, we are only informing women about these options and recommend considering using them only when the provider of standard medical care is asking for additional support. More about this issue may be found in Chap. 3.

2.4.4.1 Surgical Therapy

There are three types of surgical interventions:

- Removal of CIS, local tumor without invasion (laser, cryotherapy, LEEP, Conization)
- Removal of local tumor with limited invasion (Hysterectomy – all types)
- Palliative – reduction of tumor mass and restitution of function of other organs affected by the tumor (ureters, urethra, bowel, nerves, blood and lymph flow).

Pre-cancerous conditions are usually treated with watchful monitoring. CIS must be operated. Based upon the type, location, and size, the surgery could be local (LEEP, cryo, conization) or more extensive like removal of the cervix or the uterus.

For the invasive cancer, the treatment depends on the spread of the cancer through the lining of the cervix into deeper tissues, the extent of this spread (grade and stage of the disease, stages 1–4), age and overall health of the patient. The depth of the penetration of the tumor beyond the basement membrane is a guide to assess the extent of the primary cancer (within the cervix, local surrounding tissues and lymph nodes) and the likelihood of metastases. The treatment includes surgery (extrafascial hysterectomy, radical hysterectomy), radiation, chemotherapy and combined modalities treatment, such as applied in clinical trials. The most effective, emerging techniques include operative laparoscopy, thermo and cryoablation [93].

Hysterectomy

Hysterectomy (*hysteros* – womb in Greek) is the ultimate surgical treatment of cervical cancer. It can be limited to cervix only (cervicotomy), involve the entire uterus (hysterectomy), with an abdominal or vaginal approach; leave a piece of cervix intact (subtotal hysterectomy), or include removal of complete uterus, adnexa, ovaries, lymph nodes, part of vagina and of pelvic tissue (radical hysterectomy).

Hysterectomy is a major surgery (with all risks of general anesthesia) and leaves women with permanent damages, which pose new risks such as internal bleeding, blood clots, damage to bladder, and infection. The risk of operational death is 1/1000. Postoperative complications are changes in sex drive, weight gain, constipation and pelvic pain. Hot flushes and other peri-menopausal symptoms (if ovaries are removed), early osteoporosis and depression can occur [7].

Hysterectomy is performed for treatment of many other conditions not related to cervical cancer. The list includes endometriosis (20 %), benign growth (fibroids, myoma), prolapsed uterus, pelvic inflammatory diseases (20 %). Tumors, including cervical cancer caused only 10 % of all hysterectomies. In spite of the concerns that many hysterectomies had been performed unnecessarily there is evidence that women after hysterectomy could feel better. At least, this was suggested in the Maine Woman's Health Study [7].

Radical hysterectomy is a major surgery performed through an abdominal incision. Surgeon removes uterus along with tissues next to the uterus (parametria and the uterosacral ligaments). Sometime, it may include removal of ovaries and fallopian tubes. Regional lymph nodes are also removed. Such a radical operation has a substantial impact on woman's life and her physical, psychical and social rehabilitation.

With a purpose, we are bringing in this group of surgery two interventions that many authors consider more conservative, cryotherapy (freezing) and laser treatment (when they are performed as therapy, not as diagnostic intervention). They are both performed on the lesions seen on the cervix; both destroy cells and do not provide insight into the condition of the normal tissue surrounding the lesion. Both procedures should be reserved for definite CIN diagnosis only.

Because cryotherapy or **cryoablation** [182] is easy to perform and is of low cost, it has been recommended for prevention of cervical cancer in developing countries. The strategy "Screen & Treat," which has been discussed before, has been approved and providers (trained health personnel) has been allowed to inspect cervix under the speculum, brush with a swab swamped in vinegar and, if white patches" appear, to treat them with directed cryoablation. Obviously, this was a political decision and has no roots in health science. Although white patches could be cleared, without histological analysis of the surrounding tissue, nobody could be sure whether cancer cells were not left behind, and the woman, treated in such a way, could develop invasive cervical cancer beyond curability. Cryosurgery could be accepted only by surgeons and for removal of CIS.

Trachelectomy is a specific surgery when lower part of uterus is preserved, formed into artificial cervix and surrounded by vagina – this operation enable women to have normal sexual life and pregnancy again.

2.4.4.2 Radiotherapy of Cervical Cancer

Radiation therapy uses high energy x-rays or particles to kill cancer cells. It can be external or internal, or so called brachitherapy.

Radiotherapy or radiation therapy is the medical use of ionizing radiation as part of cancer treatment to control malignant cells; it is different from radiology where radiation is used for medical imaging and diagnosis [181]. Radiotherapy works by damaging the DNA of cells. It is important to bring a radioactive source in contact with the tumor. The beam of electrons (beta particles), protons (alpha particles) or photons (X-rays) damage DNA chains both directly and indirectly via ionization of water and forming free radicals which damage DNA. Radiation is not selective. It damages normal (healthy) and cancer cells equally. However, at sub-lethal dose, cancer cells suffer mostly because they do not posses DNA repair system as normal cells, which survive the exposure to this dose. Radiation is limited to tumor cells using oxygen for respiratory function. Anaerobic cells (most part of tumors) are less responsive [181].

Radiation therapy is helpful for therapy of cancer and certain other diseases, but it is dangerous for healthy tissues, present risk to personnel, and should be applied only in secure environments – special rooms and special instruments. Cervical cancer is treated by two radiation therapy techniques – Teletherapy (External Beam Radiation Therapy – EBRT), and Brachytherapy (sealed and unsealed source radiotherapy).

Teletherapy (photons) is applied from outside the body, brachytherapy (electrons and protons) requires installation of radioactive source inside the uterus via a catheter-like applicator. Safety of both technologies is significantly improved with Virtual Simulation (software to delineate tumor images in three-dimension and to help planning radiation therapy). As a result, there is three-Dimensional Conformal Radiotherapy (3DCRT), a technology shaping each radiation beam to fit the profile of the target (organ, tumor). This approach reduces the radiation delivered to normal tissue and enables providers to deliver more radiation to the target.

Radiation therapy is delivered in fractions for several days and with intervals. Planning radiation therapy is very personalized and each patient/tumor must have its own protocol. In spite of all precautions, side effects are present and they may limit efficiency of this therapy.

Side effects or adverse events are classified in acute (epithelial damage – soreness, redness, swelling, ulceration), medium and long term (fibrosis due to scars, local hair loss, dryness due to glandular damage, secondary cancer), and cumulative effects.

Details about patient preparation for radiation and peri- and post-operative care are published in many instructions and always given to patients. One of the comprehensive summaries is available on the Internet [34].

Radiation therapy is indicated in all cervical cancer staged 1B and above. Results are reciprocal with the grade, but at average, 5-year survival expectation rates are above 80 %. This is still not considered satisfactory; therefore, radiation therapy should be considered for combination with chemotherapy.

2.4.4.3 Chemotherapy of Cervical Cancer

Chemotherapy is therapy with drugs. This is a systemic type of therapy, different from surgery and radiotherapy, which are local types of therapy. The goal of chemotherapy is to give a drug orally or per infusion in amount sufficient that this drug, when reaching tumor tissue, will be in concentration that will enable it to enter into tumor cells and exert the expected effect – kill cells or stop their reproductive ability. The problem is that chemotherapeutics are toxic, and a balance between their beneficial and adverse effect must always be calculated for each patient before application [35].

Another problem is that there is no drug specific for cervical cancer; consequently, all anticancer drugs might be affective, but their real benefit versus toxicity must be established in prior clinical trials. Having said that, we are trying to discourage individual experiments outside the well-documented studies; the risks are too large. We would also like to discourage using alternative medicine in form of herbs, extracts, teas, or injection that has not been proven. Particularly, different sorts of "healthy herbs" marketed as food supplements may be even contra-productive. Many times, the vitamins contained in those alternative medicines may counteract the beneficial effects of anticancer drugs. The author of these lines has personal experience with unexpected failures of otherwise good chemotherapy protocols because of the counter effect produced by the food the family was bringing without physician consent to their relatives in the hospital.

Since chemotherapy is only partially effective, there are many research efforts to improve this situation by introducing new drugs (rarely), by changing drug combinations doses and schedules (frequently) and by adding supplemental (adjunct) drugs for correction of unwanted toxic effects of the chemotherapeutics. A lot of information on chemotherapy of cervical cancer is available on the Internet (PubMed site for professionals) many other sites for nonprofessionals.

One of them we may recommend is UK Cancer Research Web Site (http://www.cancerhelp.org.uk) under the topic Cervical Cancer Chemotherapy. There is a comprehensive summary of what is available for those receiving chemotherapy for cervical cancer [31].

Most of chemotherapy protocols for cervical cancer include cisplatin, ifosfamide, paclitaxel, irinotecan, and gemcitabine in combination with cisplatin.

Cisplatin is made by chemical synthesis and contains platinum core and chlor and amino groups. The drug acts by cross-linking with DNA, counteracts cell mitosis while DNA repair mechanism cannot overcome the permanent damage caused by cisplatin, and initiates apoptosis leading ultimately to cell death. Dose is adjusted to affect only rapidly dividing cells like malignant cells. However, because the cervical cancer is slow growing tumor, the potentials of cisplatin are limited.

Ifosfamide is an antimetabolite. It is chemically similar to nitrogen mustard and cyclophosphamide. The drug requires metabolic activation in the liver. Active metabolites interfere with DNA cross-linking and the cell division is aborted. Ifosfamide was recommended as threeline chemotherapy for germ tumors (testicular, ovarian) and in combination with cisplatin for other tumors including cervical cancer.

Paclitaxel is a new synthetic drug from a group known as Taxane (tradename Taxol), but it was discovered as a natural product with anticancer effects. The drug is an antimicrotubule agent that interferes with microtubule formation and disrupts cell mitosis. It is recommended for treatment of metastatic breast cancer, metastatic ovarian cancer, Kaposi's sarcoma, and in combinations with other drugs for cervical cancer [26].

Irinotecan (Camptosar) is a novel anticancer drug from the group of topoisomerase inhibitors. It requires liver transformation into an active metabolite. Its main use is in colon cancer. It is also recommended in combinations with 5-fluorouracil and leukovorin.

Gemcytabine (Gemzar) is a nucleoside analog that exhibits antitumor activity (kills cells undergoing S1 phase of mitosis). It is incorporated into DNA and blocks further synthesis. Gemzar is given in combination with cisplatin adding to this drug for treatment of NSCLC (non-small cell lung cancer) and in pancreatic cancer.

Each of these drugs has its own toxicity that is related to their activity but on healthy tissues that also have higher proliferation rate (gastrointestinal, genitourinary) and also to metabolically sensitive parenchymal cells such as liver, neural, or kidney. This toxicity is inherent with the drug structure and function and could be manipulated only by changing the dose or regime of administration. Many protocols are designed to counteract chemotherapeutic drug's toxic effects, but many of them have their own toxicity. An unbearable fatigue is the usual adverse effect of chemotherapy. All other toxicities like impairment with immune defense (infections treated with antibiotics), erosion of epithelium (total parenteral nutrition), bleeding (platelet transfusions), and similar, could be alleviated and treated, but the chemotherapy will certainly influence the quality of life – at least during the period of application. The risk/ benefit of this therapy must always be established for each single patient. Our recommendations, given in the table above are only suggestions for women in need and their doctors providing help.

This small review of drugs used for chemotherapy of cervical cancer is given to show that the early detection of cervical lesions that could develop into cervical cancer and their removal (excision biopsy) is the best possible treatment for cervical cancer. Everything else is less effective and should be avoided.

At the end of this section, we would add that combination therapy has been designed to reduce toxicity of individual drugs, and to widen the spectrum of targets

(DNA, free radicals) inside tumor cells; thus to provide conditions for more effective therapy.

Newer type is Targeted therapy for cervical cancer. It includes drug Bevacizumab (Avastin) which is an angiogenesis inhibitor and reduce blood supply feeding cancer.

None of all three types of therapy for invasive cervical cancer could cure the patients. They can provide temporary relief, postpone tumor growth, produce a gamut of side effects, but *quo ad vitam* the prognosis is poor.

2.4.4.4 Non-surgical Therapy

Therapeutic Vaccination

Vaccinia virus recombinant MVA E2 vaccine could be used to treat CIN2/3 lesions associated with HPV infection. In one study, 10^7 virus particles per dose were injected directly into the uterus once every week over a 6-week period. The lesions were eliminated in 20/34 patients, 11/34 had reduction of 50 % in lesion size. All patients developed antibodies against MVA E2 vaccine suggesting limitation of further treatment [70].

Self-Support

We strongly believe that cancer patients must fight their disease with full support of their families. As an oncologist, I have witnessed the devastating effect of depression and lack of hope – simply lives were terminated shortly after such psychological desperation occurred. On the contrary, those who were able to see "the light in the tunnel" lived much longer and their wellbeing was preserved in between the series of recurrent therapies. The choice, without exception, is in favor of psychological support before, during and after any kind of medical activity designed to prolong the life of cancer patient.

2.4.4.5 Immunotherapy

Experience from modern Africa has shown that cervical cancer incidence is higher among patients from HIV disease and that individual cases are in more advanced phase than if occurring in healthy subjects without HIV. Human immunodeficiency virus is causing breakdown of the immune system providing environment for other risk factors to promote generating cervical cancer and to support its growth. In this situation, similar to the breaks of immune system by chemotherapy, it is important to support the patient's immune system by options described as biological therapy or biotherapy. Immunotherapy works by stimulating the ailing immunize system to attack cancer cells or/and providing with appropriate antibodies – usually, specific monoclonal antibodies. This approach to cervical cancer therapy is still in developmental phase and final conclusion of its still is pending.

The prevention of cervical cancer is still the only option for cure.

2.5 2016 Estimate of the Prognosis for Cervical Cancer

Not a long ago, cancer was officially considered as a non-communicable disease because it was clear that cells cannot be transferred by simple communication between persons. Recently, the sharp increase of cancer risk factors, many of which include infectious agents as viruses, bacteria, and/or parasites; have slowly started to change this dogma.

Cervical cancer, in particular, is related to chronic inflammation which is caused by viruses and in some cases by other infectious agents. Consequently, modern epidemiologists consider cervical cancer as a sort of a communicable disease.

Because of this change of opinions, we have decided to describe the prognosis of cervical cancer dichotomically: as an individual and as a social disease. All measures, medicine is using to postpone death from cervical cancer, such as prevention, surveillance, diagnosis, therapy and palliation, are still actual and effective if applied for the benefit of individual women as well as for the societies where women present a half of the population.

The crucial change in the social aspect of this fight is the IT revolution and introduction of mobile phone telemedicine with possibility to bridge the disparity by connecting scattered points-of-care with remote expert medical centers and to provide high qualified diagnosis and guidance within hours – or while women is still on the premises. This is a novelty you will find in our book.

But, measuring the success/failure rate of medical approaches is different for individual women and for the society.

For individual women, the success is (1) early detection of lesions in removable phase before the tumor growth has reached the CIN 2 phase; (2) Diagnosis of tumor before its growth has passed 1A phase (still radically operable); (3) Availability of tools and procedures to extend life or to postpone death.

For society, the measures are epidemiological: (1) Mortality rate (proportion of women who die from cervical cancer in 1 year; (2) Prevalence rate (proportion of women with cervical cancer within 1 year in a certain society. (3) Incidence (proportion of women who get cervical cancer in a population of 100,000 women at risk).

Then other aspect of the same question is what the society is? The answer is clear. Cervical cancer is ubiquitous disease. It does not recognize territory, race, social or economic status – it attacks every women, at any time and any place. Consequently, our Fight against cervical cancer must be directed to all women worldwide. This is why we selected a New Strategy for Global Cervical Cancer Screening Application.

Cervical cancer screening is only a part of the Global Fight Against cervical cancer. But, this part is extremely important if applied for all women at risk and conducted properly.

According to American experience, which serves as a "gold" standard, social impact to target is the reversal of mortality and prevalence of cervical cancer in a country and achieving a continuous trend towards reduction (self-sustainability of the procedure per country). In the US, it was achieved only when the outreach of women at risk passed the threshold of 51 % during a period of about 50 years.

Is it possible to achieve in the world? This book is trying to provide an option instead of answering the question. We believe the answer is yes, for shorter period of time, e.g. 10–15 years, and for much less cost than in the US. Our calculations have shown that current finding is a sufficient to change the strategy only if the GDP per capita in a respected country is about $10,000. Low and Middle Income Countries must be subsidized to make the modern cervical cancer screening and prevention meeting the goal to reverse cervical cancer trends in their countries. But, a cervical cancer epidemic of mortality and prevalence is a world problem, and United Nations and World Health Organization are expected to do their part, too.

However, this strategy cannot be achieved in most of the current world unless the strategy in each country is changed, the government do not adopt goal-oriented policy, the professional societies change their guidance including the modern electronic communication devices (mobile and internet), health industry provide tools to meet the new strategy, and health care providers teach women on how to fight for wellbeing in their lives, not only how to diagnose and treat diseases.

Some of these topics are explained in details in our book, some are only presented as guidelines, and some are only mentioned as future options.

Finally, we believe, the readers of this book, will spread this challenge and will seed the new ideas that will slowly grow for the benefit of women in the whole world. But, this road is long and full of hurdles. It will need courage and will to go, not only to come to the end. This is why the book is addressed to all women – they have to fight for their own wellbeing – and we believe in them.

Chapter 3
Coping and Living with Cervical Cancer

3.1 Coping

Introduction, perception and action. Coping with a positive Pap test and coping with cervical cancer on a daily basis. Support from health providers, caregivers, family and friends. Support groups.

Cervical cancer is fearsome for those who have it or think they might get the disease in the future. It has serious emotional effect and take courage to carry on. Help is necessary and it is available. We will discuss separately how to cope with a positive Pap test (pre-cancer, cancer alert) and will devote the rest of this chapter on coping with cervical cancer on a daily basis. It is a continuation of the knowledge that you gained about medical treatment in the previous chapters. Here, we will discuss the importance of psychological factors and summarize how to use this kind of support that is available from health providers, caregivers, family and friends. Support groups and other professional support are also discussed.

Fear is a part of our lives, and we deal with fear almost on a daily basis. Health problems are among the most frequent stressors [10]. However, we differently perceive stress and react individually to stress. The same stressor may provoke quite a different reaction in different persons. For example, common sense dictates that fear of cervical cancer would motivate most women to go and take a Pap test. However, our Survey on the participation of women in Pap test and cervical cancer screening indicates that many do not take Pap test because they are afraid of the exam and even more of the result of this exam (See Sect. 3.4). These are educated women living in Washington Metro Area, but in spite of availability of medical care, they choose not to take a Pap test. They are afraid and rather do not want to know what is going on within their body. One highly educated university professor personally told me, she is so afraid that she would rather not know! This calls for education and for counseling of high school girls and women of all ages and categories. "The worst fear is from the fear itself!" (Franklin Delano Roosevelt).

N. Markovic, O. Markovic, *What Every Woman Should Know about Cervical Cancer*, DOI 10.1007/978-94-017-7560-1_3

3.1.1 How to Cope When the Result Is Abnormal Pap Test?

Another question is how to approach and help women who take the Pap test and get an abnormal/positive result (dysplasia, pre-cancer). Again, fear could paralyze a woman from acting! The attitude of the nurse, who first informs a woman about the positive Pap test is very important. Some women complain that they are informed almost a month after the test is taken, and this is the first wrong step creating resistance and declining confidence in the health provider. "Why didn't the nurse and/or the doctor inform me on time and advise me what to do? They do not care!" This is a normal defensive reaction. How different it could be if a nurse calls a woman on time, approaches her carefully explaining that there is something that is not normal, but not cancer, and advise her to schedule an appointment with her doctor who will provide more detailed information. Every woman would immediately schedule the appointment, gladly visit her doctor and follow the advice that he/she is providing. These women will certainly feel more comfortable to continue the follow-up examinations.

Small things to do that mean so much! Doctors and nurses have different attitudes and bedside manners, but kindness, patience and right information given at the right time should motivate every woman to successfully cope with the problem, not to discourage and inhibit her to actively participate in the treatment. Even the strongest women are fragile dealing specifically with gynecological diseases, which have a particular impact on their emotions and they will certainly appreciate support and help. As soon as a woman is assured that she does not have cancer and has confidence in the health provider, she is motivated to educate herself about the condition that will further increase her confidence. One positive action creates and leads to another positive action.

One of the aims of this book is to collect information about cervical cancer in one place, making this book a woman's friendly companion: Our goal is to educate, to encourage, to ignite optimism and action and to further motivate her to solve her problem. We intend to explain that pre-cancer is not yet cancer, and there are straightforward options available for immediate treatment. Depending on the grade of the abnormality, the doctor will advise different diagnostic procedures (colposcopy, biopsy), and then an appropriate treatment. Remember, the Pap test is only a screening test. Colposcopy and biopsy clarify the diagnosis. These procedures and the follow-up treatment (if cancer is excluded) are not so difficult to experience, particularly knowing that the problem will be soon removed from the first place on the priority list.

In the meantime, waiting results can be frustrating. This is where friends and family are needed to talk, encourage that most likely it is pre-cancer and that they will all help her to decide with her doctor for the best option how to proceed. You can always say: "Let us first hear about the result".

When the new result will arrive, the doctor will discuss with a woman, explaining her the meaning of the result and will suggest treatment. I would recommend going to this appointment with a member of the family or with a close friend. It is good if all involved are already educated about a positive Pap test and can help asking educated questions. This book is one-stop resource for that. Remember, you are the best advocate about your health! In rare occasions a woman, at least in the beginning, would try to handle everything alone not asking for a company – this should be respected, and family/friends should wait until she is asking for support.

Now, the recommendation depends on the level of the abnormality (level of dysplasia). The doctor may suggest different procedures (conization, LEEP, cryosurgery, laser therapy) (see Chap. 2). Some doctors may even suggest hysterectomy for a woman who does not have intention of having more children. You can immediately decide and continue with the treatment, or ask for a little bit time to consider the options. The time that you may ask for consideration depends on the level of dysplasia, and the doctor will tell you whether an immediate action is required (within 2 weeks, for example), or you can postpone the decision. If this is the case, than educate yourself further about your specific situation, read recommended literature, talk with others and you may ask for second opinion. Once you make the decision, you should act promptly so you can get beyond the problem. Again, pre-cancer is curable, the procedures are usually not so difficult, recuperation is relatively fast, and you can continue with your life. Only control follow-up will continue. This is why it is important to have Pap smear done regularly, so you can catch the disease in the early pre-cancer stage, solve the problem and continue to be a healthy and active woman.

According to the results, the doctor may even decide to wait for few months for spontaneous resolution of the problem. Instead to being stressed and nervous, you should be motivated to learn more about the abnormal Pap test, and instead of being nervous and fearful, increase your resistance lowering stress, eating healthy food, having sufficient rest, balancing your activities and carrying on an active, normal life. You can read further in this chapter how to achieve this. Please also refer to Chap. 2 (Sects. 2.3.2.1 and 2.3.4).

3.1.2 The Diagnosis Is Cervical Cancer

What if the diagnosis is already cervical cancer? Then, a woman needs all the support she can get from everybody: Family, health providers, friends, support groups. Again, fighting the fear and encouraging her that there is help available is very important. Showing kindness and compassion is critical approach from the health provider, beginning from the receptionist, to the nurse and doctors.

At this point, the most important next step is to determine the stage of the disease and make the best plan for treatment. If the cancer is only localized (carcinoma *in situ*), the chances are again excellent for recovery. If the cancer has already been spread, it is difficult, but possible to restrict its growth, improve the quality of life, and prolong life for years. Do not despair, with today's diagnostic and treatment options every woman can be treated and continue with her life. However, the treatment will take longer and will be more expensive. This situation is serious and requires lot of courage from the patient, support from family and a good health provider's team who will be leading her and helping her throughout the process.

Most doctors have a policy to be honest about the diagnosis, treatment options and prognosis. This is a good starting point for a trusted relationship. Making an immediate program for action will ignite hope that there are capable professionals to guide her during the process. Introducing her to other specialists (surgeons, specialized oncologists, radiologists) and good coordination between the primary physician and other doctors is again a confirmation for a sick woman that she is in good hands. Please read the real stories in Sect. 3.3. Also, refer to Chap. 2 (Sect. 2.3.4.1).

Otherwise, searching for second opinion is very frustrating for a patient at this moment – this is another fear that she may offend the primary physician and his team. What she will do then? One fear induces another fear and a vicious cycle is formed that can harm the patient and the prospective for treatment of the disease. Time is lost; frustrations disturb appetite, sleep and rest which further aggravate the situation. Because emotional factors are so important to cope with this hardship, mind–body connection should be directed in a positive direction to help, not to aggravate the disease (see Sect. 3.2).

3.1.3 Support from Caregivers and Close Family in Day-by-Day Coping with the Disease

The role and the support of the members of the family become extremely important. There is a saying: "If one member of the family has cancer, the whole family is ill." This is a big truth! In order to really provide support, family member who will be involved in everyday contacts with the patient (or other caregivers) should also read this book and understand the problems. There are many delicate issues to deal with, and patients may easily loose the confidence in the caregiver during these trying times. After that, the patient simply does not want to share feelings and fears anymore. That is not good for anybody. I would also suggest that caregivers avoid general statements like "Everything is going to be all right"; because this will not be the case if certain steps are not taken. Knowing that something is wrong, most women want to know the truth from the beginning.

Rarely, it might be necessary not to reveal the whole situation in the beginning, but in my opinion, the truth should be told as soon as possible, with an optimistic outcome in order to gain patient's full collaboration to participate in the battle against the disease. In any case, one member of the close family must be fully informed of the situation.

What about advanced cancer? Surgery is a mutilating procedure removing a part of the body. Radiation is tissue destruction and chemotherapy is toxic with effects of the entire body. Treating advanced cancer is not an easy task and it is difficult to achieve a substantial improvement. In these situations patients and their families easy loose hope and turn to alternative and complementary medicine options. Even doctors, who are also family members, may become wrong advisors. This is a moment when coping with the disease turns into coping with death as an inevitable outcome. It is a new situation and requires selective approach. Hope must never be destroyed; on the contrary every effort should be made to nourish it (see next paragraph – new treatments).

This book is an excellent introduction also for family members faced with the support and care of cervical cancer patient. Reading this book, the family could learn about the disease and how to approach the patient. One of the most important advices from a family will be to motivate the patient to fight the disease and to continue with further tests and treatment. If she is comfortable with her gynecologist/oncologist, the follow-up and treatment should start as soon as possible. Believe or not, when things start to happen (analysis after analysis, treatment after treatment), it is easier than the initial period immediately after receiving a bad news that you have cancer and do not know, or have not decided what to do. Denial and anger, depression and refusal to continue with tests and start the treatment (that are common in the beginning) are even more difficult to cope. There is a long way to go, different problems to deal and it is sometimes even more difficult for a caregiver than for the patient. There will be time of treatment, recovery from treatment, cancer-free period, a period when cancer returns, and the advanced stages. Constant emotional support is needed with a positive focus in the future, a hope for better, including repeatedly reminding the cancer patient that the ongoing research is constantly finding new ways for treatment and help. This is the whole truth – new diagnostic methods are being constantly discovered (particularly imaging technologies), new biomarkers are being found to lead to better and faster diagnosis, new encouraging drug treatments are being developed (targeting cancer cells only, antibody treatments, drug that do not kill the cancer cell but reprogram it, genetic treatment), new radiation therapies (more targeted), new surgical, less aggressive procedures (e.g., procedures. that do not require classic surgery, but are done with a small cut on the body, e.g., cryoablation), etc. Cancer is certainly not what it were 5–10 years ago. There is a tremendous source for hope now.

The role of the family is also to create, as much as possible, a healthy atmosphere at home. Thus the time spend between hospitals, exams and treatment will become healing time. Lowering the level of stress in the family, an optimistic outlook, a warm atmosphere of caring and love are extremely important. Mind-body connection exists and sometimes this connection may work in favor or may further harm the patient. The family has an important task in this effort to help their loved one. Engaging the patient in some work and household activities, accordingly to her current status (in consultation with the physician) is also important for the well-being of the patient. She will feel that she continues to contribute to the family and will not be occupied thinking only about the disease. This is a trying time for the family and anxious time for patients.

Cancer patients have so much anxiety in their lives (worrying about staying alive – an uncertain immediate future, financial problems, pain, job changing), that some patients transform their anxiety into harsh behavior towards caregivers. They even try to fight with caregivers who are only trying to help. Caregivers should understand that this is temporary change of behavior and should simply overlook these episodes.

Also, there are instances of recollection and analyzing what was done and patients blame themselves and others for something that has been done or should have been done differently in the past. This is again a normal reaction of regrets and apologizes. The best thing is to persuade the patient that this is past history, these actions cannot be changed now and everyone should move forward. Caregivers also should plan time to relax and should call on other members of the family to help.

The family and caregivers have to be educated on ways how to protect the cancer patient from infections, particularly during treatment and early recovery. It means, if somebody in the family gets the flu or some other type of infection, this person should be isolated from direct contact with the patient. Infections may compromise and disrupt the recovery. The same should be related to friends and visitors without exceptions.

For both patients and caregivers, it is particularly hard to cope during the period of treatment (chemotherapy, radiation). The patent suffers from the side effects of treatment, and it is so difficult for the family to see the loved one suffering. Inform the doctor about each side effect (e.g., vomiting, pain, nausea) and ask for instructions how to cope or whom you may contact for further help. These symptoms are directly related to treatment and gradually disappear. The social services department in the hospital of your doctor's office may be of some help, or may direct you to somebody else who might be able to help.

3.1.4 Support of Extended Family and Friends

What about extended family and friends? Everybody can do some good, sometimes just being a good listener. Let patient tells you about her problems. However, if she is not willing to talk, do not insist. If she decides to confine in you "listen with your heart", do not try immediately to change her feeling and behavior. Let her feel that you are there for her, she can come back to you and can count on you. Cancer is a serious disease and a complex approach is needed, but everybody in the patient's circle of friends and family could help with something. Do not be surprised that the strongest women when faced with a diagnosis of cancer will "need people" to listen and to help in many different ways. It is a long way to go! Lot of adjustments are needed at different points of time, at different types of treatment and different stages of the disease. Family must adjust to these stages and provide at all times a continuous emotional support, encouragement and hope. Emotional status of the patient is so important for the success, and this is the least a family can do. Once she is not with the family anymore, grief and condolences will not help. The help is needed when she can have benefit of it.

3.1.5 *Support Groups*

There are cases when husbands ask for divorce when women get sick or a woman may not have close family, and friends are not always available. There is other help that is available within the hospital (support groups), in the community in American Cancer Society local chapters (see Further Reading) and non-profit organizations discussion groups on-line, e.g., National Cervical Cancer Coalition, NCCC (http://www.nccc-online). The address and more can be found in Further Reading. Women who suffer from the same disease share their experiences, ask for advice, follow-up with other women in same situation, encourage and provide emotional support. "I can cope" educational programs, community classes and on line classes can be found on the ACS web site (www.cancer.gov), under ACS Support Programs and Services.

You will find also other useful links in Where to Read More. Rely primarily on ACS, FDA, NIH, NCI, other government agencies, hospitals and universities, and established organizations, like NCCC and similar.

3.2 Living with Cancer

What else can I learn and do to help myself?

Complementary and alternative medicine. Holistic view of the six dimensions of health. Strategies in stress release.

What is alternative and what is complementary medicine? Mind/body/spirit interventions and other complementary approaches. You must consult your doctor before taking any step toward using any alternative or complementary treatments.

The six dimensions of health: Physical, emotional, mental, social, spiritual and environmental health.

Stress release is one of the mind/body interventions that are recognized by both conventional and complementary medicine. In this chapter, you will learn more about stress, its mechanism in order to fight it more successfully. Different stress coping strategies are also described in sufficient details to be helpful for every woman.

An overview of eating for optimal health is given at the end of this chapter.

In the beginning of this chapter, let us explain the meaning of some frequently used terms in conventional medical practices. *Standard treatment* means that this is evidence-based medical treatment tested under strict guidelines and found to be safe and useful. *Investigational treatment* (called also *clinical trial*) is a treatment that has been studied first *in a laboratory, in vitro* (e.g., on human cultured cells), followed *by research in vivo (on* experimental animals). When proven to be safe and promising, a research treatment protocol is designed which, when approved by Food and Drug Administration (FDA, www.fda.gov), is used for humans in a controlled study. This controlled study is a clinical trial. When the results of the clinical trials show credible evidence that the treatment is safe and effective it becomes a standard treatment. The treatment is to be approved by FDA. See Sect. 3.4 and Internet links to clinical trials.

3.2.1 Complementary and Alternative Medicine

Complementary and alternative medicines are different practices. They are not a part of conventional medicine which is practiced by medical doctors (MD) or doctors of osteopathy (OD). The National Center for Complementary and Alternative Medicine at the National Institutes of Health defines *alternative and complementary medicine as "health care practices that are not integral part of the conventional medicine*" [33, 81, 86, 131]. Whatever the definition is, no alternative or complementary medicine cures cancer. It is not possible to overemphasize the need to tell your doctor if you intend to use any alternative or complementary treatment because it may be potentially harmful and interfere with the conventional medicine treatment that you are taking.

Alternative therapy is unproven therapy that is used instead of proven, standard therapy. Some alternative therapy may have dangerous, even life-threatening effects. Never replace conventional medical treatment, such as surgery, chemotherapy, radiation that has been proven for treatment of cancer and prolonging survival, for unproven alternative approaches. An example of alternative therapy is Homeopathic medicine, remedies made of very small doses of herbs, minerals, animal products, or diluted chemicals. There is no scientific evidence that homeopathic remedies are effective therapy in cancer patients [81, 110].

Complementary therapy is used in addition to standard, conventional medicine therapies. It may help alleviate side effects of chemotherapy, improve the patient sense of well-being and the quality of life by controlling pain, relieving physical distress and helping the patient improve emotionally. Some examples of complementary therapy are stress release techniques (e.g., relaxation strategies), peppermint tea for nausea or acupuncture to reduce pain. Again, you should consult your doctor before using any complementary therapy [4].

It is beyond the scope of this book to discuss in detail different complementary and alternative therapies that are available. We will provide only a general overview. Some of them are using dietary supplements, e.g., antioxidants, which are hoped to "clean" the body from oxidative damage (green tea, vitamin E), other supplements (vitamin A, D), shark cartilage, different herbs, etc. You will be directed to further readings for these issues in (Literature Cited and Where to Read More) (Annex and Literature cited). Again, talk to your doctor – even vitamins are not allowed during some chemotherapy treatment. It is also worth mentioning that it is not necessarily true that products derived from plants are "natural" and therefore safe. Have also in mind that food supplements are not always regulated, not put under rigorous testing and manufacturing procedures, so their purity, quality and content may be questionable.

Other complementary and alternative medicine modalities are acupuncture, homeopathy, natural energy restoration, naturopathy. Pease see further readings on alternative and complementary medicine in Where to Read More. We particularly recommend visiting the National Institutes of Health's Center for Alternative and Complementary Medicine and the American Cancer Society web sites provided in this part of the book [4, 137].

In any case, we suggest that you gather information, discuss your options and evaluate treatment providers. Ask for references about the practitioner who offers the treatment, check governmental listings that regulate and license health providers, consider the cost. Again, be very cautious with complementary and alternative therapies and research in details all available sources. Do not hesitate to consult your doctor! Doctors know that majority of cancer patients use some kind of complementary medicine.

Sedatives and antidepressants, as a supportive care, are also frequently used for cancer patients in different occasions.

At the end of this chapter, you will have a chance to read about issues related to healthy eating. Diet is so important in health and disease that we decided to provide an overview on this subject based on both traditional medicine and dietetic point of view.

Mind-body connection has been proven and stress does decrease our immunity to diseases and affects our organ systems. Living with cancer, stress becomes a part of our everyday lives: Being suspicious that something is wrong with us, visit a doctor to find out what is wrong, waiting for the result, cope with the result, pass through treatments, remissions and re-occurrences – these are all serious stressors. However, the stress could be controlled. Our book, we hope, will help to maneuver easier through a labyrinth of options, skills, knowledge and wisdom to find what is the best for you, to have a less stressful life and how you can help yourselves and teach others to pass through difficult times with less psychological scars.

In general, there are two main factors that contribute to the severity of stress. The imminence of the stressful event and the ignorance about strategies needed to cope. More imminent the stressful situation is and more ignorant we are, the greater the stress is. We cannot help you to change the imminence of the stressful situation, neither can you have control on that. There are situation in life when we cannot change the imminence of unpleasant situations approaching us "without invitation". However, you may try, whenever you can and as much as you can, to allow yourself some time to think, plan and decide. This rule applies to everyday normal life, but particularly in trying times of great stress like a grave disease.

Contrary, I think we can offer suggestions of ways how to cope more easily. This is why the next sections are devoted to these important issues.

3.2.2 Holistic View of Health and Wellness

Health problems are the main stressors in our lives. After realizing that we have a diagnosis of cancer, we are faced with our own mortality. Suddenly our whole life is changed. Things that were so important to us became of much lesser priority. The feelings of shock, disbelief, anxiety, depression, sadness and anger started to build up. We fall asleep and awake with the same thought: I have cancer, am I going to die and what am I going to do now?

Alleviating stress is becoming an important strategy to fight cancer. Proven stress-release techniques may become a part of standard treatment, not only the complementary treatment. Stress, particularly chronic stress (that is exactly the situation with cancer patients) is very harmful for our body. Alleviating stress we sleep and eat better, increase our immunity and think more rationally. It is time to start working on that. As for everything else in order to fight something you have to know more about what you are fighting.

I was teaching stress release strategies one-semester courses at universities for years and I saw how people struggle to relieve stress with more or less success. I will try to explain to you what is stress and it's mechanism and to inform you about some important strategies that you might use for self-help. There is not a general recipe and there is no one-strategy suggestion. It is always a combination of strategies, and you may change those strategies in time; in addition, different stressors may require different techniques for coping. Although some of these strategies are harmless (mental relaxation, mediation), you still need to inform your doctor about your intentions/efforts to release stress and check with him/her whether and how much some of them (for example exercise, yoga) you are allowed in this particular point of your disease or treatment. In many hospitals, you may find organized stress release help like courses, workshops and groups under the supervision of professionals. This is a trusted and easy resource you can use.

In order to better understand stress and plan strategies to alleviate it, you should be aware that besides physical health (that is now disturbed by your diagnosis), there are other dimensions of health, not directly affected by the cancer that you can engage to improve and become healthier (Fig. 3.1a) [25, 59, 72, 99]. This will, in turn, help you battle with the physical problems.

3.2.3 Which Are Other Dimensions of Health Described as a Holistic Health Model?

These are:

- Emotional health (feeling component, our feelings and how we deal with them)
- Mental/intellectual health (ability to learn, intellectual capabilities to process information clearly and accurately, decision making process)
- Social health (ability to have satisfying relationships)
- Spiritual health (a sense of meaning of value in life, belief in supreme being) and
- Environmental health (appreciation of the external environment)

The World Health Organization (WHO) is defining health as a complete physical, mental and social well-being. Spiritual and emotional health (and most recently environmental health), were added as dimensions of health [175].

Rule #1: People's ability to manage stress is influenced by the degree of which they function optimally in each of these dimensions.

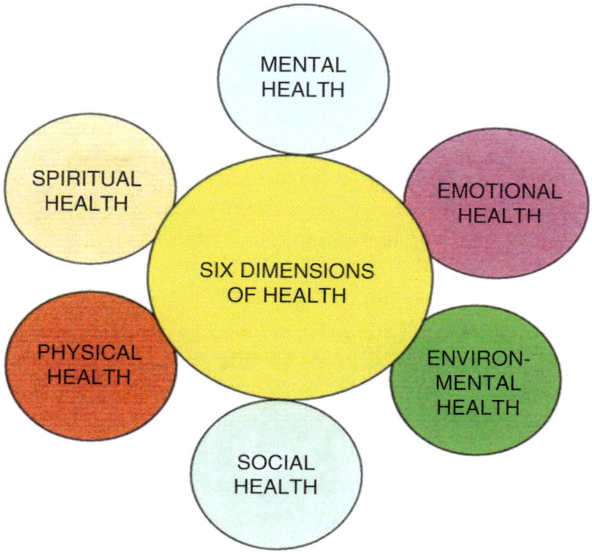

Fig. 3.1a The six dimensions of health

I will present to you some examples to better understand those others dimensions of health that you may not had a chance to concentrate on before. Again, it is time now to think of strengthening these components of your health in order to improve your physical health more efficiently.

3.2.4 How We Can Achieve a Higher Level of Wellness Across all Dimensions of Health?

For example, let's talk about improving social health. It is known that people with supportive social relationships (family, friends, coworkers) are better able to cope with problems and better manage stress; a well functioning social support network helps dispel the negative effects of stressors when you are exposed to them. We were already talking about the support of family and friends in the previous chapter. Cultivating good relationships takes compassion, energy, time, patience, nurturing and sometimes forgiveness. However, sincere, good relationships with right people help to counteract the negative effects of stressors, and the feeling that there is somebody there when you need him/her make us more stress resistant. Isolation is a serious risk factor for stress.

A key to understand spirituality is to view it as moderator of life events, daily hassles, and chronic pressures. It is one of the factors that are taken in consideration when evaluating one's ability to cope with stress. The main component of spirituality is religion, belief in a higher power, divine being – belief in God, but also includes our faith in life, nature, justice, our connectedness with the environment, and our belief in doing well for others beyond ourselves. Spirituality affects patient perceptions of their illnesses, their faith and ability to get well, their will to live, their behavior during illness. *Spiritually mature people have increased ability to cope with crises and greater ability to handle stress*. Please read the story of MM in Sect. 3.3.

Ask your health care team about the resources available at your hospital. Some members of the clergy are specially trained to help cancer patients. Big hospitals, like Mayo Clinic, have chaplains available and when you are admitted into the hospital, you may find in your room material from your religion to read. This is comforting for the patient.

Emotional and mental (intellectual) health is also a determining factors how we perceive stress and how we handle stressful situations [109]. Improving emotional health is may be the most difficult task of all. This is why we will discuss this issue in more details, pointing to some strategies that might be helpful.

Our emotional health depends very much on our personality. Personality is a collection of thoughts, attitudes, values, believes, perceptions, and behaviors defining how we see ourselves and the world around us. Briefly, there are three types of personalities (A, B, C) and many subtypes (a combination of them,) but when it comes to stress there are only two: Stress-resistant and stress-prone personality types [25, 72]. There are opinions that stress prone personality types (type C) are more susceptible to cancer. People with an attitude to give up and to develop a feeling of helplessness and hopelessness are more prone to cancer and have worse survival [10, 157, 167]. Psycho immunology, a new scientific discipline is confirming the connection of stress and diseases [67].

We cannot change our personality very much, but we can try to improve ourselves by learning more about emotional health or seeking help when needed (from family, friends and professionals) in order to put our feelings under control, and not to allow them to guide us to an inappropriate decision. Do not use drugs that may cause addiction. Do not drink alcohol. Seek help from professionals (psychologist, life coaches, social workers, psychiatrists) without shame. Some of them specialize in helping cancer patients.

Let me give you some examples of what we could do. One strategy is a very well known power of "Positive Thinking". We could learn to try finding a positive side in every event – if you try, you will find something good and useful, and even you cannot recognize it in the beginning. Usually, under stress, we simply do not see the positive side of things. Typing a word "positive thinking quotes" in the search window of the Internet, you can find lot of literature about positive thinking and powerful quotes on this subject [149]. For example "The positive thinker sees the invisible, feels the intangible and achieves the impossible"… or the famous Winston Churchill quote" A pessimist sees the difficulty in every opportunity and the optimist sees the opportunity on every difficulty". Or, you may choose to read books on the subject [125, 147].

It is also recommended to try to reduce the "Negative Self-talk" (sub-vocal talking to oneself), repeatedly torturing yourself with negative self-messages that then become secondary stressors. Particularly, if this self-talk and blaming you continue long after the stress does not exist any more. It will also help if you seek company with people who nurture your feelings, not those who hurt them.

There is another powerful strategy that could help us in improving our emotional health, emphasizing that we can keep our negative feelings, accept them, but we can learn to transform them into a productive behavior. This is the essence of Morita therapy, based on Buddhism, teaching us that that we can acknowledge distressing thoughts and feelings, but get beyond them by engaging ourselves in doing something productive [75, 150, 151]. The more creative the engagement is, the greater the success. Write, paint, create something new, or just clean the bathroom, help somebody else, finish some other obligations that you have postponed.

I use this technique myself. I acknowledge my feelings, they are realistic, based on real stressors, they are here and I do not want to just forget about them until the stressor is present. But I will not allow the stress from those feelings to paralyze me and to control me. At the time of actual stress (of course, if it is not something that requires immediate action), I just work, create a new text, plan a new experiment and conduct it, help somebody else, exercise, try to concentrate on the new task at that moment and examine my feelings just a little bit later. You will be surprised how your understanding of the feelings improves, new solutions emerge and everything seems easier than perceived before. There is a saying: "Morning is wiser than evening." The negative feelings may even slowly transform into positive feelings. This will boost our self-esteem that you can live a productive life in spite of having distressing thoughts and feelings that the life is bringing.

Also, be good to yourself, forgive yourself if you make mistakes, everybody makes them and you already learned how to forgive others. You may think now that it is easier to say than to do, but let grace and love guide your way instead of revenge, hostility and anger.

Try to enjoy life more as much as you can. We need to have fun from time to time to reach high level of emotional health. This is not a lost time, as we frequently think, contrary we will perform better if we care enough to increase our emotional wellness and emotional well-being.

How can we enrich our intellectual (mental) capabilities. This is easier than taking control of our feelings. It means expanding our general base of knowledge, particularly learning about the disease and gathering information on how to combat it. This will strengthen your capability to think rationally in stressful situations, our problem solving logic and reason to guide us through difficult times. If we are informed about the issue, we better process the information, come to better decision and perceive the stress sometimes even more as a challenge than as an immediate threat not having the ability to solve.

I suggest that you use this book as your guide for learning and to refer to it periodically, as necessary. Learn about cervical cancer. Knowledge diffuses stress and fear about unknown and gives us power. This fact has been acknowledged by women that suffered from cervical cancer, they quote "Ignorance creates fear, knowledge is a power". Please read the letters from real people who suffered from cancer how they feel about learning more about the disease and how to cope with it (Sect. 3.3). You may also expand more in the recommended selective readings provided in

Where to Read More. However, I would not encourage a patient to start reading professional medical literature aimed for medical professionals, because sometimes you may be exposed to much information and terms that you do not understand, what could be only frightening, not helpful.

The improvement of *the* environmental health depends not only on the individual, but it is more a result of collective effort. Everybody could do something to improve the environment in different ways for the benefit of all. It is easier to deal with problems when your environment is better, supportive and creates better access to services, and day-to-day better quality of life.

3.2.5 Understanding the Mechanism of Stress

In the same spirit, learning more about the enemy that is harming us and of fighting it more successfully, let us now help you learn more about stress itself. What is stress all about? Is it a normal reaction to threat? What is happening in our body during stress? Why is the stress harmful? How I can become a more stress-resistant person? Which stress release strategies are available?

Stress is a normal reaction of our body when we feel threatened and perceive that our balance is disturbed. The state of balance in our body is called homeostasis. Our body responses to change to return to homeostasis. This adaptive response is called General Adaptation Syndrome (GAS), described by Hans Selye [159]. Any event that requires a person to adjust, make changes or expend resources has potential to be stressful. Negative or unpleasant events, uncontrollable, unpredictable and ambiguous events, particularly those that are imminent are perceived as stressors. Since a positive Pap test is a perception of threat, it is normal to feel stressed; even more so with a diagnosis cervical cancer. Everybody will perceive this event as a stress, the difference being only in the stress level and the reaction to stress based on personality and the level of health in other dimensions. When you are in a hospital you may be asked to determine your level of stress on a scale of 1–10.

According to GAS there are three phases of stress response: Alarm, Resistance and Exhaustion (Fig. 3.1b) [59, 126, 159].

What happens in our body in the first moment, during the first phase of stress? This phase is called the alarm phase. It is exactly an alarm to prepare the body for action. Since extra energy is needed, adrenal glands (the glands located near the top of kidneys) release the hormone adrenalin. Adrenalin stimulates the heart to pump more blood and supply the body (particularly the brain) with extra needed blood, dilates respiratory small airways to increase air flow and oxygen needed to fight, increases breathing rate, dilates the pupils and stimulates the liver to release more sugar in the blood for more energy. As you can see, this is a signal to combat threat, a positive reaction of the body. For example, when we are driving a car and somebody is about to hit us, the alarm is helping us to act immediately and save our life. You may find in some popular books the citation "fight-or-flight" phase. It means

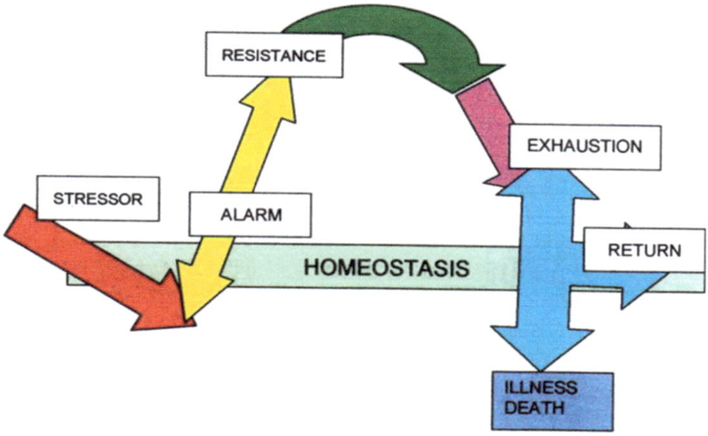

Fig. 3.1b General Adaptation Syndrome – GAS

bodily response options available in coping with stressors to either confront the stressor (fight) or to avoid it (flight).

The alarm phase is not so harmful because lasts very short time (minutes or seconds), until the stressor is removed. However, if the stressor is not removed (like hearing a bad news about an existing disease) it is followed by the second resistant phase of stress response. This phase is induced again by hormones of the suprarenal glands, glycocorticoids-cortisol, mineralocorticoids and other hormones of the outer part of the gland called cortex. These hormones are responsible for adjusting various organs and glands to produce more energy to sustain the increased demand to keep the body into balance. The body is more capable of responding, but for a price of increased demand to the body. This phase, if it is allowed to last long is very harmful and the body may enter the exhaustion phase which could actually caused illness or aggravation of the existing illness.

Stress directly affects our cardiovascular system, the endocrine system, muscles, the immune system, digestive system, and affects our mind. In reality, the stress is practically ruining our body. When we hear the bad news about cervical cancer, we probably cannot avoid experiencing the short alarm phase, but we certainly should not allow ruining our body keeping it in the resistance phase for too long. By alleviating the stress we should allow our body to slowly progress into the recovery phase that will help us to fight the cancer itself. This chapter is aimed to help you to alleviate stress, become more stress resistant and allow your body to proceed in the recovery phase and to return to homeostasis.

How Can We Alleviate Stress? At any given moment our ability to interpret and react to stressors is influenced by the level of wellness across ALL the six dimensions of health. We cannot have 100 % wellness in all these dimensions, but we should strive to increase this wellness level (as discussed earlier) as much as possible. This is the first and the most important strategy that will make us more stress resistant. If the physical health is disturbed by the disease, we should strive to increase the level of wellness in the other dimensions to help us pass through difficult time of illness. When we are functioning efficiently emotionally, we will be able to better control our emotions, and less likely to react inappropriately. When we have a proper level of social well-being, we are aware of social resources to help us in time of need. Spiritual maturity gives us fait and serves as a buffer against stress. Mental health helps us to process information properly, think rationally and logically, come to an educated decision – knowledge decreases fear from ignorance and gives us power and better control of our lives. It is also easier to deal with problems when your environment is supportive and create better quality of life. Certainly, our commitment to improve our physical health will become even more – our life-time dedication.

3.2.6 Stress Release Strategies

Although stress release techniques, particularly massage, yoga, meditation, etc. have been considered in the past as a supportive care measures, we are discussing them in the context of complementary medicine, as they tend to be recently categorized by ACS.

The stress release techniques are usually classified in four groups:

Rethink, Reduce, Relax and Reorganize (four Rs)

3.2.6.1 Rethink

Rethink means changing your thoughts about stressors [25, 75, 125, 147, 150, 151].

Rethink the pace of your life. Do we rush too much through the day that we lose track of important things and meanings of life being too busy, too preoccupied? Is it time to rethink the pace of our lives?

We were talking about the power of positive thinking in this chapter, discussing emotional health. Focusing on negative feelings may immobilize us. Being stressed we lose the capability to even see the good things that are happening. Sometimes, it is so difficult that we cannot keep going. But, it will not help if you stay in bed and feel sorry for yourself. We need not to allow us to stay longer with this attitude. It does not certainly mean denying the seriousness and the importance of the problem. No, it means acknowledging it, but not with self-pity. This will not bring us closer to the solution. Try to use Morita therapy in the moments of despair. Do something productive, continue with the things that you are doing for the rest of the day, give a chance to the negative feelings to be replaced with other feelings. You can also prove to yourself that, in spite of having distressing thoughts and feelings, you have control of your behavior and your life. It is difficult, but possible! Please see the discussion on Morita therapy earlier in the section on emotional health that is a rethink strategy at the same time.

Again, do not forget to be good to yourself, forgive yourself, make time during the day (at least half an hour) for yourself to do something just for you, and what you enjoy doing. During this time force yourself not to think of anything that is stressful. Recharge your batteries! Are we allowing this time to ourselves every day, or we are too busy for that. Find time and try to enjoy life more. This will give you extra strength. One lady with cancer in her letter suggested: "Be more with your little ones, they will give you a lot in return" (Sect. 3.3).

3.2.6.2 Reduce

Reduce is the second level of defense. There are three "A"s to reduce: Abolish, Avoid and Alter. It is an effort to downscale our lives to reduce stress, to live simpler and to concentrate to what is most important – our health [25, 61, 126]. In a situation when you are faced with your diagnosis, in order to concentrate your resources towards this most important issue you should think to reduce other stressors, make selection what you are doing and try to abolish (completely eliminate) some obligations, alter (change) some stressors, or avoid (minimize exposure) to some stressful situations.

For example, ask somebody to drive you to the hospital or doctor's appointment if driving is stressful for you; try during this time to diffuse stress and concentrate on your appointment.

Join a car pool for work if the drive is long and stressful. Drop from some classes if you attend school, cut some obligations that are stressful for some time. If you concentrate to "reduce strategy", you will see how many situations and stressors can be altered, abolished and avoided. Certainly, during the disease, lot of adjustments must be done to reduce the work that you have been doing before. Some women perceive this very stressful. Do not stress yourself about that. Just think that this is temporary, look on this just as to one of the strategies to fight the disease.

Get adequate amount of rest. Do not deprive yourself from sleep, particularly during the disease. Sleep is important for your recovery and your well-being. Forget about the alarm clock for some time. Most people need 8 h sleep for optimal functioning. However, it is a different situation when you cannot sleep well, insomnia (sleeplessness). Anxiety is one of the most common causes of sleeplessness.

Here are some tips to counteract sleeplessness, without taking sleep pills. Do not focus on your worries before bedtime; avoid drinks with caffeine in evening hours; avoid large, late meals, and drink a glass of warm milk before bedtime. Try to go to bed at the same time every evening and make your bedroom a peaceful place for rest. If you cannot fell asleep, try to reconstruct a happy event or do something else, but do not make sleeplessness a secondary stressor.

3.2.6.3 Relaxation Techniques

Relaxation strategies are usually perceived as a typical stress reduction model. But, as you can see in this book, they are only a part of overall stress reduction strategies.

Relaxation is generally defined as "having passive mental state" allowing your mind to slow down. Relaxation strategies may be passive (without involving physical activity) and active, involving different extent of physical activity [59, 142].

Passive Relaxation Techniques

I will talk about breathing to reduce stress, mediation, visual imagery accompanied with listening music/or aromatherapy.

Stress relaxation breathing is to learn to engage our whole lungs and to fill them with air. Breathing, most of us are using only the upper portions of our lungs. Find a quite place and sit strait in a chair. Slowly inhale through your nose, pushing your stomach forward and raising your shoulders, let your ribs expand. Keep your breath for few seconds and start slowly exhales through your mouth (you may produce a sound, even such as tennis players making while hitting the ball in front of the full event!). Your shoulders fall, ribs shrink and pull your stomach back. Repeat this three more times at the time. Try to practice several times during the day.

Mediation originates in India and Tibet. Mediation slows our thoughts, giving us a temporary break from many thoughts and feelings that we encounter every day. There are different types of mediation, e.g., *focused mediation*, like object mediation for example a candle, or sound meditation – listening music. Music has the ability to profoundly affect emotions. Pleasant aromas also make us feel good. The other type of meditation, non-focused mediation is just an open focused mediation, not paying attention to a focal point, but let stimuli enter and exit without paying any attention to them.

Visual Imagery – mental creation of relaxing visual images and scenes usually combined with other relaxation techniques like deep breathing, music, and aromas. Music and aromatherapy can be used as a relaxation technique not necessarily combined with other relaxation techniques. Music therapy is being used more and more in hospitals, particularly children's hospitals.

Try picturing yourself in your favorite environment; visualize a beautiful mountain lake, places with good memories. There are also low-cost audiotapes with gentle music and pleasant narrator bringing you mentally to wonderful peaceful places. Some audiotapes are only with natural sounds (bird's songs, sea waves). Reserve 15 min to half an hour to listen to the tapes in a pleasant atmosphere, and try to diffuse your worries.

Active Relaxation Strategies

These strategies require physical activity. I will briefly cover muscle relaxation techniques, yoga, massage and physical exercise. Muscle tension is a common stress reaction that we are not even aware off.

Systemic muscle relaxation teaches that you can learn to relax your muscles (facial, skeletal) if you alternate contraction and relaxation of individual muscle and group. You will soon sense the difference between when your muscles are tense or relaxed. While you practice muscle relaxation, you may choose listening to a pleasant music. Begin by concentrating on your facial muscles. Try to relax one-by-one muscle groups; you will realize how tense they were before and how much tension you were holding.

Yoga stretching helps us to combat the consequences of sedentary life style that causes "shortened" muscles, tendons and ligaments. There are several different types of yoga; and if you are interested to learn more, please see Further readings (Where to Read More). Yoga sessions are advertised in hospitals, in your community, exercise facilities, and shows are available on TV. You can also buy videotapes in stores. If performed properly only to the extent you feel comfortable, yoga is helpful in decreasing muscle tension. It also increases flexibility, loosening the connective tissues and release fatigue and pain. It may bring mental relaxation.

Massage therapy relieves muscle tension and stimulate circulation bringing oxygen and other nutrients to the tissues to make us feel better. Medical/sport massage is directing to healing muscle tissues damaged in sport activities because of damage or overexertion, or for relaxing muscle tension. Check with your doctor and inquire about massage therapy in the medical facility where you are getting your medical treatment.

Release through physical activity is one of best strategies to release stress. Physical activity may be just exercising in bed, walking, jogging, running, and working out with exercise equipment in fitness facilities. Regardless of the types of physical exercises, we feel better releasing tension after physical activity. The benefit of a physical activity, if prescribed properly, may be enormous. It increases our general physical health, strengthens our muscles, enhances cardio-respiratory function, lowers the blood pressure, decreases cholesterol levels and increases "good lipids". Releasing endorphins and increasing secretion of dopamine and serotonin in the brain is making us feel good. Physical activity un-fogs our mind, increases creativity and ability to focus, reduces anxiety improving outlook on life and enhanced self-image and self-esteem.

However, it is very important to consult your doctor about all these active relaxation techniques. Your doctor, who is aware of your disease, must advise you of the level of activity allowed for you. Do not be frustrated, the level of allowed activity is constantly changing depending on the current patient status. ACS is also providing guidelines on physical activity for cancer patients [4, 6].

3.2.6.4 Reorganize – The Last Step: Use all the Resources to Become a More Stress-Resistant Person

It means combining all stress release strategies to work together [4, 25, 59, 72]. The four Rs, Rethink, Reduce, Relax Release, should be combined into the fifth R that is Reorganize. It means to reorganize our lifestyle toward living healthier life and learning "life skills" that help in stress management. The nature of an individual stressor will guide you which strategy to use and how to combine them. This is a learning process, experience is necessary, but if you really devote your time to become a more stress resistant person, you will succeed. What you can certainly achieve, and what is the most important of all is to work hard to improve all the six dimensions of health.

Applying different stress release strategies, together with your constant effort to achieve the highest level of wellness across all dimensions of health is the way for you to become more stress-resistant person.

This was the aim of this chapter: Little everyday things that use to stress us previously, should not disturb us any more, at least not with the same intensity. We start to give priorities in life among our goals putting our health first. In this context understanding prevention, e.g., cervical cancer screening, becomes a part of our routine. This is a precious personal resource for our better health.

3.2.7 An Overview on Eating for Optimal Health in Cancer Prevention and Cervical Cancer

Researchers agree more and more that poor diets and sedentary lifestyle are contributors to cancer risks. Diets and nutrition are beyond the scope of this book and you will be guided to additional readings in the next chapter. However, because of the role of diet for our overall health well-being, what is very important for cancer patients, we will provide an outline on the subject.

Maintaining a healthy weight is important in reducing the risk of cancer and other chronic diseases (cardiovascular diseases, diabetes, etc.). Obesity increases the risks of several cancers, e.g., endometrial and breast cancer, colon, esophagus and kidney. One explanation is that excess adipose (fat) tissue produces estrogen that may increase the chances for women after menopause to become victims of cancer. To assess whether you are overweight and how much, you can calculate the relationship between your height and weight to find out about your Body Mass Index (BMI). See references and the ACS guidelines on nutrition and physical activities for cancer prevention [6].

To start a healthy diet, you need to do some planning. First, write down what you will need to eat in the following week or more. If you do not have some gastrointestinal disease that limits your diets or special requirements of the therapies that you are having, try to include more (about five servings) of fruits and vegetables, while limiting high-calories food. Fruits and vegetables will help you reduce weight plus they contain vitamins, minerals, antioxidants and other healthy components which are good for you. However, during some chemotherapy protocols you may be asked to avoid certain of these foods, so ask your health provider and follow the instructions.

We recommend that you also include foods in your diet that contains fiber. Fibers are foods that are not digested in our system, but serve to maintain the volume and help you to be regular. They are also making feel full, thus limiting the desire for overeating. Food that contains whole grains is a good source of fiber, e.g., oatmeal, whole-wheat bread, brown rice (instead of white rise). Eat whole fruit rather than drink juice in order to increase fibers in your diet. The direct preventive role of foods that contain fiber has been proven for colorectal cancer. Natural fibers supplements (e.g., Metamucil) may also be helpful.

The following is a simple guide for choosing food and planning recipes. Red meets (like beef, pork and lamb) should be avoided in favor of the white meet (chicken and turkey). Fish is a good source of unsaturated fatty acids and is good for the body, as are milk (particularly fortified skim milk) and other dairy products, unless you are intolerant for lactose. Use olive oil instead of other vegetable oils. Do not use animal fat, avoid bacon and processed food.

Check with your doctor about any diet restrictions and speak with dietitian to help you create a nutritious, balanced diet. Read more about healthy eating after cancer at the ACS web site [5]. Refer also to Chap. 2 of this book discussing nutrition of cervical cancer patients.

We hope that this chapter providing an insight in all dimensions of health and concentrating on stress releasing strategies will provide you with an additional resources to successfully confront the disease and mobilize additional inner strengths to survive the disease.

We believe, the chapter on emotional support would be useful guides not only for the patients, but also for caregivers, family and friends to learn more how to provide their best support and care.

3.3 Stories from Real People

This chapter is to honor brave women who have passed through difficult days, nights, months and years accepting the truth that they are ill, endured the pain, stress, disappointments and despair at times, but succeed to go on, confront their illness and in many case survived cancer. "Surviving cancer is a triumph" says Ms Dunn.

These women had courage to talk and to pass their wisdom to other women wanting to help. Never lose hope! There is always hope, even in darkest nights, the light can start shining from somewhere and become brighter and brighter. Do not forget that there are two most important things that are worthwhile living: These are hope and self-esteem. As long as, deep inside, we respect ourselves and we do not lose hope, we have a chance to go on and survive cervical cancer. Here are some excerpts from women's stories:

V.V. WROTE: I was 19 years old when I was first diagnosed with cervical cancer. I had a LEEP. The doctor said that I will not be able to carry a baby to full term. However, here I am now with four kids … I am regularly going for follow-up and hope that I will continue to be well…

G.H. WROTE: I was in a similar situation. It was very hard, but I got a lot of support from my family. I also got support from friends that I have never seen, but who wrote me in the darkest days of despair. May your days, dear friends, be filled with hope, your heart filled with love and your spirit with joy…

A.S. WROTE: I'm a cervical cancer survivor. I had surgery a year ago – a radical hysterectomy and then radiation. I'm constantly worried about recurrence. Once you've been diagnosed, you have a history of cancer which means there is always a possibility that cancer will come back. Doesn't mean it will, but doesn't mean it won't either. I got second opinion, and I am glad I did. I suggest you to do the same and I wish you the best. Try to always be aware but not let it eat away at you. Knowledge is power and we are strong women…

M.M. WROTE: I also had CIN 3. It was in the early stages and confined to the cervix, so I had a LEEP/cone biopsy done and it seems to have removed all the cells, as they couldn't even detect HPV being present any longer. I won't lie, the LEEP procedure is uncomfortable, but very effective treatment for CIN. I have been HPV/Cervical cancer free for more than 8 years now and haven't had a reoccurrence.

Ask your doctor. They should give you all the information so you can make an informed decision about your care. Just remember, there are a lot of women here to help you and listen if you need us!

L.P. WROTE to a lady going to surgery. May I suggest that when you see your surgeon and/or the anesthesiologist in the hospital, you let them know you're very anxious! I was also very afraid but, as soon as I answer all the pre-surgery questions, they gave me some medication. I even do not remember being wheeled into the operating room and anything after. I woke up in the recovery room. Ii hope you don't have too long to wait until surgery is scheduled. It is great that you brought relaxation tapes. They helped me, too.

It is also wonderful that you have support of your parents and your husband. It makes a difference. Please inform me how you are doing…

W.W. Wrote: Thank you very much for the positive energy and good wishes. The moral support is so important that I am not giving up. It is wonderful and is already helping me. Thank you so much again…

L.R WROTE: I have the same thing. As I understand this is the last stage before cancer or before it becomes untreatable. It will sometime become invasive. I have had this since I was about 20 years old and I thought that it was really nothing. I did have a LEEP though, but I never thought of it again, did not have regular check-up. Unfortunately, it came again but this time worst, because I let it go…So please take it serious and find out about treatment options. Learn as much as you can about cervical cancer, and ask your closest family if possible to learn more, so you could talk at home…

S.C. WROTE: I am in the same situation. I have a small child, and I understand. For me the most difficult was to hear that I couldn't have another child. With your husband and your family there to help you, you will be fine. Here are some links that may help you to learn more…. Please keep us posted; the waiting is always the hardest part.

M.Y. WROTE as an answer to a lady diagnosed with cancer. Your positive attitude is great and that will be the key in beating the cancer. Your inner strength is always going to be with you, even when you're going through difficult treatments. Certainly you're feeling alone and scared – it is scary. Do you have a support group such as in your area? It might help to have in person group support in addition to what you can get via the Internet. Please keep us up to date on your progress. Take care.

M.K. WROTE: I am so sorry to hear of your latest results. You are strong and determined. Arm yourself with information and supply your spirit with positive energy. I copied this link for you… I love listening to inspirational music, too. My thoughts and prayers are with you and your family. If you need to talk I am here for you…

FT WROTE: I was interested for years to find out about an option for a Home Pap test. This would be a gift for women. I was reading on the Internet hoping to find that you are now offering the MarkPap® Self for home testing. Please send me more information about this product, I would be willing to participate on the survey and look forward to hearing from you. Thank you.

Dr. Annie Dunn contributed with a beautiful personal story entitled "Surviving Cancer is a Triumph." She also sheared some thoughts about cultural diversity and the importance of education in improving women's health.

A diagnosis of cancer is unwelcome news and poses challenges with adjustments in many different levels of a person's life. Frequently, the initial reaction to a cancer diagnosis includes emotional responses such as fear and anxiety with a feeling of being overwhelmed. For many individuals the expectation of cancer is frequently one of lingering, pain-producing illness, followed by death. This grim view of cancer can influence attitude and perceived control and often leads to feeling of loneliness, helplessness, and hopelessness. Yet, the view of cancer as a catastrophic illness is not experienced by all who received it; thus, for them the diagnosis may be less traumatic and the reaction less extreme.

While there is no specific set of suggestions that fit each individual case, one may benefit from developing coping strategies to deal with the effects of the diagnosis. Avoiding the reality of a cancer diagnosis may temporarily reduce stress but in the long-term poses risk for a healthy future. Becoming involved, accepting responsibility in decisions regarding treatment options, and developing a positive attitude are important steps toward successfully fighting and possibly eradicating the threatening disease.

Personal experience and reaction to a cancer diagnosis involved my confidence in my physician and my motivation to participate in my treatment. Upon hearing my diagnosis of cancer, the following conversation took place between my physician and me.

> Doctor, "your tests results indicate that you have cancer".
> My reply, "what can WE do about it?"

The word WE in my reply suggested that I had a personal responsibility for participating in my treatment and possible eradication of the disease. Did I experience immediate fear and anxiety upon hearing my diagnosis, no I did not. My immediate concern was directed toward available treatment options. I followed my physician's opinion that a surgical procedure was the best choice with other treatment options to follow.

Following a successful surgical procedure, I sought a second medical opinion and made a choice to undergo additional treatment for further protection.

Decisive actions and my motivation to participate in decisions regarding my treatment choices contributed to my more than 12 years of cancer-free life. An annual check-up continues to be a reminder that responsibility for my health belongs to me. The check-ups are as much a part of my life as eating, sleeping and working.

Surviving cancer is a triumph but it imposes many emotional challenges. Stigmas associated with cancer do exist. Family friends and co-workers may fear contagion and relationships become more cautious. Some of my colleagues seemed uncomfortable in my presence when I first mentioned that my cancer treatment was scheduled for the following day. Even though I continued my normal work routine throughout my treatment, their expectation of my capacity to perform my duties was influenced by their personal fear of the horrific "CA" diagnosis. In other words, you have cancer, should you not be home taking care of yourself. Comments such as, "How are YOU doing" became less frequent. Later, I became aware that by emotionally distancing themselves from me protected them. Family members' concern, support and understanding can be costly but the sacrifice is well worth the effort. A sense of togetherness provides strength and a buffer to stress when coping with any adverse event. My social environment in the workplace changed once my treatment was completed. It seemed as though 'now we are again safe.'

The task of coping with a diagnosis of cancer is not easy and requires adaptive thinking and behavior change directed at challenging aspects of the disease. Behavior change which leads to effective coping includes psychological defenses such as making necessary decisions to protect oneself from life threatening effects of the disease. Yet, the perceived threat brings fear and anxiety, which may negatively influence our actions when we are faced with factors relating to health issues, especially cancer. These negative influences may prevent individuals from taking necessary action, thereby leading to greater stress and possible risk.

The psychological defense, positive thinking, can help reduce denial, fear and anxiety and increase one's opportunity for positive behavior. On the other hand, the opposite effect may occur when negative thinking patterns lead individuals to believe they themselves are unable to influence or control events in their lives. Persistent pessimism and a feeling of helplessness are patterns of negative thinking which may create an absence of a prospect for positive outcome. While a positive attitude does not always bring positive behavior, it does create a possible starting point for positive behavior change when one's sense of well-being is threatened. Optimism and a belief, that one is in control and has the ability to make good things happen, had a positive effect.

There is an urgent need for education and outreach programs with approaches designed to address perceptions of health care issues worldwide. Programs with goals to change negative thinking to more positive thinking and to change misperceptions can help to save lives.

Targeting at risk groups and providing information which addresses barriers to screening, diagnosis, prevention and treatment of cancer and other diseases will have positive results. While barriers to choosing to participation in healthy lifestyles may involve factors such as individual choices, there are broader considerations.

Barriers to good health include attitudes and beliefs regarding health practices and they are shaped by many factors. Some such factors include religion, individual perceptions, age, sex, culture, and socio-economic status.

For example, culture and its embodiment of traditions and values associated with beliefs and behaviors may pose questions regarding personal autonomy and serve as barrier to early detection and treatment of cancer in women, especially cervical cancer.

Philosophical values and beliefs vary from culture to culture with great variability within cultures. For example, in specific cultures, a woman's view of self as an interdependent part of a larger group may influence how she views her health and her need to take action. Denial of a health problem or tolerance of health problems can delay access to health care. Lack of orientation to preventative medical options may prevent women in some cultures from seeking health screening. In some cases medical care is sought only in the presence of symptoms or pain.

Cultural influences affect all life events and, even with intervention programs, may influence one's choosing to seek health care. Effective intervention strategies require knowledge of specific cultural barriers which may prevent women from health screening, especially cervical cancer screening. This knowledge will increase opportunities to break down such barriers in at risk groups before cervical cancer becomes a problem.

Intervention programs designed to foster increased awareness and willingness to participate in medical treatment and prevention of cancer should communicate information in a sensitive and supportive manner with respect for the individual.

Another barrier to health screening may be the individual's perception of health and wellness. Such perceptions differ from person to person within cultures and across cultures. A person's misconception of their vulnerability to cancer and its threat to their health may influence their involvement and be a barrier to their taking preventative action. This misconception may contribute to an absence of coping strategies, should a cancer threat become a reality.

Through educational programs, which promote growth in self-efficacy, the large number of at risk women who, for a number of reasons have not been screened for cancer, may become more confident. Increased confidence can lead to commitment and responsibility for taking care of self and possibly others.

Education may foster a sense of control and help women overcome barriers to treatment by increasing awareness and stressing their need to know about aspects of cancer some of which are: early detection through screening, screening options, diagnosis, treatment options, expenses involved, behavioral risks, available resources, and assistance and services. Just by knowing that one is not alone without different options, support and resources may reinforce their decision to take positive action leading to a cancer-free life. Alternate options with purpose to safe lives are forthcoming.

In the near future, a promising option for women, a home Pap test for cervical cancer screening and detection, will be available in drug stores. This preventive method will be less expensive, less uncomfortable, and more private than methods currently available. This is an opportunity for women who, in the past, have been reluctant to seek cancer screening options, to take advantage of screening and feel secure by doing so.

Finally, take responsibility for your health and remain positive. Believe in yourself, that you have some control in what happens to you and, that your survival is worth the effort.

Ms. Paula Matuskey, Instructional Dean, sent us a letter expressing a point of view from one who had not have a personal history of cervical cancer. It is an expression of deep feeling and emotion to the loss of those who lost the fight to survive, and how faith and spiritual guidance eased that sense of loss.

Spirituality is one of those concepts that are hard to grasp. Scott Peck who wrote "The Road Less Traveled" often spoke of spirituality as surrender to a higher power. And he said this knowing that for some people the higher power is God, whereas for others that higher power may be "justice" or "peace." Or even all of these.

Probably no medical diagnosis threatens to shake our faith more, be it in God or those other concepts, than a cancer diagnosis. The word "cancer" strikes terror in our hearts. Even though we realize that cancer is comprised really of many illnesses, some of which are more intractable than others, we immediately find ourselves confronted with the end of our life. In real terms. So how do we cope with the idea?

A number of years ago I read somewhere that it's not what happens to you that define you but, rather what you do with what happens to you. Never having faced my own diagnosis of cancer, but knowing closely several people that have struggled and ultimately lost the battle, I find myself wondering what I would do.

I have come to the conclusion that I would strive to stay in touch with my higher power – which for me is God. Holding out for some magical "cure" is at best illusionary if not irrational, and in the end the best we can do try to live each moment like our last; not recklessly, but in a spirit of appreciation.

In a period of three and half years, I lost both my parents, my parents-in-law, a great uncle, an aunt, my friend of 20 years, and another friend I had known for 30 years. Without my faith, I don't know how I could look forward to another day.

Ms. Teresa Bevin, psychotherapist and author, sent us a story about Carmen. Carmen had just turned 43 when she first began to feel that something was wrong with her body. At first, she felt it at an intuitive level, but later she began to notice brief, but sharp pains in her pelvic area. At first she thought that it could be an intestinal discomfort, but after addressing the pain with laxatives, natural digestive supplements and the like, she obtained no relief. At first she was able to put it all out of her mind for weeks at a time, but the intense pain eventually made itself felt with more frequency.

One morning, Carmen found some blood stains in her underwear and she became alarmed. She was still menstruating, but it wasn't time for her period yet. She debated whether she should go see a doctor, but she was not used to going to doctors and the idea scared her. Talking to her husband would bring her no relief, since they were having serious problems and the word "divorce" had been used by each of them at different times during the last few months. He was controlling, verbally abusive, and not at all sympathetic about anything that was going on in her life. He had isolated her from her friends and had tried to talk her into leaving her job and staying home. He often told her that nobody would miss her at work, that her job was unimportant. Still, she had refused to leave her job. It was her point of contact with the world, her co-workers, and it made her feel like her life had some meaning. Because of her refusal to stay at home full-time, her husband had become perpetually sullen and irritable, to the point that she avoided speaking to him for fear of his unpredictable reactions and outbursts of rage. Carmen finally spoke to a co-worker who referred her to a Dr. S. a female gynecologist with decades of experience. Carmen armed herself with courage and went to see this well-recommended doctor.

Dr. S took her time palpating Carmen's pelvic area, and asked her many questions, and wanted to know why she didn't go for regular Pap smears. Carmen had no concrete answer. She simply avoided doctors. She felt she was healthy and knew of no history of gynecological problems in her family.

It was clear to Carmen that Dr. S. didn't have a good feeling from what she had seen and heard, but it was necessary to wait for lab results, which seemed to take forever. Carmen was scared and alone. Had it not been for her co-worker she wouldn't have had any one at all to talk to during this time of uncertainty.

After a number of tests, Dr. S. sat her down and gave her the bad news. She had cervical cancer and a complete hysterectomy was in order, followed by "other measures" to prevent the spread of the disease. Carmen was aware of some of those measures. But Dr. S. didn't stop there. She asked Carmen about her personal life, and all came pouring out – her isolation, her lack of self-esteem, and her silent cohabitation with her husband. Dr. S. recommended counseling for Carmen, and that's how I got to meet her.

The day Carmen came into my office for the first time she looked as if someone had just hit her over the head with a pole. She looked down and dragged her feet, as if she were carrying the weight of the world. She had set a date for her surgery but had yet to tell her husband. It was clear to me that nobody who felt the way she felt could possibly stay healthy for long. The connection between emotions and body functioning cannot be denied, and Carmen was a palpable example of this connection.

Five years have passed since the day I met her, and I still see Carmen once a month. Her surgery and subsequent treatments were successful, but it was a long, painful ordeal. She now must be under doctors' care on a regular basis in case of a relapse, although she doesn't believe that could happen. Carmen straightened her affairs, divorced her husband and her level of stress decreased remarkably. She practices yoga and relaxation techniques, continues to work, has received a promotion, and is making new friends. She feels on top of the world. She says now that, in a way, this close encounter with cervical cancer, as scary and painful as it was, helped her change her life by forcing her to look into her emotional health as well as that of her body.

Early detection, together with strong emotional support seems to be the key to surviving cervical cancer. Any effort made in order to insure the most expedient way to screen women for this disease should be encouraged, together with education, awareness and emotional support.

3.4 Survey on What Women Think About Pap Test

This is a survey conducted by BioSciCon, Inc. in Washington Metro Area on the subject what women think about the standard Pap test and how they feel about new technologies, e.g., self-sampling for cervical cancer screening.

3.4.1 Background

Between 2001 and 2005 we conducted clinical trials intended to assess safety and effectiveness of MarkPap test in comparison with the conventional Pap smear and the ThinPrep Pap test as a representative of the liquid-based Pap technologies [122]. Twenty-five hundred subjects were enrolled and 2000 completed the study. During this period we contacted doctors and nurses at clinical sites who were involved in subject recruitment, interviews, examination and creation/maintenance of the clinical case reports forms. During these contacts we learned that women living in Washington Metro Area are sometimes reluctant to have their Pap test performed and even more hesitant to commit themselves for having a regular Pap test during the next 2 years (one of the study requirements).

3.4.2 Identifying the Problem

Planning further studies, we addressed this issue of reluctance/hesitation towards Pap test. Interestingly, the literature related to women's behavior and cervical cancer is full of studies about risk factors, educational intervention to increase the outreach, to reduce risk factors, to improve the Pap test procedure with new techniques for specimen sampling, processing, and the new criteria for specimen reading and interpretation, but very little information exists on the question "How women perceive the test?" Thinking about this issue, we came to an idea to conduct a survey to reveal women's attitude towards Pap test, but not as "the best test available" because this will leave them without choice – inevitably positive response. It was obvious that women must have a choice on order to give unbiased answers.

3.4.3 Addressing the Problem – Study

In 2006, we were ready to start our new survey. Planning the survey, we decided to ask women about their readiness to use another, noninvasive test if such is available. In searching for such an alternative we decided to ask for a home test because of the two precedent experiences, the Pregnancy Test, and Multistix test for urinalysis, which are both accepted and popular between women and men. We could ask this question because we knew about MarkPap test and the capability of this technology to, using the biomarker specific characteristics produces a reliable home test for screening healthy women for hidden signs of cervical dysplasia [52].

A simple questionnaire was developed (Table 3.1) and the survey was initiated in the beginning of 2007.

The Survey has two arms, a "conventional" performed by volunteers distributing the survey to women at different locations (particularly among those who have

Table 3.1 A survey for the improvement of Pap test outreach

	Questions	Answers	
1	Your age?	□ Under 18, □ 18–29, □ 30–44	
		□ 45–60. □ Over 60	
2	How would you describe yourself? Please mark both race and religion	□ White, non-Hispanic	□ Christian □ Jewish
		□ Hispanic □ African American	□ Islam □ Buddhism
		□ African □ Asian, □ Other	□ Other
3	What is your highest education?	□ Elementary school □ High School	
		□ Undergraduate □ Graduate	
4	Do you know what the Pap test is?	□ Yes □ No	
5	Have you had a Pap test before?	□ No □ Yes, regularly once in 1–3 years	
		□ Yes, irregularly	
6	If your answer is NO, please explain. Even if your answer is YES, you are welcome to express your opinion about Pap test	□ I feel good, I do not think I need it □ Do not have time □ Uncomfortable with the pelvic exam	
		□ Afraid of Pap test □ Expensive □ Do not know where to go □ The result is not always good and I have to wait long time for the result	
7	What would you think about taking a specimen at home? Would you buy a kit in a drug store, and take the specimen in the privacy of your home?	□ Excellent, is there a home Pap test?	
		□ Maybe	
		□ Cannot decide	
		□ Not interested	
8	Would you prefer to do the home Pap test first and then (if needed) to visit a doctor?	□ Yes, I would first do the Home Pap	□ No, I would prefer to always have a gynecologist take the sample
9	Please add your comment		

lower resources and less ability to use health services), and a "web-based electronic" questionnaire for those who have access to the Internet and web communications. You may wish to use the link below and to participate in the survey:

http://www.surveymk.com/s.aspx?sm=aKALIgzj7AwSthXcp0nI1w_3d_3d

3.4.4 Study Results and Analysis

An interim analysis was performed after first 500 responses were collected from the conventional survey. The results are presented below.

Total Number of responses: 500
Inadequate responses: 1

Although almost all women (93 %) were aware of the existence of Pap test, 22 % had never had the Pap test done.

(a) *Non-participants in Pap test screening*
They had different reasons for not participating:

28.84 % feel good and do not need to have Pap test
15.38 % the pelvic exam is not comfortable and should be avoided
11.53 % are simply afraid of Pap test (knowing results, or examination)
21.15 % consider Pap test expensive
13.46 % have identified different reasons each less than 5 %

However, 94 % of them was willing to use alternative test (home pap) if available. Their answers were distributed as follows:

17 % will immediately consider home test
76.92 % would consider it seriously but need more information
5.76 % do not have interest in home test

If home test were available, 77.88 % would prefer this test before going to a doctor, and 21.15 % will still prefer visiting the doctor first.

(b) *Participants in Pap test screening*
Majority of answers, 74.19 % came from women who had Pap test (48.98 % participate in regular Pap test screening – at least once in 3 years, and 51.01 % participate irregularly).
Among those women who participate regularly in screening (and to whom also a chance to express the complaints) a small group of about 10.06 % participated and provided the following answers:
11.76 % feel good and do not see the need to regularly have the test
5.88 % do not have time – priority for Pap test
47.05 % found pelvic exam uncomfortable
17.64 % are still afraid in spite of having the test regularly
5.88 % do not know exactly where to go for the test
11.76 % had different reasons, but not the cost of the test

Cervical cancer is a preventable disease **IF** detected on time. Regular Pap test is the best preventive method currently available. However, 20 million American women at risk do not participate in regular Pap test screening (as it is now offered), and only 6.5 % women at risk worldwide are covered with this test. Thousands of women die per year. We need your opinion on a new emerging, improved Pap test (future Home Pap test), that would allow women to get a specimen in the privacy of their home (self-sampling) and send it into the laboratory for Pap testing. Please answer the questions below. Thank you

In spite of regular participation in Pap screening, this group showed a great interest in home test (89.88 %), and wanted to know more (53.64 %). Only 10 % was indifferent. Interestingly, 50.88 % women in this group were ready to use Home test before going to a doctor.

Among those women who participate irregularly, another group of 9.09 % complained without being asked. Their complaints are about:

25.0 % feel good
6.25 % do not have time
37.5 % uncomfortable with pelvic exam
25.0 % expensive test
6.25 % do not know where to go

Majority of these women (97.72 %) were interested in home test, and 72.72 % would first use Home test, and then, if necessary, visit a doctor.

Interestingly, both groups who participate in screening (regularly or irregularly) presented a great interest in home Pap test.

In the structural analysis of women who prefer having the home Pap test first, we found 332 responses or 66.4 % of all responses. Among them, younger women were more inclined towards Home test (88.88 %) in comparison with older women who were more conservative (only 37 % were inclined to take Home test first.) Other generation (between 18 and 60 years of age) showed a moderately increased interest (between 65 % and 67 %) preferring home test prior to visiting a doctor.

African women were much more interested to take Home test first (81.21 %) then the African American (73.05 %), Hispano (69.64 %) or white (60.28 %). Religion did not play a significant role in this population of women living in the US, but the numbers are small for any conclusion. Education could play some role in women's determination for home test. The most interested were women with high school education (73.33 %); the most conservative were women with graduate education (57.53 %). This could also be a result of age difference.

3.4.5 Conclusion

Women are generally not comfortable with the current Pap test procedure (pelvic exam) to the extent of not participating in regular screening (28.21 %) and would prefer an alternative home test (77.2 %).

3.4.6 Post Survey

In 2015 we reviewed this survey and compared it with many similar public opinion assessments of the Pap test and the cervical cancer screening. During these 7 years, we were not able to find any major discrepancy from the conclusion made in our survey from 2005.

Although not very complementary for the "many improvements" advertised in between, this conclusion is one more element to our conviction that that classic opinion on cervical cancer screening, when the global application is needed, must be improved with fresh ideas. Some of them can be found in the following chapters.

Chapter 4
Cervical Cancer Screening After 2008

4.1 Current Practices

4.1.1 Afterword to 2008 Edition

The manuscript for the book *What Every Woman Should Know About Cervical Cancer* was submitted for publishing on September 30, 2007. The next month, the 2006 Consensus *Guidelines for the Management of Women with Abnormal Cervical Cancer Screening Tests* were published in the October issue of the *Journal of Lower Genital Tract Disease* and in the October 2007 issue of the *American Journal of Obstetrics and Gynecology*.

The major difference between these 2006 Guidelines and the previous 2001 Guidelines, recommended by the same consensus conferences, is (1) the introduction of HPV DNA testing in the primary screening for cervical cancer and (2) adjustments made in the management of women with HPV DNA +/− tests. The adjustments were necessary to limit the fast mounting cost of cervical cancer screening caused by the HPV testing. It is important to note that the authors of this clinical practice guidance document, in the preamble stated clearly "these guidelines should never substitute for clinical judgment" giving back the power of decision to doctors and ultimately to patients themselves. This statement is a great support to our book and to our objective to help women understand the value of testing and medical options and to become educated patients who could contribute to the right diagnosis and treatment of their own conditions.

In the follow-up, along with the promotion of HPV testing, many limitations were noted, and the regulatory agencies (FDA, CDC), professional societies (CAP, ASC, ASCP) and even manufacturers of HPV vaccines and HPV tests, indicated that the annual cytological testing should be considered as the gold standard not as an unnecessary alternative to the more complicated new testing. American Cancer Society (ASC) acknowledged the HPV testing, but did not change their 2003 *ACS*

N. Markovic, O. Markovic, *What Every Woman Should Know about Cervical Cancer*, DOI 10.1007/978-94-017-7560-1_4

Guidelines for Early Detection of Cancer, where Pap test (cytological screening) is the pivotal laboratory instrument to measure women's risk for cervical cancer.

Introduction of HPV DNA testing into the primary screening has brought one big accomplishment; the Pap test is again recognized as the best test for cervical cancer control worldwide. Together with HPV vaccination (cancer prevention) the Pap test is becoming our hope for eradication of cervical cancer in twenty-first century. This change of perception has set aside the work of WHO, IARC Cervical Cancer Screening Group, PAHO, PATH, JHPIEGO and other members of the Alliance for Cervical Cancer Prevention who considered Pap test as an unaffordable luxury for cervical cancer screening in low resource countries, and recommended alternative methods such as visual inspection with acetic acid (VIA), DNA HPV testing alone, and/or one-visit screen-and-treat approaches. Now, Pap test (cytological cervical cancer screening) is again the first priority, but the new question is what type of primary screening to be used. All of these options are addressed in our book.

Another major event, already discussed in this book, was the introduction of HPV vaccines (Merck's Gardasil, and Glaxo SmithKline's Cervarix). This accomplishment has risen hopes that cervical cancer could be prevented by global vaccination (eliminate the HPV viral strains that can cause cervical cancer by eliminating them from the population) and lot of money and effort was given to recruit people worldwide to accelerate the access of vaccines to the developing world.

The difference, between the day the manuscript for this book was submitted and the day it is published, was made by an enormous effort given to support those universal noble hopes. Supported by Melinda and Bill Gates Foundation, PATH has launched worldwide marketing to raise awareness of the preventability of cervical cancer deaths among all women in the world (1.7 billion at risk). A *Call to Stop Cervical Cancer*, which has been a logo for this campaign, is now beginning to institutionalize these activities into marketing entities coordinated by PATH. More information is available at http://www.cervicalcanceraction.org.

We have joined the campaign *Call to Stop Cervical Cancer* with a wish to contribute to this noble cause providing women with evidence-based information, which could educate them for making better decision about their own protection from cervical cancer. Namely, stopping cervical cancer with vaccination, today, is only a wish until more effective vaccines are developed. Current vaccines cover only four HPV strains (out of at least 100) and are intended only for sexually naïve girls. Once infected with HPV, a woman remains infected for life with a weak natural immunity that clears the clinical signs until reinfection or reduction of immunity occurs. The current vaccine cannot add to or change this immunity. New vaccines are necessary. We hope that in the twenty-first century this technical barriers will be overcome and there will be vaccines for all types of HPV and vaccines or other immuno-therapies for non-infected and infected women alike; but, this time has not come yet, and a caution is needed to prevent general public disappointment (with all negative repercussions) when vaccinated women will start getting cervical cancers. To prevent this disappointment, all agencies involved in cervical cancer prevention and control insist on keeping cervical cancer screening programs alive for the next 10, 20 and more years.

On the 4th of February, World Cancer Day, the International Agency for Research on Cancer (IARC) has published *2007 Annual World Cancer Data Update* and *2008 Cancer Challenges*. The first, among General Challenges is "To prevent those cancers that can be prevented." Two Specific Priorities are also related with cervical cancer, "To implement what is known to reduce risk" and "To develop concerted action against cancer of the cervix."

The call for "concerted action" was long due. Today, we have available tools for successful cervical cancer control (cytological screening in different versions), tools for cervical cancer prevention are in the beginning of promising development (HPV vaccination), but we lack a substantial progress in cervical cancer therapy – surgical removal of early lesions that could develop into cancer is still the only therapy providing cure. This is why IARC is highlighting cervical cancer prevention and control.

The *Call to Stop Cervical Cancer* is also dedicated to prevention and control. The programs for development of new vaccines and programs to increase the awareness of vaccine protection are underway and well organized. Cervical cancer control is entangled with some confusion because of different options. The major dilemma is which examining procedure and what type of laboratory technique to recommend for mass cervical cancer screening worldwide. The stance of this book is to keep the tradition until the new option proves its superiority. It means, regular annual cervical cancer screening with a biomarker-based cytological test, similar to the conventional Pap test or liquid-based Pap with HPV testing in addition (if necessary).

We see our contribution in this direction with development of Home Test and MarkPap® Digital, two options available only because of our biomarker previously discussed in this book. We also believe that the medical device industry and the health care providers will join our vision to do whatever is possible:

- To make the collection of material and primary screening more affordable and more comfortable for every woman via development of new devices (e.g., Home Test)
- To improve the accuracy of diagnosis by introducing telecytopathology digital screening procedures (based on biomarker-based cytology, digital imaging and on-line communication) between field sites where specimen is taken and processed and the remote screening sites where digital images of positive specimens are examined

In addition to the better and new HPV vaccines, we expect, these two accomplishments, Home Test and Digital Screening to become operational new tools for response to the unmet goals summarized in the *Call to Stop Cervical Cancer* in the twenty-first century.

4.1.2 What Happened with Pap Test After 2008

4.1.2.1 Dethroning the Classic Pap test

By the end of Twentieth Century, Pap test was justly proclaimed the "best anticancer screening test available" because, at that time, in the US there were about 100 million women at risk, 50 million Pap test were performed annually, one woman participated in screening at least once in 3 years, about 3.5 million specimens were found suspect (ASCUS+), almost 600,000 women are diagnosed as at higher risk (HSIL) and 40,000 were operated for cure. As a result, the cervical cancer prevalence and mortality dropped for more than 80 % in comparison with rates before the campaign [162, 209].

This trend did not continue after 2008; the classic Pap test was almost replaced with liquid-based Pap test, HPV co-testing was introduced, cost was increased, periods between subsequent screenings were prolonged – all of these "improvements" resulted in leveling the curve of prevalence and mortality, and recently (2012–2014) some increase has been noticed [135].

In parallel, the idea that Pap test ailing is developing and, without any robust statistical data (clinical outcomes), the enthusiasm of women to participate in regular screening has been decreased [228, 229].

4.1.2.2 Disappointment with the Global Outreach

There are 193 member states at the United Nations and each of them is a member of the UN General Assembly. World Health Organization is an Agency of UN with 194 members [230].

Governments and health care services in all these countries are fully aware of the cervical cancer screening and its benefit. However, they cannot easy match the cost/benefit of applying a cancer control measure to at least 51 % of the population at risk, and paying whatever is necessary for symptomatic women who will inevitably die of cervical cancer.

This issue we have addressed in this book and we have come to interesting conclusion:

> In countries where GDP PC is above $10,000, it is easy to introduce and to maintain cervical cancer screening with MarkPap Test; in countries where GDP PC is less than $10,000 there is necessity for additional funds – Government, charity, industry, private etc. Otherwise the screening can be applied but will not be efficacious – substandard screening is worse than no screening. [231] (Chap. 6)

4.1.2.3 Failure of Alternatives to Repeat the Success Results of Pap Test in the US

Pap smear, liquid-based Pap test (ThinPrep and SurePath), different version of HPV testing (HC-2, High Risk HPV (COBAS), visual assessment (VIA, VILI) and other local versions have been in practice as alternatives for the "famous" Pap test.

Unfortunately, although many of them have shown "significant" improvement based on statistical analyses of surrogate endpoints, none has changed the three robust endpoints – outreach (continues to stay within the range of 10–25 %, prevalence and mortality (both are still showing the increasing rates).

4.1.2.4 Attempts to Balance the Screening Cost with the Benefits Obtained

In the US, Pap test was introduced in the middle of the Twentieth Century by the American Cancer Society's nationwide campaign which was followed with legislative and financial regulations designed to provide a self-sustainable test delivery for 50 years to come. This fact was largely neglected by other countries in their attempts to replicate the Pap test success rates. In this chapter, we are trying to summarize the international experience and the current cost/benefit assumptions [175, 230].

4.1.2.5 Search for New Ideas to Reverse the Increasing Cervical Cancer Trends Worldwide

After reversal, the growth curve for cervical cancer prevalence and mortality rates in the US has taken a steep downward course – so, that some women's organizations, like Women in Government, had started the campaign to "eradicate cervical cancer." [178]. Unfortunately, in 2010 this trend stopped, the curves leveled and in few instances started to grow again (opposite reversal) [135, 232]. It was mostly connected with the reduction of number of Pap test screenings, and with the extension of time between two screenings from 3 to 5 years. It was obvious that not the Pap test technology, but the detection and removal of suspect lesions on time have been disturbed by the new "improvements."

To solve this problem we turned to our earlier proposal – using CAP-PAP biomarker to increase the sensitivity of testing [114–118, 202, 206, 210–212]. It happened that this biomarker is vaginal fluids resistant and that the molecular stain stays even in the cellular debris of the vaginal fluids [121, 206, 209] (Chap. 7). That was the reason why we invented a new specimen self-sampling device to give women opportunity to collect material at home, to send it to the laboratory and to receive results with almost the same accuracy as the material was collected by spatula scrapping (Chap. 7). This new specimen collecting technology, fully dependable of the MarkPap test biomarker characteristics, attracted wide attention as the solution for cervical cancer screening in rural and underdeveloped parts of many countries – with other words, it opened hopes for global mass cervical cancer screening [121, 122, 207–209] (Chap. 7 and Annex).

IT revolution has brought much improvement to the medical device area, such as telemedicine, and information image technology. Digital networking has made available easy exchange of medical information between scattered points-of-care and remote medical centers, making the consultation of experts accessible and affordable to many more centers, laboratories and small hospitals – wireless areas covered more of the space and the global medicine with mobile health became an excellent medium for fast, accurate and low cost mass cervical cancer screening. This book addresses those new tools separately [206, 208–224] (Chap. 7 and Annex).

4.1.2.6 Change of WHO Strategy

Probably the most significant change was made by the World Health Organization (WHO). After years of advocating Pap test, they concluded to change to the next strategy, Screen & Treat, and to recommend any screening technique (preferably VIA) and the same day application of therapy (cryotherapy) to small visible lesions (See Sect. 4.2 and Annex). We have analyzed their recommendation and we found that with an additional test, particularly the new biomarker, MEDYKO, this strategy could be much improved. This issue is discussed in Chap. 7.

4.1.3 Pap Test Now

The name Pap Test is now used as a descriptor for a composite medical strategy including

1. Recruitment of healthy women to participate in a voluntary screening of their genital system for hidden signs of a disorder which may develop into cervical cancer,
2. Examining woman and collecting cervical specimens for in vitro laboratory testing,
3. Preparing specimens for staining,
4. Staining with Papanicolaou stains,
5. Drying slides and mounting with permanent mount for microscopic analysis,
6. Reading slides under microscope magnification of x20 and up, for procedural quality control,
7. Selecting normal looking slides from abnormal and suspicious,
8. Reviewing abnormal specimens by qualified examiner,
9. Interpreting the clinical condition from the pathocytological diagnosis assessed from microscopic examination of the in vitro specimen,
10. Releasing women, if the examining result is negative,
11. Recommending women to further diagnosis, if the result is positive,
12. Start diagnostic procedure with colposcopy to search for visible lesions on cervix and around,
13. Performing punch or investigative biopsy on visible lesions,
14. To prepare biopsy material for histological examination,
15. To stain histological preparation with H/E stains,

16. To read and interpret histological specimens by pathologist,
17. To report final results back to the originator of the IVD examination,
18. To recommend women to further management depending upon the diagnostic results,
19. To remove cancer in situ by small surgery for cure, and
20. To recommend major surgery for invasive cervical cancers. With this final recommendation, Pap test moves from the preventive medicine (cancer control, surveillance) into another category – cancer diagnosis and treatment.

All these 20 steps are previously discussed in Chap. 2, under Cervical Cancer title. Each of the steps has several options, which are discussed above.

However, these all 20 steps are optional and the next steps are only indicated by the results of the previous steps. This is why only a few steps are needed for women with negative Pap, leaving the impression of a simple IVD method. And, this is why, if someone takes responsibility for conducting Pap test, and misses some of the steps, the service could be substandard and could make, in some cases, more harm than the benefit.

Cervical cancer was "the major killer of women from malignant diseases," because cervix is hidden inside female body making detection of early signs of this disease impossible without pelvic exam, the cervical cancer screening, as designed for the Pap test, and the results of its mass application in the US, has gained the reputation of the "best anticancer preventive measure available." Indeed in comparison with no exam, it was a great achievement.

If this was true, the question arise why such an excellent methods has not been applied worldwide immediately? There are many answers and the truth is probably among them, includes all of them or any combination.

When in the middle of Twentieth Century Pap test was introduced in Yugoslavia by appropriate health care providers, I was among those who were supposed to decide whether to make it mandatory or to allow individual women to decide. We were looking to the question why we need Pap test when colposcopy was easily available and free of charge in that country. Punch biopsy was also easy to perform and was the practice of regular health care providers in the state owned Health Houses for Mother and Child. We left decision on health care providers, either home standard or Pap test as recommended. Pap test did not gain the expected priority.

Similar thoughts occupied opinion leaders in India. They knew that Pap test begins with cervicoscopy – visual inspection of cervico-vaginal region exposed to human eyes by speculum and lights. In the US, the alternative colposcopy was combined with biopsy and histology and was expensive. India and WHO (IARC) decided for VIA or visual inspection with acid, to disclose suspect lesions and to remove them. When acetic acid (vinegar) and/or iodine solution (lugol) were added to visual inspection, cervical lesion became more visible. Because of this advantage, the visual inspection technology spread around the world – particularly in low and middle income countries [209].

Recently, again from India, came another idea. If VIA test was better than no testing, why not trying simple survey among healthy women to select those who have some gynecological complaints or fears (Tata Hospital, Mumbai, 2014). Indeed, results were favorable even for this approach [225].

However, none of these approaches could compete with the 20 steps comprehensive Pap test. Why, simply because none of them was intended to cure, all of them were only parts of the Pap test and, therefore, designed to move the procedure one or two steps further, but not to achieve the goal of Pap test – to reverse the mortality of cervical cancer in the selected country.

Another event that changes the efforts to apply Pap test worldwide was the introduction of HPV Testing in the beginning of Twenty-first Century. HPV HC2 test (by Digene) was approved by FDA as "method for detection of HPV viruses, which can be involved in developing a chronic HPV disease (warts), which, if persistent, could develop into cervical cancer." But, this fact was interpreted as "breakthrough news" – a virus is causing cervical cancer and prevention of HPV infection could reduce or even eliminate cervical cancer. Soon this enthusiasm dropped, but the insistence on immunization of girls with HPV vaccine remind until present.

We agree that HPV virus (particularly the "oncogenic" strains) is closely connected with cervical cancer. However, we believe that HPV is a tumor promoter rather than a carcinogenic agent. This concept is closer to the truth (see later) and it is opening new avenues for the use of vaccination – in HPV related tumors (including cervical cancer) for treatment – to stop or reduce the tumor growth (www.bioscicon.com).

In conclusion, in the period between the two editions of our book, it became undisputable that the cervical cancer is preventable disease, that many women lives could be saved with different cervical cancer control measures, but the big dilemma continues – what is the best method or methods for mass cervical cancer screening in populations where health care is below US standard. The new Strategy is needed for Global Cervical Cancer prevention [194, 198, 200, 202, 208, 209, 212] (see Annex).

4.1.4 *Challenges to Standard Pap Test After 2008*

4.1.4.1 Overview

Between 1950 and 2010, the classic Pap test has gained reputation of the "best cancer screening test available," but this reputation was tainted by the understanding that the test has inherited false negative rates coming from sampling and interpretation errors (NIH Consensus Conference on Cervical Cancer).

To reduce the sampling error, liquid-based Pap (LBP) specimen collection procedures were introduced by Cytyc Corp. (Thin Prep Pap Test) and by TriPath Imaging Inc. (SurePath), claiming that specimens in solution will guarantee investigation of the "total" specimen, not only a part of it as in the classic Pap smear test. The marketing success of this overstatement caused Pap smear to be almost completely replaced in the US by the specimen collecting solutions and both companies were bought by international multibillion enterprises Hologic Corp. Inc. (ThinPrep Pap test) and Becton Dickinson Corp. (SurePath test).

Unfortunately, cells collected in suspension with both systems, have to be transferred onto microscopic slides for further processing (Papanicolaou staining, reading and interpretation) and this procedure requires multiple transferring and multiple slides, a fact that increased the cost of testing. A single microscopic slide preparation meant another sampling (from the suspension now) and could not be the representative of the "total" specimen collected. This suspension sampling is aside from the problem that the specimen collection device could miss the area with abnormal cells.

Although the LBP did not meet the goal because it was developed, the solution had another advantage – cells were available in solution and could be destroyed and homogenized, thus, making specimens amenable for polymerase chain reaction (PCR) and for HPV viral particles – HPV testing bloomed using the Pap test collected material.

In the years to come (2008–2015) HPV testing was first used as accessory to LBP, than in parallel (as co-testing), and finally, with introduction of automatic HPV counters (COBAS by Roche) it is becoming to be advertized as for primary cervical cancer screening.

Some of the most recent guidelines have recommended HPV for primary screening and cytological testing as secondary – all because HPV material can be easily obtained with swab, the procedure is painless, low cost and could be repeated many times.

The idea behind this trend is obvious. If HPV test is negative, then HPV immunization with either one of two vaccines (Gardasil, Merck and Cervarix by GSK) will prevent the carcinogenic effect of HPV and the incidence of cervical cancer should be reduced. Again, some doubts are still present. First, HPV is a virus, not cervical cancer – infection with HPV can occur the next day after the test was found negative. Second, the vaccination, according to the manufacturers, is not effective after girls had been exposed to HPV infection – only HPV naïve girls develop active protection.

These facts have been mirrored in the guidelines on how to proceed with women after Pap test data are available.

Serious scientific dilemmas exist because all this data, either pro or contra, are based upon surrogate laboratory testing and statistical significance "proof." Clinical outcomes, as the most robust measuring parameters will only be available after 20–30 years of experience – such a long period is needed to assess the effects of the intervention on the occurrence (incidence and prevalence) of cervical cancer and on the mortality of this disease in a selected population.

Facing such dilemmas, the World Health Organization (WHO) in 2012–2013 has changed its recommendation for cervical cancer screening. Instead of being unequivocally in favor of Pap test, mostly under pressure from underdeveloped countries who cannot afford frequent screening by any method, WHO recommended change of the strategy into so called Screen & Treat, meaning that women should receive treatment of minor lesions, which could develop into cervical cancer, the same day when they are diagnosed by any screening method – visual inspection with acid (VIA), visual inspection with lugol (VILLI), Pap smear, LBP of HPV tests (see Sect. 4.2). The recommended treatment is with liquid nitrogen applied by field nurses specifically trained in the procedure; this is not the cryoablation, a standard surgical procedure for excision of small tissue lesions. Substandard freezing cervical tissue may result in two damages: be not deep enough to eliminate all cancer cells, and be too drastic to leave scar tissue which can close cervical channel or facilitate cervical rupture during pregnancy. Harm could be larger than benefit – dilemmas remain [208].

4.1.4.2 A Meaningful Composite Biomarker

Because in the first edition of this book (2008) we have predicted that introduction of surrogate end-points and using them for FDA approval together or instead of robust endpoints as clinical outcomes could create more dilemmas than clarity on management of women with laboratory tests (either positive or negative), in 2012, we revisited our clinical trial materials (2000 microscopic preparations obtained and processed with CAP-PAP test for detection of abnormal specimens) with several thousand cells classified in all cytopathological and TBS categories, and we have decided to introduce a new composite biomarker, which would include metabolic information about early changes (pre-cancer), ongoing cancer (DNA) and prognosis of this cancer (HPV) (Medyko, Sect. 7.3).

All three components are always present on slides stained with cervical acid phosphatase – Papanicolaou staining procedure (new name MarkPap®) and are visually recognized as ME(tabolic red granules of the acid phosphatase staining product, DY(splasia) as DNA creating nuclear shape, color, size; and KO(ilocytes) HPV derived vacuoles suggesting worse prognosis of lesions already being infected with tumor growth promotion virus. The acronym or the name of this composite biomarker was decided to be MEDYKO (Sect. 7.3).

4.1.4.3 Automatic Screening – Image Analysis

Screening vast majority of negative for a few abnormal cells Pap slides, and to accurately detect few abnormal specimens (rare events) has been a dream of every cytotechnologists or pathologist involved in mass cervical cancer screening. Two semiautomatic microscope systems have gained world reputation – ThinPrep Imager and SurePath Focal Point. Unfortunately, they both are using Papanicolaou stained slides and, because of the inherited high diagnostic error, have failed to meet the goal. Therefore, they are now used in practice to select the most likely negative cells, leaving 20 % of cells for visual examination by the personnel trained in cytopathology with Pap staining.

Both instruments are now considered as accurate with limits, but because of automation and reduction of human effort, they are also considered as economically justifiable and their use is increasing.

We have tried both instruments on slides stained with MarkPap test, and we have shown that the diagnostic accuracy can dramatically be improved; however, using our biomarker requires substantial change in the software of the image analysis programs, and the current management of the manufacturers, was not excited for changing it.

However, the challenge is still there, and antibody-based immunocytochemistry using manual examination could easily take advantage of the more accurate staining procedure based on a selective biomarker [213–219, 221–223] (Chap. 7 and Annex).

4.1.4.4 Outreach

Success of Pap test screening in the US was achieved with an outreach of above 50 % women at risk. It is not achievable in the LMIC because it requires duplicate of the American Pap test – all components: space, equipment, and supply, as well as the personnel trained in cytopathology at the point-of-care – a task unaffordable for most of these countries. Alternative to the test elements could produce only substandard testing and results with more unacceptable accuracy of results.

One of the chemical characteristics of the biomarker is that its solid stain is unsolvable in acid vaginal fluids. It means, in vaginal fluids where cellular morphology is easily disintegrated, the biomarker labels will stay untouched even in detritus. Since MarkPap test procedure can detect only cell-bound labels, we recognized it as an open door to develop a new test based upon self-collection of cervico-vaginal fluids at home of the woman at risk, sending the material to the pathology laboratory and proceed it further with slightly modified MarkPap test. In one clinical trial we tested this concept and have obtained satisfactory results. The idea for Home Pap was born and we applied for patent protection. In this book this technique is described in Chap. 7. This protection was necessary because of the huge market values of the device which can enable women to avoid health care providers for specimen collection. Many problems – social, familiar, religious etc. could be solved and women could be released to collect their specimens by themselves. We expect a dramatic increase of the outreach – at least women have said so in their responses on the Survey [121, 197, 202, 206, 207, 209] (Chap. 7 and Annex).

4.1.4.5 Screening with Biomarker

MarkPap test>digital imaging>TC protocol>IT networking>exchange of medical image information between scattered POCs and REMOTE expert centers has become a viable option with two projects: IT Telehealth System and Global ITTHC Network.

Both are described in the MarkPap Test Illustrated [119, 122, 202, 209, 213, 215–219, 221–223] (Chap. 7 and Annex).

4.1.4.6 Funding Cervical Cancer Control

Approximately 4 % of population is asking for medical help each day, only less than 1 % is asking for disorders related to cancer, and less than 2 ‰ for cervical cancer. Once cervical cancer is suspected, the diagnosis, therapy, palliation is costly and because of the ultimate fatal outcome it is considered as a necessary burden to health insurance funds.

In a population of 2.5 billion women at risk, 600,000 new cases per year and 300,000 deaths annually are small numbers; it is only 24/10e5 or 12/10e5 respectfully. These numbers also hide 40,000 patients operated from CIS (carcinoma in situ) or HSIL (high risk squamous intraepithelial lesion) meaning the same number of women lives are saved. If this number per a life is multiplied by the cost of diagnosis and treatment, the loss of reproduction potential, and the loss of economic contribution, our estimates show the countries with GDP_PC of more than $10,000 should immediately apply MarkPap test-based cervical cancer screening and will have positive cost/benefit outcomes. Countries where the GDP_PC is less than $10,000 should ask for additional funding or using the campaign tactics. Otherwise, they will not be able to implement and maintain service which will guarantee participation of more than 50 % of women at risk (See Cost/Benefit, Sect. 6.5).

4.1.5 Pap Smear Test Vs Liquid-Based Pap Test

In the middle of Twentieth Century, Dr. George Papanicolaou from Rockefeller Center in New York, NY, described his test for examination of cervical epithelium, which differed from the previous techniques by two substantially new elements: (1) a wooden spatula was used for scrapping cervix after the mucus was removed with cotton swab. The collected sample is than smeared onto microscopic slide, fixed in alcohol and sent to the laboratory for further processing. The excoriated sample contained more well preserved cells than the prior technique collecting cells already separated from the cervix and been free floating in the cervico-vaginal fluids (exfoliated cells); (2) Papanicolaou staining procedure using standard hematoxylin eosin stains but in combination with courses of alcohol cleaning to remove most of debris, bacteria and fungi and (3) adding additional stains (Orange G, EA-65) to make the images clearer, stains brighter and images more appealing to the examiners. He also described morphological changes, mostly on the nucleus, previously non visible, to which he connected characteristics seen in epithelial dysplasia, and added a new classification of specimens into test negative (no dysplasia) test suspect (mild dysplasia) and frank abnormality (severe dysplasia). Women with specimens with dysplasia were recommended for further diagnostic procedures (colposcopy, biopsy, histology) and to respectable surgical intervention, if needed.

Liquid-based Pap test is nothing else, but change of specimen sampling technology. Instead of using spatula to smear specimen onto microscopic slide, the new technology uses brush or spatula rinsed inside a cell preservative solution, and using machine to transfer cell suspension to microscopic slide. ThinPrep is using a solution based on methanol and ThinPrep Processor for preparing slide staining. SurePath is using solution based upon ethyl alcohol and density gradient to transfer suspended cells onto microscopic slides. For both technologies, Papanicolaou staining is used for visualization of cellular morphology and cytopathohisotlogical standards for reporting the clinical condition as found in the specimen.

In 1996 and again in 2001, the NIH convened Consensus Conferences to "improve" the cytopathological diagnosis of dysplasia found on Pap smear, and The Bethesda System (1996) and 2001 Bethesda System terminology for reporting results of cervical cytology have been adopted to replace the cytopathological diagnosis of no, mild, moderate and severe dysplasia. Two thresholds were also introduced: Lower between no and mild dysplasia (ASCUS+) and Higher between moderate and severe dysplasia (HSIL+) respectfully between cytohistological diagnosis between carcinoma in situ and invasive carcinoma or (CIN 2/3+) Since the new nomenclature was based on individual assessment, to bring some kind of objectivity, the FDA has used a panel of experienced cytopathologists to re-review the specimens on slides and to come with an Adjudicated Cytological Truth (ACT) as a new parameter for valuation of the results obtained by a standard and the new methods.

These two thresholds have been extensively used as the cut off endpoint measurements between success/failure estimated in clinical trials designed to statistically demonstrate that new "improved Pap tests, including HPV testing" have been at least equal if not better than the classic Pap smear test.

The story here is described to show readers that the final solution of cervical cancer problem is far from the end, Yes, preventive screening may detect early signs of lesions and lead to their removal with cure, but what screening to use when no one is completely secure not to miss false negatives and the best versions are unaffordable for the most of the population at risk, means only the additional work is necessary to improve this procedure or find another better assay, which can be fast, accurate, affordable accessible and low cost – as of 2015, it seems such solution could be found when all current methods are composed and integrated into a single system. It seems that the concept of MEDYKO is a candidate for such method that could meet all requirements and that better solution is not possible at this moment. What we think, it will be described in the next chapters, the New Strategy and the New Tools to meet this Strategy.

A parallel analysis between Pap smear test and LBP (both versions) is presented in the Annex of this book under PPP section [209, 212, 220, 226, 233] (Chap. 7 and Annex).

4.1.6 HPV Testing and Immunization

4.1.6.1 Co-testing HPV + Cytology Improved by CAP-PAP Test

Human papilloma virus testing and immunization is the new (Twenty-first Century) issue of great importance for health care providers (what to recommend), for health policy makers (whether or not to mandate immunization and for whom), for women at risk (whether, how and when to protect themselves and their female kins), and for scientists (whether a virus is carcinogenic – as some studies show, or only tumorigenic according to other studies).

Human papilloma virus is ubiquitous, more symbiotic with humans than pathogenic. Only few of its 300 strains already known, can cause a benign tumors – warts and only 4 are connected more directly with cervical cancer Strain 16 and 18 have been given name oncogenic, but definite proof (e.g., to satisfy Koch postulates with or without exceptions) is still to be presented [209].

HPV is highly infectious, but has weak pathogenic and even weaker tumorigenic effect (1 cervical cancer-like lesion in 2000 HPV positive healthy subjects) and the immunogenicity is proven, but still not completely understood (why only HPV negative young girls can produce antibodies against HPV virus, why HPV positive women cannot be protected with "buster" doses).

In our Cap-Pap (MarkPap) test slide library, we have evidence that most all (120) specimens obtained from diagnosed cervical cancer had morphological signs of koilocytosis (morphology of warts) together with acid phosphatase positivity – a biochemical marker of cervical cells abnormality, and nuclear changes showing different DNA aberration as typical for cervical cancer [195, 209; 214, 220, 224] (Chap. 7.3, Annex and Media).

However, among general population we have seen more specimens with normal DNA (no dysplasia) but with acid phosphatase positivity and koilocytosis, as well as acid phosphatase positivity without koilocytosis as well as HPV (HC2 test) positivity without either acid phosphatase or koilocytosis positive cells. These findings indicate to three stages of HPV interaction with female genital system: simple infection without causing disease, HPV disease, and cervical cancer. These stages are well known in infective disease: infection, infectious disease, and advanced disease. In the first phase, the infection can resolve by itself, in disease phase it can be resolved with some help, and in the advanced disease phase, it need substantial help and may or may not ever resolve.

If this information could be inferred to all Cap-Pap stained cervical cancer specimens, then it would be possible to examine instantly in a single run all three parameters under the microscope. It brought our attention to the possibility to create a composite biomarker with information about morphological changes (acid phosphatase), dysplasia (morphology of nuclei) and HPV disease (koilocytes) leaving HPV testing for detecting the infection. Suddenly, a new opportunity for the old cytopathomorphology has risen. This will be discussed under separate article in MEDYKO [212, 224] (Sect. 7.3).

The modern version of CAP-PAP Test is MarkPap® test. It has its an alternative way for specimen collection in solution. MarkPap solution is compatible with the solutions used for collection of cells for HPV testing. It means, if the specimen is collected in MarkPap Solution, and transferred onto microscopic slides to be stained for MarkPap test, the results can be upgraded into a combined pathocytological assessment (MEDYKO) and HPV testing (from the LBP sample). Suddenly, a cytopathology laboratory can do four testing from the same specimen: metabolism, DNA, HPV disease and HPV infection. This information, provided at the same experimental session, could provide sufficient information for the medical doctor to decide on how to proceed with the positive subject the same day the results are ready. The possibility for false negative Pap smear screening could be dramatically reduced. In our clinical trial, using MarkPap test, the false negative rate was below 4 % (acceptable error) while the control Pap smear test revealed the false negative reading in more than 20 % [195, 209, 212, 214, 220, 224] (Sect. 7.3 and Annex).

In 2015, HPV testing is entering into a more mature phase. It is now recommended for co-testing with cytological testing (see CDC guidance 2012) and HPV is described as an agent that can cause cervical epithelial cell changes similar to those which could be seen at Pap test and classified into one of the Pap positive category. This is acceptable and is favoring the use of our composite biomarker, MEDYKO, for instant diagnosis of abnormal cytology indicating potential danger of cervical cancer development and seeking for further diagnostic testing and removal of lesions creating those changes.

We believe that the new working formula could be defined as: MPT (MEDYKO) >>(PAP+HPV)>PAP or>HPV alone.

4.1.6.2 Immunization

HPV immunization is here to stay. The vaccines (quadrivalent Gardasil, and bivalent Cervarix) indeed produce immune response with development of antibodies against the viral particles towards which they are developed, and the active antibodies could effectively destroy new entries of viruses. There is nothing equivocal in this statement. It is the core of FDA approval for both vaccines.

The problem is in the interpretation, advertizing and recommendations. Does this vaccination protect from cervical cancer development in later age? Probably yes, but this is not confirmed, yet. More time and accumulated experience is needed for a final answer to this question. Consequently, the newest guidelines recommend continuous cytological screening for cervical cancer regardless of immunization. The risk of missing a suspect lesion in its removable phase is too big to overwhelm the hopes and believes into safe and sound protection.

This reduction in the initial enthusiasm, also gives the answer to the question, to mandate vaccination for sexually naïve girls or, to let parents deciding whether to weigh the risks and benefits and to decide what to do with their daughters?

Current guidance is clear. Let parents decide. But what they have to know? This is the question of assessing and judging the risk versus benefits. In our previous edition, we took stance that if the vaccine indeed protects from cervical cancer than immunize. If there are doubts about immunization efficacy or longevity of protection, than check for the frequency and severity of adverse events. If vaccine can cause death of one subject, avoid such a risk for your daughter. This stance has not been changed, but only confirmed through the years.

Now, we are challenging a still unchartered zone. If HPV immunization can protect against a new infections (which is not in doubt) and the HPV virus is responsible for tumor growth (growth promoter) then why do not explore vaccinating older women, already affected by HPV and particularly why not trying it as adjunct therapy to an advanced cervical cancer. This is an option deserving more attention that it was given in previous years. This idea is grounded on an experimental fact: the viral effect on cellular growth in vitro is directly related to the viral load. Reducing the viral load in vivo – which can be accomplished with immunization, could slow tumor growth? We would like to know the answer, which is still not given [120].

4.1.7 Management of Women After Pap Test

A woman should know that she could change her destiny, if she wishes and if she has the knowledge and tools to do so.

4.1.7.1 Background

In the middle of Twentieth Century, Pap test was introduced as an in vitro diagnostic laboratory method for screening healthy women for early detection of lesions which, if untreated, could develop into cervical cancer, and to remove it.

Initially, the emphasis was given to (1) Specimen sampling – transitional zone, (2) specimen preparation – smear or LBP with Papanicolaou staining, (3) specimen interpretation – pathocytological and Bethesda classification, and (4) removal of the lesion – any of surgical options depending upon the type and size of the lesion. Later, when more data had been acquired, the next criterion was entered, it is (5) the outreach or the percent of women at risk participating in regular cervical cancer screening programs. Closely connected is the next criterion, (6) frequency of testing – from annual (preferably), to one in 3 years (obligatory).

Later, Dr. Papanicolaou has started a School for Cytotechnologists – to standardize interpreting the results, and other cervical cancer screening health care providers, including the American Cancer Society have developed standards for all five topics. These standards were published and they became the first Guidelines for Pap test.

In the second half of the Twentieth Century, the success of prevention was measured with robust measuring endpoints: mortality and disease progress as found in consecutive Pap tests (annual screening) In 1996, a NIH Consensus Conference on Cervical Cancer (1996) has introduced a universal system for reading and interpretation of microscopic preparations (TBS) to help fast increasing practice both in the US and abroad. Unfortunately, this subjective method of assessment was conveniently used to create new success/failure measuring endpoints – this time surrogate (laboratory results).

In follow-up, when FDA approved using laboratory data as primary endpoints in clinical trials, many health professionals and health industry were encouraged to "improve" already "the best cancer screening test available," and many new methods, tests, products and procedures came on the market claiming to be at least equal, if not better, than the standard Pap test and offering new adjunctive advantages. Their appearance has not stopped yet and new guidelines must be created to guide health care providers to navigate among this increasing number of information now available.

This Chapter is designed to be a Compendium of some of that new guidance, which the authors have considered as influential on the current medical practice of cervical cancer screening.

The list includes, but is not limited to:

1. 2009, American College of Obstetricians and Gynecologists (ACOG)
2. 2012, American Cancer Society (ACS)
3. 2012, Centers for Disease Control (CDC)
4. 2012, US Preventive Service Task Force (USPSTF)
5. 2013, World Health Organization (WHO)
6. 2014, American Society for Colposcopy and Clinical Pathology (ASCCP)
7. 2014, Centers for Medicare and Medicaid (CMS)
8. 2014, National Cancer Institute (NCI) Cancer Statistics
9. 2014, American Society for Cytopathology (ASCP)

Between 2008 and 2015, a period between our two editions of this book, the major change in those guidelines was an increasing emphasis on LBP (liquid-based Pap specimen collections), and on HPV testing, which is a good prognostic parameter, but is advertized (although not fully approved) for primary screening [233] (Chap. 7 and Annex).

Those new guidelines have been influenced by financial aspects, too. Initially, Pap test cost was $15.00, but had been raised to $60.00–$100.00 in 2014. Health insurance companies, who are paying for this cost, had raised concerns of scientific value of so frequent screening of healthy women and have succeeded to extend the periods between screenings from annual to once in 3 years. Now, there are tendencies to extend even more, and to replace Pap test with less expensive alternatives which are not either approved by FDA or not evaluated in clinical practice with their effect on clinical outcomes – mortality and disease progression.

Modern, IT-based technologies, such as telemedicine, global cytopathology networking, mobile WiFi cytopathology and similar, have been mentioned, discussed, and regarded as a possible future development, but none has been introduced into the current guidelines (2015).

4.1.7.2 Critical Reading

Initial, and most respected, guidelines were very simple:

1. If Pap test is negative – repeat screening on annual basis.
2. If Pap test is suspect or positive – recommend further diagnostic procedures (colposcopy and biopsy)
3. If diagnosis is LSIL or HSIL respectfully CIN 2/3, consider removal of lesion by excision of cryoablation.
4. Everything higher than CIS 1A, recommend to hospital for further treatment – surgery, radiation and chemo-immunotherapy.

This strategy has changed by adoption of surrogate success/failure measuring endpoints, new tools and many new clinical trial results – all of them very influential to the mind setup of opinion leaders sitting at the consensus conferences – the Twentieth Century invention used to replace the individual responsibility of attending physicians and to dilute the liability for their decisions. Individual liability has been judged upon the degree of complaisance with medical protocols previously recommended by such consensuses and the actual outcomes and the critical thinking over the course of the diseases treated by a certain protocol was not strictly requested. The old Medical Oath by Hippocrates said differently – doctors are obliged to do the best they know and could without exception of who is the patient.

The modern management algorithms are like a tree with plenty of branches (see the ASCCP Guidelines in Sect. 4.2.2.3) and data of statistical probability what would happen if one or other therapy is used. It is not difficult to navigate among those branches, but, when individual patient is in question the protocols – no matter how extensive – become insufficient to give all answers necessary for successful result. The Hippocrates Oath takes care of those situations when personalized medicine approach is more important than the social medicine based protocols.

With all of this has been said, we believe that the decision about cervical cancer screening and management of women after the test should be made by individual health care providers and educated women together based upon the recommendation but modified to each individual situation. It puts much burden to the doctor's shoulders, but this is why they have been trained to carry and cope with it.

4.2 Guidelines

4.2.1 Overview of Guidelines After 2008

1. 2009 – ACOG
2. 2012 – ACS
3. 2012 – CDC
4. 2012 – USPSTF

5. 2013 – WHO
6. 2014 – ASCCP
7. 2014 – CMS
8. 2014 – NCI/NIH
9. 2014 – ASCP

Ad 1 and #6, #9

ACOG stands for the American College of Obstetricians and Gynecologists. In 2009 they published Cervical Cancer Screening Guidelines and upgraded them in 2015.

ACOG has adopted Guidelines published by ACS 2012, ASCCP and ASCP 2012, as well as USPSTF 2012 and ASCCP interim guidance for 2015 (See Sect. 4.2.2).

This College recommends equally two cytological tests, Pap smear and LBP, a HPV-co-test (cytology + HPV test administered together) and primary high risk HPV testing (as an alternative to contesting or cytology alone).

ACOG is also making selective approach to age groups, has added Risk assessment and has estimated balance between Harms and Benefits.

Ad 2 and #6 and #9

ACS stands for the American Cancer Society, the first organization that recognized the value of Pap test and has launched the nationwide campaign in 1045, which is still the most successful cancer control event in the US. ACS has since become the main authority for assessment evaluation and guidelines for further implantation of Pap test screening. However, ACS is closely collaborating with other societies working in the related fields and frequently their guidelines are jointly published.

In 2012, ACS, ASCCP, and ASCP have published Screening Guidelines for the Prevention and Early Detection of Cervical Cancer (see Sect. 4.2.2). The word "prevention" was introduced because of HPV testing and the hope that preventing HPV infection with HPV vaccines the occurrence of cervical cancer (incidence) could be reduced as well as reduction of tumor development if detected on time with the cytological testing as early signed of lesions potentially developing into cervical cancer.

This time ACS is categorical that only High Risk HPV testing (HPV types 16 and 18) is recommended, and testing for other types was rejected as "with no clinical role for cervical cancer screening or evaluation of women with abnormal cytology. This is big change to previous guidelines when standard HPV testing (HC-2) was recommended as co-testing. It is also supporting our prediction that HC-2 use should be revised and corrected.

ACS has also, like other authors of such guidelines, recommended different combination of screening for different age groups, but, again, this is more a result of statistical estimate of the prevalence of HPV infection and cervical cancer, than a selection based upon data (evidence-based medicine principles could not be applied there because it is difficult to collect true information about human sexual activity – the main route of HPV transmission of infection.

Ad 3

CDC stands for Centers for Disease Control, the US Government Agency regulating clinical practice.

Ad 4

USPSTF stands for United States Preventive Services Task Force an active group which recently was authorized to evaluate cervical cancer screening. Their primary focus was on Risk Assessment, Screening Tests, Timing for Screening, Interventions and Balance of Harms and Benefits.

Their recommendation was simple and clear: Women age 21–65: screen with cytology test every 3 years; if co-testing with HPV is included, extend screening on every 5 years; do not screen anything else (see attachment).

The original Pap test was successful when it was administered annually. Why periods between screening in the US are now to be extended to 3 or 5 years? In support of this extension there are only surrogate endpoints – no study has shown benefit by robust (clinical outcomes) endpoints. The natural development of cervical cancer from a single cell to a visible and manageable lesion (CIS, or ICC grade 1A) is 3 years at average. With 20 % inherited false negative rate of Papanicolaou staining (unchallenged method for cervical cytology) annual screening was seemingly good to detect lesions in their pre-invasive phase and to reduce the false negative rate by frequency of screening.

We are pointing to this fact only to emphasize that cervical cancer screening, although so successful, have helped health care providers to remove potential malignant lesions at early stages, but have not changed the natural course of cervical cancer development. HPV infection detection has helped to establish better knowledge of interaction between the virus and the cancer, but its application also has not changed the natural history of cervical cancer. More work and new ideas are needed in this arena.

Ad 5

WHO stands for World Health Organization and for their International Agency for research on cancer (IARC). For many years they were promoters of the classic Pap test and annual screening. After introduction of surrogate endpoints, HPV testing and VIA/VILI screening, WHO has changed their recommendation and has started to advocate a completely new strategy under the name “Screen and Treat” (see Sect. 4.2.2).

This new WHO Strategy is addressing the needs in low and middle income countries (LMIC) and is placing emphasize on clinical intervention the same day when screening is done – while a woman is still on the premises and needs diagnostic intervention. This is the same request as for the faster turn back of results for Pap test (few hours than few days or weeks), but advocating nurses to apply cryotherapy as treatment of visually identified lesions and without cytological confirmation, could be a strategy bringing more harm – cervical scar – obstruction, rupture, infection, bleeding. These possible adverse events should be avoided in healthy women.

Anyhow, WHO has recognized the lack of current practices and has opened contest for new strategy. Our next chapter will present our ideas in this direction (Media).

4.2.2 *Individual Guidelines*

4.2.2.1 ACOG

The American College of Obstetricians and Gynecologists

FREQUENTLY ASKED QUESTIONS
FAQ085
SPECIAL PROCEDURES

Cervical Cancer Screening

- What is cervical cancer screening?
- How is cervical cancer screening done?
- Who should have cervical cancer screening and how often?
- When can I stop having cervical cancer screening?
- What happens if I have an abnormal screening test result?
- Are cervical cancer screening results always accurate?
- Glossary

What is cervical cancer screening?

Cervical cancer screening is used to find changes in the cells of the cervix that could lead to cancer (see the FAQ Cervical Cancer). Screening includes the ***Pap test*** and, for some women, testing for ***human papillomavirus (HPV)*** (see the FAQ Human Papillomavirus [HPV] Infection).

How is cervical cancer screening done?

Cervical cancer screening is simple and fast. It takes less than a minute to do. With the woman lying on an exam table, a ***speculum*** is used to open the vagina. This device gives a clear view of the cervix and upper vagina.

For a Pap test, a small number of cells are removed from the cervix with a brush or other tool. The cells are put into a liquid and sent to a lab testing. For an HPV test, sometimes the same sample taken for the Pap test can be used. Sometimes, two cell samples are taken.

Who should have cervical cancer screening and how often?

You should start having cervical cancer screening at age 21 years. How often you should have cervical cancer screening depends on your age and health history:

- Women aged 21–29 years should have a Pap test every 3 years.
- Women aged 30–65 years should have a Pap test and HPV test (co-testing) every 5 years (preferred). It is acceptable to have a Pap test alone every 3 years.

When can I stop having cervical cancer screening?

You can stop having cervical cancer screening after age 65 if you do not have a history of moderate or severe cervical ***dysplasia*** or cervical cancer and if you have had either three negative Pap test results in a row or two negative co-test results in a row within the past 10 years, with the most recent test performed within the last 5 years.

What happens if I have an abnormal screening test result?

You most likely will have additional testing after an abnormal test result. This testing can be simply a repeat Pap test, An HPV test, or a more detailed examination called a ***colposcopy*** (with or without a ***biopsy***). If results of follow-up tests indicate precancerous changes, you may need treatment to remove the abnormal cells.

Are cervical cancer screening results always accurate?

As with any lab test, cervical cancer screening test results are not always accurate. Sometimes, the results show abnormal cells when the cells are normal. This is called a "false-positive" result. The tests also may not detect abnormal cells when they are present. This is called a "false-negative" result. Many factors can cause false results:

- The sample may contain too few cells.
- There may not be enough abnormal cells to study.
- An infection or blood may hide abnormal cells.
- Douching or vaginal medications may wash away or dilute abnormal cells.

To help prevent false-negative or false-positive results, you should avoid douching, sexual intercourse, and using vaginal medications or hygiene products for 2 days before your test. You also should not have cervical cancer screening if you have your menstrual period.

Glossary

Biopsy: A minor surgical procedure to remove a small piece of tissue that is then examined under a microscope in a laboratory.

Colposcopy: Viewing of the cervix, vulva, or vagina under magnification with an instrument called a colposcope.

Dysplasia: A noncancerous condition that occurs when normal cells are replaced by a layer of abnormal cells. Dysplasia can be mild, moderate, or severe.

Human Papillomavirus (HPV): The name for a group of related viruses, some of which cause genital warts and are linked to cervical changes and cervical cancer.

Pap Test: A test in which cells are taken from the cervix and vagina and examined under a microscope.

Speculum: An instrument used to hold open the walls of the vagina.

If you have further questions, contact your obstetrician–gynecologist.

FAQ085: Designed as an aid to patients, this document sets forth current information and opinions related to women's health. The information does not dictate an exclusive course of treatment or procedure to be followed and should not be construed as excluding other acceptable methods of practice. Variations, taking into account the needs of the individual patient, resources, and limitations unique to institution or type of practice, may be appropriate.

4.2.2.2 ASC 2015

Cervical Cancer Screening Guidelines for Average-Risk Women[a]

		American Cancer Society (ACS), American Society for Colposcopy and Cervical Pathology (ASCCP), and American Society for Clinical Pathology (ASCP)[1] 2012	U.S. Preventive Services Task Force (USPSTF)[2] 2012	American College of Obstetricians and Gynecologists (ACOG)[3] 2012	Society of Gynecologic Oncology (SGO) and the American Society for Colposcopy and Cervical Pathology (ASCCP): Interim clinical guidance for primary hrHPV testing[4] 2015
When to start screening[b]		Age 21. Women aged <21 years should not be screened regardless of the age of sexual initiation or other risk factors.	Age 21. *(A recommendation)* Recommend against screening women aged <21 years *(D recommendation).*	Age 21 regardless of the age of onset of sexual activity. Women aged <21 years should not be screened regardless of age at sexual initiation and other behavior-related risk factors *(Level A evidence).*	Refer to major guidelines.
Statement about annual screening		Women of any age should not be screened annually by any screening method.	Individuals and clinicians can use the annual Pap test screening visit as an opportunity to discuss other health problems and preventive measures. Individuals, clinicians, and health systems should seek effective ways to facilitate the receipt of recommended preventive services at intervals that are beneficial to the patient. Efforts also should be made to ensure that individuals are able to seek care for additional health concerns as they present.	In women aged 30–65 years, annual cervical cancer screening should not be performed. *(Level A evidence)* Patients should be counseled that annual well-woman visits are recommended even if cervical cancer screening is not performed at each visit.	Not addressed.
Screening method and intervals					
Cytology (conventional or liquid based)[c]	21–29 years of age	Every 3 years.[d]	Every 3 years *(A recommendation).*	Every 3 years *(A recommendation).*	Not addressed.
	30–65 years of age	Every 3 years.[d]	Every 3 years *(A recommendation).*	Every 3 years *(A recommendation).*	Not addressed.
HPV co-test (cytology + HPV test administered together)	21–29 years of age	HPV co-testing should not be used for women aged <30 years.	Recommend against HPV co-testing in women aged <30 years *(D recommendation).*	HPV co-testing[e] should not be performed in women aged <30 years. *(Level A evidence)*	Not addressed.
	30–65 years of age	Every 5 years; this is the preferred method.	For women who want to extend their screening interval, HPV co-testing every 5 years is an option *(A recommendation).*	Every 5 years; this is the preferred method *(Level A evidence).*	Not addressed.
Primary hrHPV testing[f] (as an alternative to cotesting or cytology alone)[g]		For women aged 30–65 years, screening by HPV testing alone is not recommended in most clinical settings.[h]	Recommend against screening for cervical cancer with HPV testing (alone or in combination with cytology) in women aged <30 years *(D recommendation).*	Not addressed.	Every 3 years. Recommend against primary hrHPV screening in women aged <25 years of age.[i]
When to stop screening		Aged >65 years with adequate screening history.[j] Women with a history of CIN2 or a more severe diagnosis should continue routine screening for at least 20 years.[k]	Aged >65 years with adequate screening history and are not otherwise at high risk for cervical cancer[j,k] *(D recommendation).*	Aged >65 years with adequate screening history.[j] Women with a history of CIN2, CIN3, or AIS should continue routine age-based screening for at least 20 years[k] *(Level A evidence).*	Not addressed.
Screening post-hysterectomy		Women who have had a total hysterectomy (removal of the uterus and cervix) should stop screening.[l] Women who have had a supra-cervical hysterectomy (cervix intact) should continue screening according to guidelines.	Recommend against screening in women who have had a hysterectomy (removal of the cervix)[m] *(D recommendation).*	Women who have had a hysterectomy (removal of the cervix) should stop screening and not restart for any reason[m,n] *(Level A evidence).*	Not addressed.

The need for a bimanual pelvic exam	Not addressed in 2012 guidelines but was addressed in 2002 ACS guidelines.[o]	Addressed in USPSTF ovarian cancer screening recommendations (draft).[p]	Addressed in 2012 well-woman visit recommendations.[q] **Aged <21 years**, no evidence supports the routine internal examination of the healthy, asymptomatic patient. An "external-only" genital examination is acceptable. **Aged ≥21 years**, no evidence supports or refutes the annual pelvic examination or speculum and bimanual examination. The decision whether or not to perform a complete pelvic examination should be a shared decision after a discussion between the patient and her health care provider. Annual examination of the external genitalia should continue.[r]	Not addressed.
Screening among those immunized against HPV 16/18	Women at any age with a history of HPV vaccination should be screened according to the age specific recommendations for the general population.	The possibility that vaccination might reduce the need for screening with cytology alone or in combination with HPV testing is not established. Given these uncertainties, women who have been vaccinated should continue to be screened.	Women who have received the HPV vaccine should be screened according to the same guidelines as women who have not been vaccinated *(Level C evidence)*.	Not addressed.

HPV = human papillomavirus; CIN = cervical intraepithelial neoplasia; AIS=adenocarcinoma in situ; hrHPV = high-risk HPV.

[a] These recommendations do not apply to women who have received a diagnosis of a high-grade precancerous cervical lesion (CIN 2 or 3) or cervical cancer, women with in utero exposure to diethylstilbestrol, or women who are immunocompromised, or are HIV positive.

[b] Since cervical cancer is believed to be caused by sexually transmissible human papillomavirus infections, women who have not had sexual exposures (e.g., virgins) are likely at low risk. Women aged >21 years who have not engaged in sexual intercourse may not need a Pap test depending on circumstances. The decision should be made at the discretion of the women and her physician. Women who have had sex with women are still at risk of cervical cancer. 10–15% of women aged 21–24 years in the United States report no vaginal intercourse (Saraiya M, Martinez G, Glaser K, et al. *Obstet Gynecol.* 2009;114(6):1213-9. doi: 10.1097/AOG.0b013e3181be3db4.). Providers should also be aware of instances of non-consensual sex among their patients.

[c] Conventional cytology and liquid-based cytology are equivalent regarding screening guidelines, and no distinction should be made by test when recommending next screening.

[d] There is insufficient evidence to support longer intervals in women aged 30–65 years, even with a screening history of negative cytology results.

[e] All ACOG references to HPV testing are for high risk HPV testing only. Tests for low risk HPV should not be performed.

[f] Primary hrHPV testing is defined as a stand-alone test for cervical cancer screening without concomitant cytology testing. It may be followed by other tests (like a Pap) for triage. This test specifically identifies HPV 16 and HPV 18, while concurrently detecting 12 other types of high-risk HPVs.

[g] Because of equivalent or superior effectiveness, primary hrHPV screening can be considered as an alternative to current US cytology-based cervical cancer screening methods. Cytology alone and cotesting remain the screening options specifically recommended in major guidelines.

[h] More experience and data analysis pertaining to the primary hrHPV screening will permit a more formal ACS evaluation.

[i] Primary hrHPV screening should begin 3 years after the last negative cytology and should not be performed only one or two years after a negative cytology result at 23 to 24 years of age.

[j] The ACS/ASCCP/ASCP/USPSTF guidelines define adequate prior screening as 3 consecutive negative cytology results or 2 consecutive negative HPV results within 10 years before cessation of screening, with the most recent test occurring within 5 years.

[k] Routine screening following recommendations for women aged 30 to 65 years should continue for at least 20 years after spontaneous regression or appropriate management of a high-grade precancerous lesion, even if this extends screening past age 65 years.

[l] Unless the hysterectomy was done as a treatment for cervical pre-cancer or cancer.

[m] And no history of CIN2 or higher in the past 20 years.

[n] Women should continue to be screened if they have had a total hysterectomy and have a history of CIN 2 or higher in the past 20 years or cervical cancer ever. Continued screening for 20 years is recommended in women who still have a cervix and a history of CIN 2 or higher. Therefore, screening with cytology alone every 3 years for 20 years after the initial post-treatment surveillance for women with a hysterectomy is reasonable *(Level B evidence)*.

[o] 2002 guidelines statement: The ACS and others should educate women, particularly teens and young women, that a pelvic exam does not equate to a cytology test and that women who may not need a cytology test still need regular health care visits including gynecologic care. Women should discuss the need for pelvic exams with their providers. Saslow D, Runowicz CD, Solomon D, et al. American Cancer Society Guideline for the Early Detection of Cervical Neoplasia and Cancer. *CA Cancer J Clin* 2002; 52:342–362.

[p] The bimanual pelvic examination is usually conducted annually in part to screen for ovarian cancer, although its effectiveness and harms are not well known and were not a focus of this review. No randomized trial has assessed the role of the bimanual pelvic examination for cancer screening. In the PLCO Trial, bimanual examination was discontinued as a screening strategy in the intervention arm because no cases of ovarian cancer were detected solely by this method and a high proportion of women underwent bimanual examination with ovarian palpation in the usual care arm.

[q] ACOG Committee Opinion No. 534: Well-Woman Visit. Committee on Gynecologic Practice. *Obstet Gynecol.* 2012;120(2)1:421–24. doi: 10.1097/AOG.0b013e3182680517.

[r] For women aged ≥21 years, annual pelvic examination is a routine part of preventive care even if they do not need cervical cytology screening, but also lacks data to support a specific time frame or frequency of such examinations. The decision to receive an internal examination can be left to the patient if she is asymptomatic and has undergone a total hysterectomy and bilateral salpingo-oophorectomy for benign indications, and is of average risk.

References:
1. Saslow D, Solomon D, Lawson HW, et al. American Cancer Society, American Society for Colposcopy and Cervical Pathology, and American Society for Clinical Pathology screening guidelines for the prevention and early detection of cervical cancer. *CA Cancer*
2. USPSTF. Screening for Cervical Cancer. 2012. Available at http://www.uspreventiveservicestaskforce.org/uspstf11/cervcancer/cervcancerrs.htm. These recommendations apply to women who have a cervix, regardless of sexual history.
3. ACOG Practice Bulletin No. 131: Screening for Cervical Cancer. ACOG Committee on Practice Bulletins-Gynecology. *Obstet Gynecol.* 2012;120(5):1222–38. doi: http://10.1097/AOG.0b013e318277c92a.
4. Huh WK, Ault, KA, Chelmow D, et al. Use of primary high-risk human papillomavirus testing for cervical cancer screening: Interim clinical guidance. *Gynecol Oncol.* 2015;125(2):330-7. doi: 10.1097/AOG.0000000000000669.

	American Cancer Society (ACS)	U.S. Preventive Services Task Force (USPSTF)	American College of Obstetricians and Gynecologists (ACOG)	Society of Gynecologic Oncology (SGO) and the American Society for Colposcopy and Cervical Pathology (ASCCP): Interim clinical guidance for primary high-risk HPV testing
Guideline committee	ACS, American Society for Colposcopy and Cervical Pathology, and American Society for Clinical Pathology-convened an expert panel.	16 volunteer members who are nationally recognized experts in prevention, evidence-based medicine, and primary care.	ACOG Committee on Practice Bulletins-Gynecology.[b]	13 experts including representatives from the Society of Gynecologic Oncology, American Society for Colposcopy and Cervical Pathology, and o ther committees convened an interim guidance panel.
Methods used to analyze the evidence	Panel is divided into six working groups to develop recommendations based on systematic review of evidence.	Recommendations are based on a systematic review of existing peer-reviewed evidence	Review of published meta-analyses and systematic review. Analysis of available evidence. When reliable research not available, consulted with experts.	Literature review, review of data from the FDA registration study, and expert opinion.
Methods used to formulate recommendations	Used the GRADE (Grading Recommendations Assessment, Development, and Evaluation) system to provide a framework for the guidelines development process. Voting on the final recommendations, with two-thirds majority constituting agreement.	The Task Force assigns each recommendation a letter grade (an A, B, C, or D grade or an I statement) based on the strength of the evidence and the balance of benefits and harms of a preventive service.	Not stated.	All voting was web-based and anonymous, with two-thirds majority constituting agreement.
Definitions of level of recommendation or evidence assigned	Not applicable.	*A recommendation:* The USPSTF recommends the service. There is high certainty that the net benefit is substantial.[a] *B recommendation*: The USPSTF recommends the service. There is high certainty that the net benefit is moderate or there is moderate certainty that the net benefit is moderate to substantial.[a] *C recommendation*: The USPSTF recommends selectively offering or providing this service to individual patients based on professional judgment and patient preferences. There is at least moderate certainty that the net benefit is small.[a] *D recommendation*: The USPSTF recommends against the service. There is moderate or high certainty that the service has no net benefit or that the harms outweigh the benefits.[a] *I statement*: The USPSTF concludes that the current evidence is insufficient to assess the balance of benefits and harms of the service. Evidence is lacking, of poor quality, or conflicting, and the balance of benefits and harms cannot be determined.[a]	*Level A evidence*: recommendations are based on good and consistent scientific evidence. *Level B evidence*: recommendations are based on limited or inconsistent scientific evidence. *Level C evidence*: based primarily on consensus and expert opinion.	Not applicable.
Source of funding	ACS, American Society for Clinical Pathology, and American Society for Colposcopy and Cervical Pathology	United States Government	American College of Obstetricians and Gynecologists	Society of Gynecologic Oncology and the American Society for Colposcopy and Cervical Pathology
Disclosures of conflict	Disclosures can be found in the document.	Disclosures can be found at www.acponline.org/authors/icmje/ConflictOfInterestForms.do?msNum=M12-0425.	Not stated.[b]	Disclosures can be found in the document..
Reference	Saslow D, Solomon D, Lawson HW, et al. American Cancer Society, American Society for Colposcopy and Cervical Pathology, and American Society for Clinical Pathology screening guidelines for the prevention and early detection of cervical cancer. *CA Cancer J Clin.* 2012; 62(3):147-72.. doi: 10.3322/caac.21139.	USPSTF. Screening for Cervical Cancer. Website: http://www.uspreventiveservicestaskforce.org/Page/Topic/recommendation-summary/cervical-cancer-screening. Accessed July 7, 2015	National Guideline Clearinghouse. Website: www.guidelines.gov. ACOG Practice Bulletin Number 131: Screening for cervical cancer. *Obstet Gynecol.* 2012;120(5):1222-38.	Huh WK, Ault KA, Chelmow D, et al. Use of primary high-risk human papillomavirus testing for cervical cancer screening: Interim clinical guidance. *Gynecol Oncol.* 2015; 125(2):330-7. doi: 10.1097/AOG.0000000000000669.

[a] These are the USPSTF grade definitions used to determine the recommendations for the 2012 guidelines.

[b] Individual members of the committees were not identified and no comment was made about conflicts of interest. (Volerman A and Cifu AS. Cervical cancer screening. *JAMA.* 2014;312(21):2279-80. doi: 10.1001/jama.2014.14992)

4.2.2.3 ASCCP

ASCCP The society for lower genital tract disorders since 1964.

Algorithms

Updated Consensus Guidelines for Managing Abnormal Cervical Cancer Screening Tests and Cancer Precursors

American Society for Colposcopy and Cervical Pathology

Reprinted – August 2014

Introduction

Cytology

Since the publication of the 2006 consensus guidelines, new cervical cancer screening guidelines have been published and new information has become available which includes key cervical cancer screening and follow up, and cervical precancer management data over a nine year period among more than 1 million women cared for at Kaiser Permanente Northern California. Moreover, women under age 21 are no longer receiving cervical cancer screening and cotesting with high-risk HPV type assays, and cervical cytology is being used to screen women 30 years of age and older.

Therefore, in 2012 the American Society for Colposcopy and Cervical Pathology (ASCCP), together with its 24 partner professional societies, Federal agencies, and international organizations, began the process of revising the 2006 management guidelines. This culminated in the consensus conference held at the National Institutes of Health in September 2012. This report provides updated recommendations for managing women with cytological abnormalities. A more comprehensive discussion of these recommendations and their supporting evidence was published in the *Journal of Lower Genital Tract Disease* and *Obstetrics and Gynecology* and is made available on the ASCCP website at www.asccp.org.

Histopathology

Appropriate management of women with histo-pathologically diagnosed cervical precancer is an important component of cervical cancer prevention programs. Although the precise number of women diagnosed with cervical precancer each year in the U.S. is not known, it appears to be a relatively common occurence. In 2001 and 2006, the American Society for Colposcopy and Cervical Pathology and 28 partner professional societies, federal agencies, and international organizations, convened processes to develop and update consensus guidelines for the management of women with cervical precancer. Since then, considerable new information has emerged about management of young women, and the impact of treatment for precursor disease on pregnancy outcomes. Progress has also been made in our understanding of the management of women with adenocarcinoma in-situ, also a human papillomavirus (HPV)—associated precursor lesion to invasive cervical adenocarcinoma. Therefore, in 2012 the ASCCP, together with its partner organizations, reconvened the consensus process of revising the guidelines. This culminated in the September 2012 Consensus Conference held at the National Institutes of Health. This report provides the recommendations developed for managing women with cervical precancer. A summary of the guidelines themselves–including the recommendations for managing women with cervical cytological abnormalities — are published in JLGTD and Obstetrics & Gynecology.

General Comments

Although the guidelines are based on evidence whenever possible, for certain clinical situations limited high-quality evidence exists. In these situations the guidelines are based on consensus expert opinion. Guidelines should never be a substitute for clinical judgment. Clinical judgment should always be used when applying a guideline to an individual patient since guidelines may not apply to all patient-related situations. Finally, both clinicians and patients need to recognize that while most cases of cervical cancer can be prevented through a program of screening and management of cervical precancer, no screening or treatment modality is 100% effective and invasive cervical cancer can develop in women participating in such programs.

The 2001 Bethesda System terminology is used for cytological classification. This terminology utilizes the terms low-grade squamous intraepithelial lesion (LSIL) and high-grade squamous intraepithelial lesion (HSIL) to refer to low-grade lesions and high-grade cervical cancer precursors respectively. For managing cervical precancer, the histopathological classification is two-tiered applying the terms cervical intraepithelial neoplasia grade 1 (CIN1) to low-grade lesions and CIN2,3 to high-grade lesions. If using the 2012 Lower Anogenital Squamous Terminology (LAST), CIN1 is equivalent to histopathological LSIL and CIN2,3 is equivalent to histopathological HSIL. Please note that cytological LSIL is not equivalent to histopathological CIN1 and cytological HSIL is not equivalent to histopathological CIN2,3. The current guidelines expand clinical indications for HPV testing based on studies using FDA-approved, validated HPV assays. Management decisions based on results using HPV tests not similarly validated may not result in outcomes intended by these guidelines. HPV testing should be restricted to high-risk (oncogenic) HPV types. Testing for low-risk (non-oncogenic) HPV types has no role in evaluating women with abnormal cervical cytological results. Therefore, whenever "HPV testing" is mentioned in the guidelines, it refers to testing for high-risk (oncogenic) HPV types only.

Comments

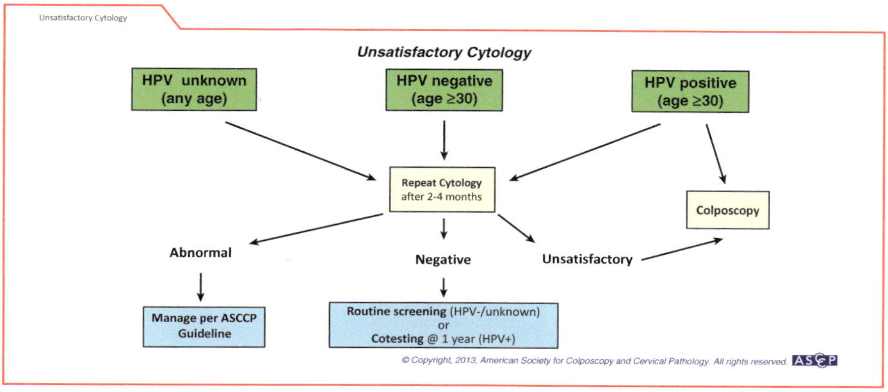
Unsatisfactory Cytology
Unsatisfactory Cytology
HPV unknown (any age)
HPV negative (age ≥30)
HPV positive (age ≥30)
Repeat Cytology after 2-4 months
Colposcopy
Abnormal
Negative
Unsatisfactory
Manage per ASCCP Guideline
Routine screening (HPV-/unknown) or Cotesting @ 1 year (HPV+)
© Copyright, 2013, American Society for Colposcopy and Cervical Pathology. All rights reserved.
ASCCP

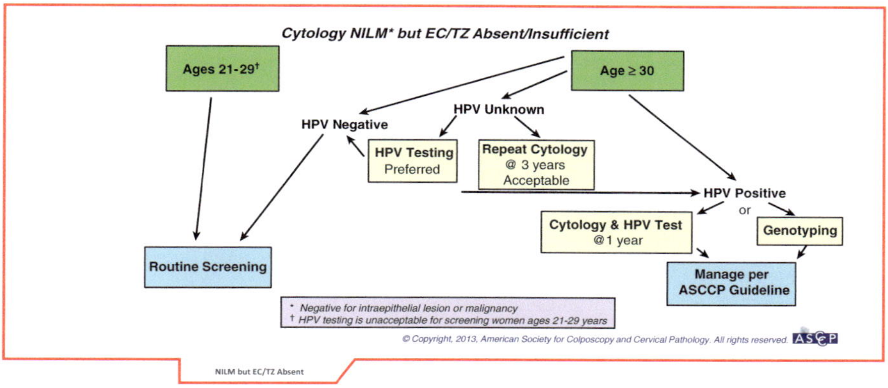
Cytology NILM* but EC/TZ Absent/Insufficient
Ages 21-29†
Age ≥ 30
HPV Unknown
HPV Negative
HPV Testing Preferred
Repeat Cytology @ 3 years Acceptable
HPV Positive
or
Cytology & HPV Test @1 year
Genotyping
Routine Screening
Manage per ASCCP Guideline
* Negative for intraepithelial lesion or malignancy
† HPV testing is unacceptable for screening women ages 21-29 years
© Copyright, 2013, American Society for Colposcopy and Cervical Pathology. All rights reserved.
ASCCP
NILM but EC/TZ Absent

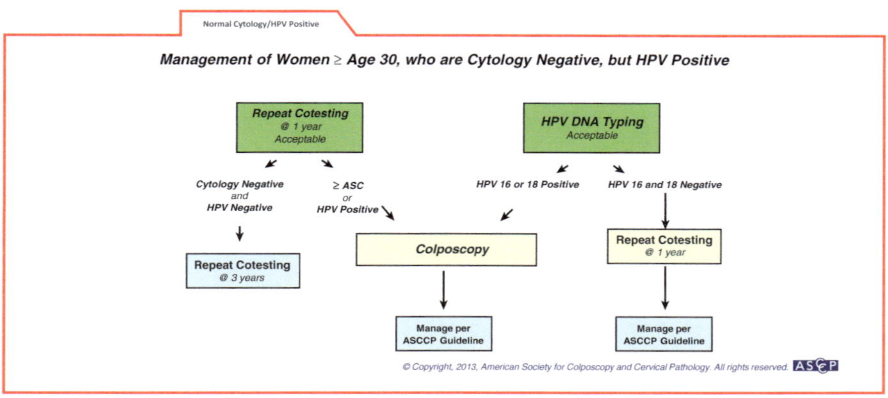
Normal Cytology/HPV Positive
Management of Women ≥ Age 30, who are Cytology Negative, but HPV Positive
Repeat Cotesting @ 1 year Acceptable
HPV DNA Typing Acceptable
Cytology Negative and HPV Negative
≥ ASC or HPV Positive
HPV 16 or 18 Positive
HPV 16 and 18 Negative
Repeat Cotesting @ 3 years
Colposcopy
Repeat Cotesting @ 1 year
Manage per ASCCP Guideline
Manage per ASCCP Guideline
© Copyright, 2013, American Society for Colposcopy and Cervical Pathology. All rights reserved.
ASCCP

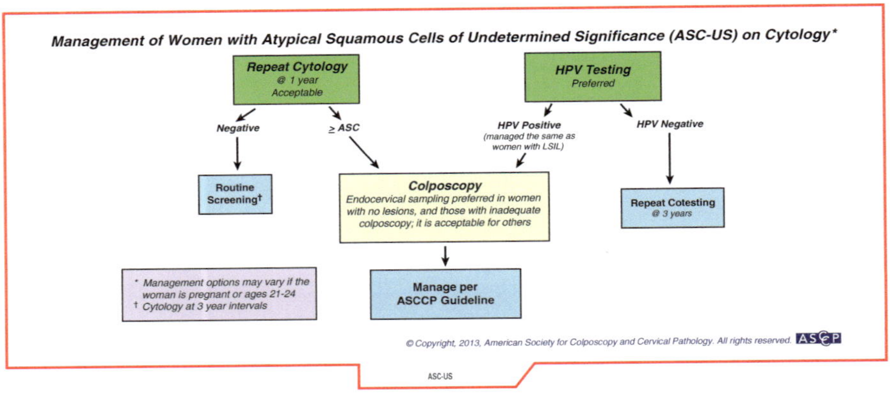
Management of Women with Atypical Squamous Cells of Undetermined Significance (ASC-US) on Cytology*
Repeat Cytology
@ 1 year
Acceptable
HPV Testing
Preferred
Negative
≥ ASC
HPV Positive
(managed the same as women with LSIL)
HPV Negative
Routine Screening†
Colposcopy
Endocervical sampling preferred in women with no lesions, and those with inadequate colposcopy; it is acceptable for others
Repeat Cotesting
@ 3 years
* Management options may vary if the woman is pregnant or ages 21-24
† Cytology at 3 year intervals
Manage per ASCCP Guideline
© Copyright, 2013, American Society for Colposcopy and Cervical Pathology. All rights reserved.
ASCCP
ASC-US

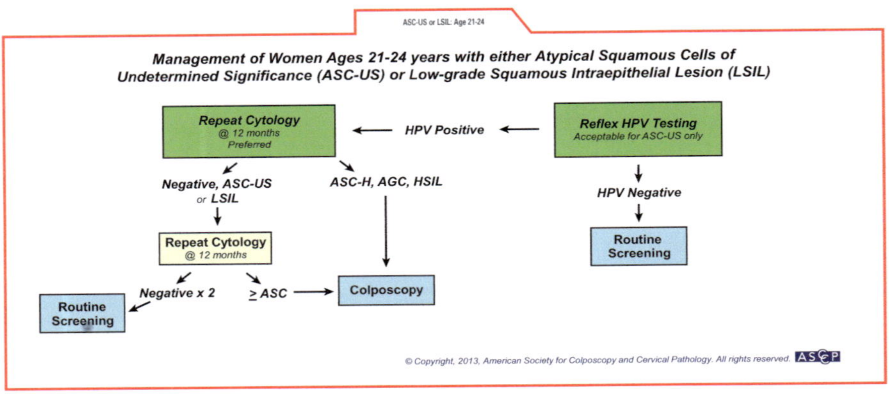
ASC-US or LSIL: Age 21-24
Management of Women Ages 21-24 years with either Atypical Squamous Cells of Undetermined Significance (ASC-US) or Low-grade Squamous Intraepithelial Lesion (LSIL)
Repeat Cytology
@ 12 months
Preferred
HPV Positive
Reflex HPV Testing
Acceptable for ASC-US only
Negative, ASC-US or LSIL
ASC-H, AGC, HSIL
HPV Negative
Repeat Cytology
@ 12 months
Routine Screening
Negative x 2
≥ ASC
Colposcopy
Routine Screening
© Copyright, 2013, American Society for Colposcopy and Cervical Pathology. All rights reserved.
ASCCP

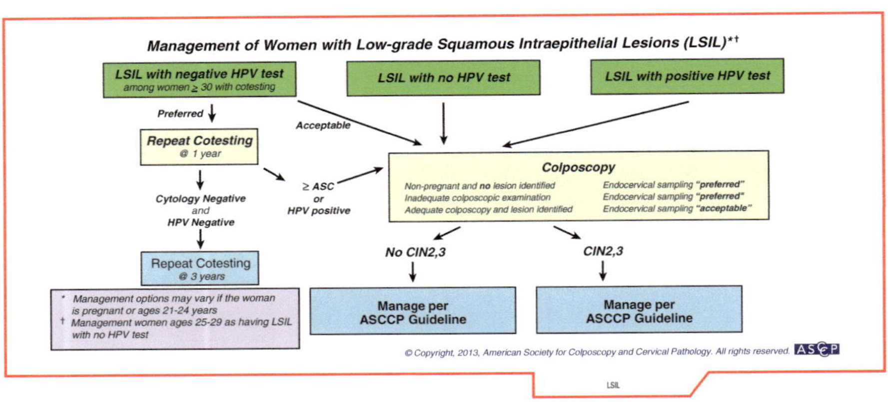
Management of Women with Low-grade Squamous Intraepithelial Lesions (LSIL)*†
LSIL with negative HPV test
among women ≥ 30 with cotesting
LSIL with no HPV test
LSIL with positive HPV test
Preferred
Acceptable
Repeat Cotesting
@ 1 year
Colposcopy
Non-pregnant and no lesion identified
Inadequate colposcopic examination
Adequate colposcopy and lesion identified
Endocervical sampling "preferred"
Endocervical sampling "preferred"
Endocervical sampling "acceptable"
Cytology Negative
and
HPV Negative
≥ ASC
or
HPV positive
No CIN2,3
CIN2,3
Repeat Cotesting
@ 3 years
* Management options may vary if the woman is pregnant or ages 21-24 years
† Management women ages 25-29 as having LSIL with no HPV test
Manage per ASCCP Guideline
Manage per ASCCP Guideline
© Copyright, 2013, American Society for Colposcopy and Cervical Pathology. All rights reserved.
ASCCP
LSIL

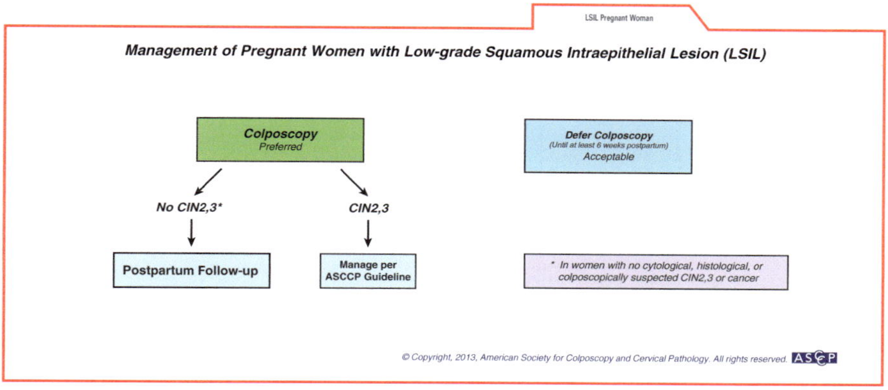
LSIL Pregnant Woman
Management of Pregnant Women with Low-grade Squamous Intraepithelial Lesion (LSIL)
Colposcopy
Preferred
Defer Colposcopy
(Until at least 6 weeks postpartum)
Acceptable
No CIN2,3*
CIN2,3
Postpartum Follow-up
Manage per ASCCP Guideline
* In women with no cytological, histological, or colposcopically suspected CIN2,3 or cancer
© Copyright, 2013, American Society for Colposcopy and Cervical Pathology. All rights reserved.
ASCCP

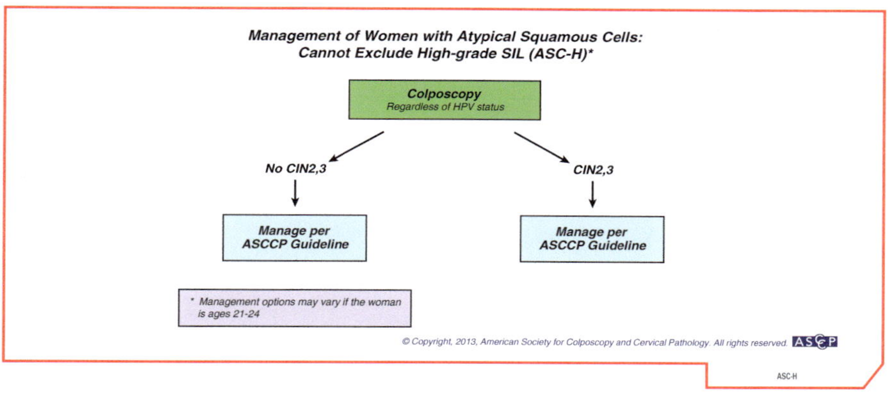
Management of Women with Atypical Squamous Cells:
Cannot Exclude High-grade SIL (ASC-H)*
Colposcopy
Regardless of HPV status
No CIN2,3
CIN2,3
Manage per ASCCP Guideline
Manage per ASCCP Guideline
* Management options may vary if the woman is ages 21-24
© Copyright, 2013, American Society for Colposcopy and Cervical Pathology. All rights reserved.
ASCCP
ASC-H

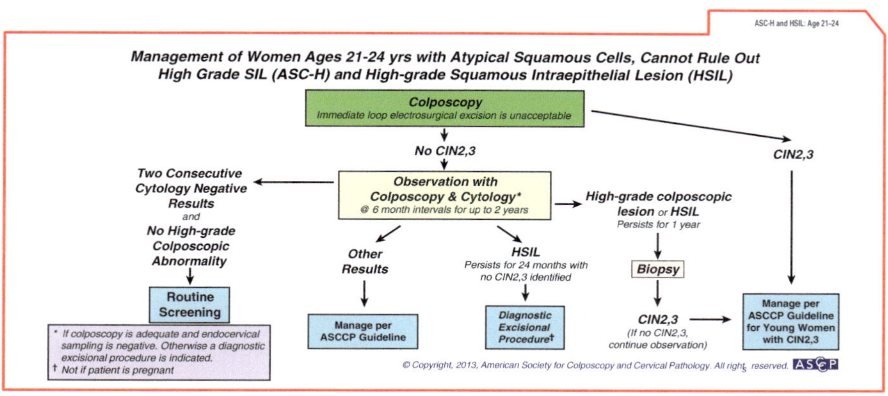
ASC-H and HSIL: Age 21–24
Management of Women Ages 21-24 yrs with Atypical Squamous Cells, Cannot Rule Out
High Grade SIL (ASC-H) and High-grade Squamous Intraepithelial Lesion (HSIL)
Colposcopy
Immediate loop electrosurgical excision is unacceptable
No CIN2,3
CIN2,3
Observation with Colposcopy & Cytology*
@ 6 month intervals for up to 2 years
Two Consecutive Cytology Negative Results and No High-grade Colposcopic Abnormality
High-grade colposcopic lesion or HSIL
Persists for 1 year
Other Results
HSIL
Persists for 24 months with no CIN2,3 identified
Biopsy
Routine Screening
Manage per ASCCP Guideline
Diagnostic Excisional Procedure†
CIN2,3
(If no CIN2,3, continue observation)
Manage per ASCCP Guideline for Young Women with CIN2,3
* If colposcopy is adequate and endocervical sampling is negative. Otherwise a diagnostic excisional procedure is indicated.
† Not if patient is pregnant
© Copyright, 2013, American Society for Colposcopy and Cervical Pathology. All rights reserved.
ASCCP

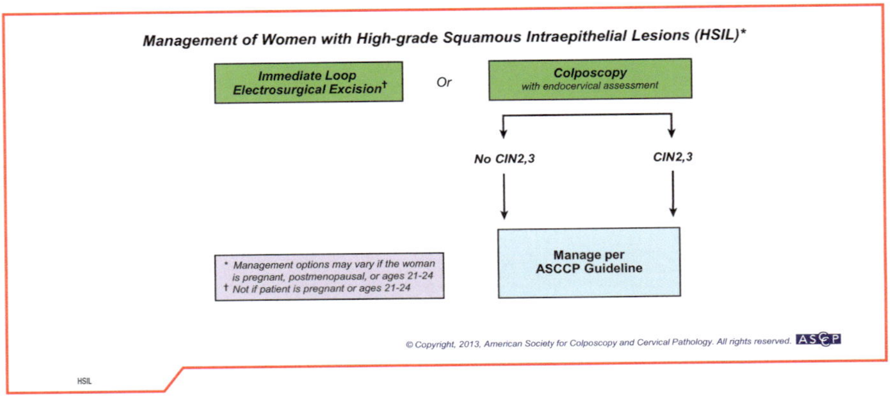
Management of Women with High-grade Squamous Intraepithelial Lesions (HSIL)*
Immediate Loop Electrosurgical Excision†
Or
Colposcopy with endocervical assessment
No CIN2,3
CIN2,3
Manage per ASCCP Guideline
* Management options may vary if the woman is pregnant, postmenopausal, or ages 21-24
† Not if patient is pregnant or ages 21-24
© Copyright, 2013, American Society for Colposcopy and Cervical Pathology. All rights reserved.
HSIL

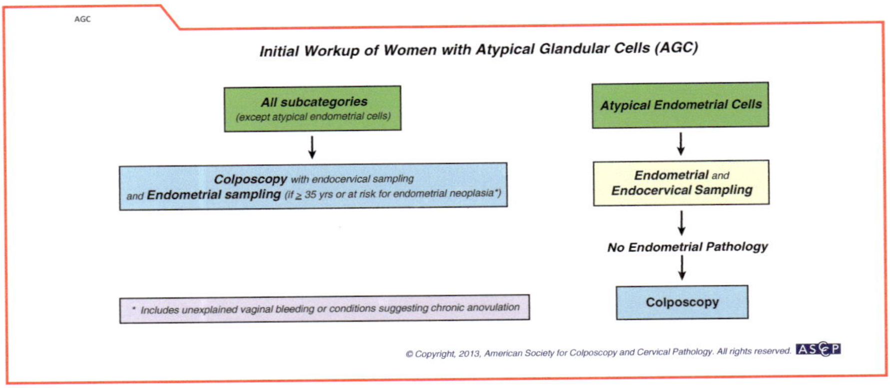
AGC
Initial Workup of Women with Atypical Glandular Cells (AGC)
All subcategories (except atypical endometrial cells)
Colposcopy with endocervical sampling and Endometrial sampling (if ≥ 35 yrs or at risk for endometrial neoplasia*)
Atypical Endometrial Cells
Endometrial and Endocervical Sampling
No Endometrial Pathology
Colposcopy
* Includes unexplained vaginal bleeding or conditions suggesting chronic anovulation
© Copyright, 2013, American Society for Colposcopy and Cervical Pathology. All rights reserved.

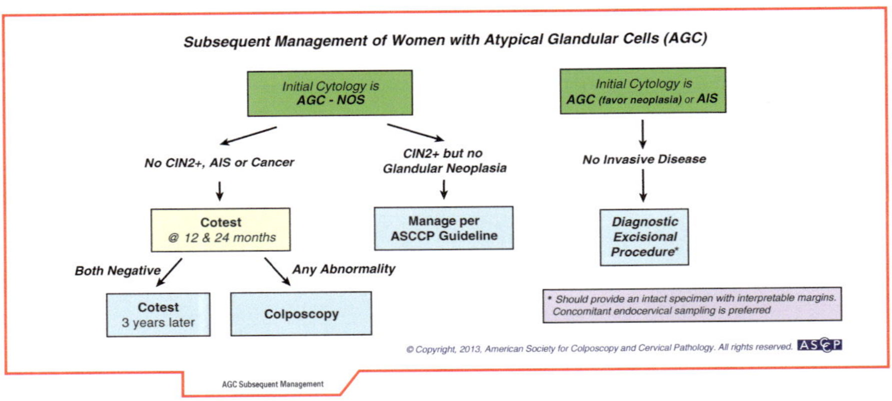
Subsequent Management of Women with Atypical Glandular Cells (AGC)
Initial Cytology is AGC - NOS
No CIN2+, AIS or Cancer
CIN2+ but no Glandular Neoplasia
Cotest @ 12 & 24 months
Manage per ASCCP Guideline
Both Negative
Any Abnormality
Cotest 3 years later
Colposcopy
Initial Cytology is AGC (favor neoplasia) or AIS
No Invasive Disease
Diagnostic Excisional Procedure*
* Should provide an intact specimen with interpretable margins. Concomitant endocervical sampling is preferred
© Copyright, 2013, American Society for Colposcopy and Cervical Pathology. All rights reserved.
AGC Subsequent Management

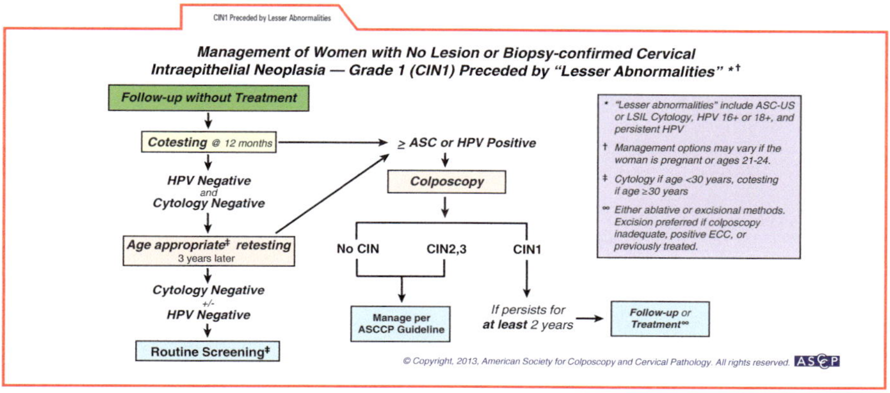
CIN1 Preceded by Lesser Abnormalities
Management of Women with No Lesion or Biopsy-confirmed Cervical Intraepithelial Neoplasia — Grade 1 (CIN1) Preceded by "Lesser Abnormalities" *†
Follow-up without Treatment
Cotesting @ 12 months
≥ ASC or HPV Positive
HPV Negative and Cytology Negative
Colposcopy
Age appropriate‡ retesting 3 years later
No CIN
CIN2,3
CIN1
Cytology Negative +/- HPV Negative
Manage per ASCCP Guideline
If persists for at least 2 years
Follow-up or Treatment∞
Routine Screening‡
* "Lesser abnormalities" include ASC-US or LSIL Cytology, HPV 16+ or 18+, and persistent HPV
† Management options may vary if the woman is pregnant or ages 21-24.
‡ Cytology if age <30 years, cotesting if age ≥30 years
∞ Either ablative or excisional methods. Excision preferred if colposcopy inadequate, positive ECC, or previously treated.
© Copyright, 2013, American Society for Colposcopy and Cervical Pathology. All rights reserved.
ASCCP

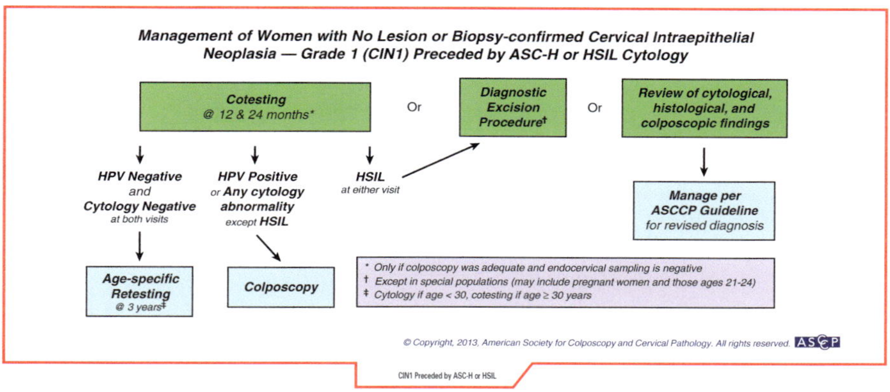
Management of Women with No Lesion or Biopsy-confirmed Cervical Intraepithelial Neoplasia — Grade 1 (CIN1) Preceded by ASC-H or HSIL Cytology
Cotesting @ 12 & 24 months*
Or
Diagnostic Excision Procedure†
Or
Review of cytological, histological, and colposcopic findings
HPV Negative and Cytology Negative at both visits
HPV Positive or Any cytology abnormality except HSIL
HSIL at either visit
Manage per ASCCP Guideline for revised diagnosis
Age-specific Retesting @ 3 years‡
Colposcopy
* Only if colposcopy was adequate and endocervical sampling is negative
† Except in special populations (may include pregnant women and those ages 21-24)
‡ Cytology if age < 30, cotesting if age ≥ 30 years
© Copyright, 2013, American Society for Colposcopy and Cervical Pathology. All rights reserved.
ASCCP
CIN1 Preceded by ASC-H or HSIL

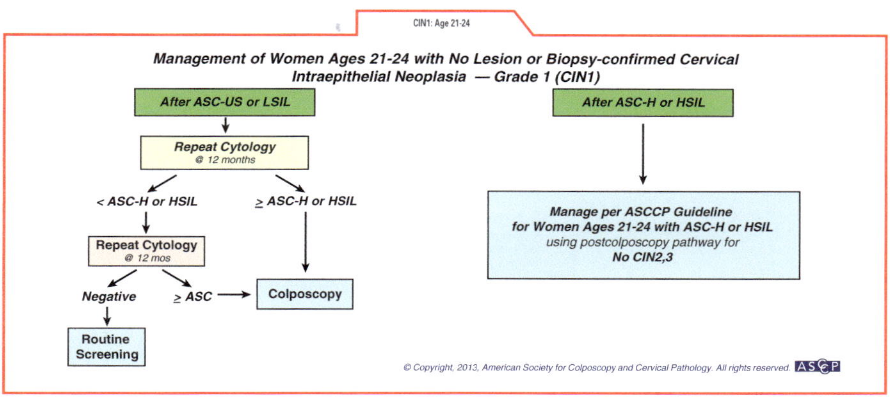
CIN1: Age 21-24
Management of Women Ages 21-24 with No Lesion or Biopsy-confirmed Cervical Intraepithelial Neoplasia — Grade 1 (CIN1)
After ASC-US or LSIL
After ASC-H or HSIL
Repeat Cytology @ 12 months
< ASC-H or HSIL
≥ ASC-H or HSIL
Manage per ASCCP Guideline for Women Ages 21-24 with ASC-H or HSIL using postcolposcopy pathway for No CIN2,3
Repeat Cytology @ 12 mos
Negative
≥ ASC
Colposcopy
Routine Screening
© Copyright, 2013, American Society for Colposcopy and Cervical Pathology. All rights reserved.
ASCCP

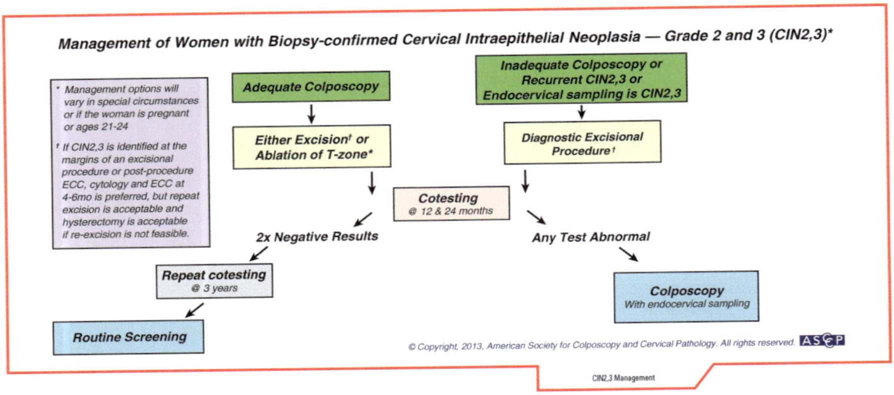
Management of Women with Biopsy-confirmed Cervical Intraepithelial Neoplasia — Grade 2 and 3 (CIN2,3)*
* Management options will vary in special circumstances or if the woman is pregnant or ages 21-24
† If CIN2,3 is identified at the margins of an excisional procedure or post-procedure ECC, cytology and ECC at 4-6mo is preferred, but repeat excision is acceptable and hysterectomy is acceptable if re-excision is not feasible.
Adequate Colposcopy
Either Excision† or Ablation of T-zone*
Inadequate Colposcopy or Recurrent CIN2,3 or Endocervical sampling is CIN2,3
Diagnostic Excisional Procedure†
Cotesting @ 12 & 24 months
2x Negative Results
Any Test Abnormal
Repeat cotesting @ 3 years
Colposcopy With endocervical sampling
Routine Screening
© Copyright, 2013, American Society for Colposcopy and Cervical Pathology. All rights reserved.
CIN2,3 Management

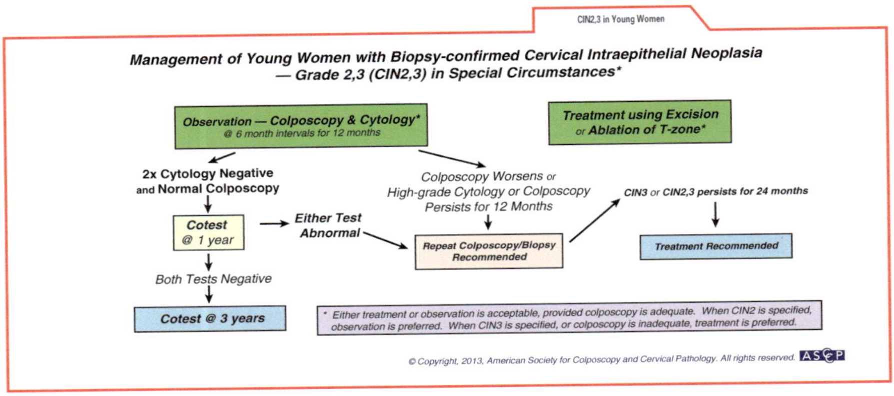
CIN2,3 in Young Women
Management of Young Women with Biopsy-confirmed Cervical Intraepithelial Neoplasia — Grade 2,3 (CIN2,3) in Special Circumstances*
Observation — Colposcopy & Cytology* @ 6 month intervals for 12 months
Treatment using Excision or Ablation of T-zone*
2x Cytology Negative and Normal Colposcopy
Colposcopy Worsens or High-grade Cytology or Colposcopy Persists for 12 Months
CIN3 or CIN2,3 persists for 24 months
Cotest @ 1 year
Either Test Abnormal
Repeat Colposcopy/Biopsy Recommended
Treatment Recommended
Both Tests Negative
Cotest @ 3 years
* Either treatment or observation is acceptable, provided colposcopy is adequate. When CIN2 is specified, observation is preferred. When CIN3 is specified, or colposcopy is inadequate, treatment is preferred.
© Copyright, 2013, American Society for Colposcopy and Cervical Pathology. All rights reserved.

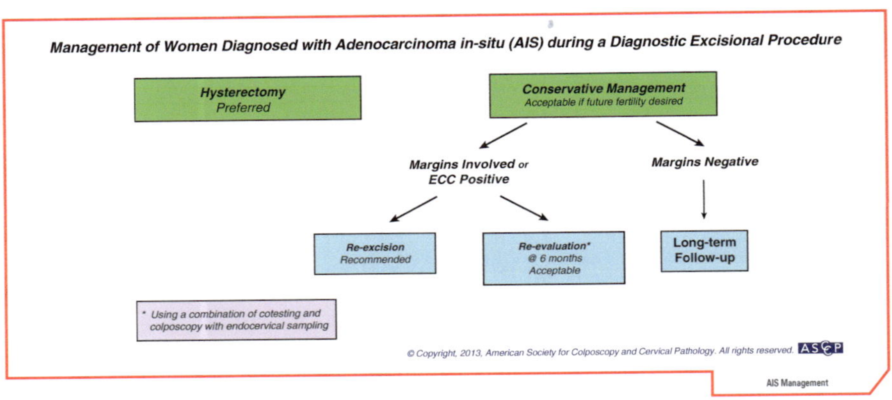
Management of Women Diagnosed with Adenocarcinoma in-situ (AIS) during a Diagnostic Excisional Procedure
Hysterectomy Preferred
Conservative Management Acceptable if future fertility desired
Margins Involved or ECC Positive
Margins Negative
Re-excision Recommended
Re-evaluation* @ 6 months Acceptable
Long-term Follow-up
* Using a combination of cotesting and colposcopy with endocervical sampling
© Copyright, 2013, American Society for Colposcopy and Cervical Pathology. All rights reserved.
AIS Management

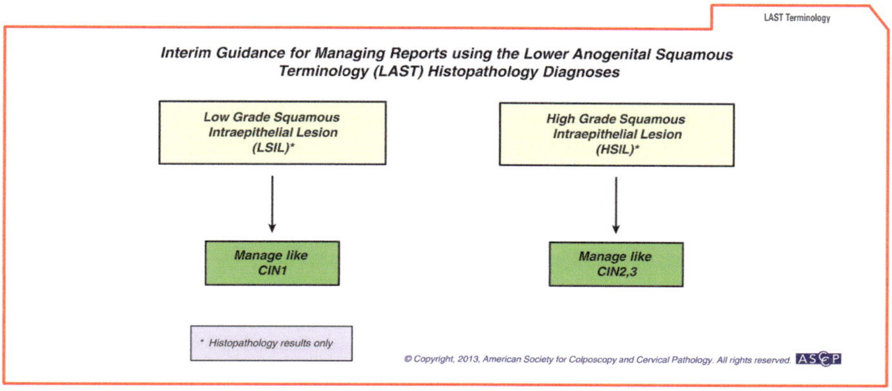

Definitions

Terms Utilized in the Consensus Guidelines

- **Colposcopy** is the examination of the cervix, vagina, and, in some instances the vulva, with the colposcope after the application of a 3-5% acetic acid solution coupled with obtaining colposcopically-directed biopsies of all lesions suspected of representing neoplasia.
- **Endocervical sampling** includes obtaining a specimen for either histopathological evaluation using an endocervical curette or a cytobrush or for cytological evaluation using a cytobrush.
- **Endocervical assessment** is the process of evaluating the endocervical canal for the presence of neoplasia using either a colposcope or endocervical sampling.
- **Diagnostic excisional procedure** is the process of obtaining a specimen from the transformation zone and endocervical canal for histopathological evaluation and includes laser conization, cold-knife conization, loop electrosurgical excision procedure (LEEP), and loop electrosurgical conization.
- **Adequate colposcopy** indicates that the entire squamocolumnar junction and the margin of any visible lesion can be visualized with the colposcope.
- **Endometrial sampling** includes obtaining a specimen for histopathological evaluation using an endometrial aspiration or biopsy device, a "dilatation and curettage" or hysteroscopy.

Acknowledgments

These guidelines were developed with funding from the American Society for Colposcopy and Cervical Pathology (ASCCP). The contents are solely the responsibility of the authors and the ASCCP.

L. Stewart Massad, M.D., Washington University School of Medicine, St. Louis, MO; Mark H. Einstein, M.D., Albert Einstein College of Medicine, Bronx, NY; Warner K. Huh, M.D., University of Alabama School of Medicine, Birmingham, AL; Hormuzd A. Katki, Ph.D., Division of Cancer Epidemiology and Genetics, National Cancer Institute, Bethesda, MD; Walter K. Kinney, M.D., The Permanente Medical Group, Sacramento, CA; Mark Schiffman, M.D., Diane Solomon, M.D., Division of Cancer Prevention, National Cancer Institute, Bethesda, MD; Nicolas Wentzensen, M.D., Division of Cancer Epidemiology and Genetics, National Cancer Institute, Bethesda, MD; Herschel W. Lawson, M.D., Emory University School of Medicine, Atlanta, GA, on behalf of the 2012 ASCCP Consensus Guidelines Conference

All copyright permission requests should be sent to the ASCCP National Office, 1530 Tilco Dr., Ste. C, Frederick, MD 21704

ASCCP
1530 Tilco Drive, Suite C
Frederick, MD 21704
(301) 733-3640 (telephone)
(800) 787-7227 (toll free)
(240) 575-9880 (fax)

For more information, or to order additional copies, please email:
administrator@asccp.org

The society for lower genital tract disorders since 1964.

www.asccp.org/Guidelines

4.2.2.4 USPSTF

New Cervical Cancer Screening Guidelines Announced

Did you know that having a Pap test annually is no longer recommended by leading medical organizations? New cervical cancer screening guidelines released separately this March by the United States Preventive Services Task Force (USPSTF) and the American Cancer Society (ACS) recommend against routine yearly testing. Instead, the guidelines recommend testing every three years for women ages 21-65; routine cervical cancer screening for women under 21 and over 65 is no longer recommended. The two groups also introduced the option of a lengthened, five-year screening interval for women ages 30-65 when screened with a combination of Pap testing and human papillomavirus (HPV) testing.

These groups routinely review the current, available scientific evidence about the benefits and harms of cancer screening and other preventive services and release guidelines for clinical practice. The Patient Protection and Affordable Care Act requires that health plans cover all preventive services rated "A" or "B" by the USPSTF, so these recommendations are particularly important.

You can find the complete USPSTF cervical cancer screening recommendation statement below. More resources including the evidence synthesis, decision analysis, clinical summary chart and a consumer fact sheet for patients can be found on the USPSTF website: http://www.uspreventiveservicestaskforce.org/uspstf/uspscerv.htm. To view the ACS recommendation statement, visit http://www.cancer.org/Cancer/news/News/new-screening-guidelines-for-cervical-cancer.

USPSTF Current Recommendation for Cervical Cancer Screening[1] Release Date: March 2012

These recommendations apply to women who have a cervix, regardless of sexual history. These recommendations do not apply to women who have received a diagnosis of a high-grade precancerous cervical lesion or cervical cancer, women with in utero exposure to diethylstilbestrol, or women who are immunocompromised (such as those who are HIV positive).

- The USPSTF recommends screening women ages 21 to 65 years with cytology every 3 years or, for women ages 30 to 65 years who want to lengthen the screening interval, screening with a combination of cytology and HPV testing every 5 years. **Grade A**
- The USPSTF recommends against screening for cervical cancer in women younger than age 21 years. **Grade D**
- The USPSTF recommends against screening for cervical cancer in women older than age 65 years who have had adequate prior screening and are not otherwise at high risk for cervical cancer. **Grade D**
- The USPSTF recommends against screening for cervical cancer in women who have had a hysterectomy with removal of the cervix and who do not have a history of CIN 2, CIN 3, or cervical cancer. **Grade D**
- The USPSTF recommends against screening for cervical cancer using HPV testing, alone or in combination with cytology, in women younger than age 30 years. **Grade D**

What do the grades mean?

Grade	Definition
A	The USPSTF recommends the service. There is high certainty that the net benefit is substantial.
B	The USPSTF recommends the service. There is high certainty that the net benefit is moderate or there is moderate certainty that the net benefit is moderate to substantial.
C	*Note: The following statement is undergoing revision.* Clinicians may provide this service to selected patients depending on individual circumstances. However, for most individuals without signs or symptoms there is likely to be only a small benefit from this service.
D	The USPSTF recommends against the service. There is moderate or high certainty that the service has no net benefit or that the harms outweigh the benefits.

1. Screening for Cervical Cancer, Topic Page. March 2012. U.S. Preventive Services Task Force. http://www.uspreventiveservicestaskforce.org/uspstf/uspscerv.htm

Clinical Summary of U.S. Preventive Services Task Force Recommendation

Population	Women ages 21 to 65	Women ages 30 to 65	Women younger than age 21	Women older than age 65 who have had adequate prior screening and are not high risk	Women after hysterectomy with removal of the cervix and with no history of high-grade precancer or cervical cancer	Women younger than age 30
Recommendation	Screen with cytology (Pap smear) every 3 years. Grade: A	Screen with cytology every 3 years or co-testing (cytology/HPV testing) every 5 years. Grade: A	Do not screen. Grade: D	Do not screen. Grade: D	Do not screen. Grade: D	Do not screen with HPV testing (alone or with cytology). Grade: D
Risk Assessment	Human papillomavirus (HPV) infection is associated with nearly all cases of cervical cancer. Other factors that put a woman at increased risk of cervical cancer include HIV infection, a compromised immune system, in utero exposure to diethylstilbestrol, and previous treatment of a high-grade precancerous lesion or cervical cancer.					
Screening Tests	Screening women ages 21 to 65 years every 3 years with cytology provides a reasonable balance between benefits and harms. Screening with cytology more often than every 3 years confers little additional benefit, with large increases in harms. HPV testing combined with cytology (co-testing) every 5 years in women ages 30 to 65 years offers a comparable balance of benefits and harms, and is therefore a reasonable alternative for women in this age group who would prefer to extend the screening interval.					
Timing of Screening	Screening earlier than age 21 years, regardless of sexual history, leads to more harms than benefits. Clinicians and patients should base the decision to end screening on whether the patient meets the criteria for adequate prior testing and appropriate follow-up, per established guidelines.					
Interventions	Screening aims to identify high-grade precancerous cervical lesions to prevent development of cervical cancer and early-stage asymptomatic invasive cervical cancer. High-grade lesions may be treated with ablative and excisional therapies, including cryotherapy, laser ablation, loop excision, and cold knife conization. Early-stage cervical cancer may be treated with surgery (hysterectomy) or chemoradiation.					
Balance of Harms and Benefits	The benefits of screening with cytology every 3 years substantially outweigh the harms.	The benefits of screening with co-testing (cytology/HPV testing) every 5 years outweigh the harms.	The harms of screening earlier than age 21 years outweigh the benefits.	The benefits of screening after age 65 years do not outweigh the potential harms.	The harms of screening after hysterectomy outweigh the benefits.	The potential harms of screening with HPV testing (alone or with cytology) outweigh the potential benefits.

Screening for Cervical Cancer: Clinical Summary of U.S. Preventive Services Task Force Recommendation. AHRQ Publication No. 1 1-05156-EF-3, March 2012.
http://www.uspreventiveservicestaskforce.org/uspstf11/cervcancer/cervcancersum.htm
More resources including the evidence synthesis, decision analysis and a consumer fact sheet for patients can be found on the USPSTF website (http://www.uspreventiveservicestaskforce.org/uspstf/uspscerv.htm). To view the ACS recommendation statement, visit http://www.cancer.org/Cancer/news/News/new-screening-guidelines-for-cervical-cancer.

4.2.2.5 WHO

WHO is the World Health Organization an agency of the United Nations.

4.2.2.6 2012 TBS Updates

2012 Updated Consensus Guidelines for the Management of Abnormal Cervical Cancer Screening Tests and Cancer Precursors

L. Stewart Massad, MD, Mark H. Einstein, MD, Warner K. Huh, MD, Hormuzd A. Katki, PhD, Walter K. Kinney, MD, Mark Schiffman, MD, Diane Solomon, MD, Nicolas Wentzensen, MD, and Herschel W. Lawson, MD, for the 2012 ASCCP Consensus Guidelines Conference

From Washington University School of Medicine, St. Louis, Missouri; Albert Einstein College of Medicine, New York, New York; University of Alabama School of Medicine, Birmingham, Alabama; Division of Cancer Epidemiology and Genetics and Division of Cancer Prevention, National Cancer Institute, Bethesda, Maryland; The Permanente Medical Group, Sacramento, California; and Emory University School of Medicine, Atlanta, Georgia

■ **ABSTRACT:** A group of 47 experts representing 23 professional societies, national and international health organizations, and federal agencies met in Bethesda, MD, September 14 15, 2012, to revise the 2006 American Society for Colposcopy and Cervical Pathology Consensus Guidelines. The group's goal was to provide revised evidence-based consensus guidelines for managing women with abnormal cervical cancer screening tests, cervical intraepithelial neoplasia (CIN) and adenocarcinoma in situ (AIS) following adoption of cervical cancer screening guidelines incorporating longer screening intervals and co-testing. In addition to literature review, data from almost 1.4 million women in the Kaiser Permanente Northern California Medical Care Plan provided evidence on risk after abnormal tests. Where data were available, guidelines prescribed similar management for women with similar risks for CIN 3, AIS, and cancer. Most prior guidelines were reaffirmed. Examples of updates include: Human papillomavirus negative atypical squamous cells of undetermined significance results are followed with co-testing at 3 years before return to routine screening and are not sufficient for exiting women from screening at age 65 years; women aged 21 24 years need less invasive management, especially for minor abnormalities; postcolposcopy management strategies incorporate co-testing; endocervical sampling reported as CIN 1 should be managed as CIN 1; unsatisfactory cytology should be repeated in most circumstances, even when HPV results from co-testing are known, while most cases of negative cytology with absent or insufficient endocervical cells or transformation zone component can be managed without intensive follow-up. ■

These guidelines are being published simultaneously in *Obstetrics & Gynecology* and the *Journal of Lower Genital Tract Disease*. The complete algorithms are published in the *Journal of Lower Genital Tract Disease* and are also available on the web site of the American Society for Colposcopy and Cervical Pathology (http://www.asccp.org/).

The contents of this article are solely the responsibility of the authors and do not necessarily represent the official views of the National Institutes of Health or U.S. federal government.

Corresponding author: L. Stewart Massad, MD Division of Gynecologic Oncology, Washington University School of Medicine, 4911 Barnes-Jewish Hospital Plaza, St. Louis, MO 63110; e-mail: massadl@wudosis.wustl.edu

Financial Disclosure

Dr. Massad has served as an expert witness. Dr. Huh has served as a consultant to Roche. Dr. Schiffman has researched reagents for Qiagen and Roche. The other authors did not report any potential conflicts of interest.

Journal of Lower Genital Tract Disease, Volume 17, Number 5, 2013, S1–S27

By 2001, revised Bethesda system terminology for reporting cervical cytology results and the availability of findings from a recent randomized trial of strategies for managing minor cervical cytologic abnormalities had created the need for a standard approach to managing women with abnormal cervical cytology and cervical cancer precursors (1–3). In response, the American Society for Colposcopy and Cervical Pathology (ASCCP) initiated a process that developed comprehensive, evidence-based consensus guidelines to aid clinicians in managing women with abnormal cervical cytology, cervical intraepithelial neoplasia (CIN), and adenocarcinoma in situ (AIS) (4, 5). Although those guidelines became the standard for managing women with abnormal cervical cytology and cancer precursors, the need for revisions became apparent. A second consensus conference in 2006 aligned management of minor cytologic abnormalities and CIN 1, incorporated follow-up results of the ASCUS-LSIL Triage Study (ALTS), identified strategies for management of positive human papillomavirus (HPV) DNA tests, and established guidelines for management of adolescents and young women (6, 7).

As updated in 2001, the Bethesda System also defined terminology for cytologic specimen adequacy, and ASCCP developed management guidelines for women with unsatisfactory cytology results and for those with negative results but limited endocervical/transformation zone (EC/TZ) component (8). These guidelines were updated in 2008 (9) but were not validated by a national consensus conference.

Previous guidelines remain valid, but knowledge has advanced. Screening has changed. In 2012, national organizations published guidelines embracing longer screening intervals and a later age to start screening (10, 11). Co-testing with cytology and HPV testing at 5-year intervals is now the preferred or acceptable strategy for cervical cancer screening for women aged 30–64 years (10, 11). Clinicians should benefit from guidance on how to incorporate co-testing into management of women with cervical abnormalities.

In addition, new evidence to guide decisions about management of abnormal screening tests and CIN and AIS emerged in 2012 from analyses of the large clinical database at the Kaiser Permanente Northern California Medical Care Plan (KPNC), conducted in collaboration with scientists from the National Cancer Institute (NCI) (12). This new evidence fills gaps in the 2006 guidelines. For example, prior management guidelines relied heavily on data from ALTS, which provided evidence on initial management of women with minor cytologic abnormalities. Results were extrapolated to provide guidelines on management of women with more severe cytologic abnormalities and post-colposcopy follow-up. The newer evidence from KPNC analyses allows validation or modification of prior guidelines in specific areas. The size of the KPNC database also allows age-based stratification of data for some types of abnormalities. While these observational data from a single U.S. region may limit generalizability and the lack of follow-up beyond 8 years may limit long-term risk estimates, publication of comparable analyses from similarly large databases soon is unlikely.

Finally, additional data have emerged in specific areas. Human papillomavirus genotyping tests have been approved; these have been recommended as an option for specific clinical scenarios to guide triage to colposcopy. More information is also available to guide management of women with unsatisfactory cytology.

In response, ASCCP conducted a consensus process to update the management of abnormal co-testing results and cytology with specimen adequacy limitations, the initial management of abnormal screening test results, options for postcolposcopy management, management of women aged 21–24 years, and other issues. This report details the consensus guidelines developed through this process.

METHODS

The process for the 2012 consensus guidelines was similar to that for the previous guidelines (4–7). Initially the ASCCP Practice Committee defined questions for the 2012 consensus process. A steering committee of nationally recognized experts in cervical cancer prevention was nominated and canvassed for additional questions. At the March 2012 ASCCP Biennial Scientific Meeting, conference attendees presented suggestions for guidelines review. Organizations that participated in the 2006 guidelines development process were solicited to nominate representatives to the revision process and also were asked to identify questions for review. Participants and participating organizations are listed in Appendix A.

A multifaceted process was used to evaluate the evidence and resolve identified issues. Five working groups were created, chaired by steering committee members and including delegates from participating organizations. For some working groups, the MEDLINE database was queried using relevant key words for English-language articles published after 2005, the date of the last consensus conference review (see Appendix 1, available online at http://links.lww.com/LGT/A9). Potentially relevant abstracts from identified articles were reviewed. Reports were rated according to the strength and quality of relevant evidence.

Other working groups focused on analyses of outcomes risk from a database of 1.4 million women cared for at KPNC and followed from January 1, 2003 to December 31, 2010. The primary outcome of interest in these analyses was CIN 3+ (CIN 3, AIS, and cancer). Cancer was used as an outcome when risk was high and CIN 2+ (CIN 3+ and

CIN 2) was used when the number of CIN 3+ events was low. Applying the concepts of "similar management for similar risks," risks were benchmarked to those for accepted management strategies. Since delegates considered zero cancer risk unattainable and CIN 3+ a reasonable proxy for cancer risk, acceptable risks were considered to be those approximating CIN 3+ risk 3 years after negative cytology or 5 years after negative co-testing. In brief, immediate colposcopy was recommended when the 5-year risk of CIN 3+ in the KPNC cohort exceeded 5%, a 6-month to 12-month return for risk of 2–5%, a 3-year return for risk of 0.1–2%, and a 5-year return interval for risk comparable to co-testing in women without a history of abnormality, or 0.1%. (12).

Draft guidelines developed by the working groups were posted to the ASCCP web site, and comments were solicited from collaborating organizations and the public. Draft guidelines revised in light of public comments were presented to a consensus conference convened September 14–15, 2012, at the Natcher Conference Center on the campus of the National Institutes of Health in Bethesda, MD. Draft guidelines and supporting evidence were presented, discussed, revised as needed, and adopted by at least 66% of voting delegates using electronic voting devices.

The terminology used in the updated guidelines is similar to prior versions, and the two-part rating system is the same (Table 1). Ratings are given in parentheses throughout the guidelines. The terms *recommended, preferred, acceptable, and unacceptable* are used in the guidelines to describe various interventions. A new term, "*not recommended*," was added to describe management strategies with weak evidence against their use but only marginal risk for adverse consequences. The strength rating of a recommendation was based on the quality of evidence supporting it but incorporated other factors, including potential for harm if an intervention did not occur and potential complications from a given intervention.

For cytologic classification and assessment of cytology specimen adequacy, the 2001 Bethesda System was used (1). For histologic classification, a two-tiered system was employed. Low-grade lesions were termed CIN 1 and high-grade lesions were termed CIN 2 or CIN 3. Some pathologists do not distinguish CIN 2 from CIN 3, and these undifferentiated high-grade lesions are termed CIN 2,3.

Table 1. Rating the Recommendations

Strength of recommendation*	
A	Good evidence for efficacy and substantial clinical benefit support recommendation for use.
B	Moderate evidence for efficacy or only limited clinical benefit supports recommendation for use.
C	Evidence for efficacy is insufficient to support a recommendation for or against use, but recommendations may be made on other grounds.
D	Moderate evidence for lack of efficacy or for adverse outcome supports a recommendation against use.
E	Good evidence for lack of efficacy or for adverse outcome supports a recommendation against use.
Quality of evidence*	
I	Evidence from at least one randomized, controlled trial.
II	Evidence from at least one clinical trial without randomization, from cohort or case-controlled analytic studies (preferably from more than one center), or from multiple time-series studies, or dramatic results from uncontrolled experiments.
III	Evidence from opinions of respected authorities based on clinical experience, descriptive studies, or reports of expert committees.
Terminology used for recommendations†	
Recommended	Good data to support use when only one option is available.
Preferred	Option is the best (or one of the best) when there are multiple options.
Acceptable	One of multiple options when there is either data indicating that another approach is superior or when there are no data to favor any single option.
Not recommended	Weak evidence against use and marginal risk for adverse consequences.
Unacceptable	Good evidence against use.

* Modified from Gross PA, Barrett TL, Dellinger EP, et al. Purpose of quality standards for infectious diseases. Infectious Diseases Society of America. Clin Infect Dis 1994;18:421. 98. Kish MA. Guide to development of practice guidelines. Clin Infect Dis 2001;32:851–4.
† The assignment of these terms represents an opinion ratified by vote during the 2012 consensus conference.

GUIDING PRINCIPLES

Participants at the consensus conference affirmed that the 2006 ASCCP guidelines for the management of abnormal cervical cancer screening tests (6) and CIN or AIS (7) remain valid, with the exception of the specific areas reviewed. Those earlier guidelines have been combined with current revisions in this document to provide comprehensive recommendations for management. Changes are summarized in Box 1.

Cervical cancer prevention is a process with benefits and harms. Risk cannot be reduced to zero with currently available strategies, and attempts to achieve zero risk may result in unbalanced harms, including overtreatment. As noted in a 2011 consensus conference on cervical cancer screening (10), optimal prevention strategies should identify those HPV-related abnormalities likely to progress to invasive cancers while avoiding destructive treatment of abnormalities not destined to become cancerous. Adopted management strategies provide what participants considered an acceptable level of risk of failing to detect high-grade neoplasia or cancer in a given clinical situation. Where data were available,

Box 1. Essential Changes From Prior Management Guidelines*

- Cytology reported as negative but lacking endocervical cells can be managed without early repeat.
- CIN 1 on endocervical curettage should be managed as CIN 1, not as a positive ECC.
- Cytology reported as unsatisfactory requires repeat even if HPV negative.
- Genotyping triages HPV-positive women with HPV type 16 or type 18 to earlier colposcopy only after negative cytology; colposcopy is indicated for all women with HPV and ASC-US, regardless of genotyping result.
- For ASC-US cytology, immediate colposcopy is not an option. The serial cytology option for ASC-US incorporates cytology at 12 months, not 6 months and 12 months, and then if negative, cytology every 3 years.
- HPV-negative and ASC-US results should be followed with co-testing at 3 years rather than 5 years.
- HPV-negative and ASC-US results are insufficient to allow exit from screening at age 65 years.
- The pathway to long-term follow-up of treated and untreated CIN 2+ is more clearly defined by incorporating co-testing.
- More strategies incorporate co-testing to reduce follow-up visits. Pap-only strategies are now limited to women younger than 30 years, but co-testing is expanded even to women younger than 30 years in some circumstances. Women aged 21-24 years are managed conservatively.

CIN, cervical intraepithelial neoplasia; ECC, endocervical curettage; HPV, human papillomavirus; ASC-US, atypical squamous cells of undetermined significance.
**Prior management guidelines were from the "2006 Consensus Guidelines for the Management of Women With Abnormal Cervical Screening Tests" (6). Prior guidelines not changed were retained.*

similar management strategies were prescribed for similar levels of risk (12, 13). Guidelines cannot be developed for all situations. Clinical judgment should always be applied when applying guidelines to individual patients. This is especially true for guidelines based on less robust evidence.

In 2012, the Lower Anogenital Squamous Terminology (LAST) Project created new terminology for HPV-related lesions of the lower genital tract (14). However, delegates to the current consensus process determined that this classification does not yet have a sufficiently robust outcomes evidence base to allow elucidation of risk-based management guidelines (see Box 2).

Algorithms detailing the different management recommendations are available at the ASCCP web site (www.asccp.org/consensus2012). A glossary of terms used in the guidelines is in Appendix B.

In the 2006 ASCCP guidelines,(6,7) several pathways concluded by returning women to "routine screening." This term was not defined, but in 2006, screening guidelines prescribed cytology at shorter intervals than now recommended. Current 2011 screening guidelines recommend either 3-year cytology intervals or, for women aged 30–64 years, 5-year co-testing intervals (10, 11). These multi-year intervals are safe only when risk for the development of CIN 3+ during the years between testing is low (10, 11). For example, women aged 30–64 years with a negative co-test have a 5-year risk of CIN 3+ of only 8/10,000 (12). Although this low level of risk can be achieved among women with negative screening histories, for those with some abnormalities, risk for CIN 3+ remains elevated for years, even after treatment and even after initial negative surveillance. After some abnormalities, current follow-up data are insufficient to define a pathway to return to 5-year routine screening intervals because even with treatment, risk does not fall to a level consistent with 5-year retesting.

When, how, and even whether to perform endocervical sampling is controversial. Endocervical brushing has better sensitivity than curettage with similar specificity, better tolerance, and fewer insufficient samples, although grading may be more difficult because stroma is rarely sampled with brushing (15, 16). Either is acceptable for endocervical sampling. In 2006, working groups assessing management of cytology reported as atypical squamous cells of undetermined significance (ASC-US) and low-grade squamous intraepithelial lesions (LSIL) defined indications for endocervical sampling, guidance that should be valid for women with cytology results of atypical squamous cells, cannot exclude high-grade squamous intraepithelial lesions (ASC-H) and high-grade squamous intraepithelial lesions (HSIL) as well.

Management strategies incorporate HPV testing based on studies using validated HPV assays. Management based on results of HPV tests not similarly validated may not result in intended outcomes and may risk patient harm. These guidelines are intended for use only with HPV tests that have been analytically and clinically validated with proven acceptable reproducibility, clinical sensitivity, specificity, and positive and negative predictive values for cervical cancer and verified precancer (CIN 2+), as documented by U.S. Food and Drug Administration (FDA) licensing and approval or publication in peer-reviewed scientific literature. Testing should be restricted to high-risk (oncogenic) HPV types (mainly 16, 18, 31, 33, 35, 39, 45, 51, 52, 56, 58, and 59), and in these guidelines "HPV testing" refers only to testing for high-risk

Box 2.

A recent consensus conference (the Lower Anogenital Squamous Terminology [LAST] Project convened by the College of American Pathologists and the American Society for Colposcopy and Cervical Pathology) adopted a two-tier terminology that incorporates ancillary tests and other criteria to distinguish indeterminate lesions as high grade or low grade. Until a comprehensive evidence review and consensus guidelines development process can be conducted, histopathology results reported as low-grade squamous intraepithelial lesions (LSIL) should be managed as cervical intraepithelial neoplasia (CIN) 1 and those reported as high-grade squamous intraepithelial lesions (HSIL) should be managed as CIN 2,3 (14).

(oncogenic) HPV types. Testing for low-risk (nononcogenic) HPV types has no role in the evaluation of women with abnormal cervical cytologic results.

Both ablation and excision effectively treat CIN. Randomized trials comparing different modalities show similar efficacy (17–20). Efficacy rates range from 90% to 95%, and most failures occur within 2 years (21), although cancers can develop up to 20 years after treatment (22). Margin status is a convenient predictor of recurrence and a traditional risk marker, although it does not appear to be an independent risk factor (23, 24). Nonsurgical therapies, including topical agents and therapeutic vaccines, remain investigational.

A wide variety of follow-up approaches have been described for women treated for CIN, incorporating cytology, HPV testing, and colposcopy alone or in combination at intervals from 3 months to annually. HPV testing is more sensitive but less specific than cytology in posttreatment follow-up and it may result in earlier diagnosis of persistent or recurrent disease (25). Protocols for follow-up after treatment of CIN have not been evaluated as primary interventions in randomized trials.

Under the 2011 screening guidelines, women followed after positive HPV tests but negative cytology were referred to colposcopy only if they had LSIL or more severe cytology or a positive HPV test during surveillance co-testing (10). However, only 0.04% of all women aged 30-64 years in the KPNC database had HPV-negative ASC-US after an HPV-positive, cytology negative result (26), so referring these women for colposcopy will burden care systems minimally. Thus, for simplicity, current guidelines recommend colposcopy for any positive HPV test or any abnormal cytology during follow-up.

Studies of the effect of treatment on future pregnancy are conflicting, although many indicate an approximately two-fold increase in preterm delivery risk (27–29). Although not proven, this is presumed to result from deficient cervical stroma, and risk appears to increase with the volume and number of excisions (30). However, many studies were done in countries where loop excisions are performed with larger loop sizes and deeper excisions than most U.S. clinicians employ. Studies linking ablative treatments to preterm delivery are even more limited and conflicting. Women with CIN may be at increased risk for preterm delivery even when untreated. Nevertheless, because pregnancy complications can be devastating, the potential benefits of treatment should be balanced against the risk to future pregnancies. Young women have high regression rates for cervical disease and low cancer risk (31–33). The term "young women" indicates those who after counseling by their clinicians consider risk to future pregnancies from treating cervical abnormalities to outweigh risk for cancer during observation of those abnormalities. No specific age threshold is intended.

In 2006, guidelines recommended less aggressive management for adolescents with cervical abnormalities (6, 34), but these are now moot because the 2011 screening guidelines recommend not screening adolescents (10, 11). Delegates to the 2012 consensus conference considered less intensive management for other young women with abnormal cytology. Cervical cancer risk remains low through age 25 years (35), HPV is common (36), and lesions often regress (37). The annual incidence of cervical cancer among U.S. women aged 21–24 years is 1.4/100,000, and almost 55,000 cytology tests must be obtained for every cervical cancer diagnosed in this age group (35). This level of risk is 10-fold higher than risk in adolescents and appears to be high enough to justify screening yet is low enough to allow observation for minor cytologic abnormalities. Guidelines for women aged 21–24 years can be extrapolated to adolescents inadvertently screened.

Interventions for abnormal screening tests and CIN or AIS have other consequences that are not easily measurable. Women experience emotional distress when receiving abnormal cytology and HPV test results, when having colposcopy even when findings are normal, and when undergoing cervical treatment. Emotional distress is usually prompted by uncertainty and anticipation of the unknown (38). Many management strategies incorporate follow-up with HPV testing, which can elicit feelings of stigma and shame when positive despite the near-ubiquitous frequency of HPV infection (39, 40). The anxiety and time required for visits to manage abnormal cytology can adversely affect relationships, work-related and school activities, and family matters (41). These potential harms reinforce the concept that colposcopy and other interventions should be avoided when risk for CIN 3+ is low and when identified lesions are likely to resolve.

In the 2001 guidelines (4), separate recommendations for ASC-US management were developed for women infected with human immunodeficiency virus and other immunosuppressive conditions. Data review in 2006 eliminated these separate guidelines. Immunosuppressed women with abnormal results should be managed in the same manner as immunocompetent women.

Chapter 5
Global Cervical Cancer Screening

This chapter contains examples of distribution of cancer in the world, with emphasis on cervical cancer.

5.1 Worldwide Application of Cervical Cancer Screening

The purpose of cervical cancer screening among healthy – asymptomatic – women is to detect the presence of lesions that could be developed into cervical cancer, and to remove them; thus, providing cure from cancer. Ultimately, cervical cancer screening test is saving lives of women in fertile periods.

There are 2.4 billion women at risk for cervical cancer world-wide. Each of them needs anticancer screening at least once in 3 years. Implementation of such policy needs substantial societal investment. Not all societies, and particularly not all governments or private enterprises are ready to invest this money without an adequate return.

But, is this true? Is mass cervical cancer screening worldwide for saving women's lives an investment without the adequate return? Is it a myth or a reality? We thought this is a question that warrants investment of resources. In this chapter we will present excerpts from our research and the summary of data collected and evaluated.

The first problem we had to solve was the valuation of a woman's life. What is the value of a woman's life? Obviously it is different among countries, states, among societies and inside each society.

First, we rejected many available data based on calculating differences between Pap test price and the cost of treating women who were missed by Pap test or never have taken one. This is not good approach because then, women who will be left to die will cost nothing, and the conclusion will be wrong. Another control group, the cost of treatment of symptomatic women, is full of confounding variables mostly depending on the site where this treatment is provided, the local philosophy of health care needs, affordability of women to participate, accessibility to health care

N. Markovic, O. Markovic, *What Every Woman Should Know about Cervical Cancer*, DOI 10.1007/978-94-017-7560-1_5

facilities and the scope of the help provided (surgery, radiation, chemotherapy, immunotherapy). This approach had to be rejected also.

Then, we decided for a completely different approach. We have tried to estimate this value using the International Monetary Fund (IMF) standard the Gross Domestic Product per Capita (GDP-PC; Sect. 5.3) assuming that one women can contribute to the GDP at least as much as ½ of a working active men, that one women at average will give birth to two children which can contribute to the wealth of the society as ¼ of a man. With these assumptions, the worth of a woman's life is at least equal, if not higher than the GDP per capita average value estimated per person in each specific state. It seemed that this approach is more realistic than the others.

Then the next part of the calculation was easy. How many women's lives can be saved with a wide campaign for cervical cancer screening? According to the US data, out 50,000,000 screened healthy women annually, 7.5 million was found Pap (+), 600,000 was diagnosed as HSIL, and 40,000 had lesions which were to be removed. This all in the country with about 100 million women at risk and the outreach of about 80 % At that time, Pap test cost in the US was $15.00 per test, and the GDP-PC was $52,000. A simple calculation could show that the saved money was more than four times the cost for this Pap test. The economic incentives were clear. But, how this calculation can be applied to other countries?

To answer this question we have surveyed the available literature and the plethora of information at the internet. The information collected was reviewed and confirmed for 57 countries. Details are presented in Sect. 6.5.2, article Economy of MPT.

The Survey questions included the total population, population of women at risk, expected number of cervical cancer screening under the scenario of one screening in 3 years, actual percent of cervical cancer screening, actual problem as measured by cervical cancer prevalence and mortality (local health statistics and WHO data), gross domestic product per capita (IMF data), and the cost of a proposed screening with the MarkPap test (BioSciCon's data) what is about $10.00 per test when integrated in a comprehensive mass cervical cancer screening in a country with established Strategy for fighting cervical cancer and network of professionals and institutions organized for this purpose.

In general, out of 2.4 billion women at risk, about 600,000 get cervical cancer annually and about 300,000 die per year. Only less than 20 % of population eligible for screening participates in regular programs; but, since 51 % is the turning point for reversal of negative trends, there is no chance that global epidemics of cervical cancer (note: cervical cancer prevalence and mortality trend is a curve rising for about 10 % annually, and population growth curve is less than 1.4 %) be prevented before the end of this century, unless some important changes are made on the global strategy for fighting cervical cancer.

Towards this goal, to change the global strategy, we devoted the next two chapters of our new edition.

Comparison among countries has revealed big differences of GDP-PC causing the value of woman's life to be estimated in a wide range between less than $1000 and more than $50,000. As much as this calculation seem speculative, it gives a solid base for assessment whether a preventive test, such as cervical cancer screening, is having economic incentives in addition to the social impact. Upon these calculations, a comprehensive cervical cancer screening including management of women with positive test (approximately $10.00 per test) is saving money to the countries with more than $10,000 GDP-PC. Other countries should seek additional funds to compensate for the cost if they need social benefit for their women. This is the point where World Health Organization, Global Health Initiative, churches and many charitable organizations and other social investors may change the outcome for women lives and the health and economic prospective of many countries with the GDP-PC less than $10.000.

Details are presented in Chap. 6, article Economy of MPT. Data in the table show that 9/11 African countries, 3/9 American, 9/15 Asian, 2/4 Australian, and 6/17 European contrives will need financial and other help, if MarkPap test is to be fully implemented, and if the New Strategy is to deliver the expected results. However, the bright sight is that the MarkPap test in this calculation is used as a comprehensive test with post-test management of women free of additional charges. The accuracy of MarkPap test could allow the health care providers to waive the cost of diagnosis and treatment of "missed" cases. This fact changes the financial balance significantly in favor of the comprehensive test combined with management of women after test.

We do not advertize MarkPap test. It could be any other biomarker with the same or similar characteristics, but we strongly recommend the utilization of IT technology, in particular, mobile phones, WiFi and Web-based networking to connect scattered points-of care with remote expert medical centers and to bring quality medical information to the network and further to each and every physician involved in prevention of cervical cancer programs.

For further reference:

1. GLOBOCAN (IARC) 2012
2. https://simple.wikipedia.ord/w/index.php?title=List_of__countries_by_GDP(PPP)_per_capita&printable, From the Internet on August_15_2015.
3. Countries selected for study review
4. Preliminary data on 57 selected countries.

5.2 Cervical Cancer Statistics - World

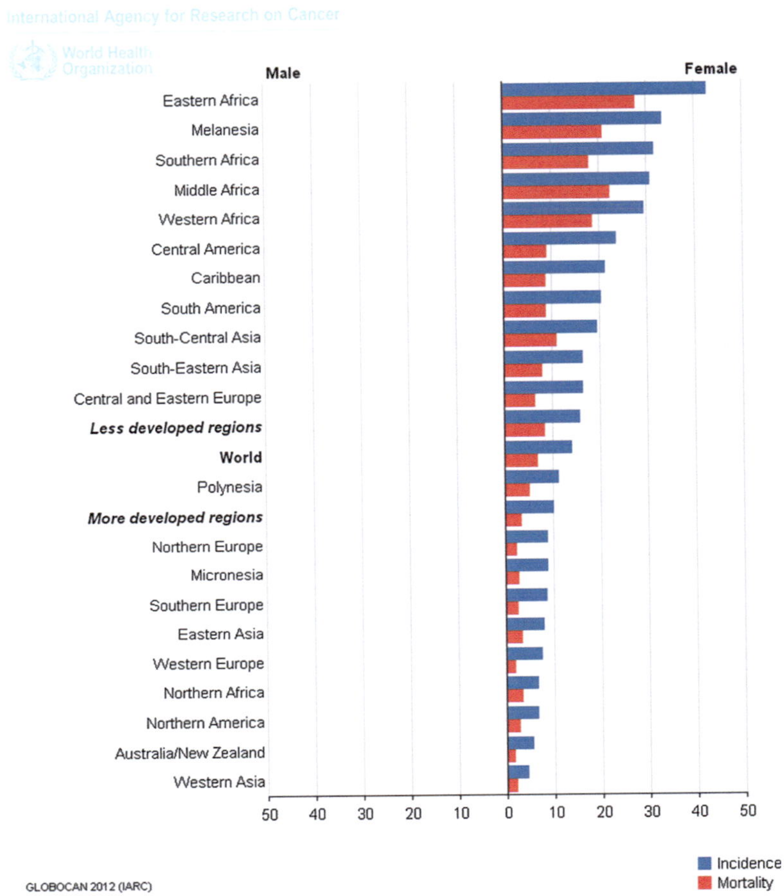

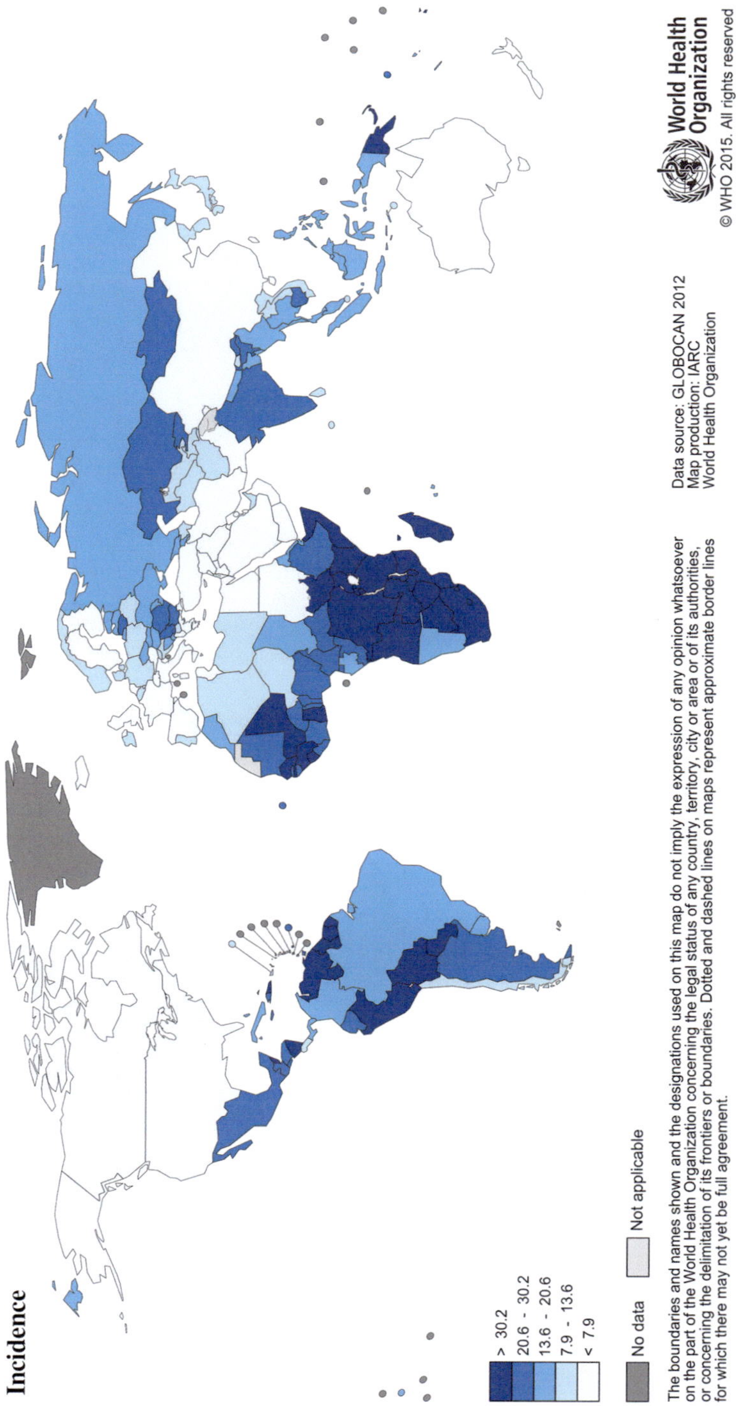
Incidence
> 30.2
20.6 - 30.2
13.6 - 20.6
7.9 - 13.6
< 7.9
No data
Not applicable
The boundaries and names shown and the designations used on this map do not imply the expression of any opinion whatsoever on the part of the World Health Organization concerning the legal status of any country, territory, city or area or of its authorities, or concerning the delimitation of its frontiers or boundaries. Dotted and dashed lines on maps represent approximate border lines for which there may not yet be full agreement.
Data source: GLOBOCAN 2012
Map production: IARC
World Health Organization
World Health Organization
© WHO 2015. All rights reserved

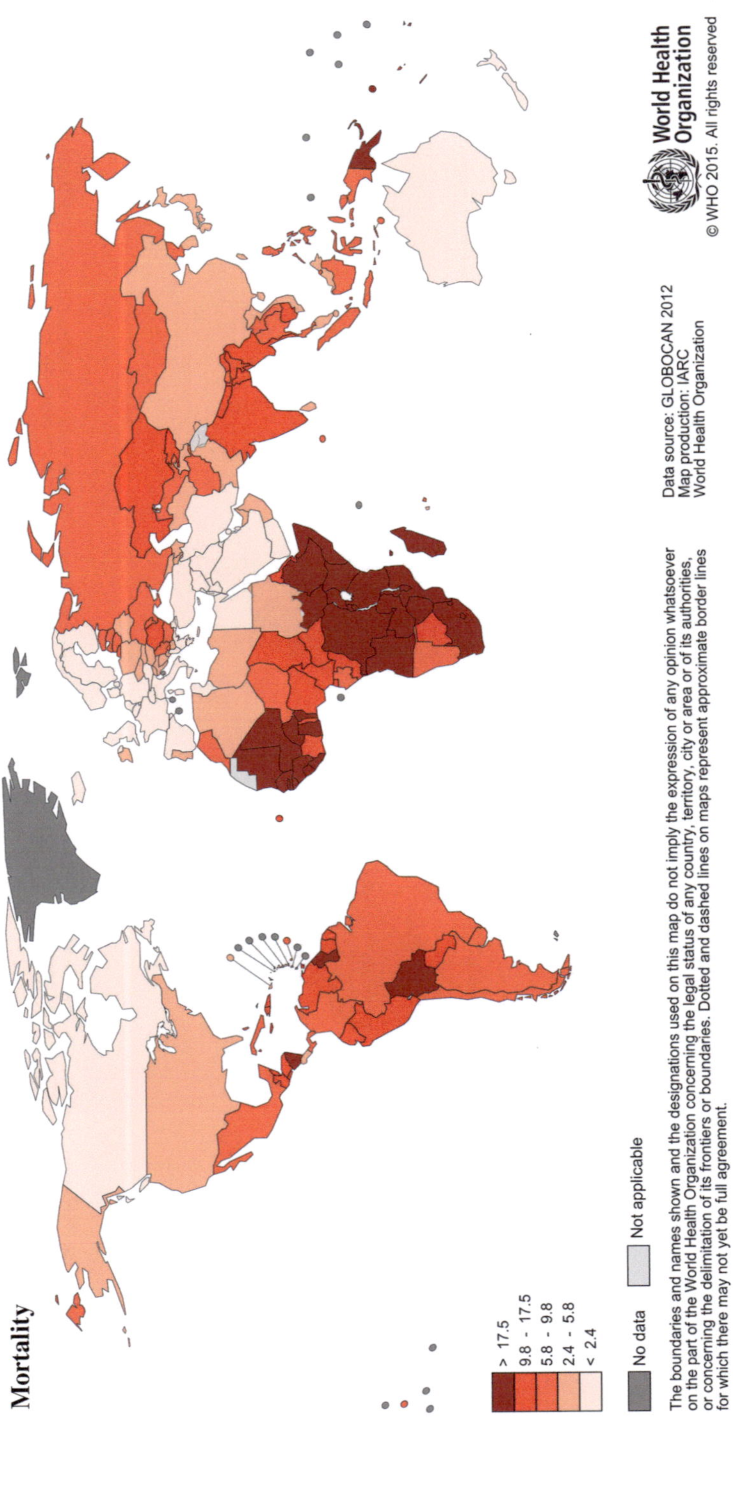
Mortality
> 17.5
9.8 - 17.5
5.8 - 9.8
2.4 - 5.8
< 2.4
No data
Not applicable
The boundaries and names shown and the designations used on this map do not imply the expression of any opinion whatsoever on the part of the World Health Organization concerning the legal status of any country, territory, city or area or of its authorities, or concerning the delimitation of its frontiers or boundaries. Dotted and dashed lines on maps represent approximate border lines for which there may not yet be full agreement.
Data source: GLOBOCAN 2012
Map production: IARC
World Health Organization
World Health Organization
© WHO 2015. All rights reserved

5.3 Preliminary Data on World Population: Health Demography

World Health Organization

Countries

Azerbaijan

Map

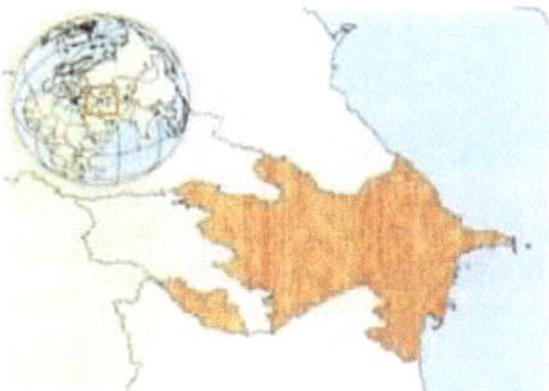

This map is an approximation of actual country borders.

Statistics

Total population (2013)	**9,413,000**
Gross national income per capita (PPP international $, 2013)	**16**
Life expectancy at birth m/f (years, 2013)	**70/75**
Probability of dying under five (per 1 000 live births, 0)	not available
Probability of dying between 15 and 60 years m/f (per 1 000 population, 2013)	**167/83**
Total expenditure on health per capita (Intl $, 2013)	**957**
Total expenditure on health as % of GDP (2013)	**5.6**

Latest data available from the Global Health Observatory

Contact information

The WHO Head of Country Office
Garakhanov, Dr Kamran

3, UN 50th Anniversary Street AZ-1001 - Baku, Azerbaijan

Telephone: +994 124 989888
Facsimile: +994124 989888 Ext 160
whoaze@euro.who.int

Country Office web site
Regional Office web site

Country profile   News and features

Health profile

Country statistics
Country profile on regional site
Country health profile
pdf

Mortality and burden of disease

Life tables
Tuberculosis
Malaria
pdf
Noncommunicable diseases
pdf

Nutrition

Child malnutrition
Nutrition

Risk factors

Alcohol
pdf
Road traffic injuries
pdf
Tobacco
pdf

World Health Organization

Countries

Benin

Map

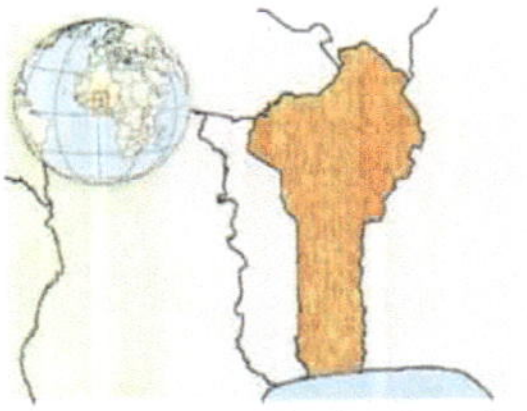

This map is an approximation of actual country borders.

Statistics

Total population (2013)	**10,323,000**
Gross national income per capita (PPP international $, 2013)	**1**
Life expectancy at birth m/f (years, 2013)	**57/60**
Probability of dying under five (per 1 000 live births, 0)	not available
Probability of dying between 15 and 60 years m/f (per 1 000 population, 2013)	**284/238**
Total expenditure on health per capita (Intl $, 2013)	**82**
Total expenditure on health as % of GDP (2013)	**4.6**

Latest data available from the Global Health Observatory

Contact information

Madame le Représentant de l'OMS par intérim
Nkurunziza, Dr Triphonie

01 BP 918 Cotonou, Benin

Telephone: +229 21301907
Facsimile: +229 21304208
afbjoms@wims.who.int

Country Office web site
Regional Office web site

Country profile News and features

Health profile

Country statistics
Country profile on regional site
Country health profile
pdf

WHO collaboration

Country cooperation strategy brief
pdf
Collaborating centres

Mortality and burden of disease

Life tables
Tuberculosis

Nutrition

Child malnutrition
Nutrition

Risk factors

Alcohol
pdf
Road traffic injuries
pdf
Tobacco
pdf

World Health Organization

Countries

Egypt

Map

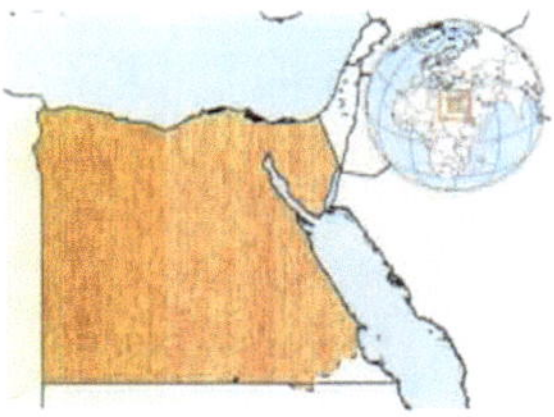

This map is an approximation of actual country borders.

Statistics

Total population (2013)	**82,056,000**
Gross national income per capita (PPP international $, 2013)	**10**
Life expectancy at birth m/f (years, 2013)	**69/74**
Probability of dying under five (per 1 000 live births, 0)	not available
Probability of dying between 15 and 60 years m/f (per 1 000 population, 2013)	**193/117**
Total expenditure on health per capita (Intl $, 2013)	**539**
Total expenditure on health as % of GDP (2013)	**5.1**

Latest data available from the Global Health Observatory

Contact information

The WHO Representative
Bekedam, Dr Hendrik Jan

PO Box No. 146 11516 - Cairo, Egypt

Telephone: +202 27957706
Facsimile: +202 27953756
emwroegy@who.int

Country Office web site
Regional Office web site

Country profile News and features

Health profile

Country statistics

Country health profile
pdf

WHO collaboration

Country cooperation strategy
pdf

Country cooperation strategy brief
pdf

Collaborating centres

Mortality and burden of disease

Life tables

Nutrition

Child malnutrition

Nutrition

Risk factors

Alcohol
pdf

Tobacco
pdf

World Health Organization

WHO African Region: Ethiopia

Countries

Ethiopia

Map

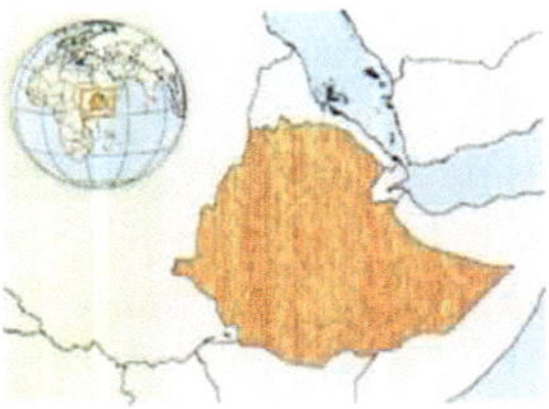

This map is an approximation of actual country borders.

Statistics

Total population (2012)	**91,729,000**
Gross national income per capita (PPP international $, 2012)	**1,110**
Life expectancy at birth m/f (years, 2012)	**62/65**
Probability of dying under five (per 1 000 live births, 2012)	**68**
Probability of dying between 15 and 60 years m/f (per 1 000 population, 2012)	**250/212**
Total expenditure on health per capita (Intl $, 2012)	**44**
Total expenditure on health as % of GDP (2012)	**3.8**

Latest data available from the Global Health Observatory

Contact information

The WHO Representative
Mpele Kilebou, Dr Pierre

PO Box 3069 Addis-Ababa, Ethiopia

Telephone: +251 115 445181
Facsimile: +251 115 514037
afwcoet@who.int

Country Office web site
Regional Office web site

Country profile News and features

Health profile

Country statistics
Country profile on regional site
Country health profile
pdf

WHO collaboration

Country cooperation strategy
pdf
Country cooperation strategy brief
pdf

Mortality and burden of disease

Nutrition

Child malnutrition
Nutrition

Risk factors

Alcohol
pdf
Tobacco
pdf

World Health Organization

Countries

Kenya

Map

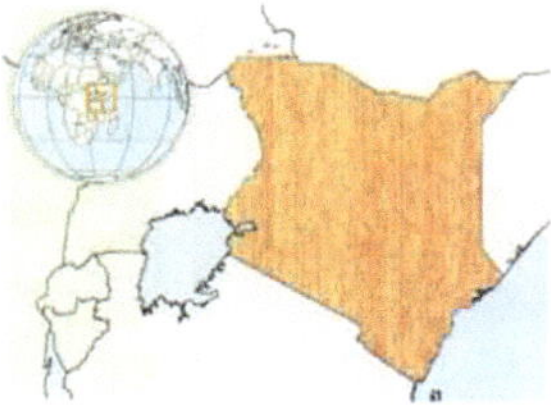

This map is an approximation of actual country borders.

Statistics

Total population (2013)	**44,354,000**
Gross national income per capita (PPP international $, 2013)	**2**
Life expectancy at birth m/f (years, 2013)	**60/63**
Probability of dying under five (per 1 000 live births, 0)	not available
Probability of dying between 15 and 60 years m/f (per 1 000 population, 2013)	**299/250**
Total expenditure on health per capita (Intl $, 2013)	**101**
Total expenditure on health as % of GDP (2013)	**4.5**

Latest data available from the Global Health Observatory

Contact information

The WHO Representative
Mandlhate, Dr Custodia

45335 Nairobi, Kenya

Telephone: +254 20 2717902
Facsimile: n/a
afkenwr@who.int

Country Office web site
Regional Office web site

Country profile News and features

Health profile

Country statistics
Country profile on regional site
Country health profile pdf

WHO collaboration

Country cooperation strategy pdf
Country cooperation strategy brief pdf
Collaborating centres

Mortality and burden of disease

Nutrition

Child malnutrition
Nutrition

Risk factors

Alcohol pdf
Tobacco pdf

World Health Organization

Countries

Nigeria

Map

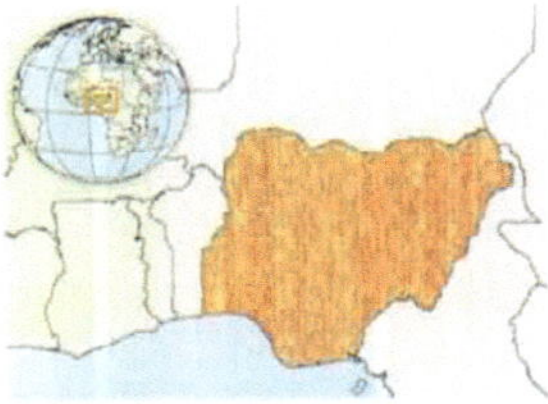

This map is an approximation of actual country borders.

Statistics

Total population (2013)	**173,615,000**
Gross national income per capita (PPP international $, 2013)	**5**
Life expectancy at birth m/f (years, 2013)	**54/55**
Probability of dying under five (per 1 000 live births, 0)	not available
Probability of dying between 15 and 60 years m/f (per 1 000 population, 2013)	**357/325**
Total expenditure on health per capita (Intl $, 2013)	**207**
Total expenditure on health as % of GDP (2013)	**3.7**

Latest data available from the Global Health Observatory

Contact information

The WHO Representative
Vaz, Dr Rui Miguel

PMB 2851 Garki 900001 - Abuja, FCT, Nigeria

Telephone: +234 8077 590066
Facsimile: +234 8077 590067
afwcongregistrystaff@who.int

Country Office web site
Regional Office web site

Country profile News and features

Health profile

Country statistics
Country profile on regional site
Country health profile
pdf

WHO collaboration

Country cooperation strategy
pdf
Country cooperation strategy brief
pdf
Collaborating centres

Mortality and burden of disease

Nutrition

Child malnutrition
Nutrition

Risk factors

Alcohol
pdf
Tobacco
pdf

World Health Organization

Countries

South Africa

Map

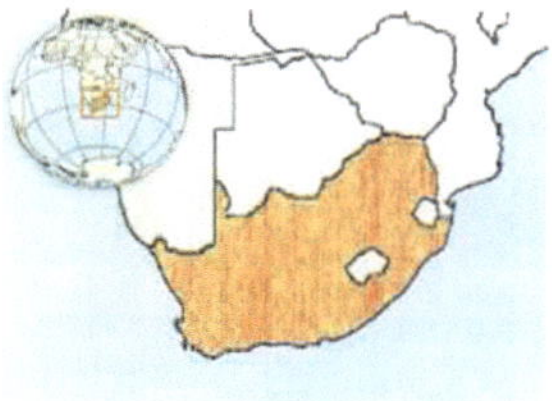

This map is an approximation of actual country borders.

Statistics

Total population (2013)	**52,776,000**
Gross national income per capita (PPP international $, 2013)	**12**
Life expectancy at birth m/f (years, 2013)	**57/64**
Probability of dying under five (per 1 000 live births, 0)	not available
Probability of dying between 15 and 60 years m/f (per 1 000 population, 2013)	**441/320**
Total expenditure on health per capita (Intl $, 2013)	**1,121**
Total expenditure on health as % of GDP (2013)	**8.9**

Latest data available from the Global Health Observatory

Contact information

The WHO Representative
Barber, Dr Sarah Louise

PO Box 13113 Tramshed 0126 - Pretoria, South Africa

Telephone: +27 12 3057709
Facsimile: +27 12 3057729
afwcozawr@who.int

Country Office web site
Regional Office web site

Country profile News and features

Health profile

Country statistics

Country profile on regional site

Country health profile
pdf

WHO collaboration

Country cooperation strategy
pdf

Country cooperation strategy brief
pdf

Collaborating centres

Mortality and burden of disease

Nutrition

Child malnutrition

Nutrition

Risk factors

Alcohol
pdf

Road traffic injuries
pdf

Tobacco
pdf

World Health Organization

Countries

Sri Lanka

Map

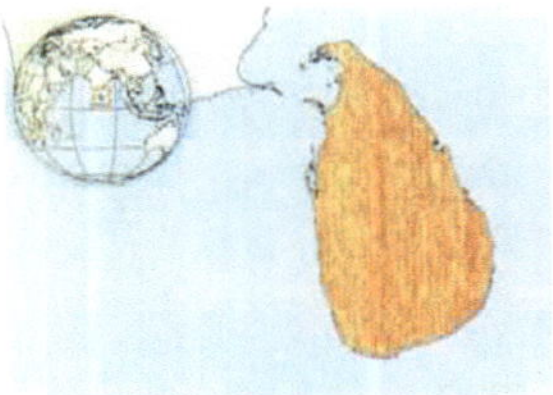

This map is an approximation of actual country borders.

Statistics

Total population (2013)	**21,273,000**
Gross national income per capita (PPP international $, 2013)	**9**
Life expectancy at birth m/f (years, 2013)	**72/78**
Probability of dying under five (per 1 000 live births, 0)	not available
Probability of dying between 15 and 60 years m/f (per 1 000 population, 2013)	**184/75**
Total expenditure on health per capita (Intl $, 2013)	**304**
Total expenditure on health as % of GDP (2013)	**3.2**

Latest data available from the Global Health Observatory

Contact information

The WHO Representative
Kumaresan, Dr Jacob

PO Box 780 Colombo 07, Sri Lanka

Telephone: +94 11 2379191
Facsimile: +94 11 2502845
srlregistry@searo.who.int

Country Office web site
Regional Office web site

Country profile News and features

Health profile

Country statistics

Country health profile
pdf

WHO collaboration

Country cooperation strategy
pdf

Country cooperation strategy brief
pdf

Collaborating centres

Mortality and burden of disease

Life tables

Nutrition

Child malnutrition

Nutrition

Risk factors

Alcohol
pdf

Road traffic injuries
pdf

Tobacco
pdf

World Health Organization

Countries

United Republic of Tanzania

Map

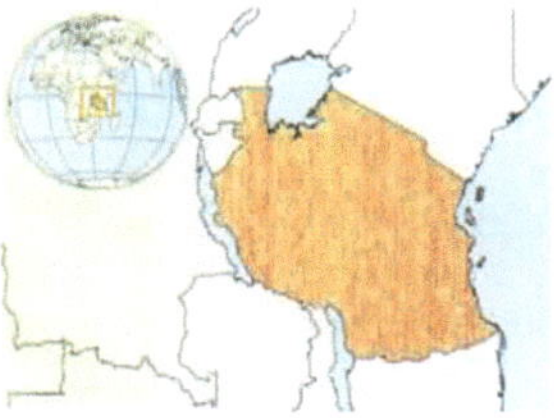

This map is an approximation of actual country borders.

Statistics

Total population (2013)	**49,253,000**
Gross national income per capita (PPP international $, 2013)	**1**
Life expectancy at birth m/f (years, 2013)	**61/65**
Probability of dying under five (per 1 000 live births, 0)	not available
Probability of dying between 15 and 60 years m/f (per 1 000 population, 2013)	**314/244**
Total expenditure on health per capita (Intl $, 2013)	**126**
Total expenditure on health as % of GDP (2013)	**7.3**

Latest data available from the Global Health Observatory

Contact information

The WHO Representative
Chatora, Dr Rufaro

PO Box 9292 Dar es Salaam,
United Republic of Tanzania

Telephone: +255 22 2111718
Facsimile: +255 22 2113180
afwcotz@who.int

Country Office web site
Regional Office web site

Country profile News and features

Health profile

Country statistics
Country profile on regional site
Country health profile
pdf

WHO collaboration

Country cooperation strategy
pdf
Country cooperation strategy brief
pdf
Collaborating centres

Mortality and burden of disease

Nutrition

Child malnutrition
Nutrition

Risk factors

Alcohol
pdf
Road traffic injuries
pdf
Tobacco
pdf

World Health Organization

Countries

Uganda

Map

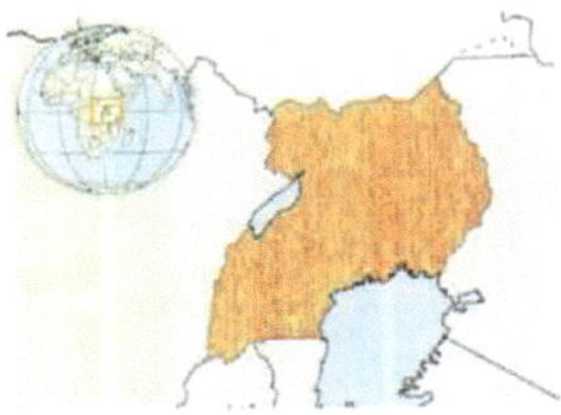

This map is an approximation of actual country borders.

Statistics

Total population (2013)	**37,579,000**
Gross national income per capita (PPP international $, 2013)	1
Life expectancy at birth m/f (years, 2013)	**57/61**
Probability of dying under five (per 1 000 live births, 0)	not available
Probability of dying between 15 and 60 years m/f (per 1 000 population, 2013)	**380/307**
Total expenditure on health per capita (Intl $, 2013)	**146**
Total expenditure on health as % of GDP (2013)	**9.8**

Latest data available from the Global Health Observatory

Contact information

The WHO Representative
Alemu, Dr Wondimagegnehu

PO Box 24578 Kampala, Uganda

Telephone: +256 414 335500
Facsimile: +256 414 335569
nyangomao@who.int

Country Office web site
Regional Office web site

Country profile News and features

Health profile

Country statistics
Country profile on regional site
Country health profile
pdf

WHO collaboration

Country cooperation strategy
pdf
Country cooperation strategy brief
pdf
Collaborating centres

Mortality and burden of disease

Nutrition

Child malnutrition
Nutrition

Risk factors

Alcohol
pdf
Tobacco
pdf

World Health Organization

Countries

Argentina

Map

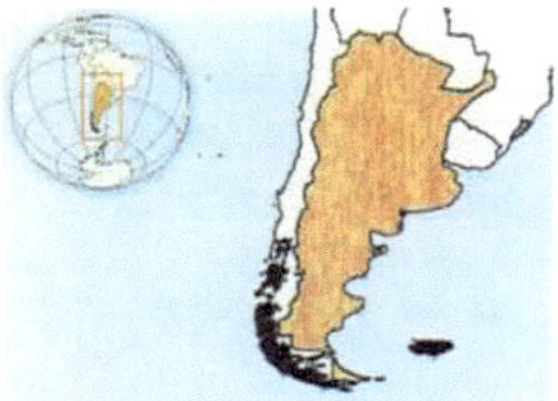

This map is an approximation of actual country borders.

Statistics

Total population (2013)	**41,446,000**
Gross national income per capita (PPP international $, 0)	not available
Life expectancy at birth m/f (years, 2013)	**73/80**
Probability of dying under five (per 1 000 live births, 0)	not available
Probability of dying between 15 and 60 years m/f (per 1 000 population, 2013)	**151/83**
Total expenditure on health per capita (Intl $, 2013)	**1,725**
Total expenditure on health as % of GDP (2013)	**7.3**

Latest data available from the Global Health Observatory

Contact information

Señora Representante de la OPS/OMS
Birmingham, Dr Maureen

Marcelo T. de Alvear 684 - 4° Piso
C1058AAH - Buenos Aires,
Argentina

Telephone: +5411 4319 4200
Facsimile: +5411 4319 4201
pwr@arg.ops-oms.org

Country Office web site
Regional Office web site

Country profile   **News and features**

Health profile

Country statistics

Country health profile
pdf

WHO collaboration

Country cooperation strategy brief
pdf

Collaborating centres

Mortality and burden of disease

Life tables

Tuberculosis

Nutrition

Child malnutrition

Nutrition

Risk factors

Alcohol
pdf

Road traffic injuries
pdf

Tobacco
pdf

World Health Organization

Countries

Brazil

Map

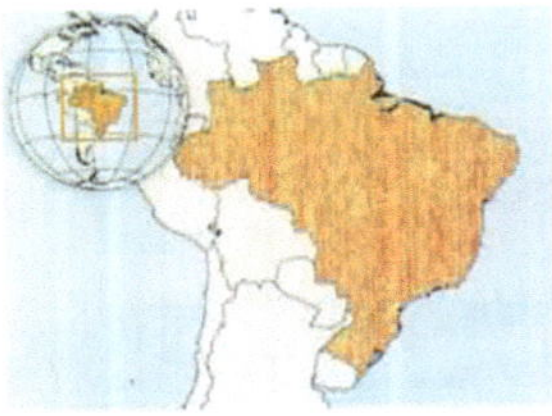

This map is an approximation of actual country borders.

Statistics

Total population (2013)	**200,362,000**
Gross national income per capita (PPP international $, 2013)	**14**
Life expectancy at birth m/f (years, 2013)	**72/79**
Probability of dying under five (per 1 000 live births, 0)	not available
Probability of dying between 15 and 60 years m/f (per 1 000 population, 2013)	**197/97**
Total expenditure on health per capita (Intl $, 2013)	**1,454**
Total expenditure on health as % of GDP (2013)	**9.7**

Latest data available from the Global Health Observatory

Contact information

The PAHO/WHO Representative
Molina, Dr Joaquin

Caixa Postal 08729 70312-970 -
Brasília, DF, Brazil

Telephone: +55 61 32519500
Facsimile: +55 61 32230269
geral@paho.org

Country Office web site
Regional Office web site

Country profile News and features

Health profile

Country statistics

Country health profile
pdf

WHO collaboration

Country cooperation strategy
pdf

Country cooperation strategy brief
pdf

Collaborating centres

Mortality and burden of disease

Life tables

Nutrition

Child malnutrition

Nutrition

Risk factors

Alcohol
pdf

Tobacco
pdf

World Health Organization

Countries

Canada

Map

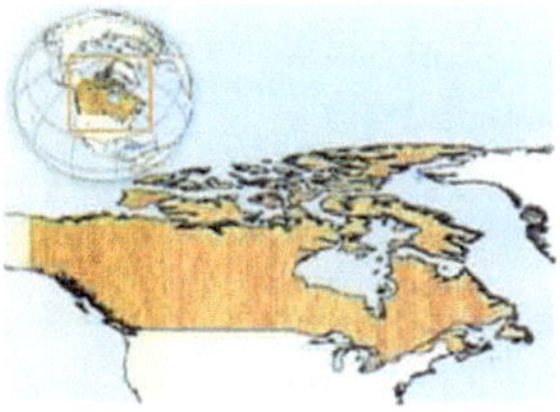

This map is an approximation of actual country borders.

Statistics

Total population (2013)	**35,182,000**
Gross national income per capita (PPP international $, 2013)	**42**
Life expectancy at birth m/f (years, 2013)	**80/84**
Probability of dying under five (per 1 000 live births, 0)	not available
Probability of dying between 15 and 60 years m/f (per 1 000 population, 2013)	**81/52**
Total expenditure on health per capita (Intl $, 2013)	**4,759**
Total expenditure on health as % of GDP (2013)	**10.9**

Latest data available from the Global Health Observatory

Contact information

Regional Office web site

Country profile News and features

Health profile

Country statistics

Country health profile
pdf

WHO collaboration

Collaborating centres

Mortality and burden of disease

Life tables

Tuberculosis

Noncommunicable diseases
pdf

Nutrition

Child malnutrition

Nutrition

Risk factors

Alcohol
pdf

Tobacco
pdf

World Health Organization

Countries

Chile

Map

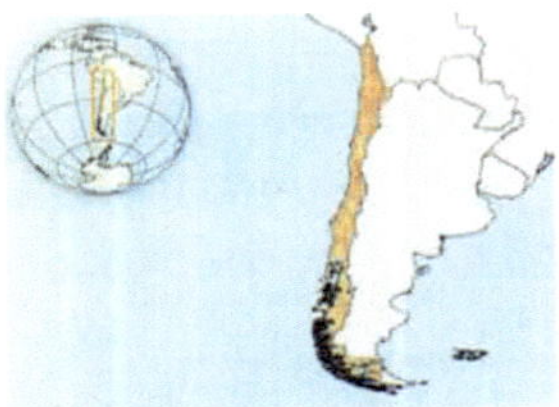

This map is an approximation of actual country borders.

Statistics

Total population (2013)	**17,620,000**
Gross national income per capita (PPP international $, 2013)	**21**
Life expectancy at birth m/f (years, 2013)	**77/83**
Probability of dying under five (per 1 000 live births, 0)	not available
Probability of dying between 15 and 60 years m/f (per 1 000 population, 2013)	**107/55**
Total expenditure on health per capita (Intl $, 2013)	**1,678**
Total expenditure on health as % of GDP (2013)	**7.7**

Latest data available from the Global Health Observatory

Contact information

Señora Representante de la OPS/OMS
Cuchi, Dr Paloma

Avenida Dag Hammarskjold 3269, Piso 1 Vitacura 7630412 - Santiago, Chile

Telephone: +56 2 24374600
Facsimile: +56 2 2074717
e-mail@chi.ops-oms.org

Country Office web site
Regional Office web site

Country profile News and features

Health profile

Country statistics

Country health profile
pdf

WHO collaboration

Collaborating centres

Mortality and burden of disease

Life tables

Tuberculosis

Noncommunicable diseases
pdf

Nutrition

Child malnutrition

Nutrition

Risk factors

Alcohol
pdf

Tobacco
pdf

World Health Organization

Countries

Colombia

Map

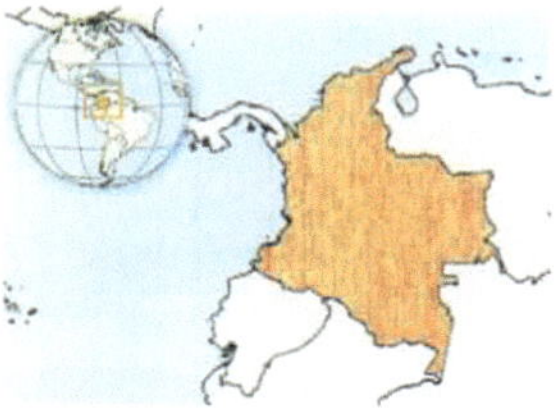

This map is an approximation of actual country borders.

Statistics

Total population (2013)	**48,321,000**
Gross national income per capita (PPP international $, 2013)	**11**
Life expectancy at birth m/f (years, 2013)	**75/81**
Probability of dying under five (per 1 000 live births, 0)	not available
Probability of dying between 15 and 60 years m/f (per 1 000 population, 2013)	**148/73**
Total expenditure on health per capita (Intl $, 2013)	**843**
Total expenditure on health as % of GDP (2013)	**6.8**

Latest data available from the Global Health Observatory

Contact information

Señora Representante de la OPS/OMS
Watson, Dr Gina

APDO 253367 Calle 66 Nr. 11 ? 50,
Piso 6 Edificio Villorio (Chapinero)
Bogota, DC, Colombia

Telephone: +57 13144141
Facsimile: +57 17455381
colmail@paho.org

Country Office web site
Regional Office web site

Country profile

Health profile

Country statistics

Country health profile
pdf

WHO collaboration

Country cooperation strategy brief
pdf

Collaborating centres

Mortality and burden of disease

Life tables

Tuberculosis

Nutrition

Child malnutrition

Nutrition

Risk factors

Alcohol
pdf

Tobacco
pdf

World Health Organization

Countries

Guatemala

Map

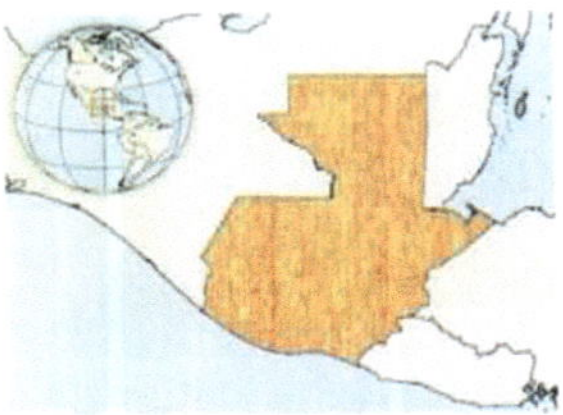

This map is an approximation of actual country borders.

Statistics

Total population (2013)	**15,468,000**
Gross national income per capita (PPP international $, 2013)	**7**
Life expectancy at birth m/f (years, 2013)	**68/75**
Probability of dying under five (per 1 000 live births, 0)	not available
Probability of dying between 15 and 60 years m/f (per 1 000 population, 2013)	**236/126**
Total expenditure on health per capita (Intl $, 2013)	**467**
Total expenditure on health as % of GDP (2013)	**6.4**

Latest data available from the Global Health Observatory

Contact information

Señora Representante de la OPS/OMS
Verdejo Pivet, Dr Guadalupe

Apartado Postal 383 Guatemala City, Guatemala

Telephone: +502 2 3322032
Facsimile: +502 2 3343804
pwr@gut.ops-oms.org

Country Office web site
Regional Office web site

Country profile News and features

Health profile

Country statistics

Country health profile
pdf

WHO collaboration

Country cooperation strategy brief
pdf

Mortality and burden of disease

Life tables

Tuberculosis

Noncommunicable diseases
pdf

Nutrition

Child malnutrition

Nutrition

Risk factors

Alcohol
pdf

Tobacco
pdf

World Health Organization

Countries

Mexico

Map

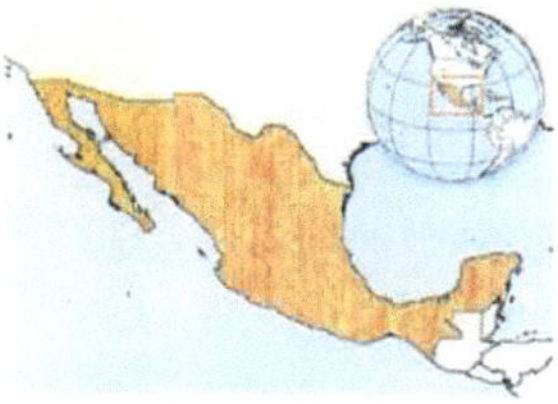

This map is an approximation of actual country borders.

Statistics

Total population (2013)	**122,332,000**
Gross national income per capita (PPP international $, 2013)	**16**
Life expectancy at birth m/f (years, 2013)	**73/78**
Probability of dying under five (per 1 000 live births, 0)	not available
Probability of dying between 15 and 60 years m/f (per 1 000 population, 2013)	**174/93**
Total expenditure on health per capita (Intl $, 2013)	**1,061**
Total expenditure on health as % of GDP (2013)	**6.2**

Latest data available from the Global Health Observatory

Contact information

Señor Representante de la OPS/OMS (interino)
González Machin, Dr Diego

Horacio N° 1855 , Piso 3, Oficina 305 Colonia Los Morales Polanco
11510 - México City, Mexico

Telephone: +52 55 59800871 - CISCO 40871
Facsimile: +52 55 53955681
pwr.mex@paho.org

Country Office web site
Regional Office web site

Country profile   **News and features**

Health profile

Country statistics

Country health profile
pdf

WHO collaboration

Country cooperation strategy brief
pdf

Collaborating centres

Mortality and burden of disease

Life tables

Tuberculosis

Nutrition

Child malnutrition

Nutrition

Risk factors

Alcohol
pdf

Tobacco
pdf

World Health Organization

Countries

Venezuela (Bolivarian Republic of)

Map

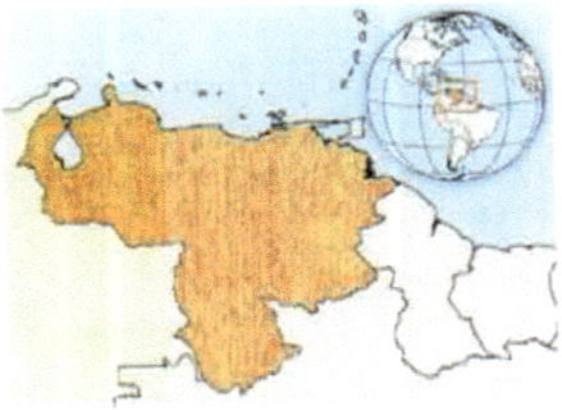

This map is an approximation of actual country borders.

Statistics

Total population (2013)	**30,405,000**
Gross national income per capita (PPP international $, 2013)	**17**
Life expectancy at birth m/f (years, 2013)	**72/80**
Probability of dying under five (per 1 000 live births, 0)	not available
Probability of dying between 15 and 60 years m/f (per 1 000 population, 2013)	**198/88**
Total expenditure on health per capita (Intl $, 2013)	**656**
Total expenditure on health as % of GDP (2013)	**3.6**

Latest data available from the Global Health Observatory

Contact information

Señora Representante de la OPS/OMS
Riera, Dr Celia

6722 Carmelitas-Caracas 1010
1060 - Caracas, Venezuela
(Bolivarian Republic of)

Telephone: +58 212 2065001
Facsimile: +58 212 2616069
webmasters@ven.ops-oms.org

Country Office web site
Regional Office web site

Country profile

Health profile

Country statistics

Country health profile
pdf

Mortality and burden of disease

Life tables

Tuberculosis

Noncommunicable diseases
pdf

Nutrition

Child malnutrition

Nutrition

Risk factors

Alcohol
pdf

Tobacco
pdf

World Health Organization

Countries

United States of America

Map

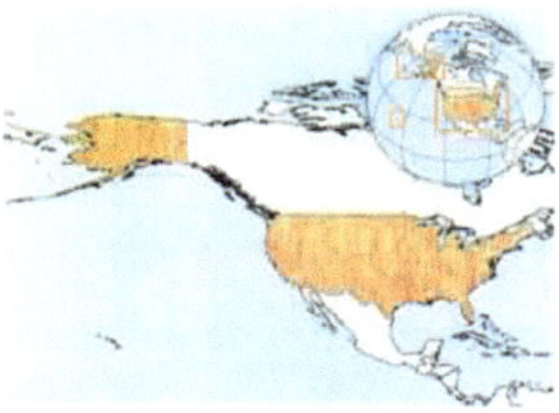

This map is an approximation of actual country borders.

Statistics

Total population (2013)	**320,051,000**
Gross national income per capita (PPP international $, 2013)	**53**
Life expectancy at birth m/f (years, 2013)	**76/81**
Probability of dying under five (per 1 000 live births, 0)	not available
Probability of dying between 15 and 60 years m/f (per 1 000 population, 2013)	**128/76**
Total expenditure on health per capita (Intl $, 2013)	**9,146**
Total expenditure on health as % of GDP (2013)	**17.1**

Latest data available from the Global Health Observatory

Contact information

Regional Office web site

Country profile News and features

Health profile

Country statistics

Country health profile
pdf

Mortality and burden of disease

Life tables

Tuberculosis

Noncommunicable diseases
pdf

Nutrition

Child malnutrition

Nutrition

Risk factors

Alcohol
pdf

Road traffic injuries
pdf

Tobacco
pdf

World Health Organization

Countries

Afghanistan

Map

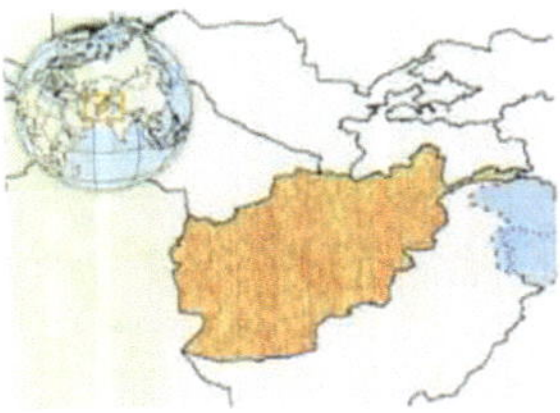

This map is an approximation of actual country borders.

Statistics

Total population (2013)	**30,552,000**
Gross national income per capita (PPP international $, 2013)	**2**
Life expectancy at birth m/f (years, 2013)	**61/62**
Probability of dying under five (per 1 000 live births, 0)	not available
Probability of dying between 15 and 60 years m/f (per 1 000 population, 2013)	**252/232**
Total expenditure on health per capita (Intl $, 2013)	**161**
Total expenditure on health as % of GDP (2013)	**8.1**

Latest data available from the Global Health Observatory

Contact information

The WHO Representative
Peeperkorn, Dr Richard

UNOCA Compound, Jalalabad Road Pul-e-Charkhi Kabul, Afghanistan

Telephone: +93700045276
Facsimile: n/a
emacoafgwr@who.int

Country Office web site
Regional Office web site

Country profile News and features

Health profile

Country statistics

Country health profile
pdf

WHO collaboration

Country cooperation strategy
pdf

Country cooperation strategy brief
pdf

Mortality and burden of disease

Life tables

Tuberculosis

Nutrition

Child malnutrition

Nutrition

Risk factors

Alcohol
pdf

Road traffic injuries
pdf

Tobacco
pdf

World Health Organization

Countries

China

Map

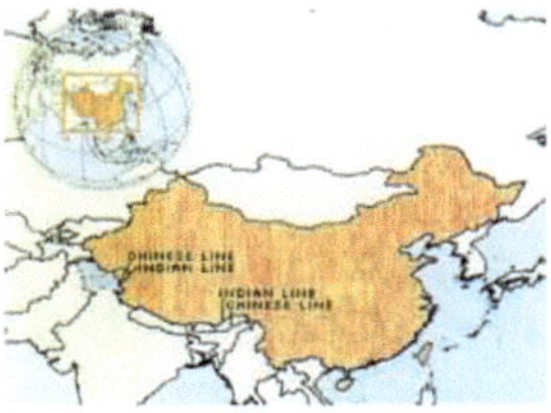

This map is an approximation of actual country borders.

Statistics

Total population (2013)	**1,393,337,000**
Gross national income per capita (PPP international $, 2013)	**11**
Life expectancy at birth m/f (years, 2013)	**74/77**
Probability of dying under five (per 1 000 live births, 0)	not available
Probability of dying between 15 and 60 years m/f (per 1 000 population, 2013)	**103/76**
Total expenditure on health per capita (Intl $, 2013)	**646**
Total expenditure on health as % of GDP (2013)	**5.6**

Latest data available from the Global Health Observatory

Contact information

WHO Representative in the People's Republic of China

401, Dongwai Diplomatic Office
Building 23
Dongzhimenwai Dajie
Chaoyang District
Beijing
100600

who@chn.wpro.who.int

Country Office web site
Regional Office web site

Country profile News and features

Health profile

Country statistics
Country profile on regional site
Country health profile
pdf

WHO collaboration

Country cooperation strategy
pdf
Country cooperation strategy brief
pdf
Collaborating centres

Mortality and burden of disease

Life tables

Nutrition

Child malnutrition
Nutrition

Risk factors

Alcohol
pdf
Tobacco
pdf

World Health Organization

Countries

India

Map

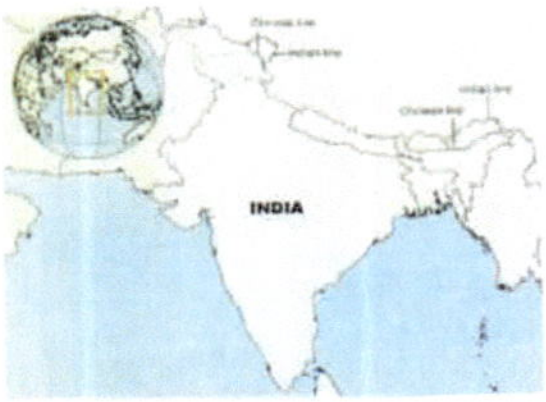

This map is an approximation of actual country borders.

Statistics

Total population (2013)	**1,252,140,000**
Gross national income per capita (PPP international $, 2013)	**5**
Life expectancy at birth m/f (years, 2013)	**65/68**
Probability of dying under five (per 1 000 live births, 0)	not available
Probability of dying between 15 and 60 years m/f (per 1 000 population, 2013)	**239/158**
Total expenditure on health per capita (Intl $, 2013)	**215**
Total expenditure on health as % of GDP (2013)	**4.0**

Latest data available from the Global Health Observatory

Contact information

WHO Country Office

Rooms 533-537, 'A' Wing
Nirman Bhawan
Maulana Azad Road
New Delhi
110011

wrindia@searo.who.int

Country Office web site
Regional Office web site

Country profile News and features

Health profile

Country statistics

Country health profile
pdf

WHO collaboration

Country cooperation strategy
pdf

Country cooperation strategy brief
pdf

Collaborating centres

Mortality and burden of disease

Life tables

Tuberculosis

Nutrition

Child malnutrition

Nutrition

Risk factors

Alcohol
pdf

Tobacco
pdf

World Health Organization

Countries

Myanmar

Map

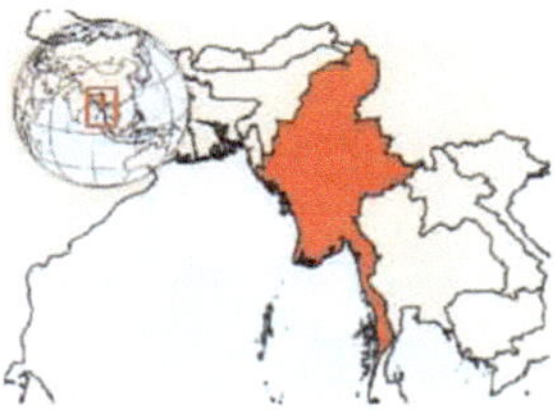

This map is an approximation of actual country borders.

Statistics

Total population (2013)	**53,259,000**
Gross national income per capita (PPP international $, 0)	not available
Life expectancy at birth m/f (years, 2013)	**64/68**
Probability of dying under five (per 1 000 live births, 0)	not available
Probability of dying between 15 and 60 years m/f (per 1 000 population, 2013)	**240/183**
Total expenditure on health per capita (Intl $, 2013)	**37**
Total expenditure on health as % of GDP (2013)	**1.8**

Latest data available from the Global Health Observatory

Country profile News and features

Contact information

The WHO Representative
Luna, Dr Jorge Mario

PO Box 14 11061 - Yangon, Myanmar

Telephone: +95 1 650386
Facsimile: +95 1 650408- 409
whommr@searo.who.int

Country Office web site
Regional Office web site

Health profile

Country statistics

Country health profile
pdf

WHO collaboration

Country cooperation strategy
pdf

Country cooperation strategy brief
pdf

Collaborating centres

Mortality and burden of disease

Nutrition

Child malnutrition

Nutrition

Risk factors

Alcohol
pdf

Tobacco
pdf

Countries

Lao People's Democratic Republic

Map

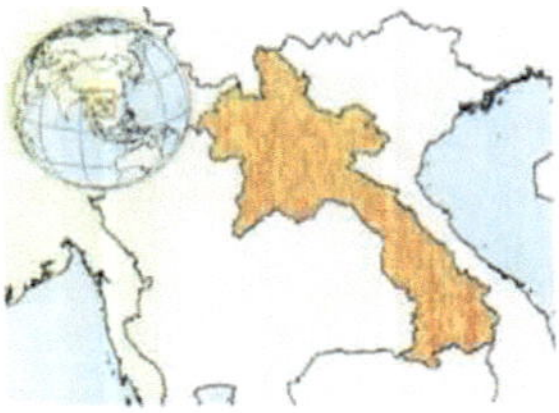

This map is an approximation of actual country borders.

Statistics

Total population (2013)	**6,770,000**
Gross national income per capita (PPP international $, 2013)	**4**
Life expectancy at birth m/f (years, 2013)	**65/68**
Probability of dying under five (per 1 000 live births, 0)	not available
Probability of dying between 15 and 60 years m/f (per 1 000 population, 2013)	**197/158**
Total expenditure on health per capita (Intl $, 2013)	**95**
Total expenditure on health as % of GDP (2013)	**2.0**

Latest data available from the Global Health Observatory

Contact information

The WHO Representative
Fleischl, Dr Juliet

PO Box 343 Vientiane, Lao People's Democratic Republic

Telephone: +856 21 353902
Facsimile: +856 21 353905
who.lao@wpro.who.int

Country Office web site
Regional Office web site

Country profile News and features

Health profile

Country statistics
Country profile on regional site
Country health profile
pdf

WHO collaboration

Country cooperation strategy
pdf
Country cooperation strategy brief
pdf

Mortality and burden of disease

Life tables
Tuberculosis

Nutrition

Child malnutrition
Nutrition

Risk factors

Alcohol
pdf
Road traffic injuries
pdf
Tobacco
pdf

World Health Organization

Countries

Cambodia

Map

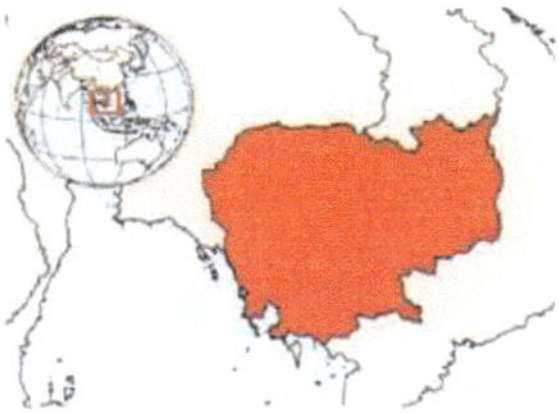

This map is an approximation of actual country borders.

Statistics

Total population (2013)	**15,135,000**
Gross national income per capita (PPP international $, 2013)	**2**
Life expectancy at birth m/f (years, 2013)	**70/75**
Probability of dying under five (per 1 000 live births, 0)	not available
Probability of dying between 15 and 60 years m/f (per 1 000 population, 2013)	**210/157**
Total expenditure on health per capita (Intl $, 2013)	**229**
Total expenditure on health as % of GDP (2013)	**7.5**

Latest data available from the Global Health Observatory

Country profile News and features

Contact information

The WHO Representative
Ahn, Dr Dong-Il

1217 Phnom Penh, Cambodia

Telephone: +855 23 216610
Facsimile: +855 23 216211
who.cam@wpro.who.int

Country Office web site
Regional Office web site

Health profile

Country statistics

Country health profile
pdf

WHO collaboration

Country cooperation strategy
pdf

Country cooperation strategy brief
pdf

Mortality and burden of disease

Life tables

Nutrition

Child malnutrition

Nutrition

Risk factors

Alcohol
pdf

Tobacco
pdf

World Health Organization

Countries

Thailand

Map

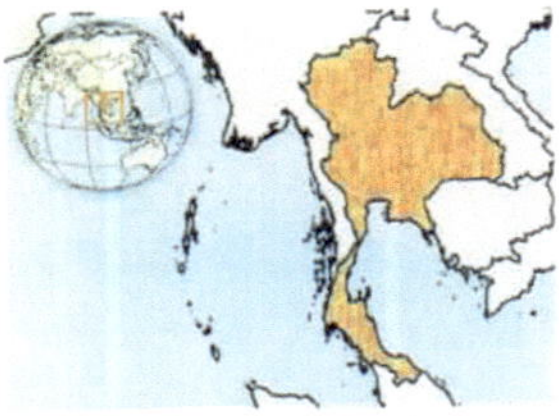

This map is an approximation of actual country borders.

Statistics

Total population (2013)	**67,010,000**
Gross national income per capita (PPP international $, 2013)	**13**
Life expectancy at birth m/f (years, 2013)	**71/79**
Probability of dying under five (per 1 000 live births, 0)	not available
Probability of dying between 15 and 60 years m/f (per 1 000 population, 2013)	**177/90**
Total expenditure on health per capita (Intl $, 2013)	**658**
Total expenditure on health as % of GDP (2013)	**4.6**

Latest data available from the Global Health Observatory

Contact information

The Acting WHO Representative
Brown, Dr Richard

88/20 Permanent Secretary
Building Ministry of Public Health
Tiwanon Road 11000 - Nonthaburi,
Thailand

Telephone: +66 25470100
Facsimile: +66 25918199
setharegistry@who.int

Country Office web site
Regional Office web site

Country profile News and features

Health profile

Country statistics

Country health profile
pdf

WHO collaboration

Country cooperation strategy
pdf

Country cooperation strategy brief
pdf

Collaborating centres

Mortality and burden of disease

Life tables

Nutrition

Child malnutrition

Nutrition

Risk factors

Alcohol
pdf

Tobacco
pdf

World Health Organization

Countries

Iran (Islamic Republic of)

Map

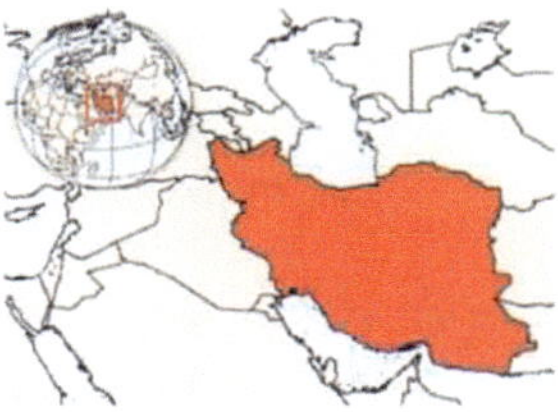

This map is an approximation of actual country borders.

Statistics

Total population (2013)	**77,447,000**
Gross national income per capita (PPP international $, 2013)	**15**
Life expectancy at birth m/f (years, 2013)	**72/76**
Probability of dying under five (per 1 000 live births, 0)	not available
Probability of dying between 15 and 60 years m/f (per 1 000 population, 2013)	**153/83**
Total expenditure on health per capita (Intl $, 2013)	**1,414**
Total expenditure on health as % of GDP (2013)	**6.7**

Latest data available from the Global Health Observatory

Country profile News and features

Contact information

WHO Representative

PO Box 14665-1565
Tehran

whoteh@ira.emro.who.int

Regional Office web site

Health profile

Country statistics

Country health profile
pdf

WHO collaboration

Country cooperation strategy
pdf

Country cooperation strategy brief
pdf

Collaborating centres

Mortality and burden of disease

Nutrition

Child malnutrition

Nutrition

Risk factors

Alcohol
pdf

Tobacco
pdf

Countries

Japan

Map

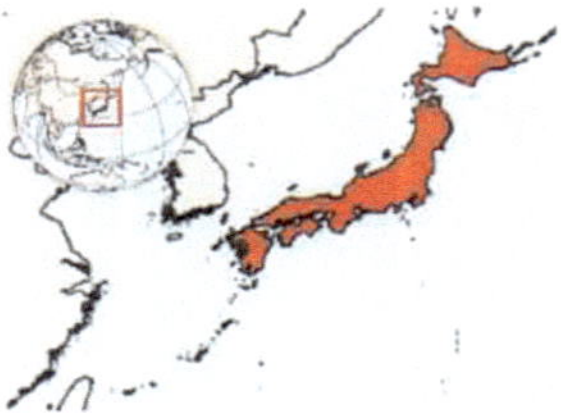

This map is an approximation of actual country borders.

Statistics

Total population (2013)	**127,144,000**
Gross national income per capita (PPP international $, 2013)	**37**
Life expectancy at birth m/f (years, 2013)	**80/87**
Probability of dying under five (per 1 000 live births, 0)	not available
Probability of dying between 15 and 60 years m/f (per 1 000 population, 2013)	**81/42**
Total expenditure on health per capita (Intl $, 2013)	**3,741**
Total expenditure on health as % of GDP (2013)	**10.3**

Latest data available from the Global Health Observatory

Contact information

Regional Office web site

Country profile News and features

Health profile

Country statistics

Country profile on regional site

Country health profile
pdf

WHO collaboration

Collaborating centres

Mortality and burden of disease

Life tables

Tuberculosis

Noncommunicable diseases
pdf

Nutrition

Child malnutrition

Nutrition

Risk factors

Alcohol
pdf

Tobacco
pdf

World Health Organization

Countries

Kazakhstan

Map

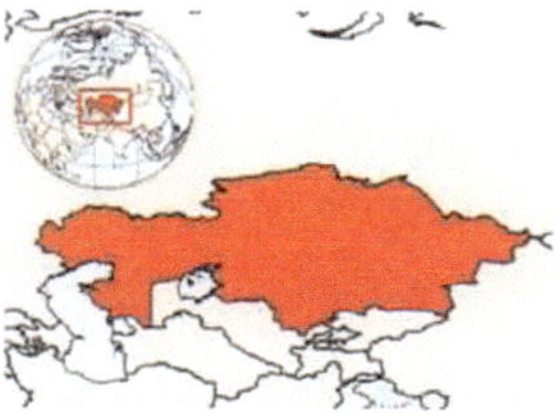

This map is an approximation of actual country borders.

Statistics

Total population (2013)	**16,441,000**
Gross national income per capita (PPP international $, 2013)	**20**
Life expectancy at birth m/f (years, 2013)	**63/73**
Probability of dying under five (per 1 000 live births, 0)	not available
Probability of dying between 15 and 60 years m/f (per 1 000 population, 2013)	**322/146**
Total expenditure on health per capita (Intl $, 2013)	**1,023**
Total expenditure on health as % of GDP (2013)	**4.3**

Latest data available from the Global Health Observatory

Contact information

The WHO Representative and Head of Country Office
Vujnovic, Dr Melita

20, Orynbor street, office 306
010000 - Astana, Kazakhstan

Telephone: +7 7172 696534
whokaz@euro.who.int

Country Office web site
Regional Office web site

Country profile   News and features

Health profile

Country statistics
Country profile on regional site
Country health profile
pdf

WHO collaboration

Collaborating centres

Mortality and burden of disease

Life tables
Tuberculosis

Nutrition

Child malnutrition
Nutrition

Risk factors

Alcohol
pdf
Tobacco
pdf

World Health Organization

Countries

Kuwait

Map

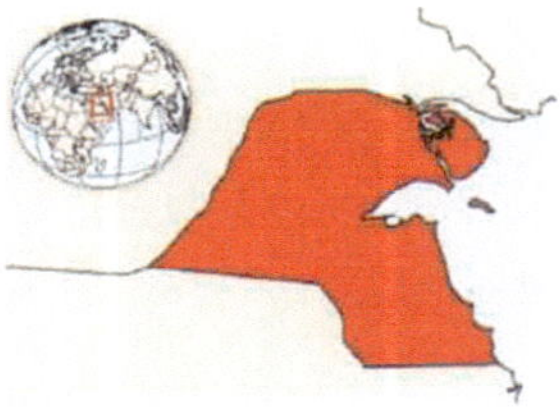

This map is an approximation of actual country borders.

Statistics

Total population (2013)	**3,369,000**
Gross national income per capita (PPP international $, 2011)	**88,170**
Life expectancy at birth m/f (years, 2013)	**78/79**
Probability of dying under five (per 1 000 live births, 0)	not available
Probability of dying between 15 and 60 years m/f (per 1 000 population, 2013)	**59/42**
Total expenditure on health per capita (Intl $, 2013)	**2,375**
Total expenditure on health as % of GDP (2013)	**2.9**

Latest data available from the Global Health Observatory

Country profile   News and features

Contact information

Regional Office web site

Health profile

Country statistics

Country health profile
pdf

WHO collaboration

Country cooperation strategy
pdf

Country cooperation strategy brief
pdf

Collaborating centres

Nutrition

Child malnutrition

Nutrition

Risk factors

Alcohol
pdf

Tobacco
pdf

Mortality and burden of disease

World Health Organization

Countries

Mongolia

Map

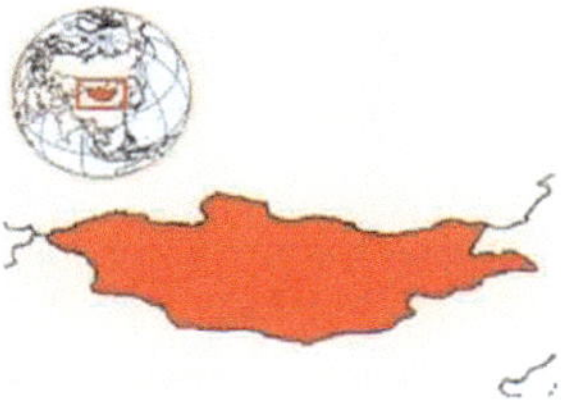

This map is an approximation of actual country borders.

Statistics

Total population (2013)	**2,839,000**
Gross national income per capita (PPP international $, 2013)	**8**
Life expectancy at birth m/f (years, 2013)	**64/72**
Probability of dying under five (per 1 000 live births, 0)	not available
Probability of dying between 15 and 60 years m/f (per 1 000 population, 2013)	**309/148**
Total expenditure on health per capita (Intl $, 2013)	**567**
Total expenditure on health as % of GDP (2013)	**6.0**

Latest data available from the Global Health Observatory

Contact information

The WHO Representative

PO Box 663 976
Ulaanbaatar 13

who.mog@wpro.who.int

Country Office web site
Regional Office web site

Country profile News and features

Health profile

Country statistics

Country health profile
pdf

WHO collaboration

Country cooperation strategy
pdf

Country cooperation strategy brief
pdf

Mortality and burden of disease

Life tables

Nutrition

Child malnutrition

Nutrition

Risk factors

Alcohol
pdf

Tobacco
pdf

World Health Organization

Countries

Russian Federation

Map

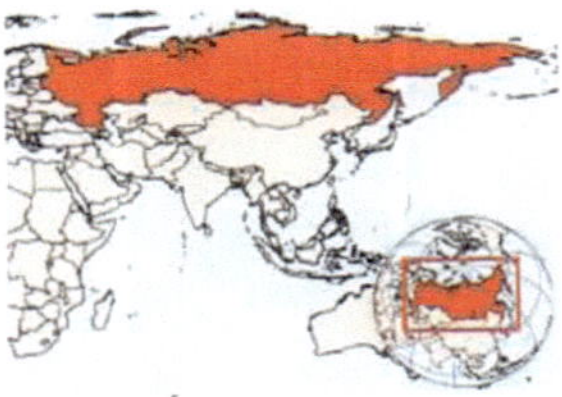

This map is an approximation of actual country borders.

Statistics

Total population (2013)	**142,834,000**
Gross national income per capita (PPP international $, 2013)	**23**
Life expectancy at birth m/f (years, 2013)	**63/75**
Probability of dying under five (per 1 000 live births, 0)	not available
Probability of dying between 15 and 60 years m/f (per 1 000 population, 2013)	**339/126**
Total expenditure on health per capita (Intl $, 2013)	**1,587**
Total expenditure on health as % of GDP (2013)	**6.5**

Latest data available from the Global Health Observatory

Country profile News and features

Contact information

The Acting WHO Representative and Head of Country Office
Nikogosian, Mr Haik

9 Leontyevsky pereulok 125009 - Moscow, Russian Federation

Telephone: +7 4957872108
Facsimile: +7 4957872119
moscow@whorussia.org

Country Office web site
Regional Office web site

Health profile

Country statistics

Country profile on regional site

Country health profile
pdf

WHO collaboration

Collaborating centres

Mortality and burden of disease

Life tables

Tuberculosis

Noncommunicable diseases
pdf

Nutrition

Nutrition

Risk factors

Road traffic injuries
pdf

World Health Organization

Countries

Pakistan

Map

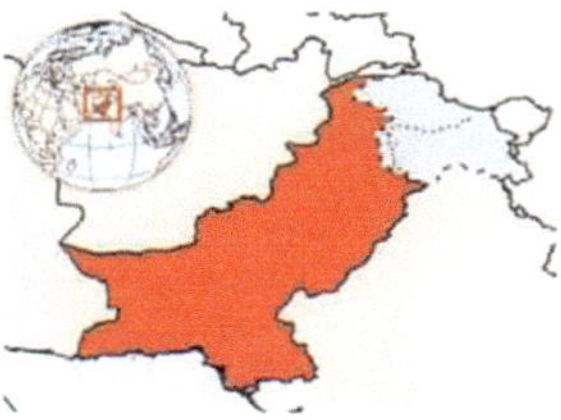

This map is an approximation of actual country borders.

Statistics

Total population (2013)	**182,143,000**
Gross national income per capita (PPP international $, 2013)	**4**
Life expectancy at birth m/f (years, 2013)	**65/67**
Probability of dying under five (per 1 000 live births, 0)	not available
Probability of dying between 15 and 60 years m/f (per 1 000 population, 2013)	**189/155**
Total expenditure on health per capita (Intl $, 2013)	**126**
Total expenditure on health as % of GDP (2013)	**2.8**

Latest data available from the Global Health Observatory

Contact information

The WHO Representative
Thieren, Dr Michel

PO Box 1013 Islamabad, Pakistan

Telephone: +92 51 843 2451
Facsimile: +92 51 925 5083
emacopakwr@who.int

Country Office web site
Regional Office web site

Country profile News and features

Health profile

Country statistics

Country health profile
pdf

WHO collaboration

Country cooperation strategy
pdf

Country cooperation strategy brief
pdf

Collaborating centres

Mortality and burden of disease

Nutrition

Child malnutrition

Nutrition

Risk factors

Alcohol
pdf

Tobacco
pdf

World Health Organization

Countries

Australia

Map

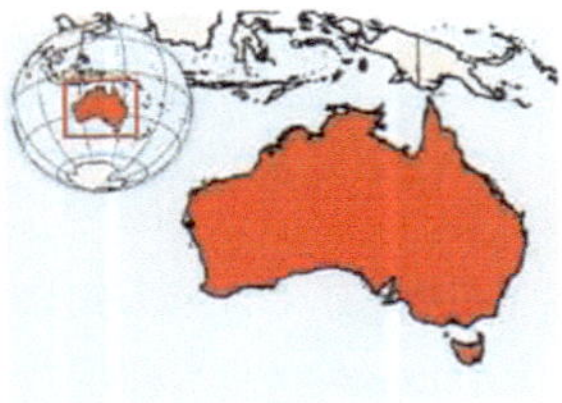

This map is an approximation of actual country borders.

Statistics

Total population (2013)	**23,343,000**
Gross national income per capita (PPP international $, 2013)	**42**
Life expectancy at birth m/f (years, 2013)	**80/85**
Probability of dying under five (per 1 000 live births, 0)	not available
Probability of dying between 15 and 60 years m/f (per 1 000 population, 2013)	**78/45**
Total expenditure on health per capita (Intl $, 2013)	**4,191**
Total expenditure on health as % of GDP (2013)	**9.4**

Latest data available from the Global Health Observatory

Contact information

Regional Office web site

Country profile News and features

Health profile

Country statistics

Country profile on regional site

Country health profile
pdf

WHO collaboration

Collaborating centres

Mortality and burden of disease

Life tables

Tuberculosis

Nutrition

Child malnutrition

Nutrition

Risk factors

Alcohol
pdf

Road traffic injuries
pdf

Tobacco
pdf

World Health Organization

Countries

New Zealand

Map

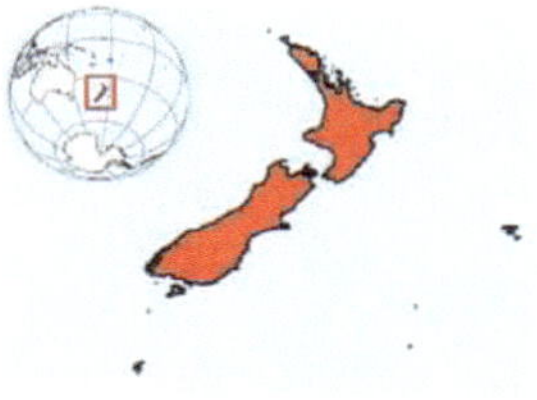

This map is an approximation of actual country borders.

Statistics

Total population (2013)	**4,506,000**
Gross national income per capita (PPP international $, 2012)	**30,750**
Life expectancy at birth m/f (years, 2013)	**80/84**
Probability of dying under five (per 1 000 live births, 0)	not available
Probability of dying between 15 and 60 years m/f (per 1 000 population, 2013)	**80/52**
Total expenditure on health per capita (Intl $, 2013)	**3,405**
Total expenditure on health as % of GDP (2013)	**9.7**

Latest data available from the Global Health Observatory

Contact information

Regional Office web site

Country profile News and features

Health profile

Country statistics

Country health profile
pdf

WHO collaboration

Collaborating centres

Mortality and burden of disease

Life tables

Tuberculosis

Noncommunicable diseases
pdf

Nutrition

Child malnutrition

Nutrition

Risk factors

Alcohol
pdf

Road traffic injuries
pdf

Tobacco
pdf

World Health Organization

Countries

Indonesia

Map

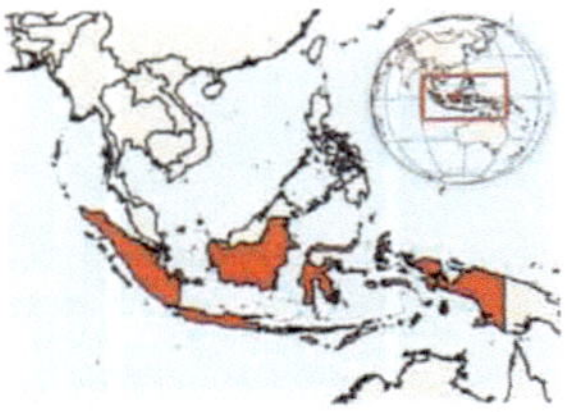

This map is an approximation of actual country borders.

Statistics

Total population (2013)	**249,866,000**
Gross national income per capita (PPP international $, 2013)	**9**
Life expectancy at birth m/f (years, 2013)	**69/73**
Probability of dying under five (per 1 000 live births, 0)	not available
Probability of dying between 15 and 60 years m/f (per 1 000 population, 2013)	**176/121**
Total expenditure on health per capita (Intl $, 2013)	**293**
Total expenditure on health as % of GDP (2013)	**3.1**

Latest data available from the Global Health Observatory

Country profile News and features

Contact information

The WHO Representative
Limpakarnjanarat, Dr Khanchit

PO Box 1302 12950 - Jakarta, Indonesia

Telephone: +62 21 5204349
Facsimile: +62 21 5201164
whoindonesia@searo.who.int

Country Office web site
Regional Office web site

Health profile

Country statistics

WHO collaboration

Collaborating centres

Mortality and burden of disease

Life tables

Tuberculosis

Noncommunicable diseases
pdf

Nutrition

Child malnutrition

Nutrition

Risk factors

Alcohol
pdf

Tobacco
pdf

World Health Organization

Countries

Philippines

Map

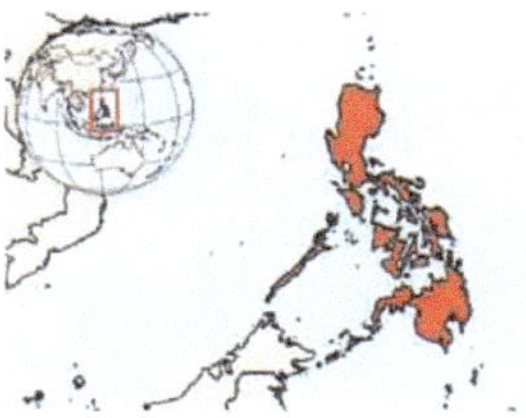

This map is an approximation of actual country borders.

Statistics

Total population (2013)	**98,394,000**
Gross national income per capita (PPP international $, 2013)	**7**
Life expectancy at birth m/f (years, 2013)	**65/72**
Probability of dying under five (per 1 000 live births, 0)	not available
Probability of dying between 15 and 60 years m/f (per 1 000 population, 2013)	**255/136**
Total expenditure on health per capita (Intl $, 2013)	**287**
Total expenditure on health as % of GDP (2013)	**4.4**

Latest data available from the Global Health Observatory

Country profile   News and features

Contact information

WHO Representative

c/o WHO Regional Office for the Western Pacific
PO Box 2932
Manila
1003

who@phl.wpro.who.int

Country Office web site
Regional Office web site

Health profile

Country statistics
Country profile on regional site
Country health profile
pdf

WHO collaboration

Country cooperation strategy
pdf
Country cooperation strategy brief
pdf
Collaborating centres

Nutrition

Child malnutrition
Nutrition

Risk factors

Alcohol
pdf
Tobacco
pdf

Countries

Denmark

Map

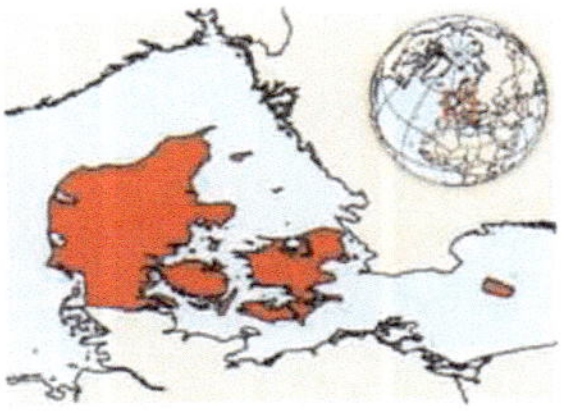

This map is an approximation of actual country borders.

Statistics

Total population (2013)	**5,619,000**
Gross national income per capita (PPP international $, 2013)	**44**
Life expectancy at birth m/f (years, 2013)	**78/82**
Probability of dying under five (per 1 000 live births, 0)	not available
Probability of dying between 15 and 60 years m/f (per 1 000 population, 2013)	**100/60**
Total expenditure on health per capita (Intl $, 2013)	**4,552**
Total expenditure on health as % of GDP (2013)	**10.6**

Latest data available from the Global Health Observatory

Contact information

Regional Office web site

Country profile

Health profile

Country profile on regional site

Country statistics

Country health profile
pdf

WHO collaboration

Collaborating centres

Mortality and burden of disease

Life tables

Tuberculosis

Noncommunicable diseases
pdf

Nutrition

Child malnutrition

Nutrition

Risk factors

Alcohol
pdf

Tobacco
pdf

World Health Organization

Countries

France

Map

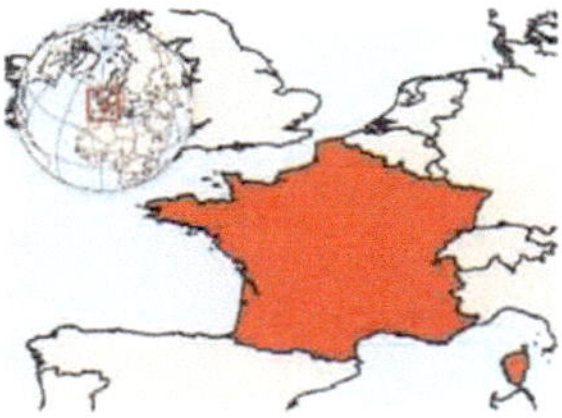

This map is an approximation of actual country borders.

Statistics

Total population (2013)	**64,291,000**
Gross national income per capita (PPP international $, 2013)	**37**
Life expectancy at birth m/f (years, 2013)	**79/85**
Probability of dying under five (per 1 000 live births, 0)	not available
Probability of dying between 15 and 60 years m/f (per 1 000 population, 2013)	**109/52**
Total expenditure on health per capita (Intl $, 2013)	**4,334**
Total expenditure on health as % of GDP (2013)	**11.7**

Latest data available from the Global Health Observatory

Country profile News and features

Contact information

Regional Office web site

Health profile

Country statistics

Country profile on regional site

Country health profile
pdf

WHO collaboration

Collaborating centres

Mortality and burden of disease

Life tables

Tuberculosis

Nutrition

Child malnutrition

Nutrition

Risk factors

Alcohol
pdf

Tobacco
pdf

World Health Organization

Countries

Germany

Map

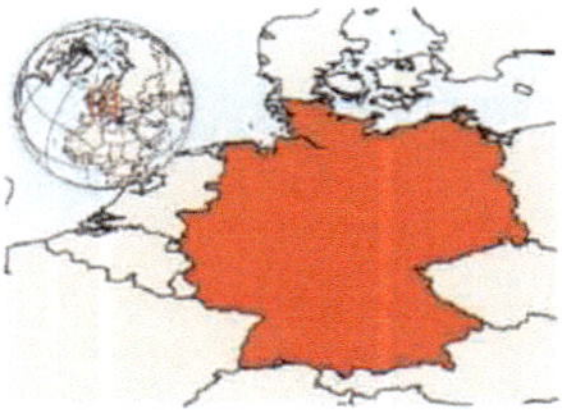

This map is an approximation of actual country borders.

Statistics

Total population (2013)	**82,727,000**
Gross national income per capita (PPP international $, 2013)	**44**
Life expectancy at birth m/f (years, 2013)	**79/83**
Probability of dying under five (per 1 000 live births, 0)	not available
Probability of dying between 15 and 60 years m/f (per 1 000 population, 2013)	**92/50**
Total expenditure on health per capita (Intl $, 2013)	**4,812**
Total expenditure on health as % of GDP (2013)	**11.3**

Latest data available from the Global Health Observatory

Contact information

Regional Office web site

Country profile News and features

Health profile

Country statistics

Country profile on regional site

Country health profile
pdf

WHO collaboration

Collaborating centres

Mortality and burden of disease

Life tables

Tuberculosis

Nutrition

Child malnutrition

Nutrition

Risk factors

Alcohol
pdf

Tobacco
pdf

World Health Organization

Countries

Greece

Map

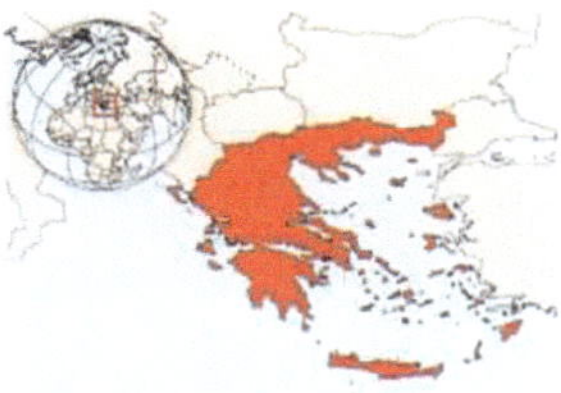

This map is an approximation of actual country borders.

Statistics

Total population (2013)	**11,128,000**
Gross national income per capita (PPP international $, 2013)	**25**
Life expectancy at birth m/f (years, 2013)	**79/84**
Probability of dying under five (per 1 000 live births, 0)	not available
Probability of dying between 15 and 60 years m/f (per 1 000 population, 2013)	**98/41**
Total expenditure on health per capita (Intl $, 2013)	**2,513**
Total expenditure on health as % of GDP (2013)	**9.8**

Latest data available from the Global Health Observatory

Contact information

Regional Office web site

Country profile News and features

Health profile

Country statistics
Country profile on regional site
Country health profile
pdf

WHO collaboration

Collaborating centres

Mortality and burden of disease

Life tables
Tuberculosis

Nutrition

Child malnutrition
Nutrition

Risk factors

Alcohol
pdf
Tobacco
pdf

World Health Organization

Countries

Hungary

Map

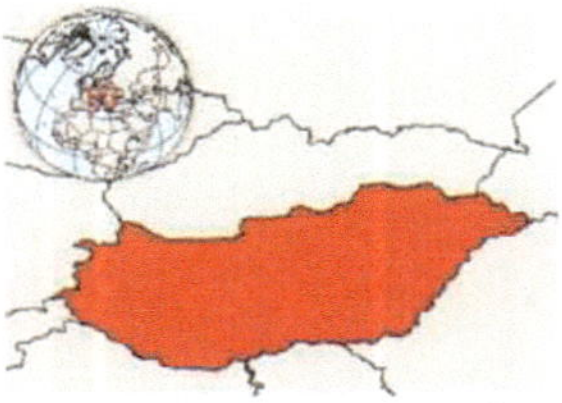

This map is an approximation of actual country borders.

Statistics

Total population (2013)	**9,955,000**
Gross national income per capita (PPP international $, 2012)	**21,000**
Life expectancy at birth m/f (years, 2013)	**71/79**
Probability of dying under five (per 1 000 live births, 0)	not available
Probability of dying between 15 and 60 years m/f (per 1 000 population, 2013)	**201/91**
Total expenditure on health per capita (Intl $, 2013)	**1,839**
Total expenditure on health as % of GDP (2013)	**8.0**

Latest data available from the Global Health Observatory

Country profile News and features

Contact information

The WHO Head of Country Office
Pusztai, Dr Zsofia

c/o National Institute of Pharmacy
Zrinyi utca 3 - 1st floor H-1051 -
Budapest, Hungary

Telephone: +36 1 3286081
Facsimile: +36 1 3286086
whohun@euro.who.int

Country Office web site
Regional Office web site

Health profile

Country statistics
Country profile on regional site
Country health profile
pdf

WHO collaboration

Collaborating centres

Mortality and burden of disease

Life tables
Tuberculosis
Noncommunicable diseases
pdf

Nutrition

Child malnutrition
Nutrition

Risk factors

Alcohol
pdf
Tobacco
pdf

World Health Organization

Countries

Italy

Map

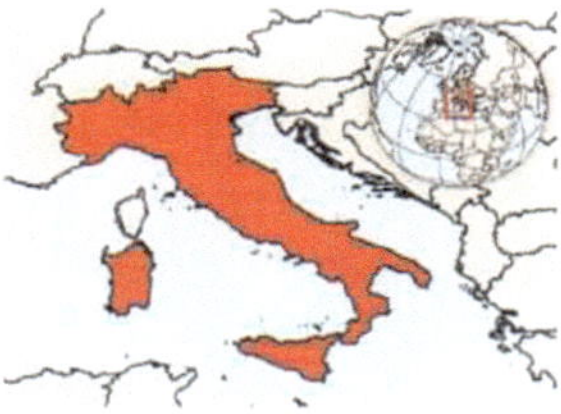

This map is an approximation of actual country borders.

Statistics

Total population (2013)	**60,990,000**
Gross national income per capita (PPP international $, 2013)	**34**
Life expectancy at birth m/f (years, 2013)	**80/85**
Probability of dying under five (per 1 000 live births, 0)	not available
Probability of dying between 15 and 60 years m/f (per 1 000 population, 2013)	**69/38**
Total expenditure on health per capita (Intl $, 2013)	**3,126**
Total expenditure on health as % of GDP (2013)	**9.1**

Latest data available from the Global Health Observatory

Contact information

Regional Office web site

Country profile News and features

Health profile

Country statistics

Country profile on regional site

Country health profile
pdf

WHO collaboration

Collaborating centres

Mortality and burden of disease

Life tables

Tuberculosis

Nutrition

Child malnutrition

Nutrition

Risk factors

Alcohol
pdf

Tobacco
pdf

World Health Organization

Countries

The former Yugoslav Republic of Macedonia

Map

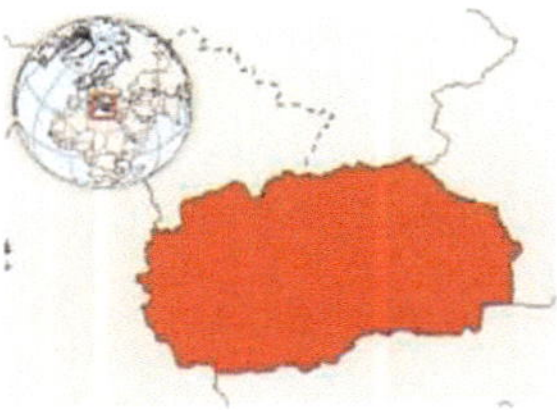

This map is an approximation of actual country borders.

Statistics

Total population (2013)	**2,107,000**
Gross national income per capita (PPP international $, 2013)	**11**
Life expectancy at birth m/f (years, 2013)	**74/78**
Probability of dying under five (per 1 000 live births, 0)	not available
Probability of dying between 15 and 60 years m/f (per 1 000 population, 2013)	**134/71**
Total expenditure on health per capita (Intl $, 2013)	**759**
Total expenditure on health as % of GDP (2013)	**6.4**

Latest data available from the Global Health Observatory

Contact information

The WHO Head of Country Office
Chichevalieva, Ms Snezhana

"Drezdenska" No. 22 1000 - Skopje, The former Yugoslav Republic of Macedonia

Telephone: +389 2306 4299
Facsimile: +389 2306 3710
whomkd@euro.who.int

Country Office web site
Regional Office web site

Country profile

Health profile

Country profile on regional site

Country statistics

Country health profile
pdf

Mortality and burden of disease

Life tables

Tuberculosis

Noncommunicable diseases
pdf

Nutrition

Child malnutrition

Nutrition

Risk factors

Alcohol
pdf

Road traffic injuries
pdf

Tobacco
pdf

World Health Organization

Countries

Norway

Map

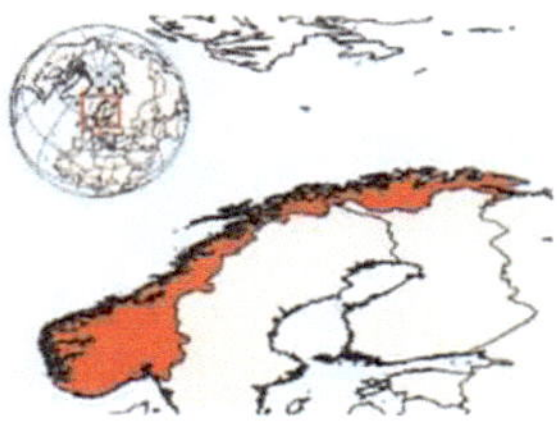

This map is an approximation of actual country borders.

Statistics

Total population (2013)	**5,043,000**
Gross national income per capita (PPP international $, 2013)	**66**
Life expectancy at birth m/f (years, 2013)	**80/84**
Probability of dying under five (per 1 000 live births, 0)	not available
Probability of dying between 15 and 60 years m/f (per 1 000 population, 2013)	**73/47**
Total expenditure on health per capita (Intl $, 2013)	**6,308**
Total expenditure on health as % of GDP (2013)	**9.6**

Latest data available from the Global Health Observatory

Contact information

Regional Office web site

Country profile

Health profile

Country statistics

Country profile on regional site

Country health profile
pdf

WHO collaboration

Collaborating centres

Mortality and burden of disease

Life tables

Tuberculosis

Noncommunicable diseases
pdf

Nutrition

Child malnutrition

Nutrition

Risk factors

Alcohol
pdf

Tobacco
pdf

World Health Organization

Countries

Netherlands

Map

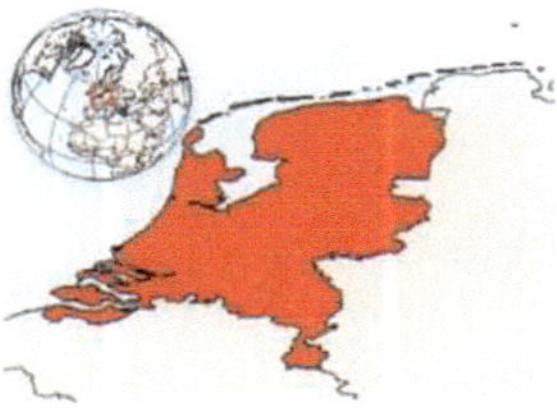

This map is an approximation of actual country borders.

Statistics

Total population (2013)	**16,759,000**
Gross national income per capita (PPP international $, 2013)	**43**
Life expectancy at birth m/f (years, 2013)	**79/83**
Probability of dying under five (per 1 000 live births, 0)	not available
Probability of dying between 15 and 60 years m/f (per 1 000 population, 2013)	**69/54**
Total expenditure on health per capita (Intl $, 2013)	**5,601**
Total expenditure on health as % of GDP (2013)	**12.9**

Latest data available from the Global Health Observatory

Contact information

Regional Office web site

Country profile News and features

Health profile

Country statistics

Country profile on regional site

Country health profile pdf

WHO collaboration

Collaborating centres

Mortality and burden of disease

Life tables

Tuberculosis

Nutrition

Child malnutrition

Nutrition

Risk factors

Alcohol pdf

Tobacco pdf

World Health Organization

Countries

Poland

Map

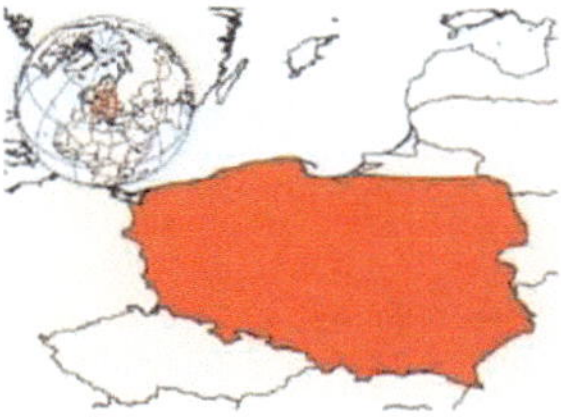

This map is an approximation of actual country borders.

Statistics

Total population (2013)	**38,217,000**
Gross national income per capita (PPP international $, 2013)	**22**
Life expectancy at birth m/f (years, 2013)	**73/81**
Probability of dying under five (per 1 000 live births, 0)	not available
Probability of dying between 15 and 60 years m/f (per 1 000 population, 2013)	**186/70**
Total expenditure on health per capita (Intl $, 2013)	**1,551**
Total expenditure on health as % of GDP (2013)	**6.7**

Latest data available from the Global Health Observatory

Country profile News and features

Contact information

The WHO Head of Country Office
Miskiewicz, Dr Paulina Marianna

WHO Country Office for Poland Al. Jerozolimskie 155 02-326 - Warsaw, Poland

Telephone: +48 22 6359496
Facsimile: +48 22 8310892
whopol@euro.who.int

Country Office web site
Regional Office web site

Health profile

Country statistics

Country profile on regional site

Country health profile
pdf

WHO collaboration

Collaborating centres

Mortality and burden of disease

Life tables

Tuberculosis

Nutrition

Child malnutrition

Nutrition

Risk factors

Alcohol
pdf

Tobacco
pdf

World Health Organization

Countries

Portugal

Map

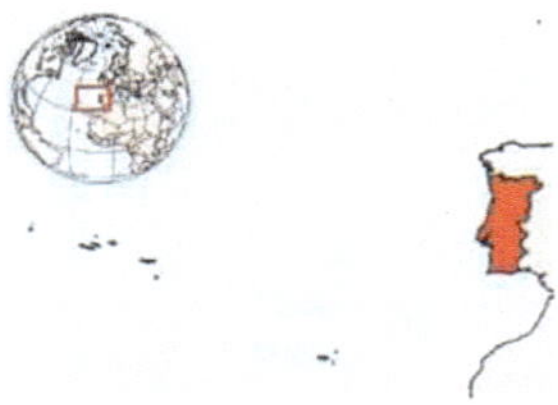

This map is an approximation of actual country borders.

Statistics

Total population (2013)	**10,608,000**
Gross national income per capita (PPP international $, 2013)	**25**
Life expectancy at birth m/f (years, 2013)	**78/84**
Probability of dying under five (per 1 000 live births, 0)	not available
Probability of dying between 15 and 60 years m/f (per 1 000 population, 2013)	**111/48**
Total expenditure on health per capita (Intl $, 2013)	**2,508**
Total expenditure on health as % of GDP (2013)	**9.7**

Latest data available from the Global Health Observatory

Country profile News and features

Contact information

Regional Office web site

Health profile

Country profile on regional site

Country statistics

Country health profile
pdf

Mortality and burden of disease

Life tables

Tuberculosis

Noncommunicable diseases
pdf

Nutrition

Child malnutrition

Nutrition

Risk factors

Alcohol
pdf

Tobacco
pdf

World Health Organization

Countries

Romania

Map

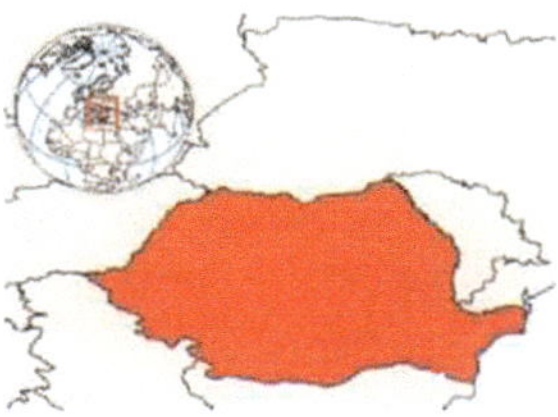

This map is an approximation of actual country borders.

Statistics

Total population (2013)	**21,699,000**
Gross national income per capita (PPP international $, 2013)	**18**
Life expectancy at birth m/f (years, 2013)	**71/78**
Probability of dying under five (per 1 000 live births, 0)	not available
Probability of dying between 15 and 60 years m/f (per 1 000 population, 2013)	**205/81**
Total expenditure on health per capita (Intl $, 2013)	**988**
Total expenditure on health as % of GDP (2013)	**5.3**

Latest data available from the Global Health Observatory

Contact information

The WHO Head of Country Office
Olsavszky, Dr Victor

UN House 48A Primaverii Blvd. R-011975 - Bucharest, Romania

Telephone: +40 21 2017891
Facsimile: +40 21 2017889
whorom@euro.who.int

Country Office web site
Regional Office web site

Country profile   News and features

Health profile

Country statistics

Country profile on regional site

WHO collaboration

Collaborating centres

Mortality and burden of disease

Life tables

Tuberculosis

Nutrition

Nutrition

World Health Organization

Countries

Serbia

Map

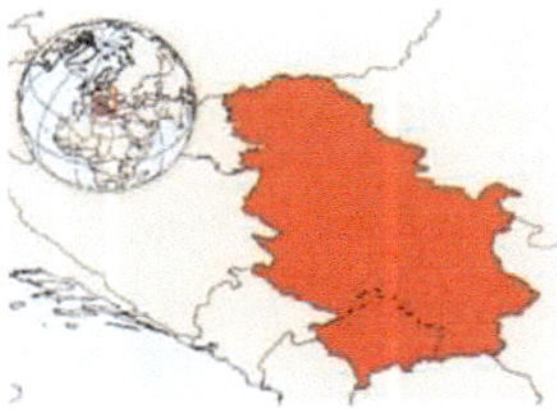

This map is an approximation of actual country borders.

Statistics

Total population (2013)	**9,511,000**
Gross national income per capita (PPP international $, 2013)	**12**
Life expectancy at birth m/f (years, 2013)	**72/77**
Probability of dying under five (per 1 000 live births, 0)	not available
Probability of dying between 15 and 60 years m/f (per 1 000 population, 2013)	**172/84**
Total expenditure on health per capita (Intl $, 2013)	**987**
Total expenditure on health as % of GDP (2013)	**10.6**

Latest data available from the Global Health Observatory

Country profile News and features

Contact information

The WHO Head of Country Office
Grbic, Dr Miljana

Hadzi Melentijeva 30 11000 -
Belgrade, Serbia

Telephone: +3811 1243 2651
Facsimile: +3811 1243 2572
whosrb@euro.who.int

Country Office web site
Regional Office web site

Health profile

Country statistics

Country health profile
pdf

Mortality and burden of disease

Life tables

Tuberculosis

Noncommunicable diseases
pdf

Nutrition

Child malnutrition

Nutrition

Risk factors

Alcohol
pdf

Tobacco
pdf

World Health Organization

Countries

Spain

Map

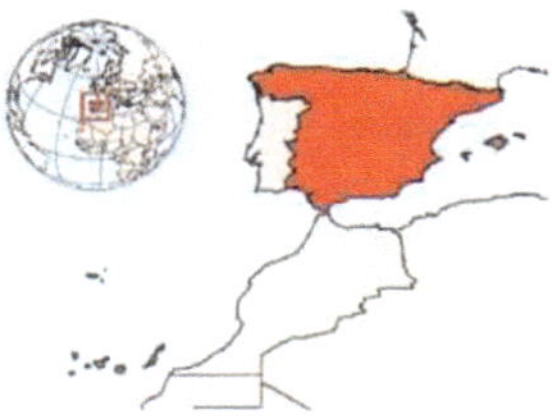

This map is an approximation of actual country borders.

Statistics

Total population (2013)	**46,927,000**
Gross national income per capita (PPP international $, 2013)	**31**
Life expectancy at birth m/f (years, 2013)	**80/86**
Probability of dying under five (per 1 000 live births, 0)	not available
Probability of dying between 15 and 60 years m/f (per 1 000 population, 2013)	**86/40**
Total expenditure on health per capita (Intl $, 2013)	**2,846**
Total expenditure on health as % of GDP (2013)	**8.9**

Latest data available from the Global Health Observatory

Contact information

Regional Office web site

Country profile   News and features

Health profile

Country statistics

Country profile on regional site

Country health profile
pdf

WHO collaboration

Collaborating centres

Mortality and burden of disease

Life tables

Tuberculosis

Nutrition

Child malnutrition

Nutrition

Risk factors

Alcohol
pdf

Tobacco
pdf

World Health Organization

Countries

Sweden

Map

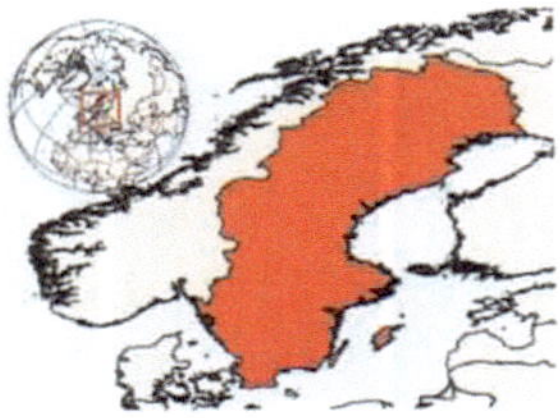

This map is an approximation of actual country borders.

Statistics

Total population (2013)	**9,571,000**
Gross national income per capita (PPP international $, 2013)	**44**
Life expectancy at birth m/f (years, 2013)	**80/84**
Probability of dying under five (per 1 000 live births, 0)	not available
Probability of dying between 15 and 60 years m/f (per 1 000 population, 2013)	**69/43**
Total expenditure on health per capita (Intl $, 2013)	**4,244**
Total expenditure on health as % of GDP (2013)	**9.7**

Latest data available from the Global Health Observatory

Country profile News and features

Contact information

Regional Office web site

Health profile

Country statistics

Country profile on regional site

Country health profile
pdf

WHO collaboration

Collaborating centres

Mortality and burden of disease

Life tables

Tuberculosis

Noncommunicable diseases
pdf

Nutrition

Child malnutrition

Nutrition

Risk factors

Alcohol
pdf

Tobacco
pdf

World Health Organization

Countries

Turkey

Map

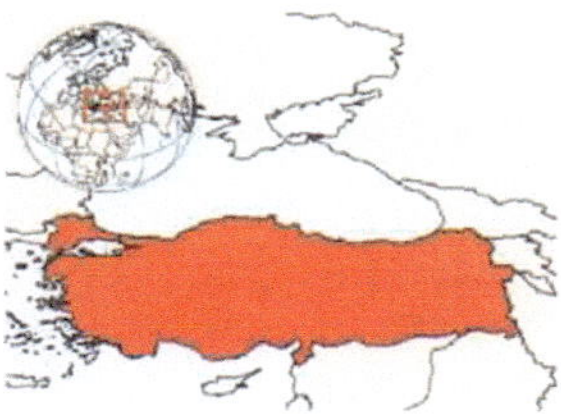

This map is an approximation of actual country borders.

Statistics

Total population (2013)	**74,933,000**
Gross national income per capita (PPP international $, 2013)	**18**
Life expectancy at birth m/f (years, 2013)	**72/79**
Probability of dying under five (per 1 000 live births, 0)	not available
Probability of dying between 15 and 60 years m/f (per 1 000 population, 2013)	**147/73**
Total expenditure on health per capita (Intl $, 2013)	**1,053**
Total expenditure on health as % of GDP (2013)	**5.6**

Latest data available from the Global Health Observatory

Contact information

The WHO Representative and Head of Country Office
Ursu, Dr Pavel

UN House - Birlik Mahallesi 415
Cadde N° 11 06610 - Cankaya,
Ankara, Turkey

Telephone: +90 312 4541083
Facsimile: +90 312 4961488
whotur@euro.who.int

Country Office web site
Regional Office web site

Country profile   News and features

Health profile

Country statistics

Country profile on regional site

Country health profile
pdf

WHO collaboration

Country cooperation strategy brief
pdf

Collaborating centres

Mortality and burden of disease

Nutrition

Child malnutrition

Nutrition

Risk factors

Alcohol
pdf

Tobacco
pdf

World Health Organization

Countries

United Kingdom

Map

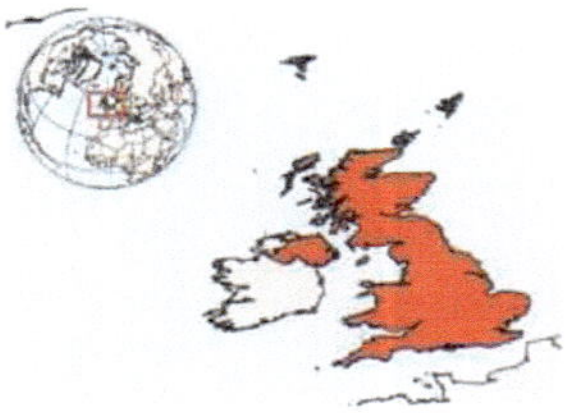

This map is an approximation of actual country borders.

Statistics

Total population (2013)	**63,136,000**
Gross national income per capita (PPP international $, 2013)	**35**
Life expectancy at birth m/f (years, 2013)	**79/83**
Probability of dying under five (per 1 000 live births, 0)	not available
Probability of dying between 15 and 60 years m/f (per 1 000 population, 2013)	**88/55**
Total expenditure on health per capita (Intl $, 2013)	**3,311**
Total expenditure on health as % of GDP (2013)	**9.1**

Latest data available from the Global Health Observatory

Country profile News and features

Contact information

Regional Office web site

Health profile

Country statistics
Country profile on regional site
Country health profile
pdf

WHO collaboration

Collaborating centres

Mortality and burden of disease

Life tables
Tuberculosis

Nutrition

Child malnutrition
Nutrition

Risk factors

Alcohol
pdf
Road traffic injuries
pdf
Tobacco
pdf

5.4 Cancer in the World

5.4.1 Continents – World Summary

5.4.1.1 Overview – Cervical Cancer in the World

	Cervical cancer in the world
35	**Africa**: 1. Algeria, 2. Azerbaijan, 3. Benin, 4. Egypt, 5. Ethiopia, 6. Kenya, 7. Nigeria, 8. South Africa, 9. Sri Lanka, 10. Tanzania, 11. Uganda.
36	**America:** 1. Argentina, 2. Brazil, 3. Canada, 4. Chile, 5. Colombia, 6. Guatemala, 7. Mexico, 8. Venezuela, 9. U.S.A.
37	**Asia:** 1. Afghanistan, 2. Burma/Myanmar, 3. China, 4. India, 5. Indochina, 6. Iran, 7. Japan, 8. Kazakhstan, 9. Korea South, 10. Kuwait, 11. Mongolia, 12. Russia, 13. Pakistan, 14. Taiwan, 15. Thailand.
38	**Australia:** 1. Australia, 2. New Zealand, 3. Indonesia, 4. Philippines.
39	**Europe:** 1. Denmark, 2. France, 3. Germany, 4. Greece, 5. Hungary, 6. Italy, 7. Macedonia, 8. Norway, 9. Netherland, 10. Poland 11. Portugal, 12. Romania, 13. Serbia, 14. Spain, 15. Sweden, 16. Turkey, 17. United Kingdom.

Cervical cancer is a global health problem needing resolution

					Population	BDP	BDP/P	Annual MPT
	#1	Region	#2	State	X10e6	*10e6	X10e3	In 10e6 need
1	1	Africa	1	Algeria	40	210.2	5360	7
2			2	Azerbaijan	9.59	73.56	7911	1.5
3			3	Benin	10.3	8.307	804	1.7
4			4	Egypt	82	272	3314	14
5			5	Ethiopia	96	47.56	505	17
6			6	Kenya	44	55.24	1245	8
7			7	Nigeria	177	522	3000	30
8			8	South Africa	53	350	6617	8.5
9			9	Sri Lanka	21	67	3300	4
10			10	Tanzania	50	33.23	695	8.5
11			11	Uganda	38	22	572	6
					<621>	1661	30,023	**106.2**
							2729	
12	2	America	1	Argentina	42	610	14,500	8
13			2	Brazil	202	2500	12,500	34
14			3	Canada	35.2	1825	52,000	6
15			4	Chile	18	225	12,500	3.5
16			5	Colombia	48	378	7830	8.5
17			6	Guatemala	16	54	3375	2.7
18			7	Mexico	123	1260	1383	21
19			8	Venezuela	30	438	24,600	6
20			9	U.S.A.	325	16,800	52,000	55

(continued)

					Population	BDP	BDP/P	Annual MPT
	#1	Region	#2	State	X10e6	*10e6	X10e3	In 10e6 need
					<831>	24,090	180,688	14.47
							20,070	**159.17**
21	3	Asia	1	Afganistan	31	21	674	5.2
22			2	Burma/Myanmar	56	53	1000	10
23			3	China	1374	11,000	8000	230
24			4	India	1280	1800	1480	215
25			5	Indochina	105	315	3000	18
26			6	Iran	80	528	6600	14
27			7	Japan	127	5900	47,000	22
28			8	Kazakhstan	17	232	13,700	3
29			9	Korea South	51	1304	26,000	9
30			10	Kuwait	4	176	52,200	0.7
31			11	Mongolia	3	17	5900	0.6
32			12	Russia	143.5	2097	14,611	25
33			13	Pakistan	190	237	1250	32
34			14	Taiwan	23.5	474	32,000	5
35			15	Thailand	66	387	5900	12
					<3551>	24,551	180,688	**601.5**
							20,070	
36	4	Australia	1	Australia	23	11,300	43,000	4
37			2	New Zealand	4.4	136	31,500	0.74
38			3	Indonesia	250	868	3500	42
39			4	Philippines	103	456,460	4500	12
					<381>	12,760	82.500	**58.74**
							20,625	
40	5	Europe	1	Denmark	6	344	58,000	1.5
41			2	France	66	2700	41,000	11.5
42			3	Germany	81	3364	42,000	14
43			4	Greece	11	341	31,000	1.9
44			5	Hungary	10	134	13,500	1.7
45			6	Italy	61	2307	38,000	21
46			7	Macedonia	2.1	10.4	5.000	0.36
47			8	Norway	5	500	100,000	0.9
48			9	Netherland	17	854	51,000	6.5
49			10	Poland	39	526	13,500	7
50			11	Portugal	11	252	23,000	1.9
51			12	Romania	22	285	13,000	3.6
52			13	Serbia	9.5	42	4500	1.6
53			14	Spain	48	1593	33,000	8.5
54			15	Sweden	10	580	59,000	1.7
55			16	Turkey	76	677	8900	12.7
56			17	United Kingdom	64	2857	45,000	11
					<539>	17,366	433,533	**105.66**
							25,502	**1031.27**
Total World			**In Billions**		**5.931**	**81 %**		

5.4.2 *Examples from Individual Countries*

5.4.2.1 Cervical Cancer in the World

B2/CH.5

According to the World Population Clock in July 2015, there was 7.33 billion population on the earth. Upon assumption that 2/3 of all women are at risk for cervical cancer, the estimated number of women at risk worldwide is about 2.6 billion.

According to the World Cancer Statistics, about 600,000 new cases of cervical cancer are registered each year, and about 300,000 women die annually of this disease. Each minute one woman gets cervical cancer and each 2 min one women die. This is unacceptable for a fully preventable disease. Ten years earlier, these numbers were different: each 2 min one woman got cancer, and each 3 min one woman died. The increase is substantial (above 50 %), but it could be also related to a better diagnosis and outreach statistics.

Anyhow, the world population is growing with a rate above 1.2 % annually, but the cervical cancer prevalence is groining almost ten times faster. It is an alarming epidemiological situation and WHO is actively engaged to find new strategies to stop this trend.

Still, the major global problem is low outreach – only about 20 % of women at risk participate in regular screening in spite of all efforts by countries to increase this number. There are no tools to help new strategies to be implemented. Search for new tools has not been discontinued in spite of many new devices and methods for measurement of HPV, collection devices and procedures, pathocytological classifications and criteria for better diagnosis of clinical conditions, cytology imaging analyzers, and lot of philanthropic aids given to LMIC.

Cervical cancer is ubiquitous disease, but is distributed unequivocally among the countries around the world. The following pages, Cervical Cancer Worldwide, illustrate these differences. The information is organized per regions (continents) countries and most frequent cancers.

Because of this difference, we have looked for a single non-medical parameter to see is there any relation with the medical cervical cancer distribution. This unique parameter is the Gross Domestic Product per Capita as measured by the International Monetary Fund.

However, before using this parameter, it was of utmost importance to determine the monetary value of a woman's life around the word. This was important to estimate the financial impact on the country what can be expected by achieving the most important social impact of the cervical cancer screening, saving women's lives.

What is the value of women's life calculated as GDP per capita. We have used that a man dur8ng his lifespan contributes to this product with an index of 100, a woman of 50 and a child of 50. In the contemporary world one woman at average delivers two children. It means that her contribution to the GDP per Capita is 50 + 2*50 or 100, or it is at least equal to a man's contribution. After this assumption was made, the calculations were easy. They are presented on the following tables Economy of MPT.

Afghanistan

Total population: 29,825,000
Income group: Low

Total deaths: 250,000
Life expectancy at birth: Total:60 Males:58 Females:61

Cancer Mortality Profile*

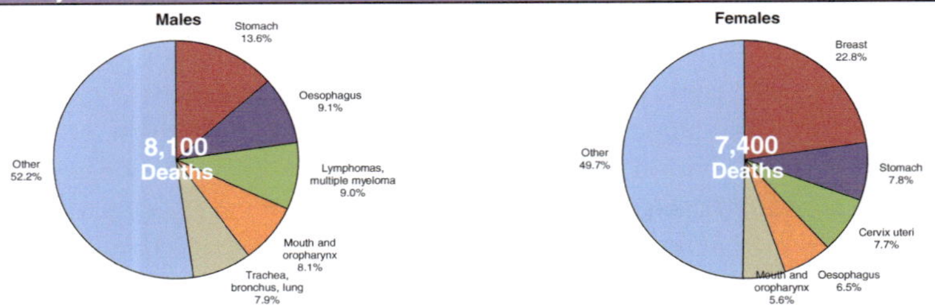

Age-Standardized Cancer Mortality Trends*

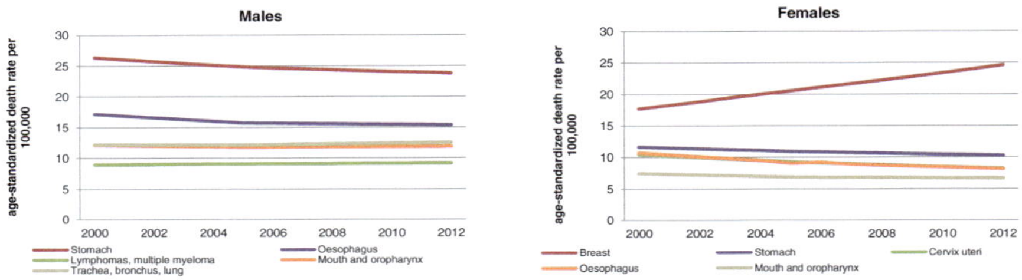

Cancer Incidence**

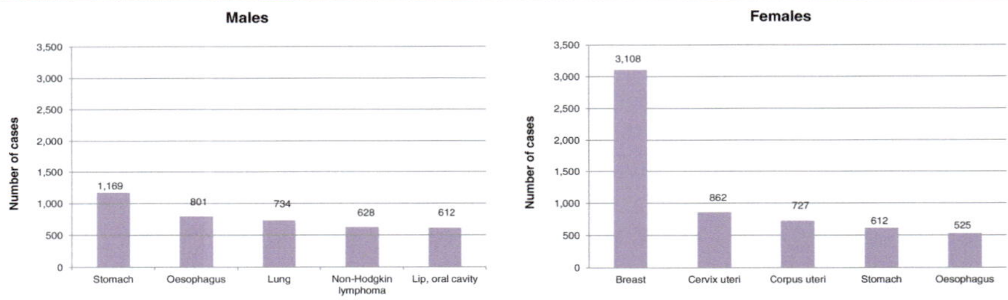

Adult Risk Factors

	Males	Females	Total
Current tobacco smoking (2011)	...	...	...
Total alcohol per capita consumption, in litres of pure alcohol (2010)	1.2	0.1	0.7
Physical inactivity (2010)	...	...	...
Obesity (2014)	1.5%	3.3%	2.4%
Household solid fuel use (2012)	-	-	81.0%

World Health Organization - Cancer Country Profiles, 2014.

Cancer Plans, Monitoring and Surveillance

Has an operational cancer policy/strategy/action plan	No
Has a cancer registry	No
Scope	
Coverage	
Last year of data	

Cancer Primary Prevention Policies

Tobacco control

Has an operational policy, strategy or action plan to reduce the burden of tobacco use	No
Smoke-free legislation	Three to five public places completely smoke-free
Tobacco dependence treatment	NRT and/or some cessation services (neither cost-covered)
Warning labels	No warnings or small warnings
Bans on advertising, promotion and sponsorship	Ban on national television, radio and print media as well as on some but not all other forms of direct and/or indirect advertising
Tobacco taxes	≤25% of retail price is tax

Overweight and obesity prevention and control

Has an operational policy, strategy or action plan for reducing overweight/obesity	No

Physical inactivity prevention and control

Has an operational policy, strategy or action plan to reduce physical inactivity and/or promote physical activity	No

Harmful use of alcohol prevention and control

Has an operational policy, strategy or action plan to reduce the harmful use of alcohol	No

National immunization

Human Papillomavirus vaccination schedule	...
Hepatitis B vaccination schedule	...
Hepatitis B vaccination coverage, infants	71%

Cancer Screening and Early Detection

Cervical cancer

Cervical cytology (PAP)	Not generally available at the public primary health care level
Acetic acid visualization (VIA)	Not generally available at the public primary health care level

Breast cancer

Breast palpation / clinical breast exam (CBE)	Not generally available at the public primary health care level
Mammogram	Not generally available at the public primary health care level

Colorectal cancer

Faecal occult blood test or faecal immunological test	Not generally available at the public primary health care level
Bowel cancer screening by exam or colonoscopy	Not generally available at the public primary health care level

Cancer Treatment and Palliative Care

Radiotherapy	Not generally available in the public health system
Total high energy teletherapy units / million inhabitants	0.0
Number of radiotherapy centres	...
Number of radiation oncologists	...
Chemotherapy (medicines not specified)	Not generally available in the public health system
Oral morphine (formulation not specified)	Generally available in the public health system
Non-methadone morphine equivalent consumption per cancer death (mg)	...
Community/home care for people with advanced stage cancer and other NCDs	Not generally available

* No mortality data available. Figures are based on national incidence estimates and modelled survival.
** No incidence data available. Figures are based on national incidence estimates from neighbouring countries.
... = No data available

World Health Organization - Cancer Country Profiles, 2014.

Argentina

Total population: 41,087,000
Income group: Upper middle

Total deaths: 314,000
Life expectancy at birth: Total:76 Males:73 Females:79

Cancer Mortality Profile

Males

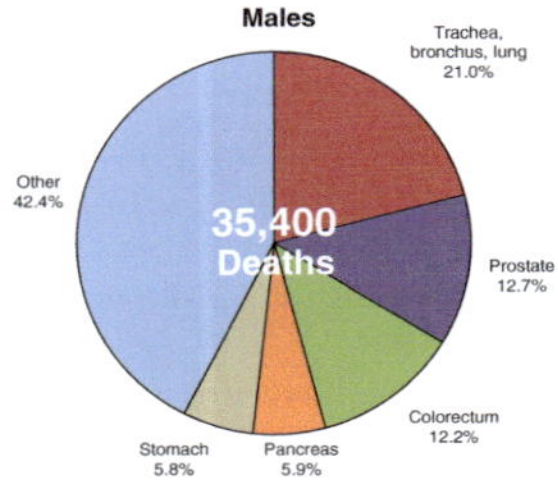

Females

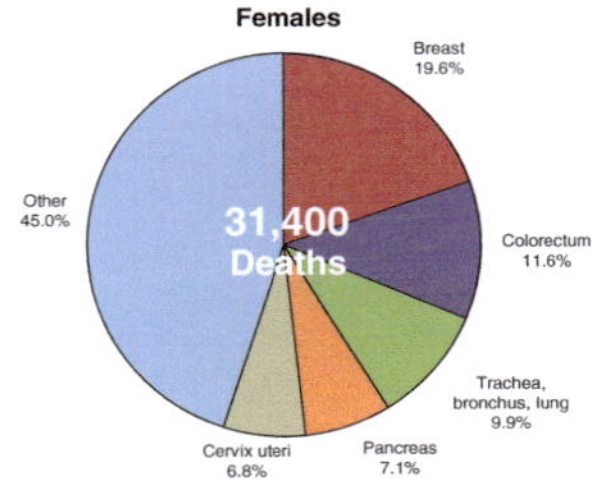

Age-Standardized Cancer Mortality Trends

Males

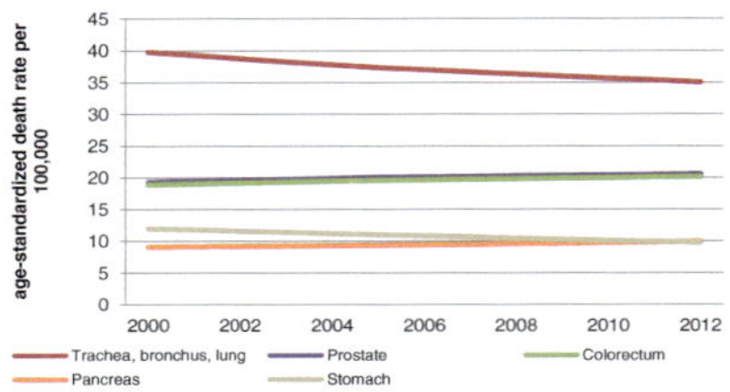

Females

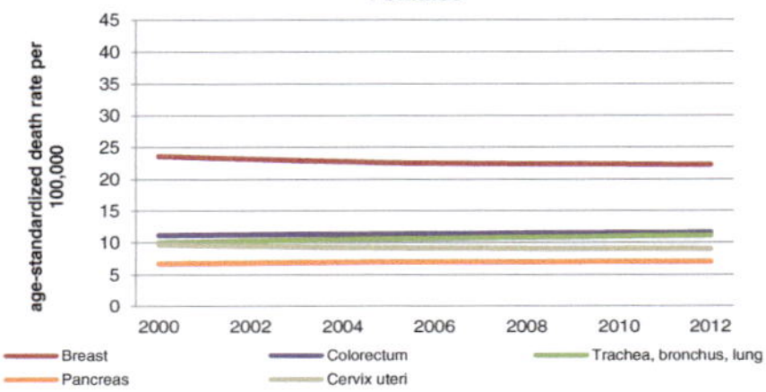

Cancer Incidence

Males

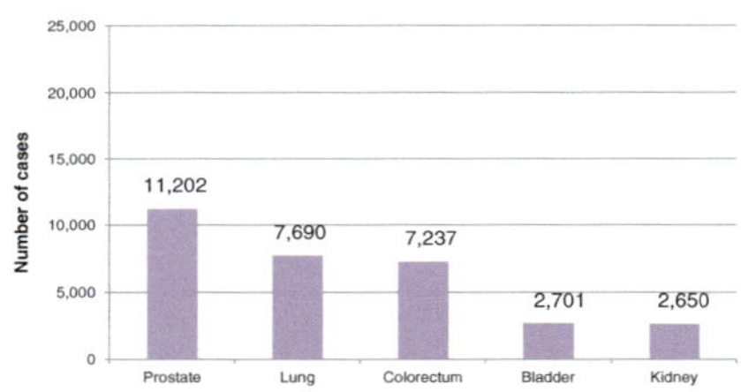

Females

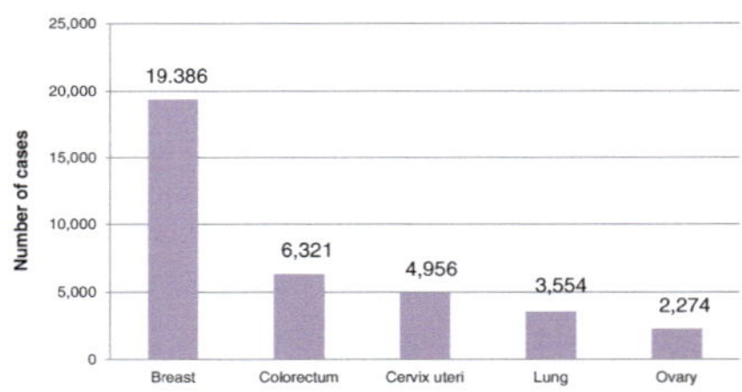

Adult Risk Factors

	Males	Females	Total
Current tobacco smoking (2011)	29.9%	16%	22.7%
Total alcohol per capita consumption, in litres of pure alcohol (2010)	13.6	5.2	9.3
Physical inactivity (2010)	35.7%	44.1%	40.1%
Obesity (2014)	23.6%	29.4%	26.5%
Household solid fuel use (2012)	-	-	1.0%

World Health Organization - Cancer Country Profiles, 2014.

Cancer Plans, Monitoring and Surveillance	
Has an operational cancer policy/strategy/action plan	Yes
Has a cancer registry	Yes
Scope	Population-based
Coverage	National and Subnational
Last year of data	2012

Cancer Primary Prevention Policies	
Tobacco control	
Has an operational policy, strategy or action plan to reduce the burden of tobacco use	Yes
Smoke-free legislation	All public places completely smoke-free (or at least 90% of the population covered by complete subnational smoke-free legislation)*
Tobacco dependence treatment	NRT and/or some cessation services (at least one of which is cost-covered)
Warning labels	Large warnings with all appropriate characteristics*
Bans on advertising, promotion and sponsorship	Ban on national television, radio and print media as well as on some but not all other forms of direct and/or indirect advertising
Tobacco taxes	51–75% of retail price is tax
Overweight and obesity prevention and control	
Has an operational policy, strategy or action plan for reducing overweight/obesity	Yes
Physical inactivity prevention and control	
Has an operational policy, strategy or action plan to reduce physical inactivity and/or promote physical activity	Yes
Harmful use of alcohol prevention and control	
Has an operational policy, strategy or action plan to reduce the harmful use of alcohol	Yes
National immunization	
Human Papillomavirus vaccination schedule	11 years (x3)
Hepatitis B vaccination schedule	Birth
Hepatitis B vaccination coverage, infants	87%

Cancer Screening and Early Detection	
Cervical cancer	
Cervical cytology (PAP)	Generally available at the public primary health care level
Acetic acid visualization (VIA)	Generally available at the public primary health care level
Breast cancer	
Breast palpation / clinical breast exam (CBE)	Generally available at the public primary health care level
Mammogram	Generally available at the public primary health care level
Colorectal cancer	
Faecal occult blood test or faecal immunological test	Generally available at the public primary health care level
Bowel cancer screening by exam or colonoscopy	Generally available at the public primary health care level

Cancer Treatment and Palliative Care	
Radiotherapy	Generally available in the public health system
Total high energy teletherapy units / million inhabitants	2.8
Number of radiotherapy centres	82
Number of radiation oncologists	176
Chemotherapy (medicines not specified)	Generally available in the public health system
Oral morphine (formulation not specified)	Generally available in the public health system
Non-methadone morphine equivalent consumption per cancer death (mg)	...
Community/home care for people with advanced stage cancer and other NCDs	Generally available

* Indicates highest possible level of achievement ... = No data available

World Health Organization - Cancer Country Profiles, 2014.

Bolivia (Plurinational State of)

Total population: 10,496,000
Income group: Lower middle

Total deaths: 72,000
Life expectancy at birth: Total:68 Males:65 Females:70

Cancer Mortality Profile*

Males

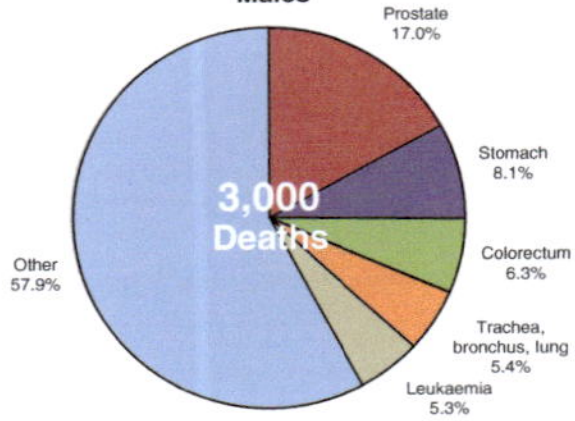

Females

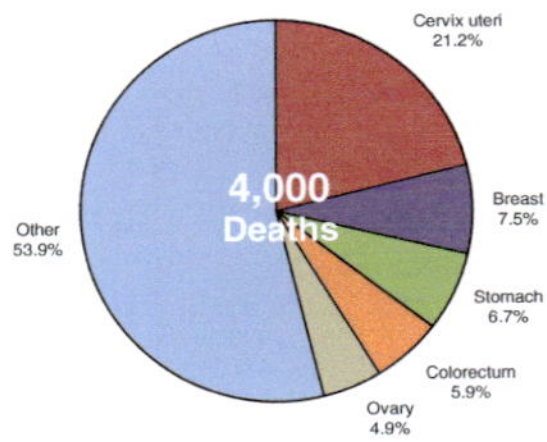

Age-Standardized Cancer Mortality Trends*

Males

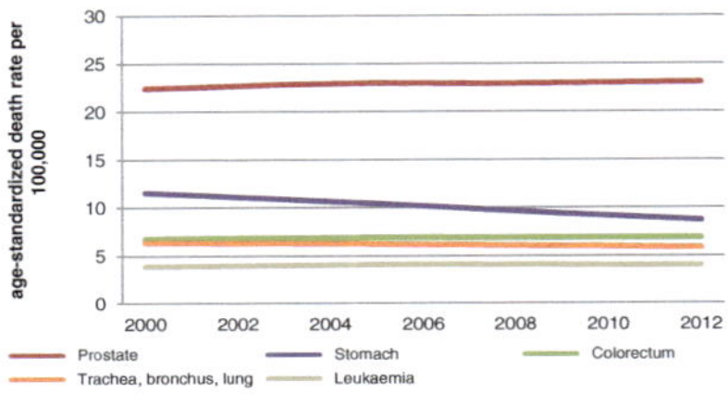

Females

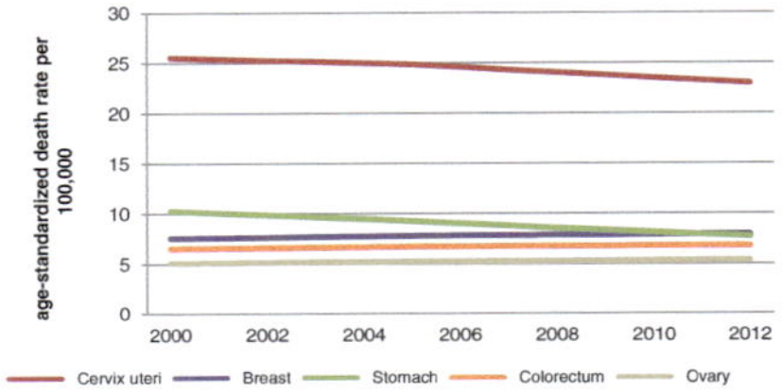

Cancer Incidence**

Males

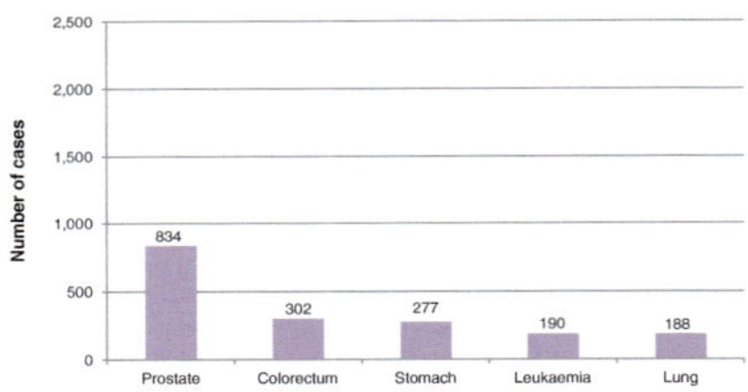

Females

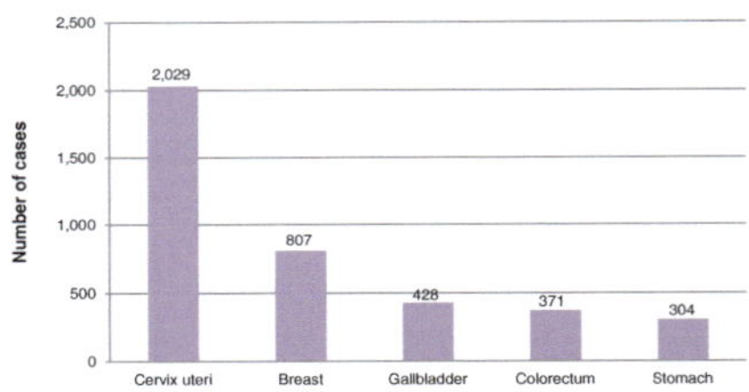

Adult Risk Factors

	Males	Females	Total
Current tobacco smoking (2011)	41.7%	18.4%	29.9%
Total alcohol per capita consumption, in litres of pure alcohol (2010)	9.1	2.7	5.9
Physical inactivity (2010)	...	...	...
Obesity (2014)	11.1%	20.6%	15.8%
Household solid fuel use (2012)	-	-	25.0%

World Health Organization - Cancer Country Profiles, 2014.

Cancer Plans, Monitoring and Surveillance

Has an operational cancer policy/strategy/action plan	Yes
Has a cancer registry	Yes
Scope	Population-based
Coverage	Subnational
Last year of data	2011

Cancer Primary Prevention Policies

Tobacco control

Has an operational policy, strategy or action plan to reduce the burden of tobacco use	Yes
Smoke-free legislation	Three to five public places completely smoke-free
Tobacco dependence treatment	NRT and/or some cessation services (at least one of which is cost-covered)
Warning labels	Large warnings with all appropriate characteristics***
Bans on advertising, promotion and sponsorship	Ban on national television, radio and print media as well as on some but not all other forms of direct and/or indirect advertising
Tobacco taxes	26–50% of retail price is tax

Overweight and obesity prevention and control

Has an operational policy, strategy or action plan for reducing overweight/obesity	Yes

Physical inactivity prevention and control

Has an operational policy, strategy or action plan to reduce physical inactivity and/or promote physical activity	Yes

Harmful use of alcohol prevention and control

Has an operational policy, strategy or action plan to reduce the harmful use of alcohol	Yes

National immunization

Human Papillomavirus vaccination schedule	...
Hepatitis B vaccination schedule	...
Hepatitis B vaccination coverage, infants	94%

Cancer Screening and Early Detection

Cervical cancer

Cervical cytology (PAP)	Generally available at the public primary health care level
Acetic acid visualization (VIA)	Not generally available at the public primary health care level

Breast cancer

Breast palpation / clinical breast exam (CBE)	Generally available at the public primary health care level
Mammogram	Not generally available at the public primary health care level

Colorectal cancer

Faecal occult blood test or faecal immunological test	Generally available at the public primary health care level
Bowel cancer screening by exam or colonoscopy	Not generally available at the public primary health care level

Cancer Treatment and Palliative Care

Radiotherapy	Generally available in the public health system
Total high energy teletherapy units / million inhabitants	0.6
Number of radiotherapy centres	5
Number of radiation oncologists	11
Chemotherapy (medicines not specified)	Generally available in the public health system
Oral morphine (formulation not specified)	Not generally available in the public health system
Non-methadone morphine equivalent consumption per cancer death (mg)	...
Community/home care for people with advanced stage cancer and other NCDs	Not generally available

* No mortality data available. Figures are based on national incidence estimates and modelled survival.
** No incidence data available. Figures are based on national incidence estimates from neighbouring countries.
*** Indicates highest possible level of achievement

... = No data available

World Health Organization - Cancer Country Profiles, 2014.

Brazil

Total population: 199,000,000
Income group: Upper middle

Total deaths: 1,318,000
Life expectancy at birth: Total:74 Males:70 Females:77

Cancer Mortality Profile

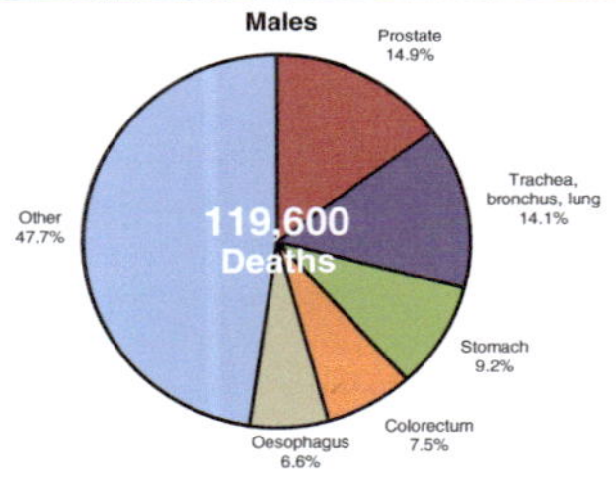

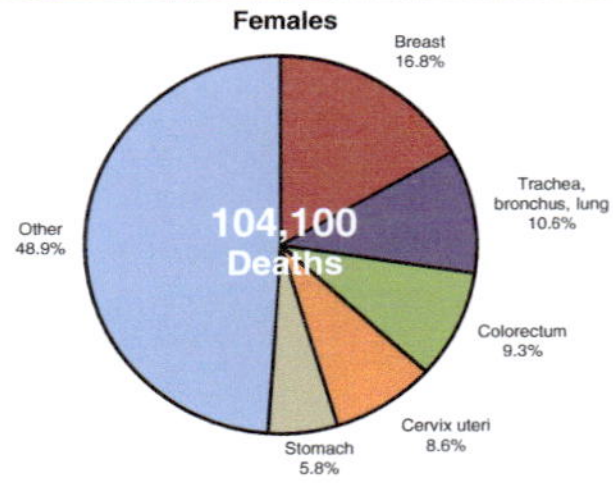

Age-Standardized Cancer Mortality Trends

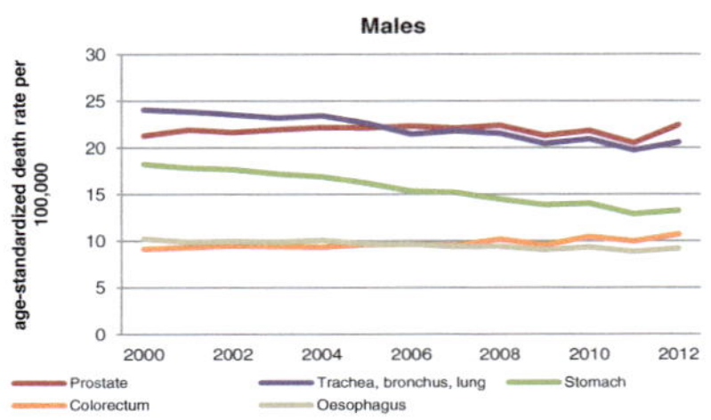

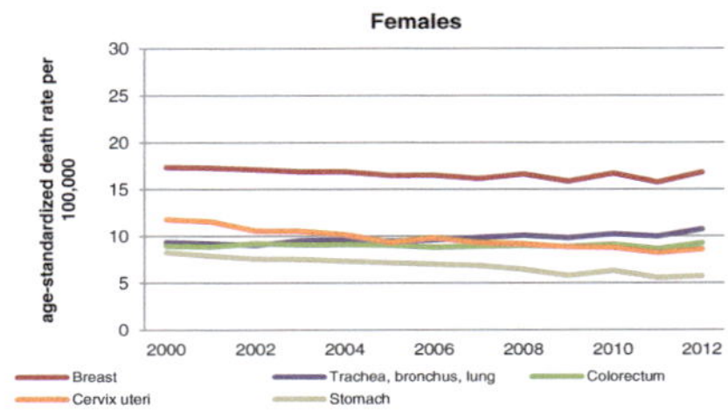

Cancer Incidence

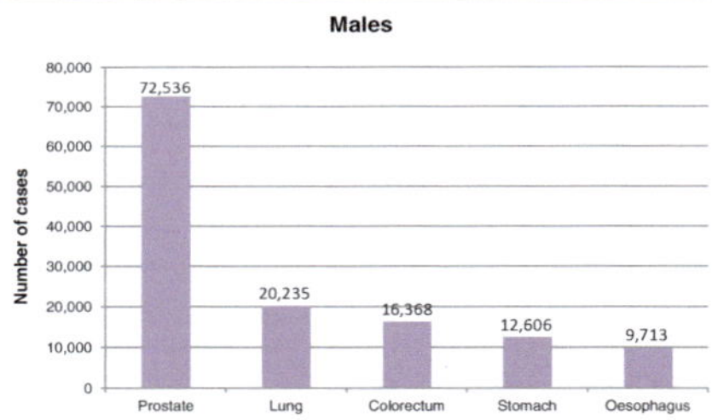

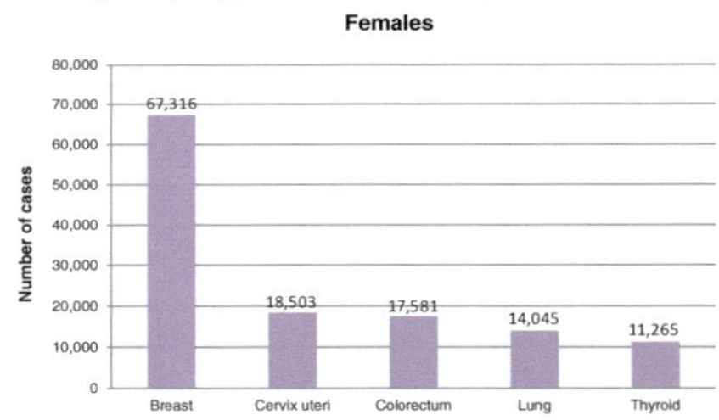

Adult Risk Factors

	Males	Females	Total
Current tobacco smoking (2011)	21.6%	13%	17.3%
Total alcohol per capita consumption, in litres of pure alcohol (2010)	13.6	4.2	8.7
Physical inactivity (2010)	24.9%	29.4%	27.2%
Obesity (2014)	17.2%	22.9%	20.1%
Household solid fuel use (2012)	-	-	6.0%

World Health Organization - Cancer Country Profiles, 2014.

Cancer Plans, Monitoring and Surveillance

Has an operational cancer policy/strategy/action plan	Yes
Has a cancer registry	Yes
Scope	Population-based
Coverage	Subnational
Last year of data	2008

Cancer Primary Prevention Policies

Tobacco control

Has an operational policy, strategy or action plan to reduce the burden of tobacco use	Yes
Smoke-free legislation	All public places completely smoke-free (or at least 90% of the population covered by complete subnational smoke-free legislation)*
Tobacco dependence treatment	National quit line, and both NRT and some cessation services cost-covered*
Warning labels	Large warnings with all appropriate characteristics*
Bans on advertising, promotion and sponsorship	Ban on all forms of direct and indirect advertising*
Tobacco taxes	51–75% of retail price is tax

Overweight and obesity prevention and control

Has an operational policy, strategy or action plan for reducing overweight/obesity	No

Physical inactivity prevention and control

Has an operational policy, strategy or action plan to reduce physical inactivity and/or promote physical activity	Yes

Harmful use of alcohol prevention and control

Has an operational policy, strategy or action plan to reduce the harmful use of alcohol	No

National immunization

Human Papillomavirus vaccination schedule	(starting in 2014)
Hepatitis B vaccination schedule	Birth, +3 doses between 20-29 years
Hepatitis B vaccination coverage, infants	95%

Cancer Screening and Early Detection

Cervical cancer

Cervical cytology (PAP)	Generally available at the public primary health care level
Acetic acid visualization (VIA)	Not generally available at the public primary health care level

Breast cancer

Breast palpation / clinical breast exam (CBE)	Generally available at the public primary health care level
Mammogram	Generally available at the public primary health care level

Colorectal cancer

Faecal occult blood test or faecal immunological test	Generally available at the public primary health care level
Bowel cancer screening by exam or colonoscopy	Generally available at the public primary health care level

Cancer Treatment and Palliative Care

Radiotherapy	Generally available in the public health system
Total high energy teletherapy units / million inhabitants	1.7
Number of radiotherapy centres	222
Number of radiation oncologists	391
Chemotherapy (medicines not specified)	Generally available in the public health system
Oral morphine (formulation not specified)	Generally available in the public health system
Non-methadone morphine equivalent consumption per cancer death (mg)	6,821.5
Community/home care for people with advanced stage cancer and other NCDs	Generally available

* Indicates highest possible level of achievement

World Health Organization - Cancer Country Profiles, 2014.

Central African Republic

Total population: 4,525,000
Income group: Low

Total deaths: 65,000
Life expectancy at birth: Total:51 Males:50 Females:52

Cancer Mortality Profile*

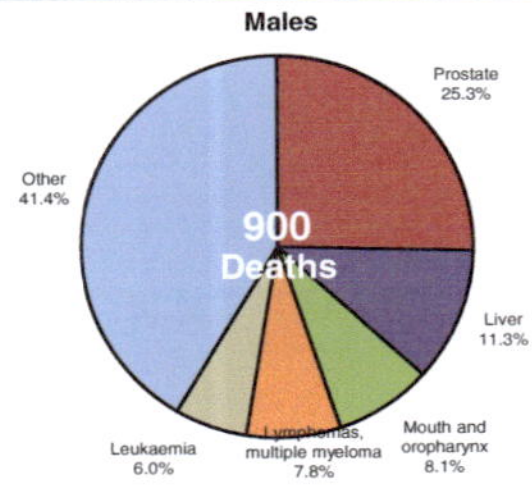

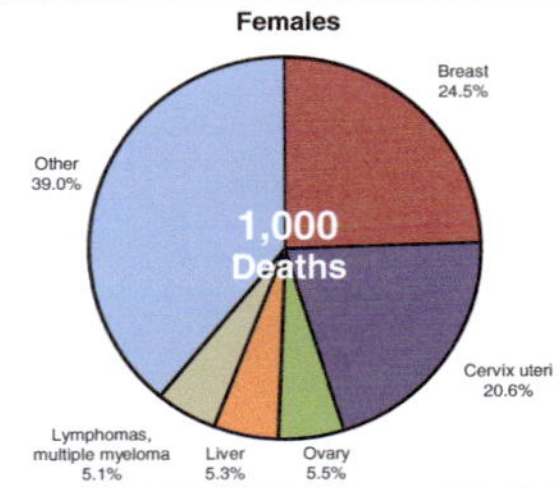

Age-Standardized Cancer Mortality Trends*

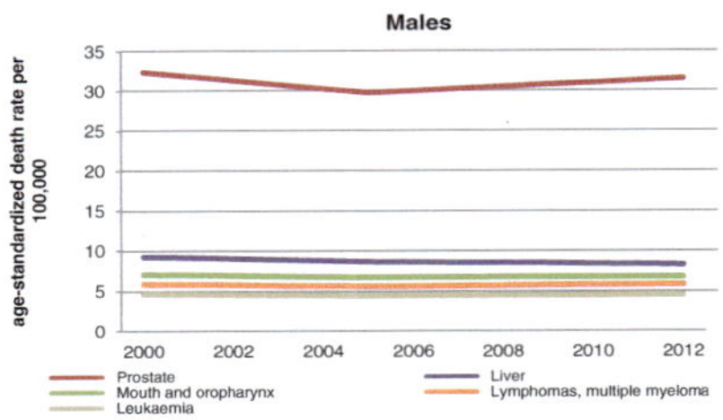

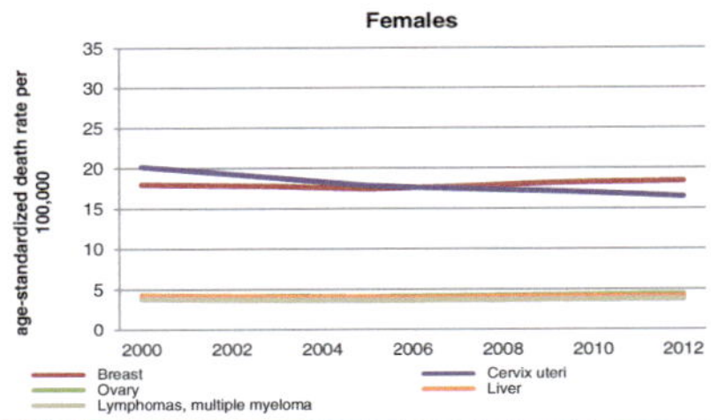

Cancer Incidence**

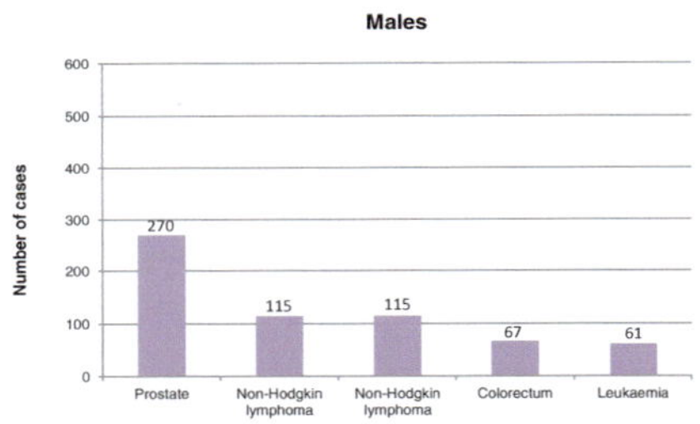

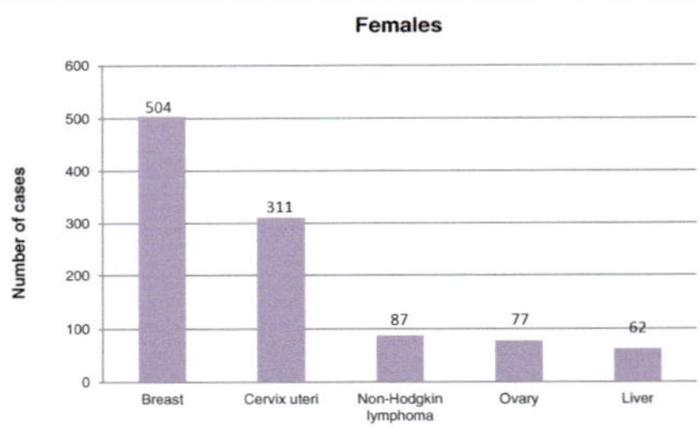

Adult Risk Factors

	Males	Females	Total
Current tobacco smoking (2011)	...	...	...
Total alcohol per capita consumption, in litres of pure alcohol (2010)	5.7	1.9	3.8
Physical inactivity (2010)	8.9%	12.0%	10.5%
Obesity (2014)	1.9%	6.7%	4.4%
Household solid fuel use (2012)	-	-	97.0%

World Health Organization - Cancer Country Profiles, 2014.

Cancer Plans, Monitoring and Surveillance

Has an operational cancer policy/strategy/action plan	No
Has a cancer registry	No
Scope	
Coverage	
Last year of data	

Cancer Primary Prevention Policies

Tobacco control

Has an operational policy, strategy or action plan to reduce the burden of tobacco use	DK
Smoke-free legislation	Up to two public places completely smoke-free
Tobacco dependence treatment	NRT and/or some cessation services (neither cost-covered)
Warning labels	No warnings or small warnings
Bans on advertising, promotion and sponsorship	Complete absence of ban, or ban that does not cover national television, radio and print media
Tobacco taxes	Data not reported

Overweight and obesity prevention and control

Has an operational policy, strategy or action plan for reducing overweight/obesity	No

Physical inactivity prevention and control

Has an operational policy, strategy or action plan to reduce physical inactivity and/or promote physical activity	No

Harmful use of alcohol prevention and control

Has an operational policy, strategy or action plan to reduce the harmful use of alcohol	No

National immunization

Human Papillomavirus vaccination schedule	...
Hepatitis B vaccination schedule	...
Hepatitis B vaccination coverage, infants	23%

Cancer Screening and Early Detection

Cervical cancer

Cervical cytology (PAP)	Generally available at the public primary health care level
Acetic acid visualization (VIA)	Not generally available at the public primary health care level

Breast cancer

Breast palpation / clinical breast exam (CBE)	Generally available at the public primary health care level
Mammogram	Not generally available at the public primary health care level

Colorectal cancer

Faecal occult blood test or faecal immunological test	Not generally available at the public primary health care level
Bowel cancer screening by exam or colonoscopy	Not generally available at the public primary health care level

Cancer Treatment and Palliative Care

Radiotherapy	Not generally available in the public health system
Total high energy teletherapy units / million inhabitants	0.0
Number of radiotherapy centres	...
Number of radiation oncologists	...
Chemotherapy (medicines not specified)	Not generally available in the public health system
Oral morphine (formulation not specified)	Not generally available in the public health system
Non-methadone morphine equivalent consumption per cancer death (mg)	...
Community/home care for people with advanced stage cancer and other NCDs	Not generally available

* No mortality data available. Figures are based on national incidence estimates and modelled survival.
** No incidence data available. Figures are based on national incidence estimates from neighbouring countries.

... = No data available
DK = Country responded "don't know"

World Health Organization - Cancer Country Profiles, 2014.

Chile

Total population: 17,465,000
Income group: High

Total deaths: 94,000
Life expectancy at birth: Total:80 Males:77 Females:83

Cancer Mortality Profile

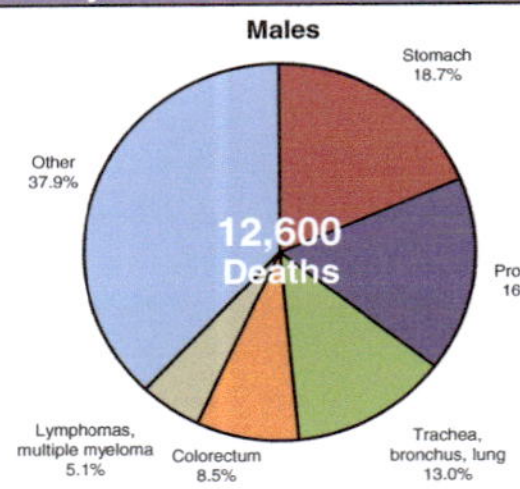

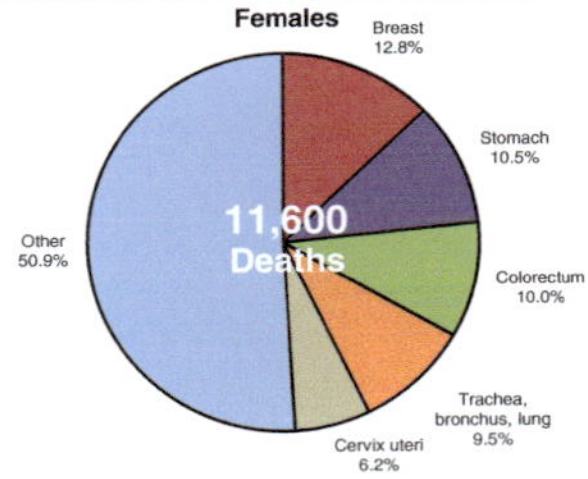

Age-Standardized Cancer Mortality Trends

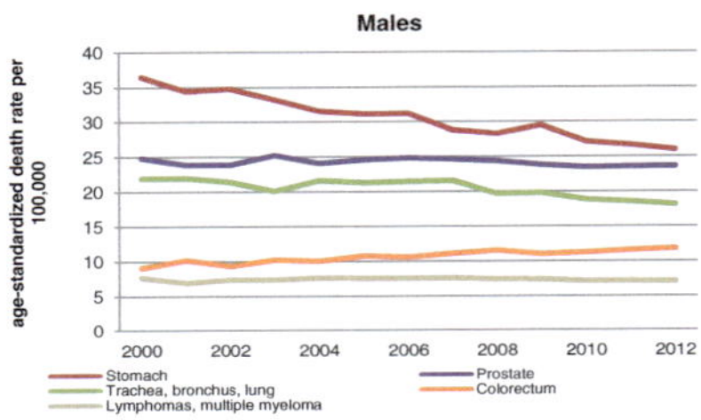

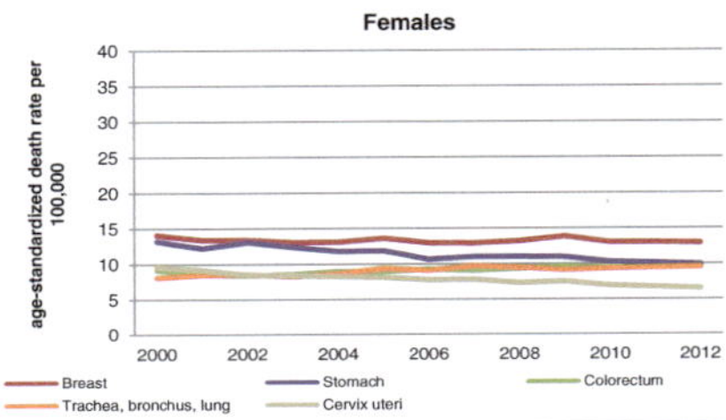

Cancer Incidence

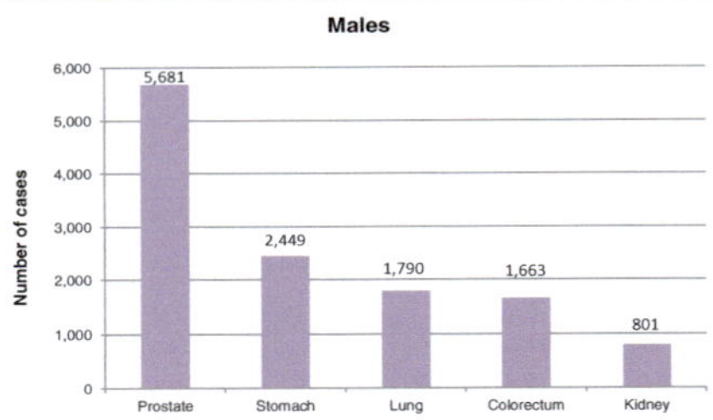

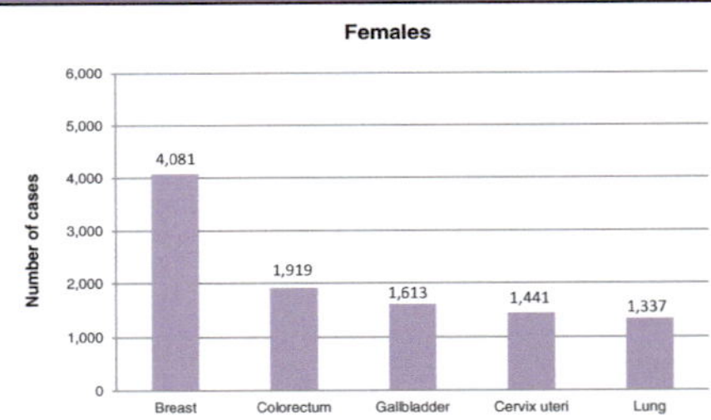

Adult Risk Factors

	Males	Females	Total
Current tobacco smoking (2011)	43.9%	37.8%	40.8%
Total alcohol per capita consumption, in litres of pure alcohol (2010)	13.9	5.5	9.6
Physical inactivity (2010)	17.6%	25.5%	21.6%
Obesity (2014)	23.7%	33.1%	28.5%
Household solid fuel use (2012)	-	-	7.0%

World Health Organization - Cancer Country Profiles, 2014.

Cancer Plans, Monitoring and Surveillance

Has an operational cancer policy/strategy/action plan	Yes
Has a cancer registry	Yes
Scope	Population-based
Coverage	Subnational
Last year of data	2011

Cancer Primary Prevention Policies

Tobacco control

Has an operational policy, strategy or action plan to reduce the burden of tobacco use	Yes
Smoke-free legislation	Three to five public places completely smoke-free
Tobacco dependence treatment	NRT and/or some cessation services (neither cost-covered)
Warning labels	Large warnings with all appropriate characteristics*
Bans on advertising, promotion and sponsorship	Ban on national television, radio and print media as well as on some but not all other forms of direct and/or indirect advertising
Tobacco taxes	>75% of retail price is tax*

Overweight and obesity prevention and control

Has an operational policy, strategy or action plan for reducing overweight/obesity	Yes

Physical inactivity prevention and control

Has an operational policy, strategy or action plan to reduce physical inactivity and/or promote physical activity	Yes

Harmful use of alcohol prevention and control

Has an operational policy, strategy or action plan to reduce the harmful use of alcohol	Yes

National immunization

Human Papillomavirus vaccination schedule	(starting July 2014)
Hepatitis B vaccination schedule	...
Hepatitis B vaccination coverage, infants	90%

Cancer Screening and Early Detection

Cervical cancer

Cervical cytology (PAP)	Generally available at the public primary health care level
Acetic acid visualization (VIA)	Not generally available at the public primary health care level

Breast cancer

Breast palpation / clinical breast exam (CBE)	Generally available at the public primary health care level
Mammogram	Generally available at the public primary health care level

Colorectal cancer

Faecal occult blood test or faecal immunological test	Generally available at the public primary health care level
Bowel cancer screening by exam or colonoscopy	Generally available at the public primary health care level

Cancer Treatment and Palliative Care

Radiotherapy	Generally available in the public health system
Total high energy teletherapy units / million inhabitants	0.9
Number of radiotherapy centres	27
Number of radiation oncologists	55
Chemotherapy (medicines not specified)	Generally available in the public health system
Oral morphine (formulation not specified)	Generally available in the public health system
Non-methadone morphine equivalent consumption per cancer death (mg)	...
Community/home care for people with advanced stage cancer and other NCDs	Generally available

* Indicates highest possible level of achievement ... = No data available

World Health Organization - Cancer Country Profiles, 2014.

Colombia

Total population: 47,704,000
Income group: Upper middle

Total deaths: 202,000
Life expectancy at birth: Total:79 Males:76 Females:83

Cancer Mortality Profile

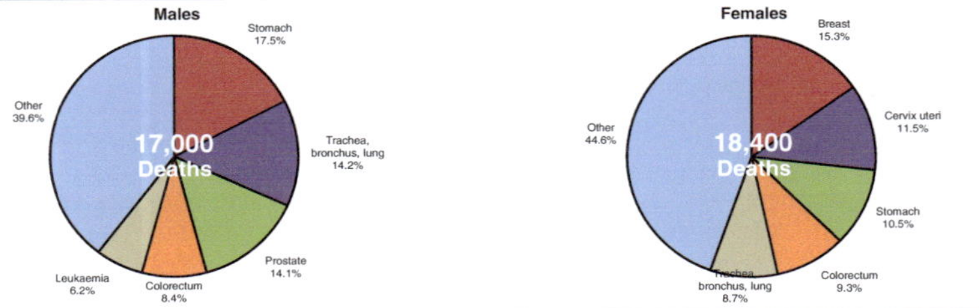

Age-Standardized Cancer Mortality Trends

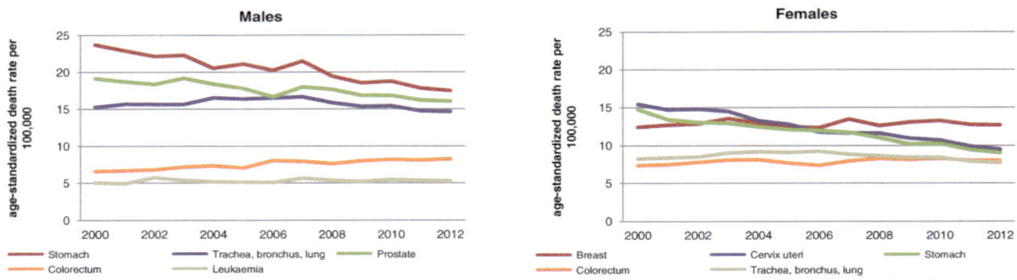

Cancer Incidence

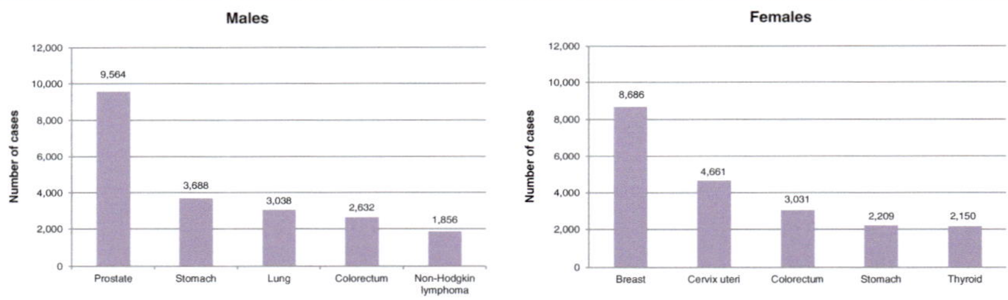

Adult Risk Factors

	Males	Females	Total
Current tobacco smoking (2011)	30.7%	5%	17.5%
Total alcohol per capita consumption, in litres of pure alcohol (2010)	9.1	3.5	6.2
Physical inactivity (2010)	53.4%	72.9%	63.5%
Obesity (2014)	15.7%	25.5%	20.7%
Household solid fuel use (2012)	-	-	15.0%

World Health Organization - Cancer Country Profiles, 2014.

Cancer Plans, Monitoring and Surveillance

Has an operational cancer policy/strategy/action plan	Yes
Has a cancer registry	Yes
Scope	Population-based
Coverage	Subnational
Last year of data	2008

Cancer Primary Prevention Policies

Tobacco control

Has an operational policy, strategy or action plan to reduce the burden of tobacco use	Yes
Smoke-free legislation	All public places completely smoke-free (or at least 90% of the population covered by complete subnational smoke-free legislation)*
Tobacco dependence treatment	NRT and/or some cessation services (neither cost-covered)
Warning labels	Medium size warnings with all appropriate characteristics OR large warnings missing some appropriate characteristics
Bans on advertising, promotion and sponsorship	Ban on all forms of direct and indirect advertising*
Tobacco taxes	26–50% of retail price is tax

Overweight and obesity prevention and control

Has an operational policy, strategy or action plan for reducing overweight/obesity	Yes

Physical inactivity prevention and control

Has an operational policy, strategy or action plan to reduce physical inactivity and/or promote physical activity	Yes

Harmful use of alcohol prevention and control

Has an operational policy, strategy or action plan to reduce the harmful use of alcohol	Yes

National immunization

Human Papillomavirus vaccination schedule	9-17 years, +11 months and 29 days
Hepatitis B vaccination schedule	Birth
Hepatitis B vaccination coverage, infants	91%

Cancer Screening and Early Detection

Cervical cancer

Cervical cytology (PAP)	Generally available at the public primary health care level
Acetic acid visualization (VIA)	Generally available at the public primary health care level

Breast cancer

Breast palpation / clinical breast exam (CBE)	Generally available at the public primary health care level
Mammogram	Generally available at the public primary health care level

Colorectal cancer

Faecal occult blood test or faecal immunological test	Generally available at the public primary health care level
Bowel cancer screening by exam or colonoscopy	Generally available at the public primary health care level

Cancer Treatment and Palliative Care

Radiotherapy	Generally available in the public health system
Total high energy teletherapy units / million inhabitants	1.4
Number of radiotherapy centres	55
Number of radiation oncologists	87
Chemotherapy (medicines not specified)	Generally available in the public health system
Oral morphine (formulation not specified)	Generally available in the public health system
Non-methadone morphine equivalent consumption per cancer death (mg)	7,954.2
Community/home care for people with advanced stage cancer and other NCDs	Generally available

* Indicates highest possible level of achievement

World Health Organization - Cancer Country Profiles, 2014.

Cuba

Total population: 11,271,000
Income group: Upper middle

Total deaths: 89,000
Life expectancy at birth: Total:79 Males:76 Females:81

Cancer Mortality Profile

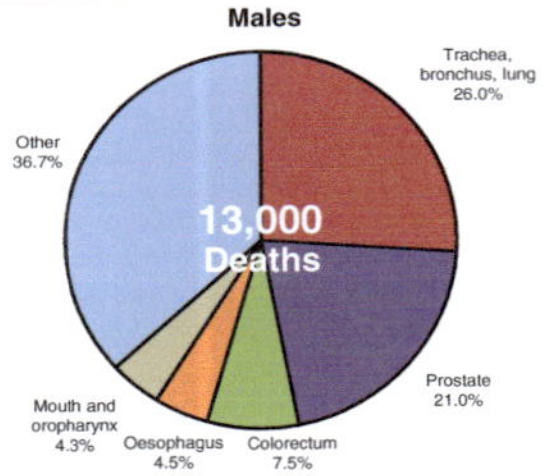

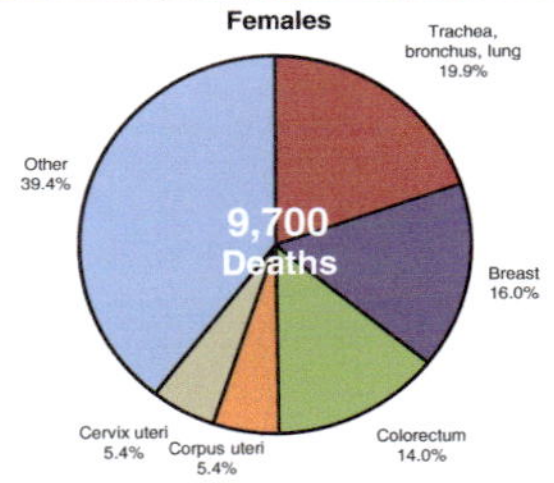

Age-Standardized Cancer Mortality Trends

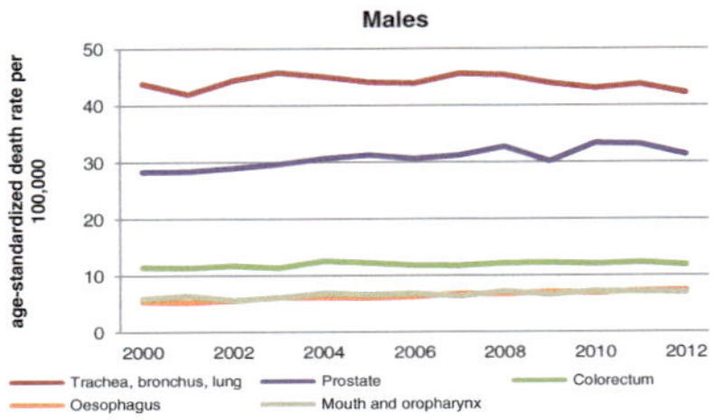

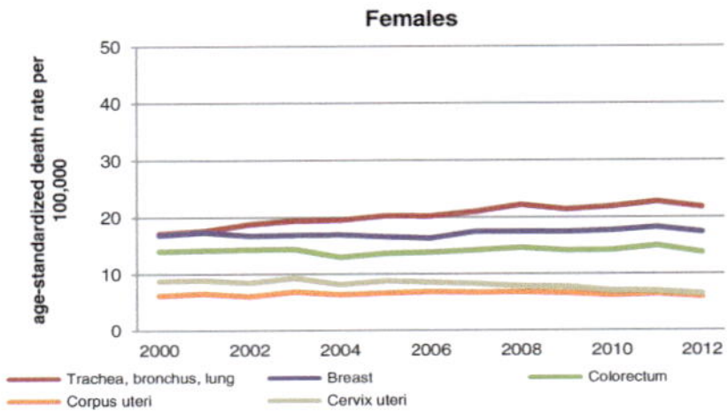

Cancer Incidence

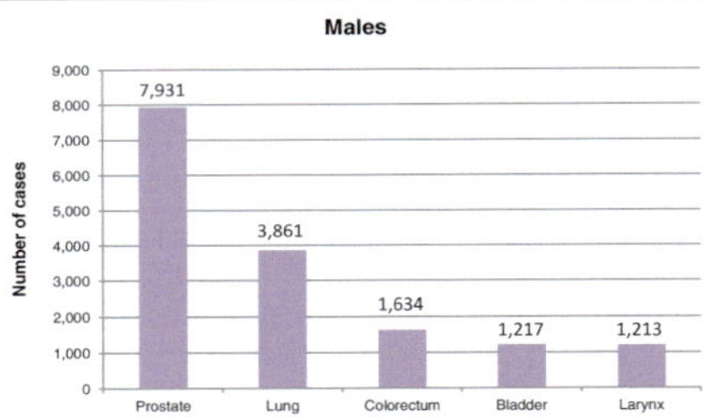

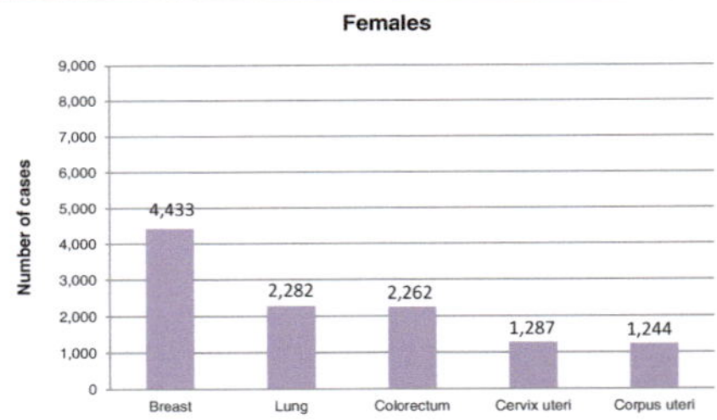

Adult Risk Factors

	Males	Females	Total
Current tobacco smoking (2011)	...	...	...
Total alcohol per capita consumption, in litres of pure alcohol (2010)	8.8	1.6	5.2
Physical inactivity (2010)	...	...	...
Obesity (2014)	20.4%	34.0%	27.2%
Household solid fuel use (2012)	-	-	7.0%

World Health Organization - Cancer Country Profiles, 2014.

Cancer Plans, Monitoring and Surveillance

Has an operational cancer policy/strategy/action plan	Yes
Has a cancer registry	Yes
Scope	Population-based
Coverage	National
Last year of data	2009

Cancer Primary Prevention Policies

Tobacco control

Has an operational policy, strategy or action plan to reduce the burden of tobacco use	Yes
Smoke-free legislation	Three to five public places completely smoke-free
Tobacco dependence treatment	NRT and/or some cessation services (at least one of which is cost-covered)
Warning labels	Medium size warnings missing some appropriate characteristics OR large warnings missing many appropriate characteristics
Bans on advertising, promotion and sponsorship	Complete absence of ban, or ban that does not cover national television, radio and print media
Tobacco taxes	>75% of retail price is tax*

Overweight and obesity prevention and control

Has an operational policy, strategy or action plan for reducing overweight/obesity	Yes

Physical inactivity prevention and control

Has an operational policy, strategy or action plan to reduce physical inactivity and/or promote physical activity	Yes

Harmful use of alcohol prevention and control

Has an operational policy, strategy or action plan to reduce the harmful use of alcohol	Yes

National immunization

Human Papillomavirus vaccination schedule	...
Hepatitis B vaccination schedule	Birth
Hepatitis B vaccination coverage, infants	96%

Cancer Screening and Early Detection

Cervical cancer

Cervical cytology (PAP)	Generally available at the public primary health care level
Acetic acid visualization (VIA)	Not generally available at the public primary health care level

Breast cancer

Breast palpation / clinical breast exam (CBE)	Generally available at the public primary health care level
Mammogram	Generally available at the public primary health care level

Colorectal cancer

Faecal occult blood test or faecal immunological test	Generally available at the public primary health care level
Bowel cancer screening by exam or colonoscopy	Generally available at the public primary health care level

Cancer Treatment and Palliative Care

Radiotherapy	Generally available in the public health system
Total high energy teletherapy units / million inhabitants	1.2
Number of radiotherapy centres	9
Number of radiation oncologists	38
Chemotherapy (medicines not specified)	Generally available in the public health system
Oral morphine (formulation not specified)	Not generally available in the public health system
Non-methadone morphine equivalent consumption per cancer death (mg)	...
Community/home care for people with advanced stage cancer and other NCDs	Generally available

* Indicates highest possible level of achievement ... = No data available

World Health Organization - Cancer Country Profiles, 2014.

Dominican Republic

Total population: 10,277,000
Income group: Upper middle

Total deaths: 49,000
Life expectancy at birth: Total:77 Males:76 Females:78

Cancer Mortality Profile

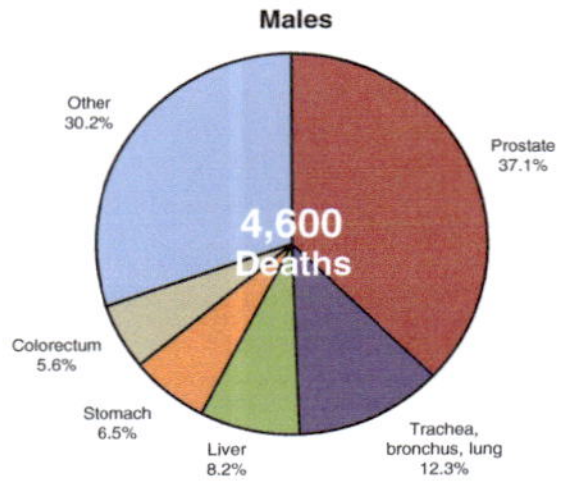

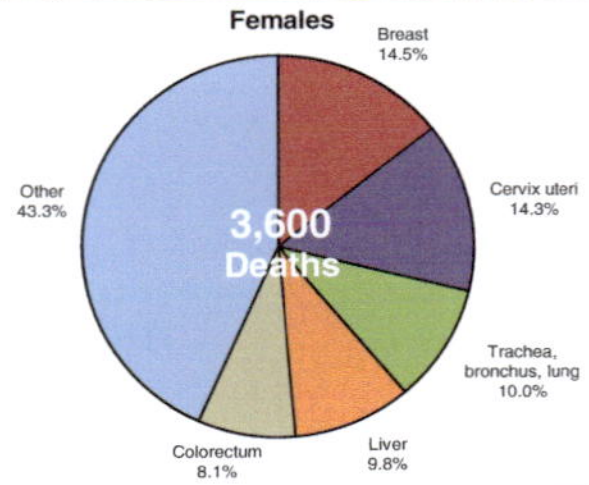

Age-Standardized Cancer Mortality Trends

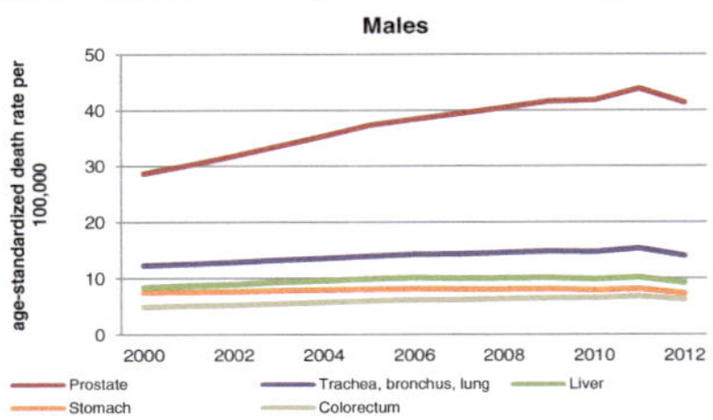

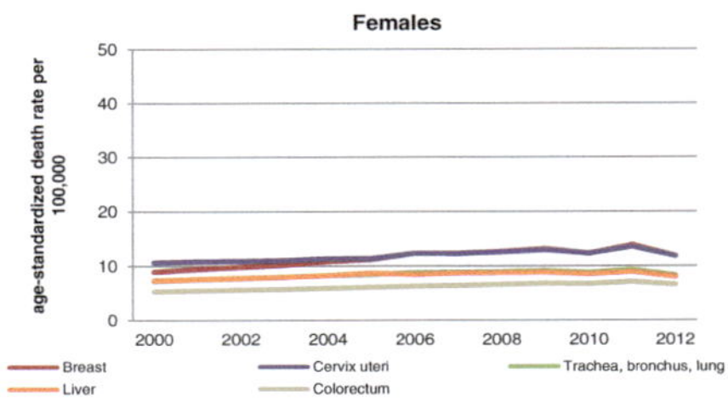

Cancer Incidence*

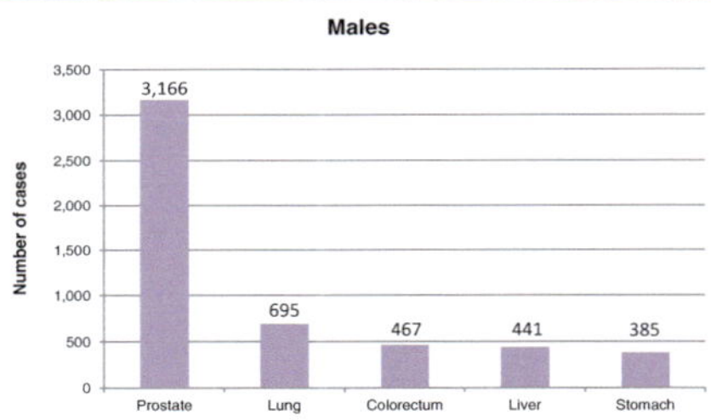

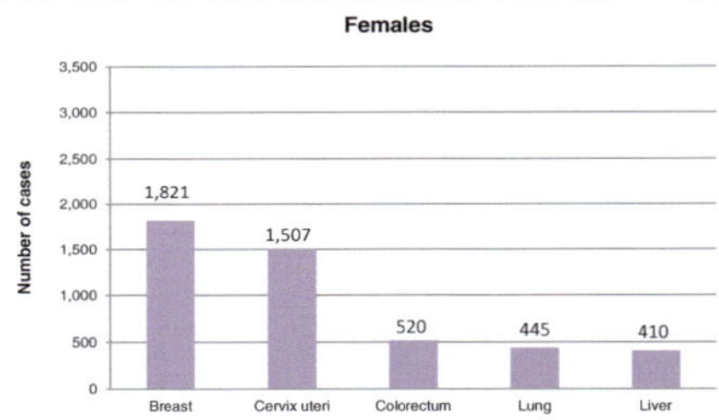

Adult Risk Factors

	Males	Females	Total
Current tobacco smoking (2011)	16.6%	15.6%	16.1%
Total alcohol per capita consumption, in litres of pure alcohol (2010)	9.8	4.0	6.9
Physical inactivity (2010)	30.5%	39.4%	35.0%
Obesity (2014)	17.6%	28.4%	23.0%
Household solid fuel use (2012)	-	-	8.0%

World Health Organization - Cancer Country Profiles, 2014.

Cancer Plans, Monitoring and Surveillance

Has an operational cancer policy/strategy/action plan	Yes
Has a cancer registry	Yes
Scope	Population-based
Coverage	Subnational
Last year of data	2013

Cancer Primary Prevention Policies

Tobacco control

Has an operational policy, strategy or action plan to reduce the burden of tobacco use	Yes
Smoke-free legislation	Up to two public places completely smoke-free
Tobacco dependence treatment	NRT and/or some cessation services (neither cost-covered)
Warning labels	No warnings or small warnings
Bans on advertising, promotion and sponsorship	Complete absence of ban, or ban that does not cover national television, radio and print media
Tobacco taxes	51–75% of retail price is tax

Overweight and obesity prevention and control

Has an operational policy, strategy or action plan for reducing overweight/obesity	Yes

Physical inactivity prevention and control

Has an operational policy, strategy or action plan to reduce physical inactivity and/or promote physical activity	Yes

Harmful use of alcohol prevention and control

Has an operational policy, strategy or action plan to reduce the harmful use of alcohol	Yes

National immunization

Human Papillomavirus vaccination schedule	(starting September 2014)
Hepatitis B vaccination schedule	Birth
Hepatitis B vaccination coverage, infants	80%

Cancer Screening and Early Detection

Cervical cancer

Cervical cytology (PAP)	Generally available at the public primary health care level
Acetic acid visualization (VIA)	Not generally available at the public primary health care level

Breast cancer

Breast palpation / clinical breast exam (CBE)	Generally available at the public primary health care level
Mammogram	Not generally available at the public primary health care level

Colorectal cancer

Faecal occult blood test or faecal immunological test	Generally available at the public primary health care level
Bowel cancer screening by exam or colonoscopy	Not generally available at the public primary health care level

Cancer Treatment and Palliative Care

Radiotherapy	Not generally available in the public health system
Total high energy teletherapy units / million inhabitants	1.2
Number of radiotherapy centres	9
Number of radiation oncologists	12
Chemotherapy (medicines not specified)	Not generally available in the public health system
Oral morphine (formulation not specified)	Not generally available in the public health system
Non-methadone morphine equivalent consumption per cancer death (mg)	...
Community/home care for people with advanced stage cancer and other NCDs	Not generally available

* No incidence data available. Figures are based on national mortality estimates and modelled survival. ... = No data available

World Health Organization - Cancer Country Profiles, 2014.

Ethiopia

Total population: 91,729,000
Income group: Low

Total deaths: 691,000
Life expectancy at birth: Total:64 Males:62 Females:65

Cancer Mortality Profile*

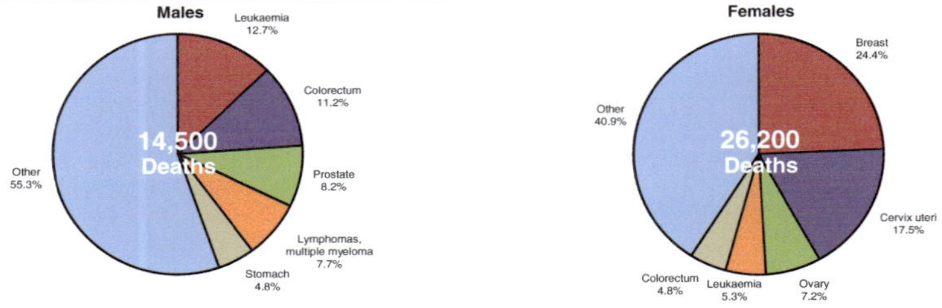

Age-Standardized Cancer Mortality Trends*

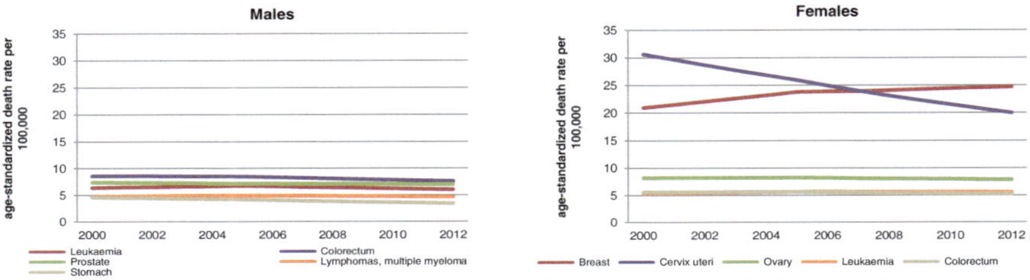

Cancer Incidence

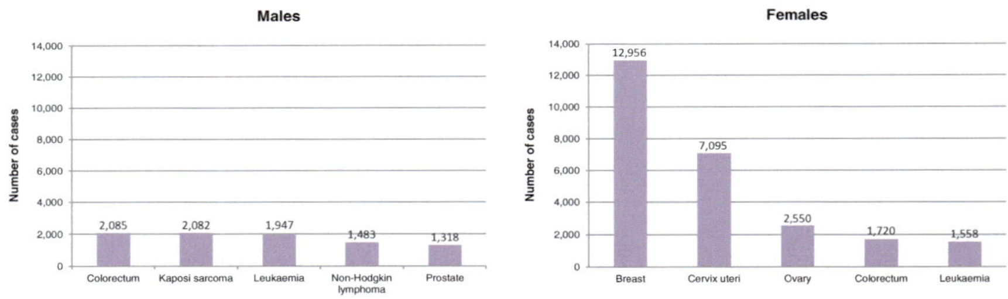

Adult Risk Factors

	Males	Females	Total
Current tobacco smoking (2011)	...	...	...
Total alcohol per capita consumption, in litres of pure alcohol (2010)	6.2	2.2	4.2
Physical inactivity (2010)	12.6%	21.5%	17.1%
Obesity (2014)	1.3%	5.4%	3.3%
Household solid fuel use (2012)	-	-	98.0%

World Health Organization - Cancer Country Profiles, 2014.

Cancer Plans, Monitoring and Surveillance

Has an operational cancer policy/strategy/action plan	ND
Has a cancer registry	ND
Scope	ND
Coverage	ND
Last year of data	ND

Cancer Primary Prevention Policies

Tobacco control

Has an operational policy, strategy or action plan to reduce the burden of tobacco use	ND
Smoke-free legislation	Up to two public places completely smoke-free
Tobacco dependence treatment	NRT and/or some cessation services (at least one of which is cost-covered)
Warning labels	No warnings or small warnings
Bans on advertising, promotion and sponsorship	Ban on national television, radio and print media as well as on some but not all other forms of direct and/or indirect advertising
Tobacco taxes	26–50% of retail price is tax

Overweight and obesity prevention and control

Has an operational policy, strategy or action plan for reducing overweight/obesity	ND

Physical inactivity prevention and control

Has an operational policy, strategy or action plan to reduce physical inactivity and/or promote physical activity	ND

Harmful use of alcohol prevention and control

Has an operational policy, strategy or action plan to reduce the harmful use of alcohol	ND

National immunization

Human Papillomavirus vaccination schedule	...
Hepatitis B vaccination schedule	...
Hepatitis B vaccination coverage, infants	72%

Cancer Screening and Early Detection

Cervical cancer

Cervical cytology (PAP)	ND
Acetic acid visualization (VIA)	ND

Breast cancer

Breast palpation / clinical breast exam (CBE)	ND
Mammogram	ND

Colorectal cancer

Faecal occult blood test or faecal immunological test	ND
Bowel cancer screening by exam or colonoscopy	ND

Cancer Treatment and Palliative Care

Radiotherapy	ND
Total high energy teletherapy units / million inhabitants	0.0
Number of radiotherapy centres	1
Number of radiation oncologists	3
Chemotherapy (medicines not specified)	ND
Oral morphine (formulation not specified)	ND
Non-methadone morphine equivalent consumption per cancer death (mg)	...
Community/home care for people with advanced stage cancer and other NCDs	ND

* No mortality data available. Figures are based on national incidence estimates and modelled survival.

... = No data available
ND = Country did not respond to country capacity survey

World Health Organization - Cancer Country Profiles, 2014.

Guatemala

Total population: 15,083,000
Income group: Lower middle

Total deaths: 80,000
Life expectancy at birth: Total:72 Males:68 Females:75

Cancer Mortality Profile

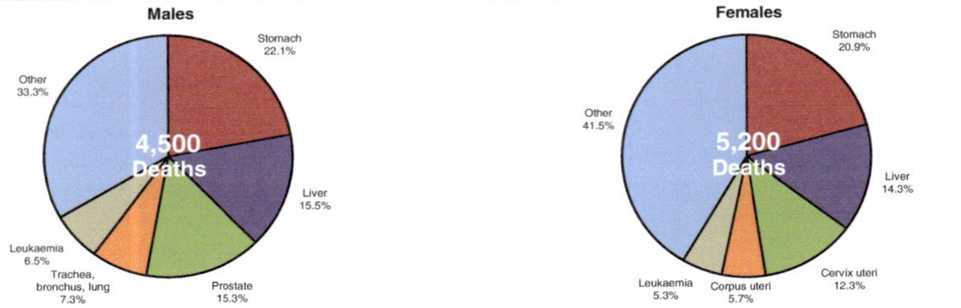

Age-Standardized Cancer Mortality Trends

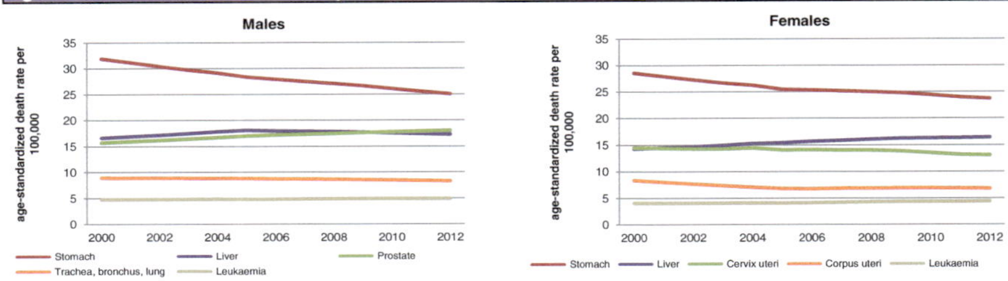

Cancer Incidence*

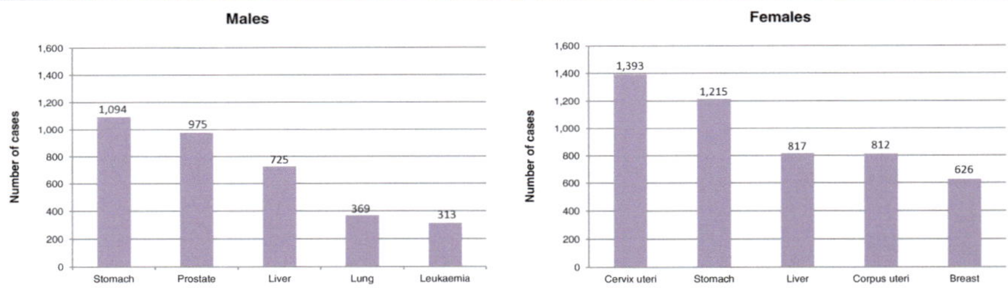

Adult Risk Factors

	Males	Females	Total
Current tobacco smoking (2011)	20%	1.7%	10.4%
Total alcohol per capita consumption, in litres of pure alcohol (2010)	7.5	0.5	3.8
Physical inactivity (2010)	10.5%	14.1%	12.4%
Obesity (2014)	11.3%	21.2%	16.4%
Household solid fuel use (2012)	-	-	64.0%

World Health Organization - Cancer Country Profiles, 2014.

Cancer Plans, Monitoring and Surveillance

Has an operational cancer policy/strategy/action plan	Yes
Has a cancer registry	Yes
Scope	Hospital-based
Coverage	Subnational
Last year of data	2010

Cancer Primary Prevention Policies

Tobacco control

Has an operational policy, strategy or action plan to reduce the burden of tobacco use	Yes
Smoke-free legislation	All public places completely smoke-free (or at least 90% of the population covered by complete subnational smoke-free legislation)**
Tobacco dependence treatment	NRT and/or some cessation services (at least one of which is cost-covered)
Warning labels	No warnings or small warnings
Bans on advertising, promotion and sponsorship	Complete absence of ban, or ban that does not cover national television, radio and print media
Tobacco taxes	26–50% of retail price is tax

Overweight and obesity prevention and control

Has an operational policy, strategy or action plan for reducing overweight/obesity	Yes

Physical inactivity prevention and control

Has an operational policy, strategy or action plan to reduce physical inactivity and/or promote physical activity	Yes

Harmful use of alcohol prevention and control

Has an operational policy, strategy or action plan to reduce the harmful use of alcohol	Yes

National immunization

Human Papillomavirus vaccination schedule	...
Hepatitis B vaccination schedule	Birth
Hepatitis B vaccination coverage, infants	85%

Cancer Screening and Early Detection

Cervical cancer

Cervical cytology (PAP)	Not generally available at the public primary health care level
Acetic acid visualization (VIA)	Generally available at the public primary health care level

Breast cancer

Breast palpation / clinical breast exam (CBE)	Generally available at the public primary health care level
Mammogram	Not generally available at the public primary health care level

Colorectal cancer

Faecal occult blood test or faecal immunological test	Not generally available at the public primary health care level
Bowel cancer screening by exam or colonoscopy	Not generally available at the public primary health care level

Cancer Treatment and Palliative Care

Radiotherapy	Generally available in the public health system
Total high energy teletherapy units / million inhabitants	0.6
Number of radiotherapy centres	8
Number of radiation oncologists	10
Chemotherapy (medicines not specified)	Generally available in the public health system
Oral morphine (formulation not specified)	Not generally available in the public health system
Non-methadone morphine equivalent consumption per cancer death (mg)	...
Community/home care for people with advanced stage cancer and other NCDs	Not generally available

* No incidence data available. Figures are based on national mortality estimates and modelled survival. ... = No data available
** Indicates highest possible level of achievement

World Health Organization - Cancer Country Profiles, 2014.

Indonesia

Total population: 247,000,000

Income group: Lower middle

Total deaths: 1,551,000

Life expectancy at birth: Total:71 Males:69 Females:73

Cancer Mortality Profile*

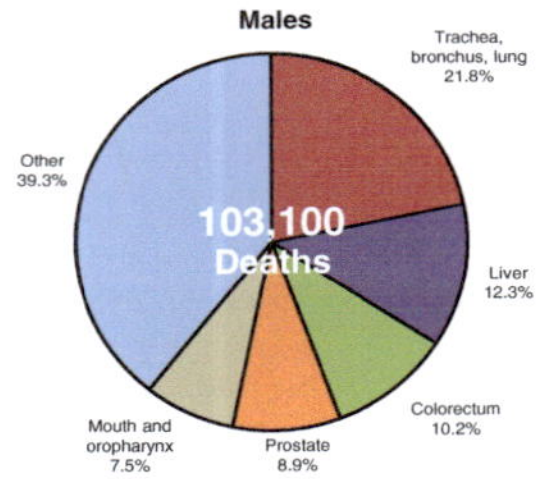

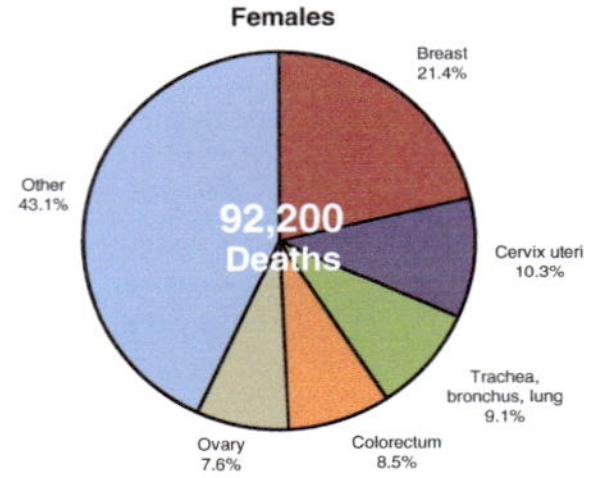

Age-Standardized Cancer Mortality Trends*

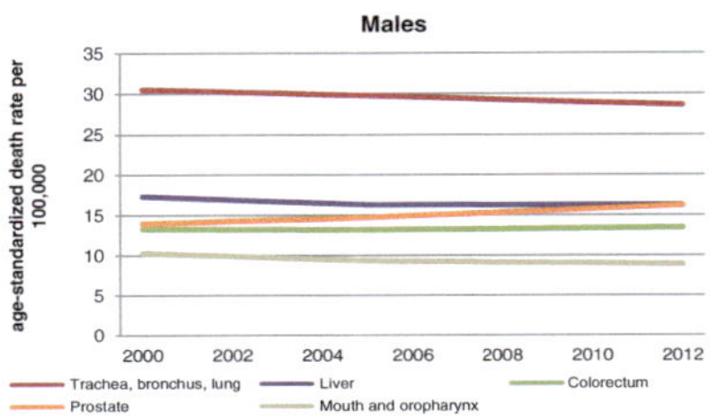

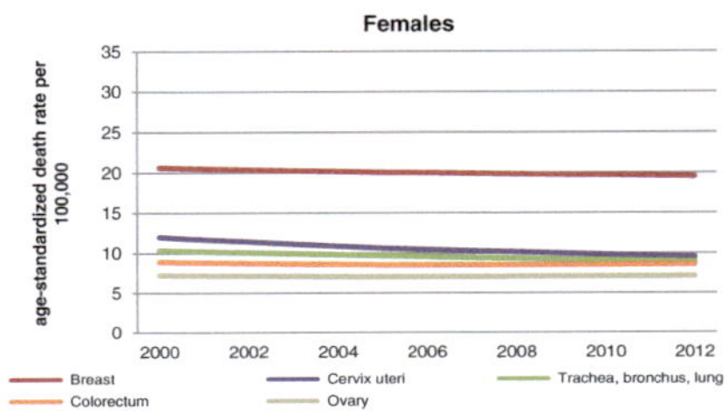

Cancer Incidence

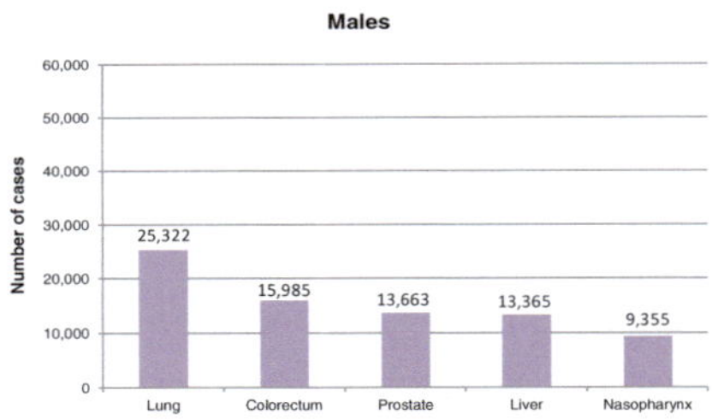

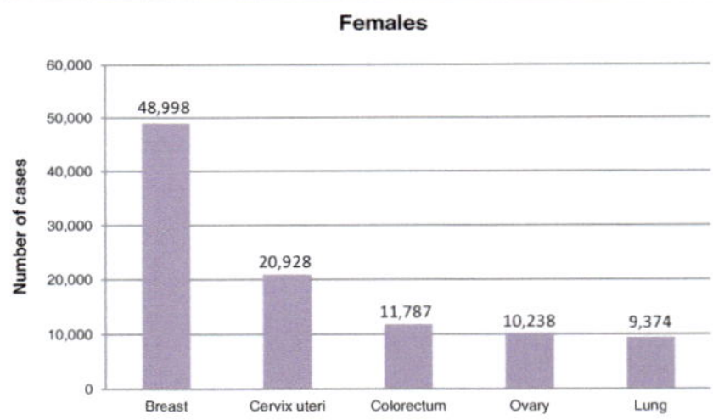

Adult Risk Factors

	Males	Females	Total
Current tobacco smoking (2011)	66.8%	3%	34.9%
Total alcohol per capita consumption, in litres of pure alcohol (2010)	1.1	0.1	0.6
Physical inactivity (2010)	24.4%	21.1%	22.8%
Obesity (2014)	3.6%	7.8%	5.7%
Household solid fuel use (2012)	-	-	47.0%

World Health Organization - Cancer Country Profiles, 2014.

Cancer Plans, Monitoring and Surveillance

Has an operational cancer policy/strategy/action plan	Yes
Has a cancer registry	Yes
Scope	Population-based
Coverage	Subnational
Last year of data	2007

Cancer Primary Prevention Policies

Tobacco control

Has an operational policy, strategy or action plan to reduce the burden of tobacco use	Yes
Smoke-free legislation	Three to five public places completely smoke-free
Tobacco dependence treatment	NRT and/or some cessation services (neither cost-covered)
Warning labels	Medium size warnings with all appropriate characteristics OR large warnings missing some appropriate characteristics
Bans on advertising, promotion and sponsorship	Complete absence of ban, or ban that does not cover national television, radio and print media
Tobacco taxes	51–75% of retail price is tax

Overweight and obesity prevention and control

Has an operational policy, strategy or action plan for reducing overweight/obesity	Yes

Physical inactivity prevention and control

Has an operational policy, strategy or action plan to reduce physical inactivity and/or promote physical activity	Yes

Harmful use of alcohol prevention and control

Has an operational policy, strategy or action plan to reduce the harmful use of alcohol	Yes

National immunization

Human Papillomavirus vaccination schedule	...
Hepatitis B vaccination schedule	0-7 days
Hepatitis B vaccination coverage, infants	85%

Cancer Screening and Early Detection

Cervical cancer

Cervical cytology (PAP)	Not generally available at the public primary health care level
Acetic acid visualization (VIA)	Not generally available at the public primary health care level

Breast cancer

Breast palpation / clinical breast exam (CBE)	Not generally available at the public primary health care level
Mammogram	Not generally available at the public primary health care level

Colorectal cancer

Faecal occult blood test or faecal immunological test	Not generally available at the public primary health care level
Bowel cancer screening by exam or colonoscopy	Not generally available at the public primary health care level

Cancer Treatment and Palliative Care

Radiotherapy	Not generally available in the public health system
Total high energy teletherapy units / million inhabitants	0.1
Number of radiotherapy centres	23
Number of radiation oncologists	41
Chemotherapy (medicines not specified)	Not generally available in the public health system
Oral morphine (formulation not specified)	Not generally available in the public health system
Non-methadone morphine equivalent consumption per cancer death (mg)	...
Community/home care for people with advanced stage cancer and other NCDs	Not generally available

* No mortality data available. Figures are based on national incidence estimates and modelled survival.   ... = No data available

World Health Organization - Cancer Country Profiles, 2014.

India

Total population: 1240000000
Income group: Lower middle

Total deaths: 9,816,000
Life expectancy at birth: Total:66 Males:64 Females:68

Cancer Mortality Profile

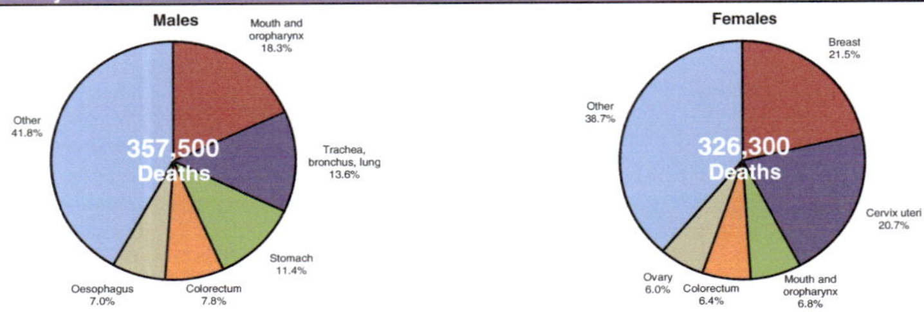

Age-Standardized Cancer Mortality Trends

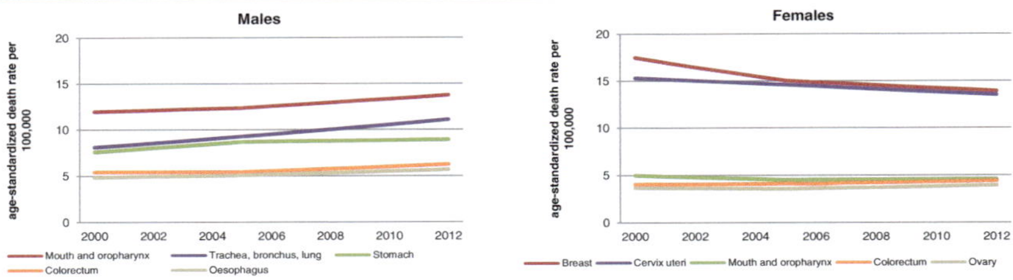

Cancer Incidence

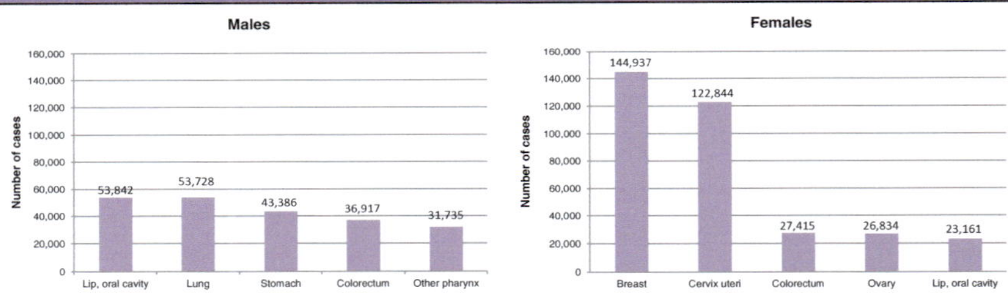

Adult Risk Factors

	Males	Females	Total
Current tobacco smoking (2011)	25%	3.9%	14.7%
Total alcohol per capita consumption, in litres of pure alcohol (2010)	8.0	0.5	4.3
Physical inactivity (2010)	9.2%	15.1%	12.1%
Obesity (2014)	3.1%	6.5%	4.7%
Household solid fuel use (2012)	-	-	63.0%

World Health Organization - Cancer Country Profiles, 2014.

Cancer Plans, Monitoring and Surveillance

Has an operational cancer policy/strategy/action plan	Yes
Has a cancer registry	Yes
Scope	Population-based
Coverage	Subnational
Last year of data	2008

Cancer Primary Prevention Policies

Tobacco control

Has an operational policy, strategy or action plan to reduce the burden of tobacco use	Yes
Smoke-free legislation	Data not categorized
Tobacco dependence treatment	NRT and/or some cessation services (at least one of which is cost-covered)
Warning labels	No warnings or small warnings
Bans on advertising, promotion and sponsorship	Ban on national television, radio and print media as well as on some but not all other forms of direct and/or indirect advertising
Tobacco taxes	26–50% of retail price is tax

Overweight and obesity prevention and control

Has an operational policy, strategy or action plan for reducing overweight/obesity	Yes

Physical inactivity prevention and control

Has an operational policy, strategy or action plan to reduce physical inactivity and/or promote physical activity	Yes

Harmful use of alcohol prevention and control

Has an operational policy, strategy or action plan to reduce the harmful use of alcohol	Yes

National immunization

Human Papillomavirus vaccination schedule	...
Hepatitis B vaccination schedule	Birth, +6 weeks, +10 weeks, +14 weeks
Hepatitis B vaccination coverage, infants	67%

Cancer Screening and Early Detection

Cervical cancer

Cervical cytology (PAP)	Generally available at the public primary health care level
Acetic acid visualization (VIA)	Generally available at the public primary health care level

Breast cancer

Breast palpation / clinical breast exam (CBE)	Generally available at the public primary health care level
Mammogram	Generally available at the public primary health care level

Colorectal cancer

Faecal occult blood test or faecal immunological test	Not generally available at the public primary health care level
Bowel cancer screening by exam or colonoscopy	Not generally available at the public primary health care level

Cancer Treatment and Palliative Care

Radiotherapy	Generally available in the public health system
Total high energy teletherapy units / million inhabitants	0.4
Number of radiotherapy centres	314
Number of radiation oncologists	353
Chemotherapy (medicines not specified)	Generally available in the public health system
Oral morphine (formulation not specified)	Not generally available in the public health system
Non-methadone morphine equivalent consumption per cancer death (mg)	...
Community/home care for people with advanced stage cancer and other NCDs	Not generally available

... = No data available

World Health Organization - Cancer Country Profiles, 2014.

Libya

Total population: 6,155,000
Income group: Upper middle

Total deaths: 26,000
Life expectancy at birth: Total:75 Males:73 Females:77

Cancer Mortality Profile*

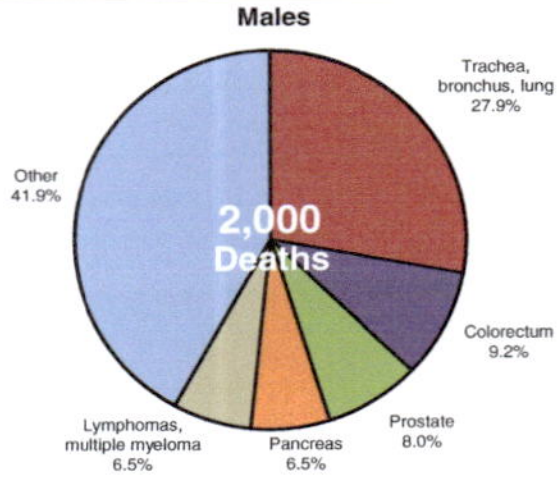

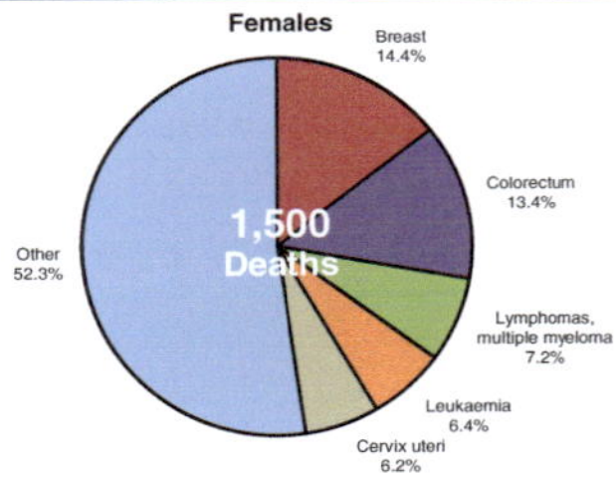

Age-Standardized Cancer Mortality Trends*

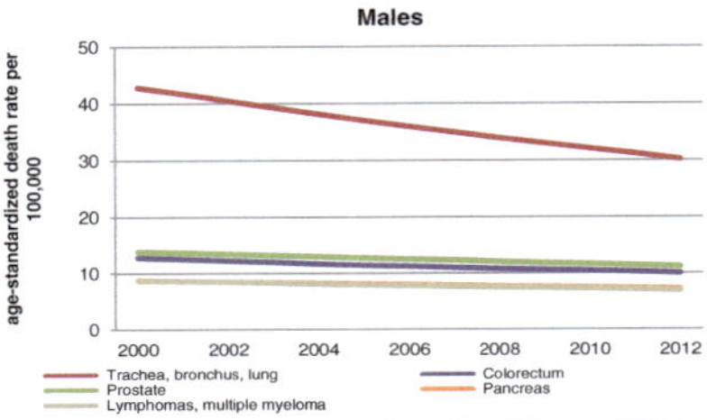

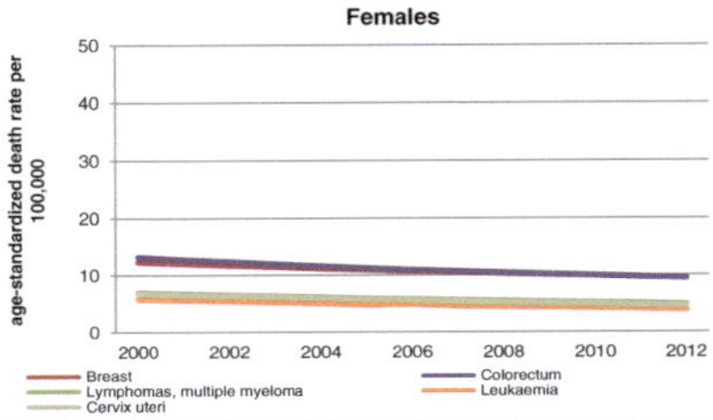

Cancer Incidence

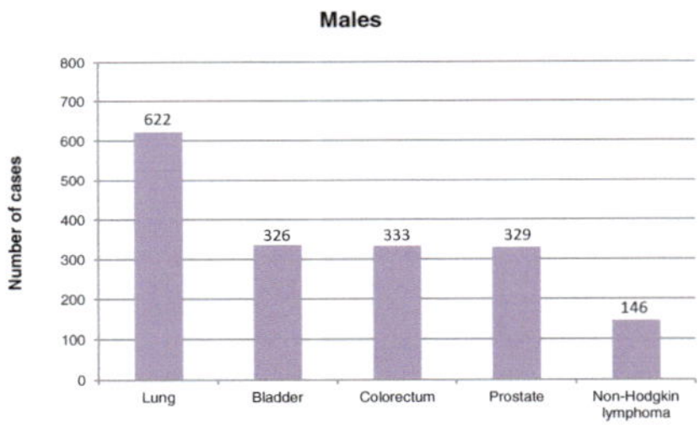

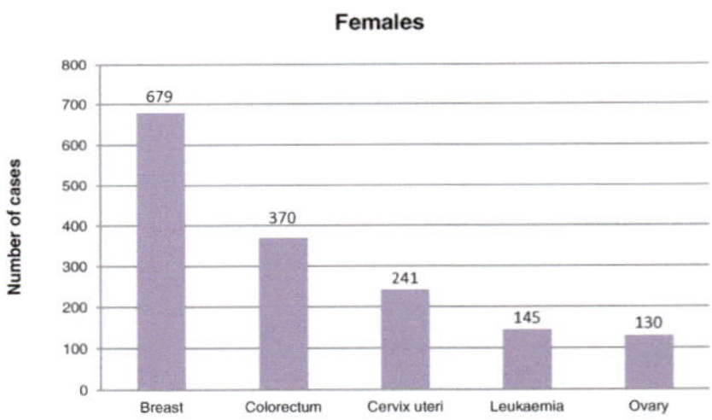

Adult Risk Factors

	Males	Females	Total
Current tobacco smoking (2011)	44.7%	<1%	22.5%
Total alcohol per capita consumption, in litres of pure alcohol (2010)	0.1	0.0	0.1
Physical inactivity (2010)	31.0%	42.3%	36.6%
Obesity (2014)	25.8%	38.0%	31.9%
Household solid fuel use (2012)	-	-	0.0%

World Health Organization - Cancer Country Profiles, 2014.

Cancer Plans, Monitoring and Surveillance

Has an operational cancer policy/strategy/action plan	No
Has a cancer registry	No
Scope	
Coverage	
Last year of data	

Cancer Primary Prevention Policies

Tobacco control

Has an operational policy, strategy or action plan to reduce the burden of tobacco use	No
Smoke-free legislation	All public places completely smoke-free (or at least 90% of the population covered by complete subnational smoke-free legislation)**
Tobacco dependence treatment	NRT and/or some cessation services (at least one of which is cost-covered)
Warning labels	No warnings or small warnings
Bans on advertising, promotion and sponsorship	Ban on all forms of direct and indirect advertising**
Tobacco taxes	≤25% of retail price is tax

Overweight and obesity prevention and control

Has an operational policy, strategy or action plan for reducing overweight/obesity	No

Physical inactivity prevention and control

Has an operational policy, strategy or action plan to reduce physical inactivity and/or promote physical activity	No

Harmful use of alcohol prevention and control

Has an operational policy, strategy or action plan to reduce the harmful use of alcohol	No

National immunization

Human Papillomavirus vaccination schedule	15 years (x3)
Hepatitis B vaccination schedule	Birth
Hepatitis B vaccination coverage, infants	98%

Cancer Screening and Early Detection

Cervical cancer

Cervical cytology (PAP)	Not generally available at the public primary health care level
Acetic acid visualization (VIA)	Not generally available at the public primary health care level

Breast cancer

Breast palpation / clinical breast exam (CBE)	Not generally available at the public primary health care level
Mammogram	Not generally available at the public primary health care level

Colorectal cancer

Faecal occult blood test or faecal immunological test	Not generally available at the public primary health care level
Bowel cancer screening by exam or colonoscopy	Not generally available at the public primary health care level

Cancer Treatment and Palliative Care

Radiotherapy	Generally available in the public health system
Total high energy teletherapy units / million inhabitants	1.0
Number of radiotherapy centres	4
Number of radiation oncologists	7
Chemotherapy (medicines not specified)	Generally available in the public health system
Oral morphine (formulation not specified)	Not generally available in the public health system
Non-methadone morphine equivalent consumption per cancer death (mg)	...
Community/home care for people with advanced stage cancer and other NCDs	Not generally available

* No mortality data available. Figures are based on national incidence estimates and modelled survival.
** Indicates highest possible level of achievement

... = No data available

World Health Organization - Cancer Country Profiles, 2014.

Sri Lanka

Total population: 21,098,000
Income group: Lower middle

Total deaths: 138,000
Life expectancy at birth: Total:75 Males:71 Females:78

Cancer Mortality Profile*

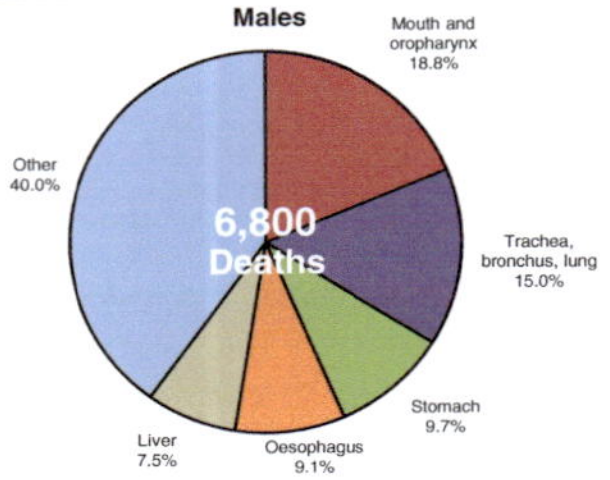

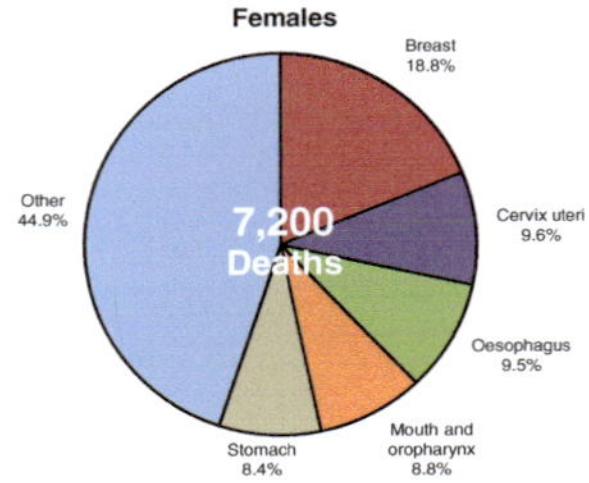

Age-Standardized Cancer Mortality Trends*

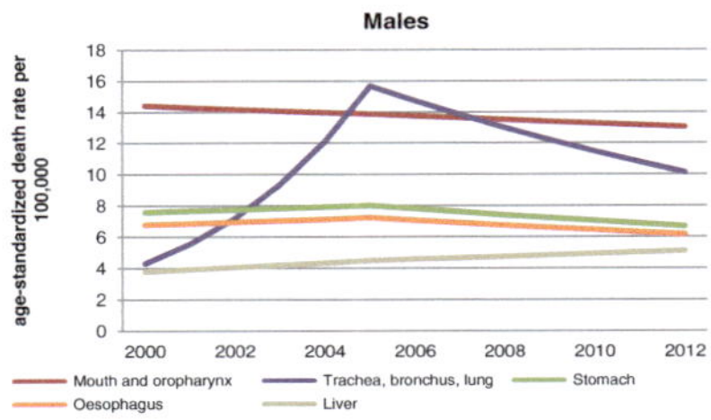

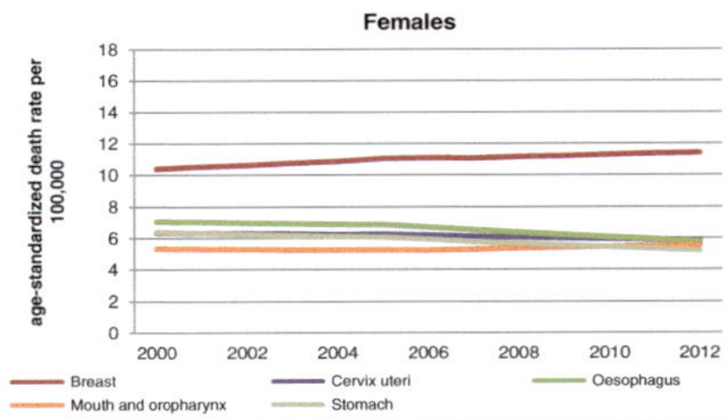

Cancer Incidence

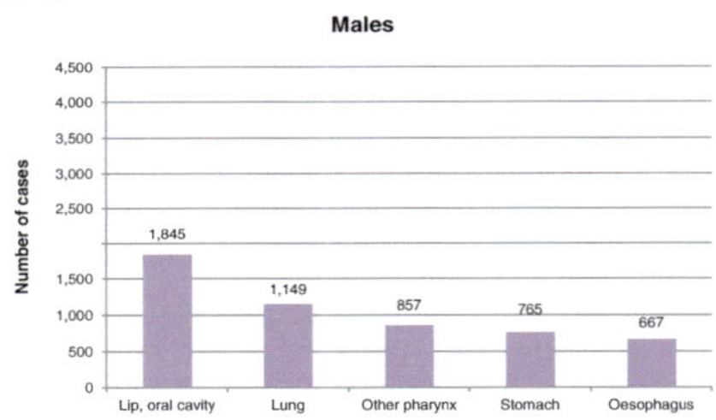

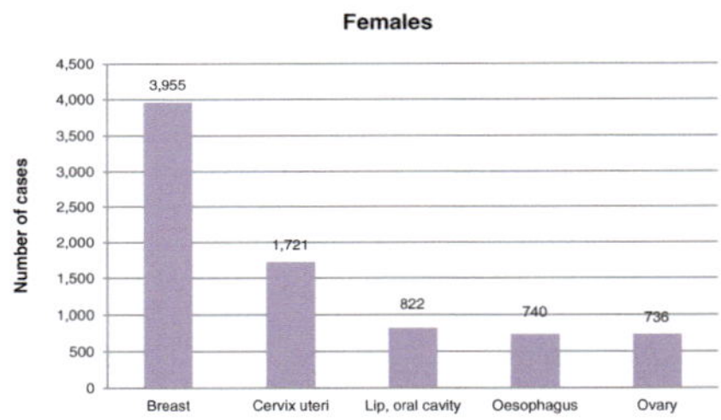

Adult Risk Factors

	Males	Females	Total
Current tobacco smoking (2011)	31.1%	<1%	15.2%
Total alcohol per capita consumption, in litres of pure alcohol (2010)	7.3	0.3	3.7
Physical inactivity (2010)	16.9%	30.2%	23.7%
Obesity (2014)	3.5%	10.0%	6.8%
Household solid fuel use (2012)	-	-	74.0%

World Health Organization - Cancer Country Profiles, 2014.

Cancer Plans, Monitoring and Surveillance

Has an operational cancer policy/strategy/action plan	Yes
Has a cancer registry	Yes
Scope	Hospital-based
Coverage	Subnational
Last year of data	2007

Cancer Primary Prevention Policies

Tobacco control

Has an operational policy, strategy or action plan to reduce the burden of tobacco use	Yes
Smoke-free legislation	Six to seven public places completely smoke-free
Tobacco dependence treatment	NRT and/or some cessation services (neither cost-covered)
Warning labels	Large warnings with all appropriate characteristics**
Bans on advertising, promotion and sponsorship	Ban on national television, radio and print media as well as on some but not all other forms of direct and/or indirect advertising
Tobacco taxes	51–75% of retail price is tax

Overweight and obesity prevention and control

Has an operational policy, strategy or action plan for reducing overweight/obesity	Yes

Physical inactivity prevention and control

Has an operational policy, strategy or action plan to reduce physical inactivity and/or promote physical activity	Yes

Harmful use of alcohol prevention and control

Has an operational policy, strategy or action plan to reduce the harmful use of alcohol	Yes

National immunization

Human Papillomavirus vaccination schedule	...
Hepatitis B vaccination schedule	...
Hepatitis B vaccination coverage, infants	99%

Cancer Screening and Early Detection

Cervical cancer

Cervical cytology (PAP)	Not generally available at the public primary health care level
Acetic acid visualization (VIA)	Not generally available at the public primary health care level

Breast cancer

Breast palpation / clinical breast exam (CBE)	Generally available at the public primary health care level
Mammogram	Not generally available at the public primary health care level

Colorectal cancer

Faecal occult blood test or faecal immunological test	Not generally available at the public primary health care level
Bowel cancer screening by exam or colonoscopy	Not generally available at the public primary health care level

Cancer Treatment and Palliative Care

Radiotherapy	Generally available in the public health system
Total high energy teletherapy units / million inhabitants	0.1
Number of radiotherapy centres	7
Number of radiation oncologists	18
Chemotherapy (medicines not specified)	Generally available in the public health system
Oral morphine (formulation not specified)	Not generally available in the public health system
Non-methadone morphine equivalent consumption per cancer death (mg)	...
Community/home care for people with advanced stage cancer and other NCDs	Not generally available

* No mortality data available. Figures are based on national incidence estimates and modelled survival.

... = No data available

** Indicates highest possible level of achievement

World Health Organization - Cancer Country Profiles, 2014.

Mali

Total population: 14,854,000
Income group: Low

Total deaths: 170,000
Life expectancy at birth: Total:57 Males:57 Females:57

Cancer Mortality Profile*

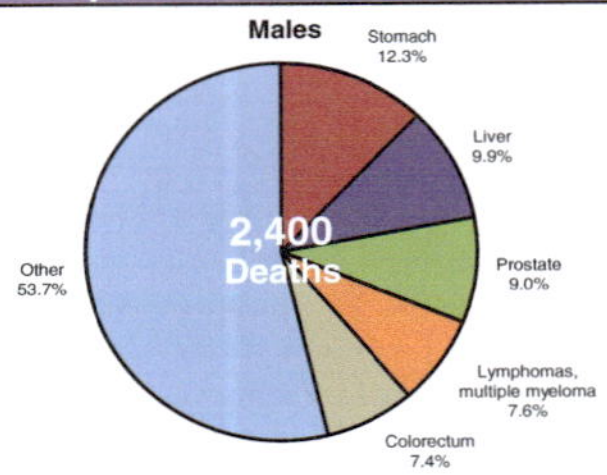

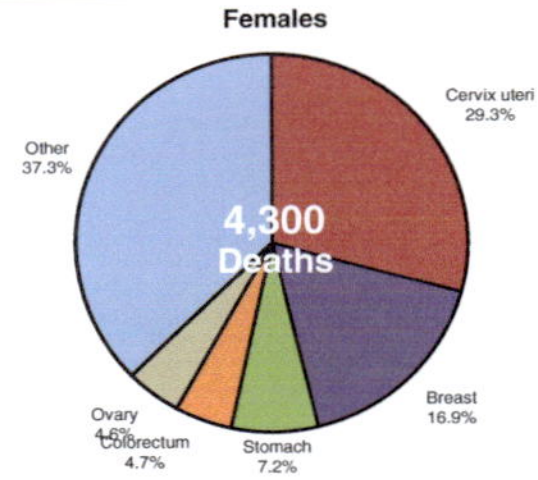

Age-Standardized Cancer Mortality Trends*

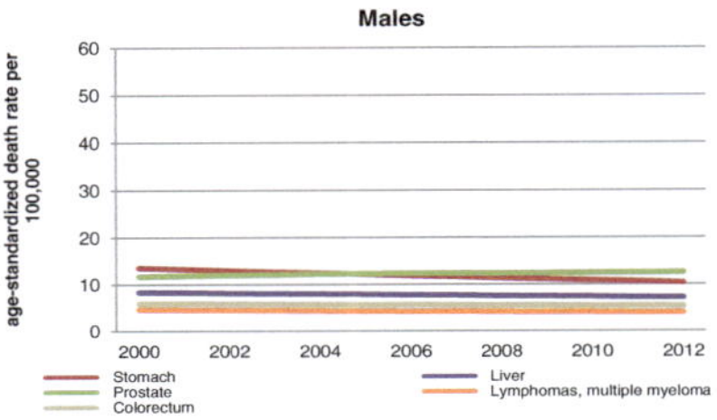

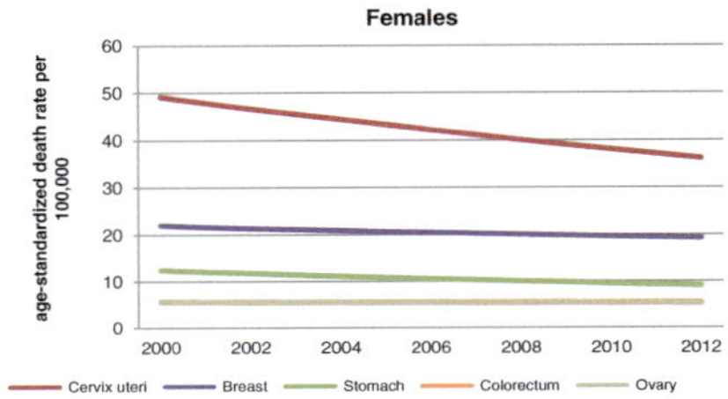

Cancer Incidence

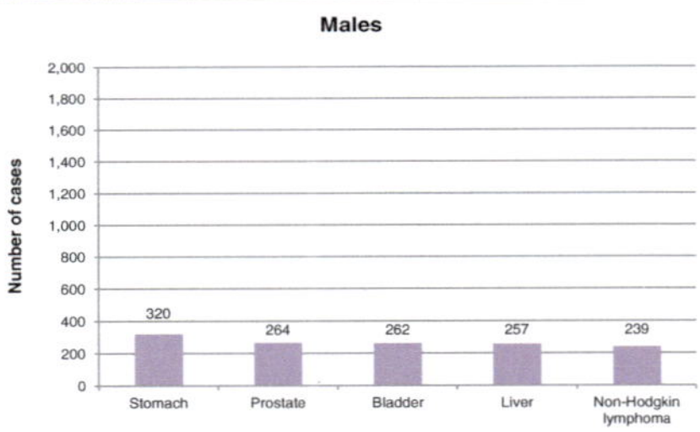

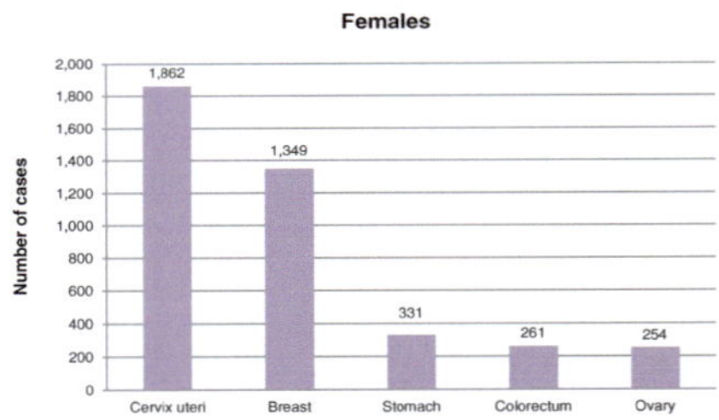

Adult Risk Factors

	Males	Females	Total
Current tobacco smoking (2011)	28.5%	2.2%	15.3%
Total alcohol per capita consumption, in litres of pure alcohol (2010)	2.2	0.0	1.1
Physical inactivity (2010)	16.2%	26.0%	21.2%
Obesity (2014)	3.2%	8.2%	5.7%
Household solid fuel use (2012)	-	-	98.0%

World Health Organization - Cancer Country Profiles, 2014.

Cancer Plans, Monitoring and Surveillance

Has an operational cancer policy/strategy/action plan	DK
Has a cancer registry	Yes
Scope	Population-based
Coverage	Subnational
Last year of data	2010

Cancer Primary Prevention Policies

Tobacco control

Has an operational policy, strategy or action plan to reduce the burden of tobacco use	No
Smoke-free legislation	Up to two public places completely smoke-free
Tobacco dependence treatment	NRT and/or some cessation services (neither cost-covered)
Warning labels	Medium size warnings missing some appropriate characteristics OR large warnings missing many appropriate characteristics
Bans on advertising, promotion and sponsorship	Ban on national television, radio and print media as well as on some but not all other forms of direct and/or indirect advertising
Tobacco taxes	≤25% of retail price is tax

Overweight and obesity prevention and control

Has an operational policy, strategy or action plan for reducing overweight/obesity	No

Physical inactivity prevention and control

Has an operational policy, strategy or action plan to reduce physical inactivity and/or promote physical activity	No

Harmful use of alcohol prevention and control

Has an operational policy, strategy or action plan to reduce the harmful use of alcohol	No

National immunization

Human Papillomavirus vaccination schedule	(starting October 2014)
Hepatitis B vaccination schedule	...
Hepatitis B vaccination coverage, infants	74%

Cancer Screening and Early Detection

Cervical cancer

Cervical cytology (PAP)	Generally available at the public primary health care level
Acetic acid visualization (VIA)	Generally available at the public primary health care level

Breast cancer

Breast palpation / clinical breast exam (CBE)	Generally available at the public primary health care level
Mammogram	Generally available at the public primary health care level

Colorectal cancer

Faecal occult blood test or faecal immunological test	Not generally available at the public primary health care level
Bowel cancer screening by exam or colonoscopy	Not generally available at the public primary health care level

Cancer Treatment and Palliative Care

Radiotherapy	Not generally available in the public health system
Total high energy teletherapy units / million inhabitants	0.1
Number of radiotherapy centres	1
Number of radiation oncologists	...
Chemotherapy (medicines not specified)	Generally available in the public health system
Oral morphine (formulation not specified)	Generally available in the public health system
Non-methadone morphine equivalent consumption per cancer death (mg)	...
Community/home care for people with advanced stage cancer and other NCDs	Not generally available

* No mortality data available. Figures are based on national incidence estimates and modelled survival.

... = No data available
DK = Country responded "don't know"

World Health Organization - Cancer Country Profiles, 2014.

Myanmar

Total population: 52,797,000
Income group: Low

Total deaths: 441,000
Life expectancy at birth: Total:66 Males:64 Females:68

Cancer Mortality Profile*

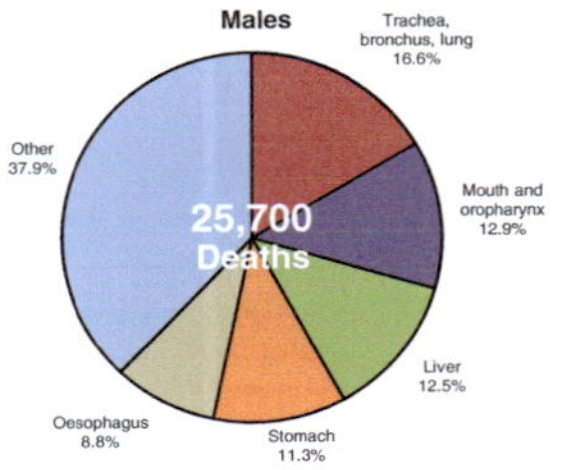

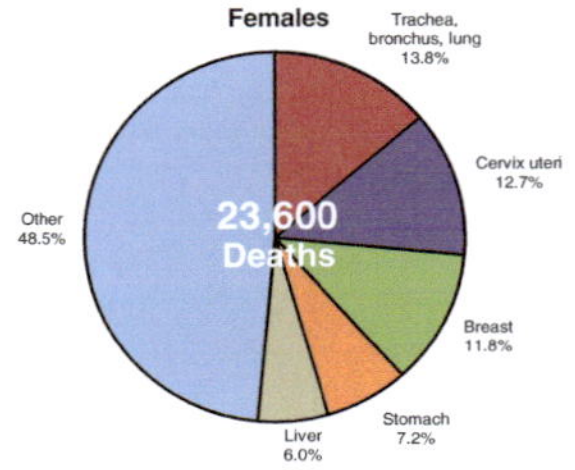

Age-Standardized Cancer Mortality Trends*

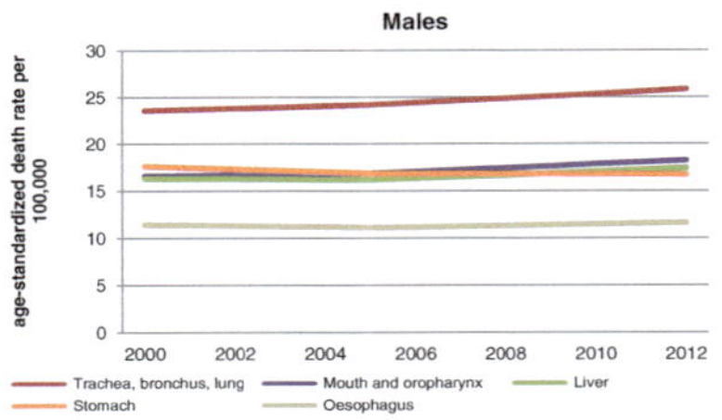

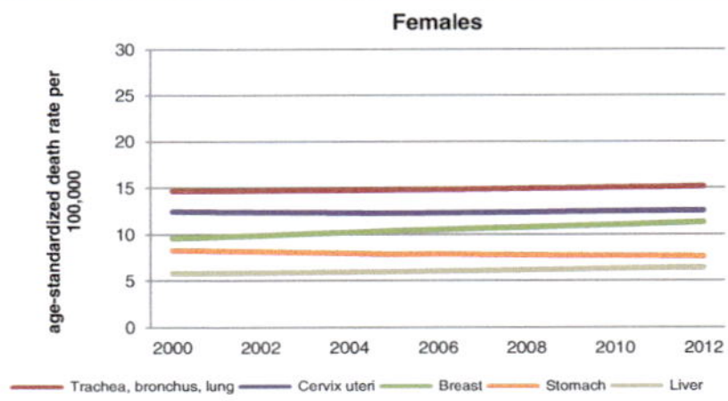

Cancer Incidence**

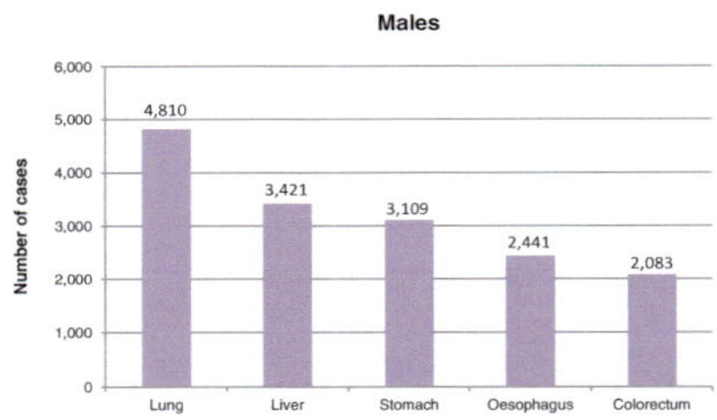

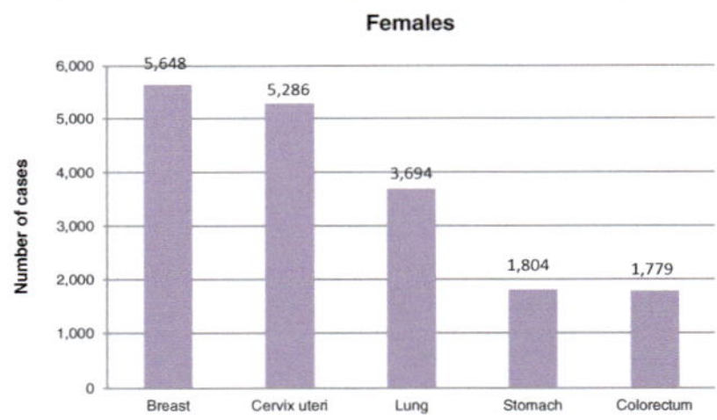

Adult Risk Factors

	Males	Females	Total
Current tobacco smoking (2011)	38.2%	6.6%	22%
Total alcohol per capita consumption, in litres of pure alcohol (2010)	1.4	0.0	0.7
Physical inactivity (2010)	7.2%	10.7%	9.0%
Obesity (2014)	1.4%	4.2%	2.9%
Household solid fuel use (2012)	-	-	93.0%

World Health Organization - Cancer Country Profiles, 2014.

Cancer Plans, Monitoring and Surveillance

Has an operational cancer policy/strategy/action plan	Yes
Has a cancer registry	No
Scope	
Coverage	
Last year of data	

Cancer Primary Prevention Policies

Tobacco control

Has an operational policy, strategy or action plan to reduce the burden of tobacco use	Yes
Smoke-free legislation	Three to five public places completely smoke-free
Tobacco dependence treatment	NRT and/or some cessation services (neither cost-covered)
Warning labels	No warnings or small warnings
Bans on advertising, promotion and sponsorship	Ban on national television, radio and print media as well as on some but not all other forms of direct and/or indirect advertising
Tobacco taxes	26–50% of retail price is tax

Overweight and obesity prevention and control

Has an operational policy, strategy or action plan for reducing overweight/obesity	Yes

Physical inactivity prevention and control

Has an operational policy, strategy or action plan to reduce physical inactivity and/or promote physical activity	Yes

Harmful use of alcohol prevention and control

Has an operational policy, strategy or action plan to reduce the harmful use of alcohol	Yes

National immunization

Human Papillomavirus vaccination schedule	...
Hepatitis B vaccination schedule	...
Hepatitis B vaccination coverage, infants	72%

Cancer Screening and Early Detection

Cervical cancer

Cervical cytology (PAP)	Not generally available at the public primary health care level
Acetic acid visualization (VIA)	Not generally available at the public primary health care level

Breast cancer

Breast palpation / clinical breast exam (CBE)	Generally available at the public primary health care level
Mammogram	Not generally available at the public primary health care level

Colorectal cancer

Faecal occult blood test or faecal immunological test	Not generally available at the public primary health care level
Bowel cancer screening by exam or colonoscopy	Not generally available at the public primary health care level

Cancer Treatment and Palliative Care

Radiotherapy	Not generally available in the public health system
Total high energy teletherapy units / million inhabitants	0.1
Number of radiotherapy centres	4
Number of radiation oncologists	23
Chemotherapy (medicines not specified)	Not generally available in the public health system
Oral morphine (formulation not specified)	Not generally available in the public health system
Non-methadone morphine equivalent consumption per cancer death (mg)	...
Community/home care for people with advanced stage cancer and other NCDs	Not generally available

* No mortality data available. Figures are based on national incidence estimates and modelled survival.
** No incidence data available. Figures are based on national incidence estimates from neighbouring countries.

... = No data available

World Health Organization - Cancer Country Profiles, 2014.

Nigeria

Total population: 169,000,000 **Total deaths: 2,083,000**

Income group: Lower middle **Life expectancy at birth: Total:54 Males:53 Females:55**

Cancer Mortality Profile*

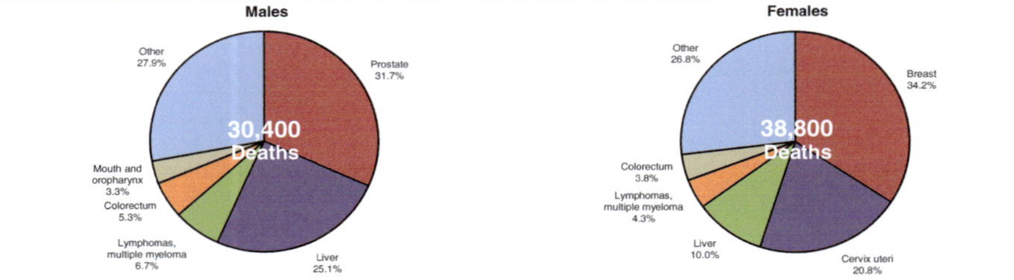

Age-Standardized Cancer Mortality Trends*

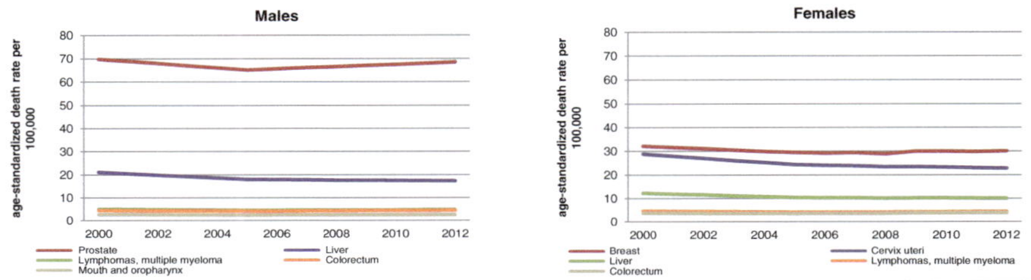

Cancer Incidence

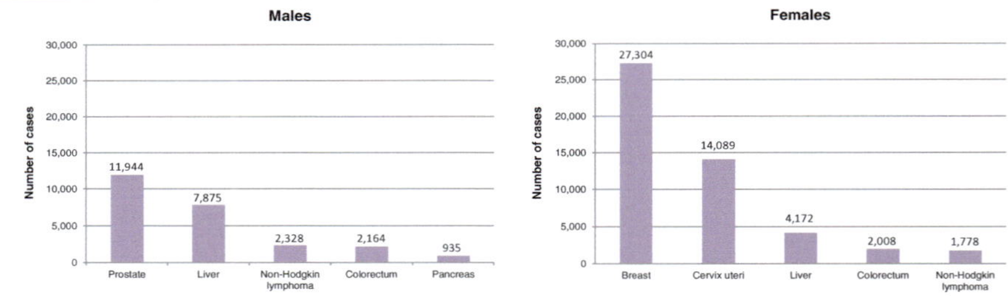

Adult Risk Factors

	Males	Females	Total
Current tobacco smoking (2011)	9.8%	2.3%	6.1%
Total alcohol per capita consumption, in litres of pure alcohol (2010)	14.9	5.1	10.1
Physical inactivity (2010)	17.7%	21.9%	19.8%
Obesity (2014)	5.3%	14.3%	9.7%
Household solid fuel use (2012)	-	-	75.0%

World Health Organization - Cancer Country Profiles, 2014.

Cancer Plans, Monitoring and Surveillance

Has an operational cancer policy/strategy/action plan	No
Has a cancer registry	Yes
Scope	Population-based
Coverage	Subnational
Last year of data	2006

Cancer Primary Prevention Policies

Tobacco control

Has an operational policy, strategy or action plan to reduce the burden of tobacco use	No
Smoke-free legislation	Three to five public places completely smoke-free
Tobacco dependence treatment	NRT and/or some cessation services (at least one of which is cost-covered)
Warning labels	No warnings or small warnings
Bans on advertising, promotion and sponsorship	Complete absence of ban, or ban that does not cover national television, radio and print media
Tobacco taxes	≤25% of retail price is tax

Overweight and obesity prevention and control

Has an operational policy, strategy or action plan for reducing overweight/obesity	No

Physical inactivity prevention and control

Has an operational policy, strategy or action plan to reduce physical inactivity and/or promote physical activity	No

Harmful use of alcohol prevention and control

Has an operational policy, strategy or action plan to reduce the harmful use of alcohol	No

National immunization

Human Papillomavirus vaccination schedule	...
Hepatitis B vaccination schedule	Birth, +6 weeks, +14 weeks
Hepatitis B vaccination coverage, infants	63%

Cancer Screening and Early Detection

Cervical cancer

Cervical cytology (PAP)	Not generally available at the public primary health care level
Acetic acid visualization (VIA)	Not generally available at the public primary health care level

Breast cancer

Breast palpation / clinical breast exam (CBE)	Not generally available at the public primary health care level
Mammogram	Not generally available at the public primary health care level

Colorectal cancer

Faecal occult blood test or faecal immunological test	Not generally available at the public primary health care level
Bowel cancer screening by exam or colonoscopy	Not generally available at the public primary health care level

Cancer Treatment and Palliative Care

Radiotherapy	Not generally available in the public health system
Total high energy teletherapy units / million inhabitants	0.1
Number of radiotherapy centres	9
Number of radiation oncologists	30
Chemotherapy (medicines not specified)	Not generally available in the public health system
Oral morphine (formulation not specified)	Not generally available in the public health system
Non-methadone morphine equivalent consumption per cancer death (mg)	...
Community/home care for people with advanced stage cancer and other NCDs	Not generally available

* No mortality data available. Figures are based on national incidence estimates and modelled survival.

... = No data available

World Health Organization - Cancer Country Profiles, 2014.

Pakistan

Total population: 179,000,000
Income group: Lower middle

Total deaths: 1,332,000
Life expectancy at birth: Total:65 Males:64 Females:66

Cancer Mortality Profile*

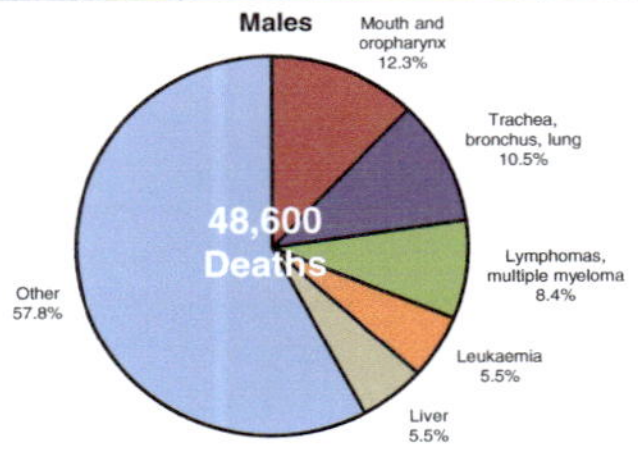

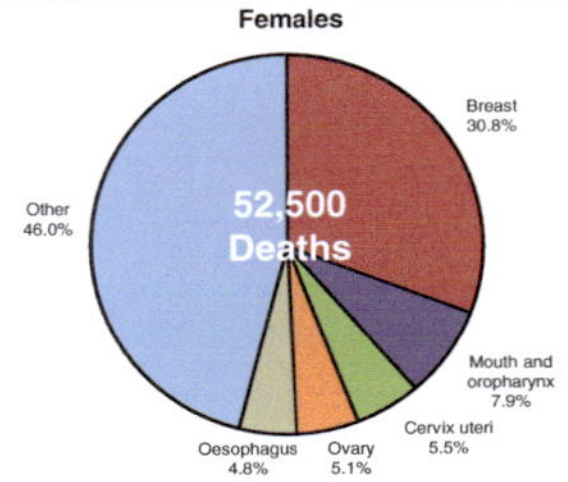

Age-Standardized Cancer Mortality Trends*

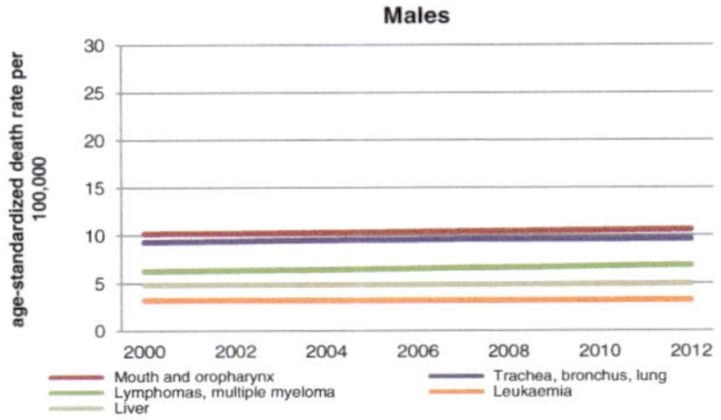

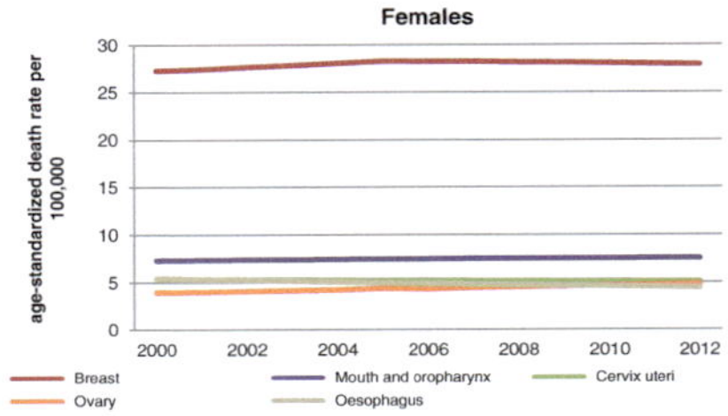

Cancer Incidence

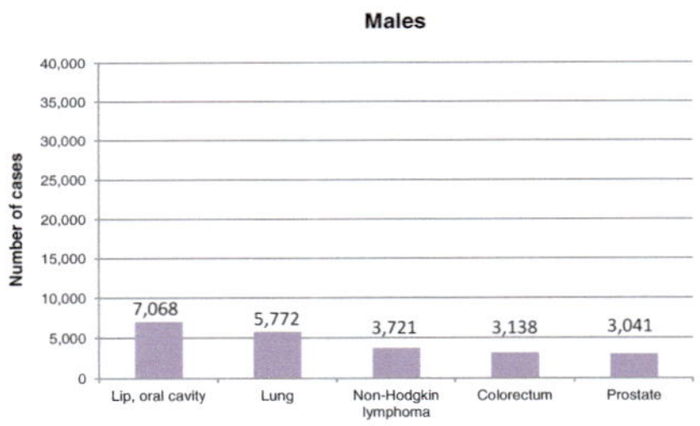

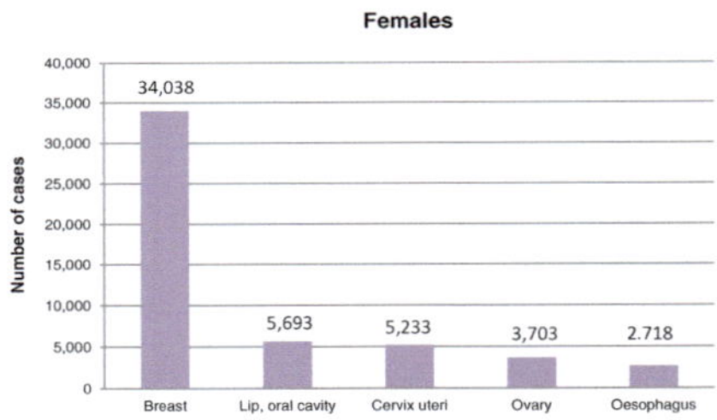

Adult Risk Factors

	Males	Females	Total
Current tobacco smoking (2011)	37.6%	7.4%	22.7%
Total alcohol per capita consumption, in litres of pure alcohol (2010)	0.1	0.0	0.1
Physical inactivity (2010)	18.5%	29.7%	24.0%
Obesity (2014)	3.3%	6.4%	4.8%
Household solid fuel use (2012)	-	-	62.0%

World Health Organization - Cancer Country Profiles, 2014.

Cancer Plans, Monitoring and Surveillance

Has an operational cancer policy/strategy/action plan	No
Has a cancer registry	No
Scope	
Coverage	
Last year of data	

Cancer Primary Prevention Policies

Tobacco control

Has an operational policy, strategy or action plan to reduce the burden of tobacco use	No
Smoke-free legislation	All public places completely smoke-free (or at least 90% of the population covered by complete subnational smoke-free legislation)**
Tobacco dependence treatment	NRT and/or some cessation services (neither cost-covered)
Warning labels	Medium size warnings with all appropriate characteristics OR large warnings missing some appropriate characteristics
Bans on advertising, promotion and sponsorship	Complete absence of ban, or ban that does not cover national television, radio and print media
Tobacco taxes	51–75% of retail price is tax

Overweight and obesity prevention and control

Has an operational policy, strategy or action plan for reducing overweight/obesity	No

Physical inactivity prevention and control

Has an operational policy, strategy or action plan to reduce physical inactivity and/or promote physical activity	No

Harmful use of alcohol prevention and control

Has an operational policy, strategy or action plan to reduce the harmful use of alcohol	No

National immunization

Human Papillomavirus vaccination schedule	...
Hepatitis B vaccination schedule	...
Hepatitis B vaccination coverage, infants	72%

Cancer Screening and Early Detection

Cervical cancer

Cervical cytology (PAP)	Not generally available at the public primary health care level
Acetic acid visualization (VIA)	Not generally available at the public primary health care level

Breast cancer

Breast palpation / clinical breast exam (CBE)	Not generally available at the public primary health care level
Mammogram	Not generally available at the public primary health care level

Colorectal cancer

Faecal occult blood test or faecal immunological test	Not generally available at the public primary health care level
Bowel cancer screening by exam or colonoscopy	Not generally available at the public primary health care level

Cancer Treatment and Palliative Care

Radiotherapy	Not generally available in the public health system
Total high energy teletherapy units / million inhabitants	0.1
Number of radiotherapy centres	26
Number of radiation oncologists	31
Chemotherapy (medicines not specified)	Not generally available in the public health system
Oral morphine (formulation not specified)	Not generally available in the public health system
Non-methadone morphine equivalent consumption per cancer death (mg)	...
Community/home care for people with advanced stage cancer and other NCDs	Not generally available

* No mortality data available. Figures are based on national incidence estimates and modelled survival. ... = No data available

** Indicates highest possible level of achievement

World Health Organization - Cancer Country Profiles, 2014.

Panama

Total population: 3,802,000
Income group: Upper middle

Total deaths: 19,000
Life expectancy at birth: Total:77 Males:74 Females:80

Cancer Mortality Profile

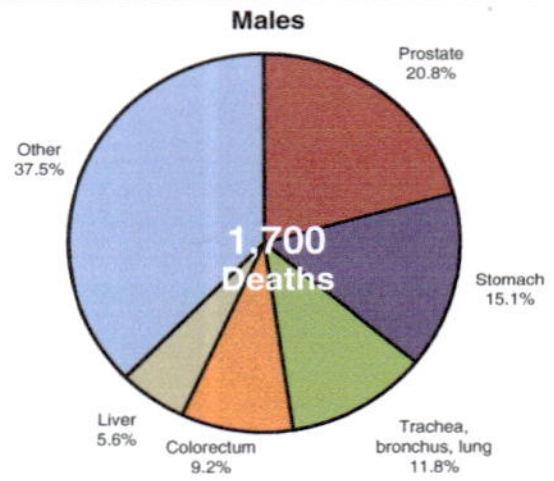

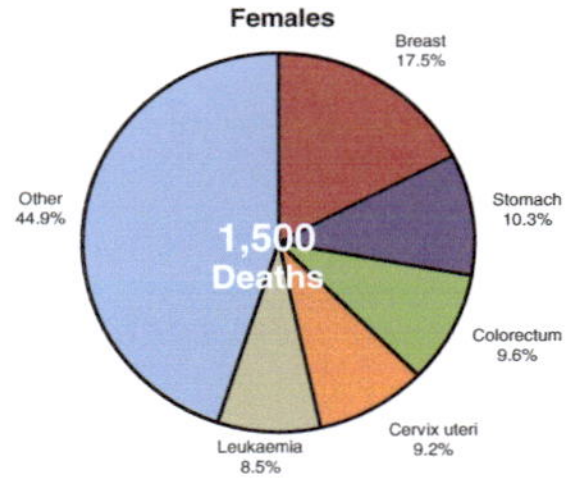

Age-Standardized Cancer Mortality Trends

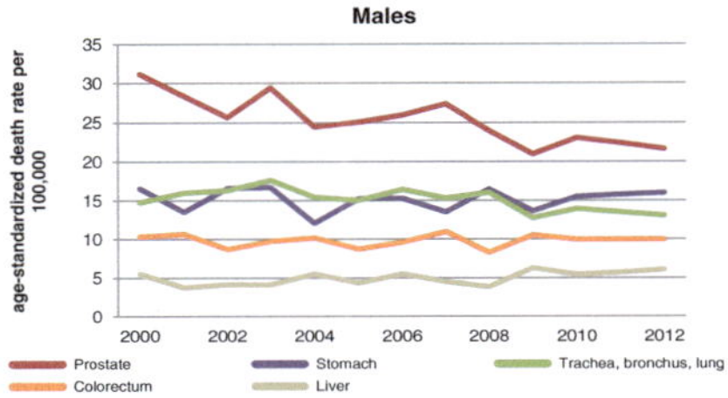

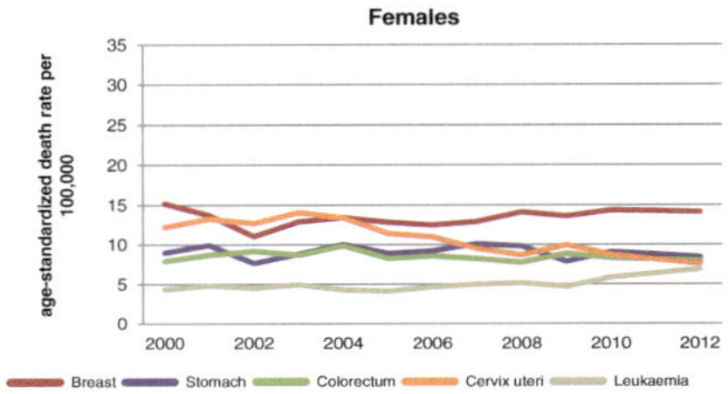

Cancer Incidence*

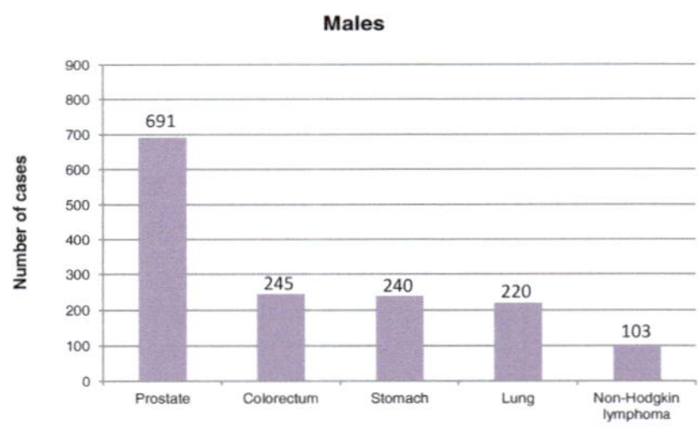

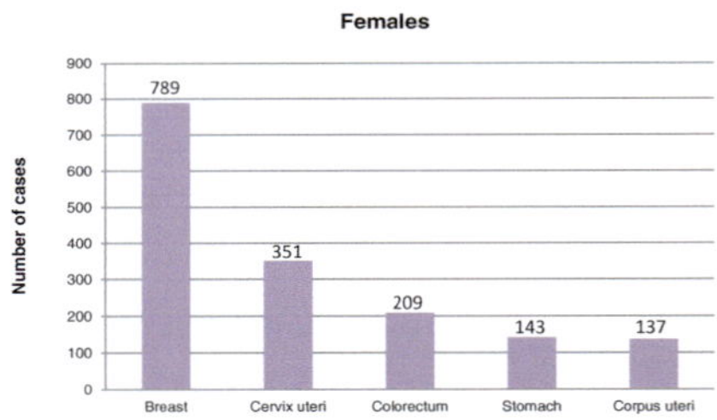

Adult Risk Factors

	Males	Females	Total
Current tobacco smoking (2011)	23.1%	4%	13.6%
Total alcohol per capita consumption, in litres of pure alcohol (2010)	11.2	4.7	8.0
Physical inactivity (2010)	...	...	...
Obesity (2014)	20.3%	32.8%	26.5%
Household solid fuel use (2012)	-	-	17.0%

World Health Organization - Cancer Country Profiles, 2014.

Cancer Plans, Monitoring and Surveillance

Has an operational cancer policy/strategy/action plan	No
Has a cancer registry	Yes
Scope	Population-based
Coverage	National
Last year of data	2011

Cancer Primary Prevention Policies

Tobacco control

Has an operational policy, strategy or action plan to reduce the burden of tobacco use	Yes
Smoke-free legislation	All public places completely smoke-free (or at least 90% of the population covered by complete subnational smoke-free legislation)**
Tobacco dependence treatment	National quit line, and both NRT and some cessation services cost-covered**
Warning labels	Large warnings with all appropriate characteristics**
Bans on advertising, promotion and sponsorship	Ban on all forms of direct and indirect advertising**
Tobacco taxes	51–75% of retail price is tax

Overweight and obesity prevention and control

Has an operational policy, strategy or action plan for reducing overweight/obesity	Yes

Physical inactivity prevention and control

Has an operational policy, strategy or action plan to reduce physical inactivity and/or promote physical activity	Yes

Harmful use of alcohol prevention and control

Has an operational policy, strategy or action plan to reduce the harmful use of alcohol	Yes

National immunization

Human Papillomavirus vaccination schedule	10 years, +1 month, +6 month
Hepatitis B vaccination schedule	Birth
Hepatitis B vaccination coverage, infants	80%

Cancer Screening and Early Detection

Cervical cancer

Cervical cytology (PAP)	Generally available at the public primary health care level
Acetic acid visualization (VIA)	Not generally available at the public primary health care level

Breast cancer

Breast palpation / clinical breast exam (CBE)	Generally available at the public primary health care level
Mammogram	Not generally available at the public primary health care level

Colorectal cancer

Faecal occult blood test or faecal immunological test	Generally available at the public primary health care level
Bowel cancer screening by exam or colonoscopy	Not generally available at the public primary health care level

Cancer Treatment and Palliative Care

Radiotherapy	Generally available in the public health system
Total high energy teletherapy units / million inhabitants	1.6
Number of radiotherapy centres	2
Number of radiation oncologists	11
Chemotherapy (medicines not specified)	Generally available in the public health system
Oral morphine (formulation not specified)	Not generally available in the public health system
Non-methadone morphine equivalent consumption per cancer death (mg)	...
Community/home care for people with advanced stage cancer and other NCDs	Generally available

* No incidence data available. Figures are based on national mortality estimates and modelled survival.
** Indicates highest possible level of achievement

... = No data available

World Health Organization - Cancer Country Profiles, 2014.

Philippines

Total population: 96,707,000
Income group: Lower middle

Total deaths: 571,000
Life expectancy at birth: Total:69 Males:65 Females:72

Cancer Mortality Profile

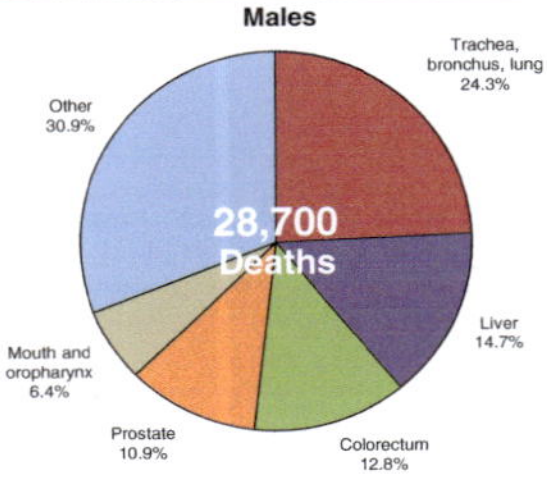

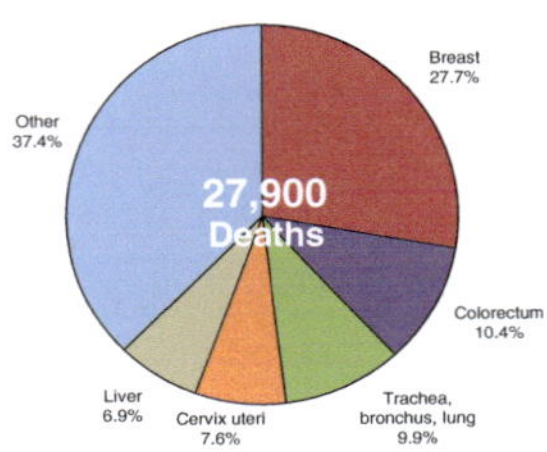

Age-Standardized Cancer Mortality Trends

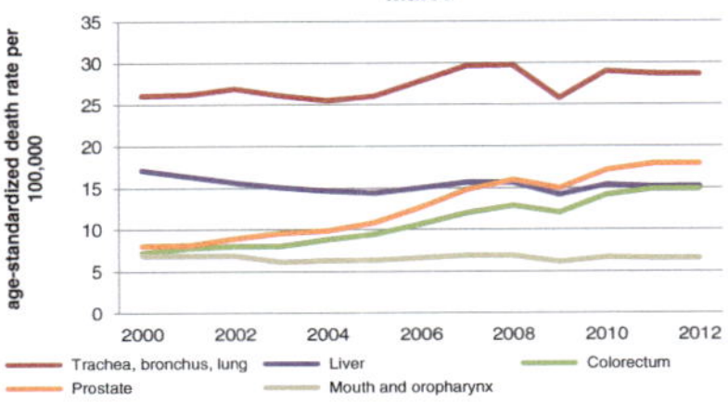

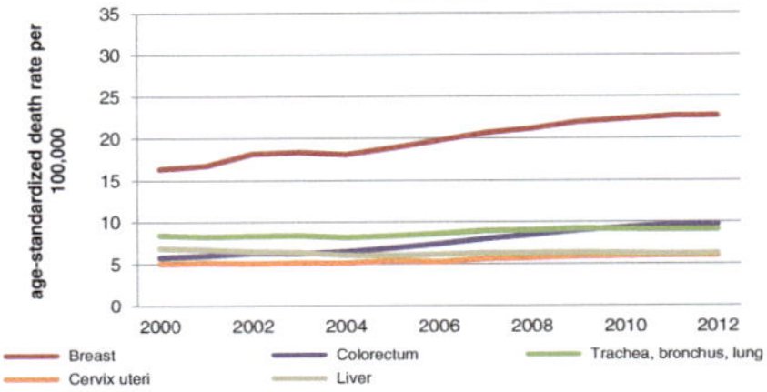

Cancer Incidence

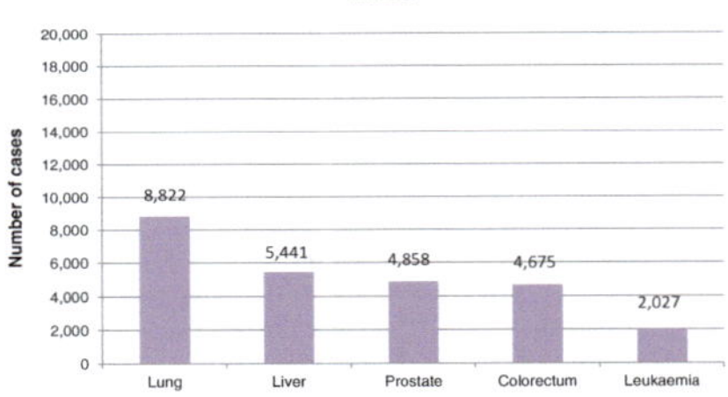

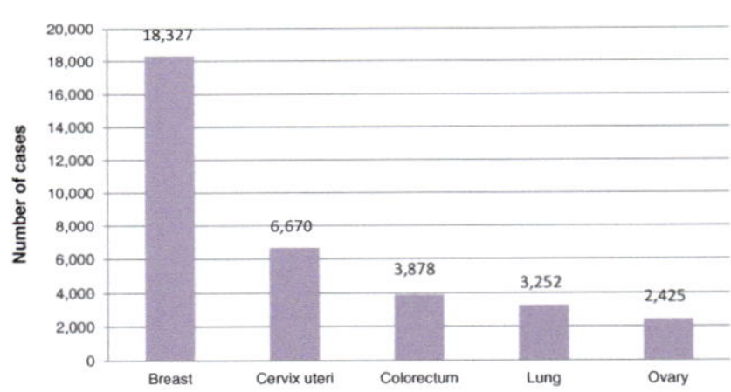

Adult Risk Factors

	Males	Females	Total
Current tobacco smoking (2011)	43.7%	9.5%	26.5%
Total alcohol per capita consumption, in litres of pure alcohol (2010)	9.2	1.7	5.4
Physical inactivity (2010)	11.5%	17.3%	14.4%
Obesity (2014)	3.4%	6.1%	4.7%
Household solid fuel use (2012)	-	-	49.0%

World Health Organization - Cancer Country Profiles, 2014.

Cancer Plans, Monitoring and Surveillance

Has an operational cancer policy/strategy/action plan	Yes
Has a cancer registry	Yes
Scope	Population-based
Coverage	Subnational
Last year of data	2003

Cancer Primary Prevention Policies

Tobacco control

Has an operational policy, strategy or action plan to reduce the burden of tobacco use	Yes
Smoke-free legislation	Three to five public places completely smoke-free
Tobacco dependence treatment	NRT and/or some cessation services (at least one of which is cost-covered)
Warning labels	No warnings or small warnings
Bans on advertising, promotion and sponsorship	Ban on national television, radio and print media as well as on some but not all other forms of direct and/or indirect advertising
Tobacco taxes	26–50% of retail price is tax

Overweight and obesity prevention and control

Has an operational policy, strategy or action plan for reducing overweight/obesity	Yes

Physical inactivity prevention and control

Has an operational policy, strategy or action plan to reduce physical inactivity and/or promote physical activity	Yes

Harmful use of alcohol prevention and control

Has an operational policy, strategy or action plan to reduce the harmful use of alcohol	Yes

National immunization

Human Papillomavirus vaccination schedule	...
Hepatitis B vaccination schedule	Birth
Hepatitis B vaccination coverage, infants	94%

Cancer Screening and Early Detection

Cervical cancer

Cervical cytology (PAP)	Not generally available at the public primary health care level
Acetic acid visualization (VIA)	Not generally available at the public primary health care level

Breast cancer

Breast palpation / clinical breast exam (CBE)	Generally available at the public primary health care level
Mammogram	Not generally available at the public primary health care level

Colorectal cancer

Faecal occult blood test or faecal immunological test	Not generally available at the public primary health care level
Bowel cancer screening by exam or colonoscopy	Not generally available at the public primary health care level

Cancer Treatment and Palliative Care

Radiotherapy	Generally available in the public health system
Total high energy teletherapy units / million inhabitants	0.2
Number of radiotherapy centres	34
Number of radiation oncologists	183
Chemotherapy (medicines not specified)	Generally available in the public health system
Oral morphine (formulation not specified)	Not generally available in the public health system
Non-methadone morphine equivalent consumption per cancer death (mg)	...
Community/home care for people with advanced stage cancer and other NCDs	Not generally available

... = No data available

World Health Organization - Cancer Country Profiles, 2014.

Rwanda

Total population: 11,458,000
Income group: Low

Total deaths: 78,000
Life expectancy at birth: Total:65 Males:63 Females:66

Cancer Mortality Profile*

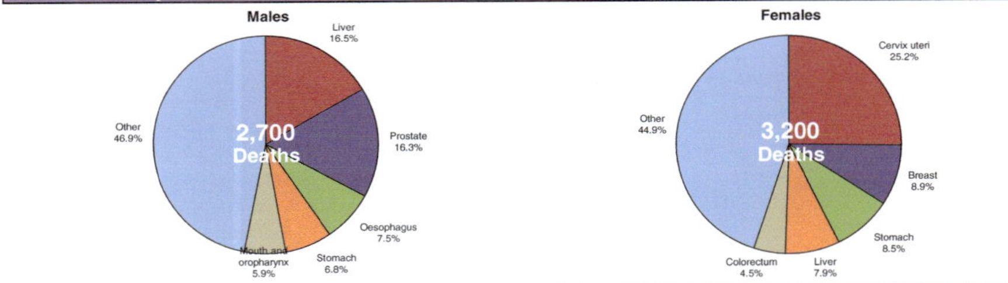

Age-Standardized Cancer Mortality Trends*

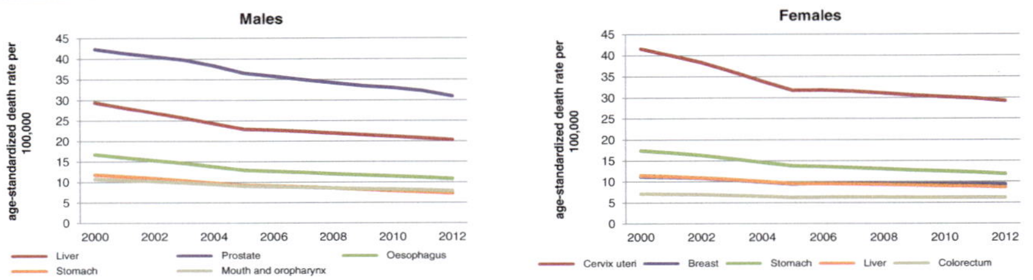

Cancer Incidence

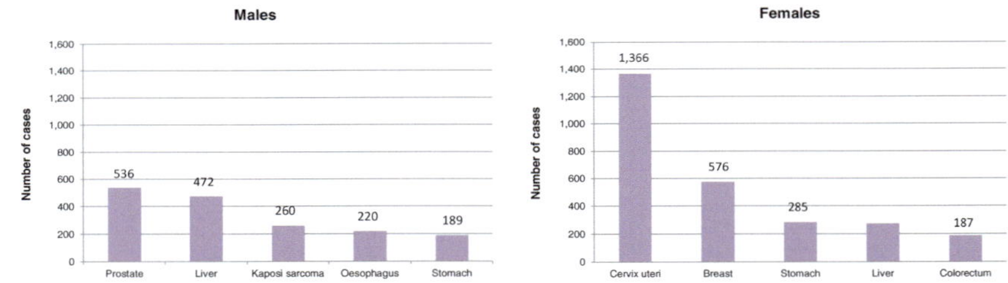

Adult Risk Factors

	Males	Females	Total
Current tobacco smoking (2011)	...	...	...
Total alcohol per capita consumption, in litres of pure alcohol (2010)	15.1	5.0	9.8
Physical inactivity (2010)	10.0%	17.0%	13.6%
Obesity (2014)	1.0%	5.4%	3.3%
Household solid fuel use (2012)	-	-	98.0%

World Health Organization - Cancer Country Profiles, 2014.

Cancer Plans, Monitoring and Surveillance

Has an operational cancer policy/strategy/action plan	Yes
Has a cancer registry	No
Scope	
Coverage	
Last year of data	

Cancer Primary Prevention Policies

Tobacco control

Has an operational policy, strategy or action plan to reduce the burden of tobacco use	No
Smoke-free legislation	Up to two public places completely smoke-free
Tobacco dependence treatment	None
Warning labels	No warnings or small warnings
Bans on advertising, promotion and sponsorship	Complete absence of ban, or ban that does not cover national television, radio and print media
Tobacco taxes	51–75% of retail price is tax

Overweight and obesity prevention and control

Has an operational policy, strategy or action plan for reducing overweight/obesity	No

Physical inactivity prevention and control

Has an operational policy, strategy or action plan to reduce physical inactivity and/or promote physical activity	No

Harmful use of alcohol prevention and control

Has an operational policy, strategy or action plan to reduce the harmful use of alcohol	No

National immunization

Human Papillomavirus vaccination schedule	9-15 years, +2 months, +6 months
Hepatitis B vaccination schedule	1st contact, +1 month, +5 months
Hepatitis B vaccination coverage, infants	98%

Cancer Screening and Early Detection

Cervical cancer

Cervical cytology (PAP)	Not generally available at the public primary health care level
Acetic acid visualization (VIA)	Not generally available at the public primary health care level

Breast cancer

Breast palpation / clinical breast exam (CBE)	Not generally available at the public primary health care level
Mammogram	Not generally available at the public primary health care level

Colorectal cancer

Faecal occult blood test or faecal immunological test	Not generally available at the public primary health care level
Bowel cancer screening by exam or colonoscopy	Not generally available at the public primary health care level

Cancer Treatment and Palliative Care

Radiotherapy	Not generally available in the public health system
Total high energy teletherapy units / million inhabitants	...
Number of radiotherapy centres	...
Number of radiation oncologists	...
Chemotherapy (medicines not specified)	Not generally available in the public health system
Oral morphine (formulation not specified)	Generally available in the public health system
Non-methadone morphine equivalent consumption per cancer death (mg)	...
Community/home care for people with advanced stage cancer and other NCDs	Not generally available

* No mortality data available. Figures are based on national incidence estimates and modelled survival. ... = No data available

World Health Organization - Cancer Country Profiles, 2014.

Somalia

Total population: 10,195,000
Income group: Low

Total deaths: 140,000
Life expectancy at birth: Total:53 Males:51 Females:55

Cancer Mortality Profile*

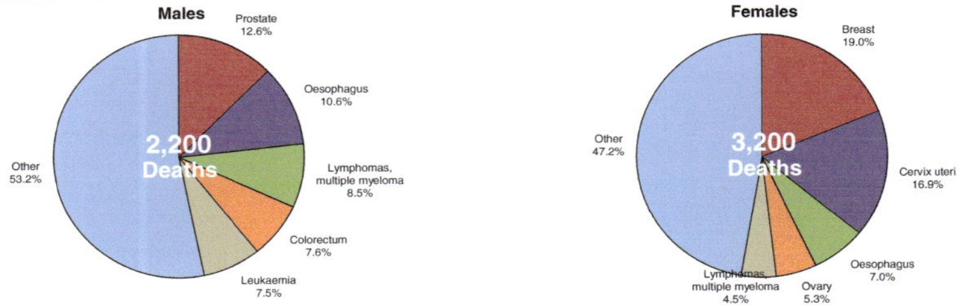

Age-Standardized Cancer Mortality Trends*

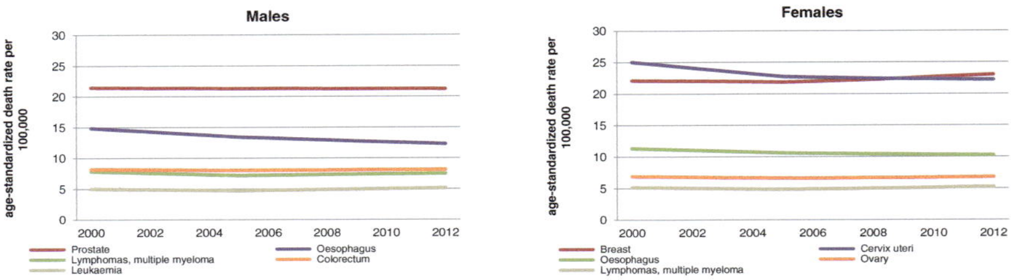

Cancer Incidence**

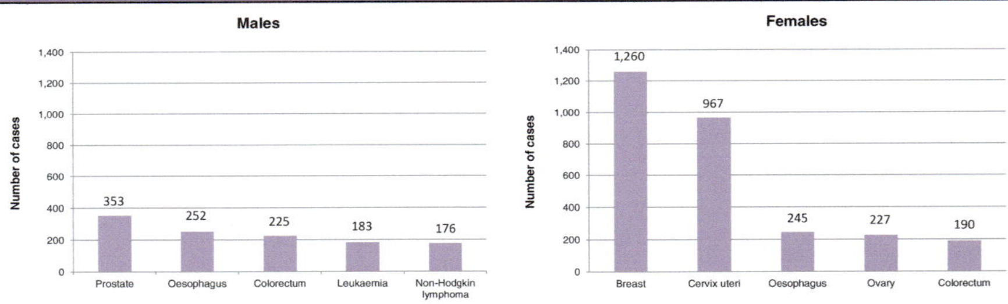

Adult Risk Factors

	Males	Females	Total
Current tobacco smoking (2011)	...	...	...
Total alcohol per capita consumption, in litres of pure alcohol (2010)	0.9	0.1	0.5
Physical inactivity (2010)	...	...	...
Obesity (2014)	1.8%	6.0%	3.9%
Household solid fuel use (2012)	-	-	96.0%

World Health Organization - Cancer Country Profiles, 2014.

Cancer Plans, Monitoring and Surveillance

Has an operational cancer policy/strategy/action plan	No
Has a cancer registry	No
Scope	
Coverage	
Last year of data	

Cancer Primary Prevention Policies

Tobacco control

Has an operational policy, strategy or action plan to reduce the burden of tobacco use	No
Smoke-free legislation	Up to two public places completely smoke-free
Tobacco dependence treatment	None
Warning labels	No warnings or small warnings
Bans on advertising, promotion and sponsorship	Complete absence of ban, or ban that does not cover national television, radio and print media
Tobacco taxes	≤25% of retail price is tax

Overweight and obesity prevention and control

Has an operational policy, strategy or action plan for reducing overweight/obesity	No

Physical inactivity prevention and control

Has an operational policy, strategy or action plan to reduce physical inactivity and/or promote physical activity	No

Harmful use of alcohol prevention and control

Has an operational policy, strategy or action plan to reduce the harmful use of alcohol	No

National immunization

Human Papillomavirus vaccination schedule	...
Hepatitis B vaccination schedule	...
Hepatitis B vaccination coverage, infants	34%

Cancer Screening and Early Detection

Cervical cancer

Cervical cytology (PAP)	Not generally available at the public primary health care level
Acetic acid visualization (VIA)	Not generally available at the public primary health care level

Breast cancer

Breast palpation / clinical breast exam (CBE)	Generally available at the public primary health care level
Mammogram	Not generally available at the public primary health care level

Colorectal cancer

Faecal occult blood test or faecal immunological test	Not generally available at the public primary health care level
Bowel cancer screening by exam or colonoscopy	Not generally available at the public primary health care level

Cancer Treatment and Palliative Care

Radiotherapy	Not generally available in the public health system
Total high energy teletherapy units / million inhabitants	...
Number of radiotherapy centres	...
Number of radiation oncologists	...
Chemotherapy (medicines not specified)	Not generally available in the public health system
Oral morphine (formulation not specified)	Not generally available in the public health system
Non-methadone morphine equivalent consumption per cancer death (mg)	...
Community/home care for people with advanced stage cancer and other NCDs	Not generally available

* No mortality data available. Figures are based on national incidence estimates and modelled survival.
** No incidence data available. Figures are based on national incidence estimates from neighbouring countries.
... = No data available

World Health Organization - Cancer Country Profiles, 2014.

Serbia

Total population: 9,553,000
Income group: Upper middle

Total deaths: 113,000
Life expectancy at birth: Total:75 Males:72 Females:77

Cancer Mortality Profile

Males

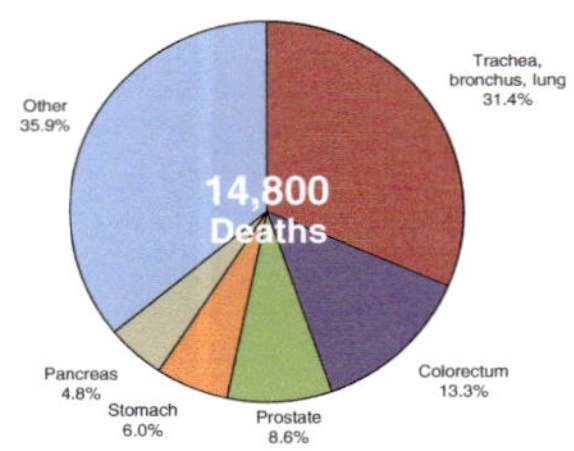

Females

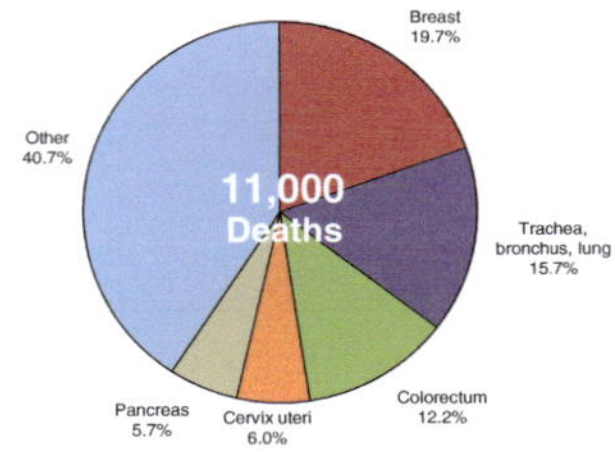

Age-Standardized Cancer Mortality Trends

Males

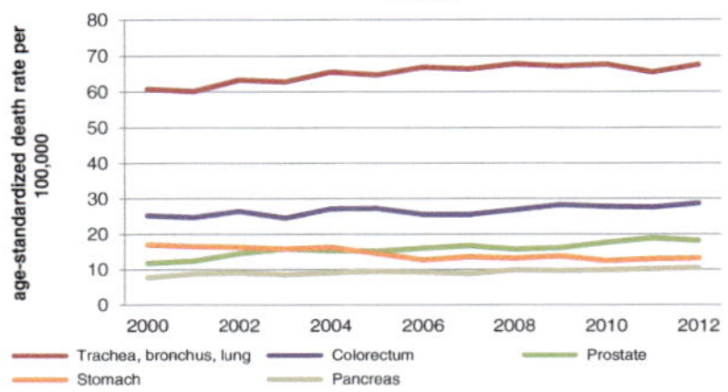

Females

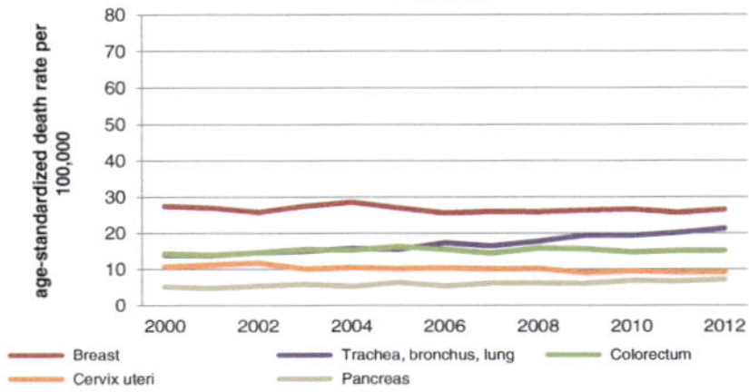

Cancer Incidence

Males

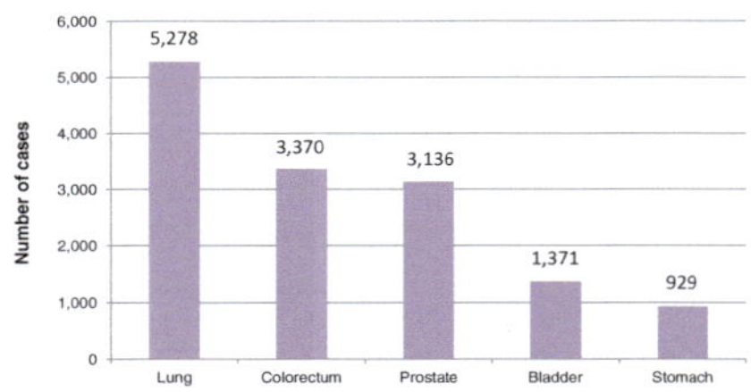

Females

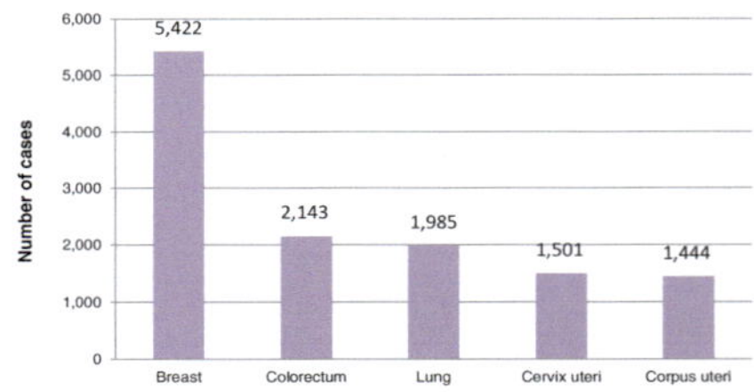

Adult Risk Factors

	Males	Females	Total
Current tobacco smoking (2011)	37.6%	27.2%	32.4%
Total alcohol per capita consumption, in litres of pure alcohol (2010)	19.7	5.9	12.6
Physical inactivity (2010)	35.3%	47.1%	41.4%
Obesity (2014)	19.7%	22.5%	21.1%
Household solid fuel use (2012)	-	-	32.0%

World Health Organization - Cancer Country Profiles, 2014.

Cancer Plans, Monitoring and Surveillance

Has an operational cancer policy/strategy/action plan	No
Has a cancer registry	Yes
Scope	Population-based
Coverage	Subnational
Last year of data	2010

Cancer Primary Prevention Policies

Tobacco control

Has an operational policy, strategy or action plan to reduce the burden of tobacco use	Yes
Smoke-free legislation	Three to five public places completely smoke-free
Tobacco dependence treatment	NRT and/or some cessation services (at least one of which is cost-covered)
Warning labels	Medium size warnings missing some appropriate characteristics OR large warnings missing many appropriate characteristics
Bans on advertising, promotion and sponsorship	Ban on national television, radio and print media as well as on some but not all other forms of direct and/or indirect advertising
Tobacco taxes	>75% of retail price is tax*

Overweight and obesity prevention and control

Has an operational policy, strategy or action plan for reducing overweight/obesity	No

Physical inactivity prevention and control

Has an operational policy, strategy or action plan to reduce physical inactivity and/or promote physical activity	No

Harmful use of alcohol prevention and control

Has an operational policy, strategy or action plan to reduce the harmful use of alcohol	No

National immunization

Human Papillomavirus vaccination schedule	...
Hepatitis B vaccination schedule	Birth, +4 weeks, +5 months, +12 years
Hepatitis B vaccination coverage, infants	91%

Cancer Screening and Early Detection

Cervical cancer

Cervical cytology (PAP)	Generally available at the public primary health care level
Acetic acid visualization (VIA)	Generally available at the public primary health care level

Breast cancer

Breast palpation / clinical breast exam (CBE)	Generally available at the public primary health care level
Mammogram	Generally available at the public primary health care level

Colorectal cancer

Faecal occult blood test or faecal immunological test	Generally available at the public primary health care level
Bowel cancer screening by exam or colonoscopy	Generally available at the public primary health care level

Cancer Treatment and Palliative Care

Radiotherapy	Generally available in the public health system
Total high energy teletherapy units / million inhabitants	1.5
Number of radiotherapy centres	6
Number of radiation oncologists	55
Chemotherapy (medicines not specified)	Generally available in the public health system
Oral morphine (formulation not specified)	Generally available in the public health system
Non-methadone morphine equivalent consumption per cancer death (mg)	...
Community/home care for people with advanced stage cancer and other NCDs	Generally available

* Indicates highest possible level of achievement ... = No data available

World Health Organization - Cancer Country Profiles, 2014.

South Sudan

Total population: 10,838,000
Income group: Low

Total deaths: 126,000
Life expectancy at birth: Total:55 Males:54 Females:56

Cancer Mortality Profile*

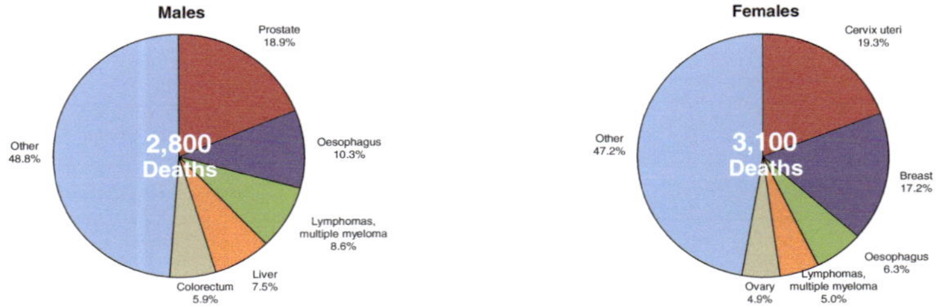

Age-Standardized Cancer Mortality Trends*

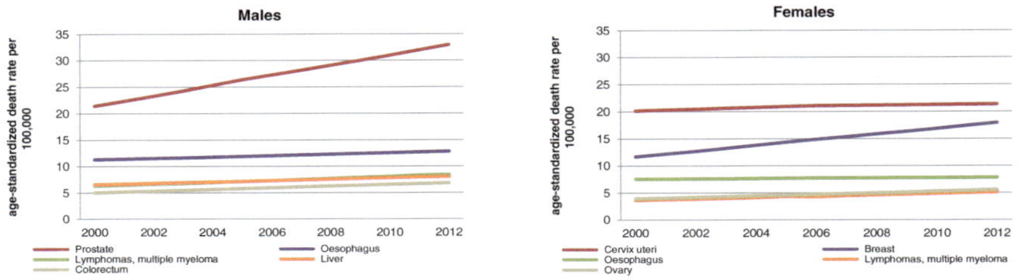

Cancer Incidence**

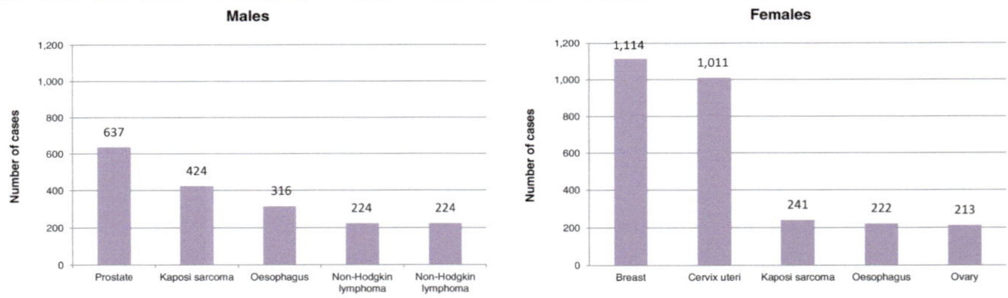

Adult Risk Factors

	Males	Females	Total
Current tobacco smoking (2011)	...	...	...
Total alcohol per capita consumption, in litres of pure alcohol (2010)	...	...	...
Physical inactivity (2010)	...	...	...
Obesity (2014)	...	...	...
Household solid fuel use (2012)	-	-	97.0%

World Health Organization - Cancer Country Profiles, 2014.

Cancer Plans, Monitoring and Surveillance

Has an operational cancer policy/strategy/action plan	ND
Has a cancer registry	ND
Scope	ND
Coverage	ND
Last year of data	ND

Cancer Primary Prevention Policies

Tobacco control

Has an operational policy, strategy or action plan to reduce the burden of tobacco use	ND
Smoke-free legislation	Up to two public places completely smoke-free
Tobacco dependence treatment	Data not reported
Warning labels	No warnings or small warnings
Bans on advertising, promotion and sponsorship	Complete absence of ban, or ban that does not cover national television, radio and print media
Tobacco taxes	Data not reported

Overweight and obesity prevention and control

Has an operational policy, strategy or action plan for reducing overweight/obesity	ND

Physical inactivity prevention and control

Has an operational policy, strategy or action plan to reduce physical inactivity and/or promote physical activity	ND

Harmful use of alcohol prevention and control

Has an operational policy, strategy or action plan to reduce the harmful use of alcohol	ND

National immunization

Human Papillomavirus vaccination schedule	...
Hepatitis B vaccination schedule	...
Hepatitis B vaccination coverage, infants	...

Cancer Screening and Early Detection

Cervical cancer

Cervical cytology (PAP)	ND
Acetic acid visualization (VIA)	ND

Breast cancer

Breast palpation / clinical breast exam (CBE)	ND
Mammogram	ND

Colorectal cancer

Faecal occult blood test or faecal immunological test	ND
Bowel cancer screening by exam or colonoscopy	ND

Cancer Treatment and Palliative Care

Radiotherapy	ND
Total high energy teletherapy units / million inhabitants	...
Number of radiotherapy centres	...
Number of radiation oncologists	...
Chemotherapy (medicines not specified)	ND
Oral morphine (formulation not specified)	ND
Non-methadone morphine equivalent consumption per cancer death (mg)	...
Community/home care for people with advanced stage cancer and other NCDs	ND

* No mortality data available. Figures are based on national incidence estimates and modelled survival.
** No incidence data available. Figures are based on national incidence estimates from neighbouring countries.

... = No data available
ND = Country did not respond to country capacity survey

World Health Organization - Cancer Country Profiles, 2014.

Togo

Total population: 6,643,000
Income group: Low

Total deaths: 65,000
Life expectancy at birth: Total:58 Males:57 Females:59

Cancer Mortality Profile*

Males

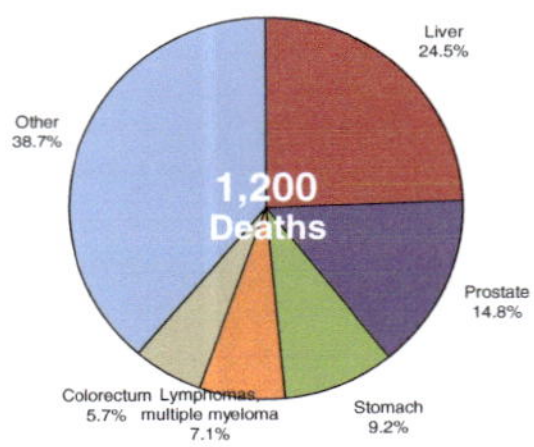

Females

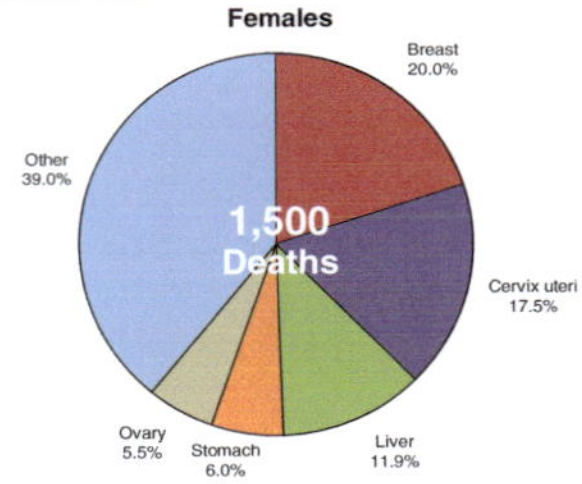

Age-Standardized Cancer Mortality Trends*

Males

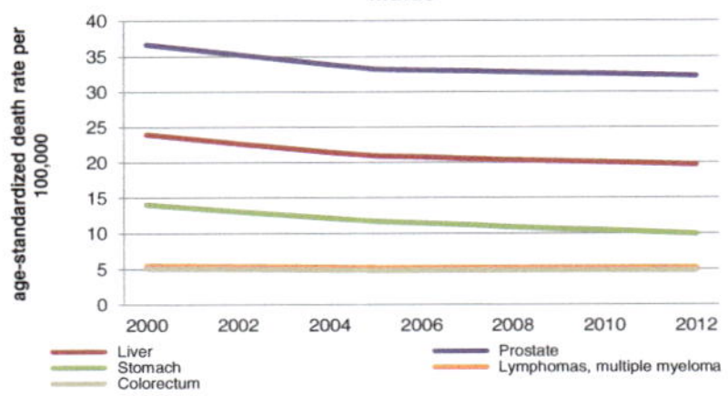

Females

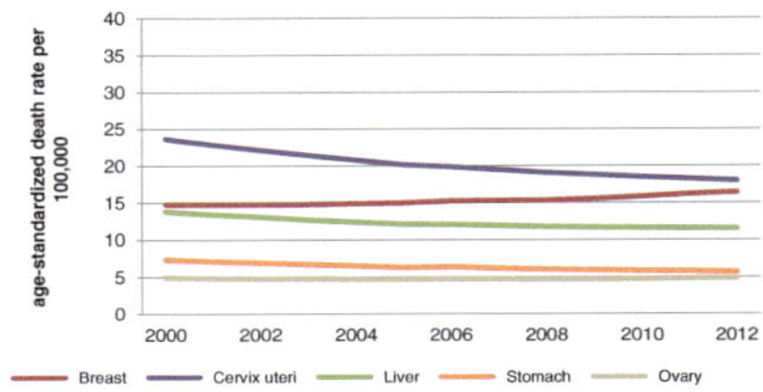

Cancer Incidence

Males

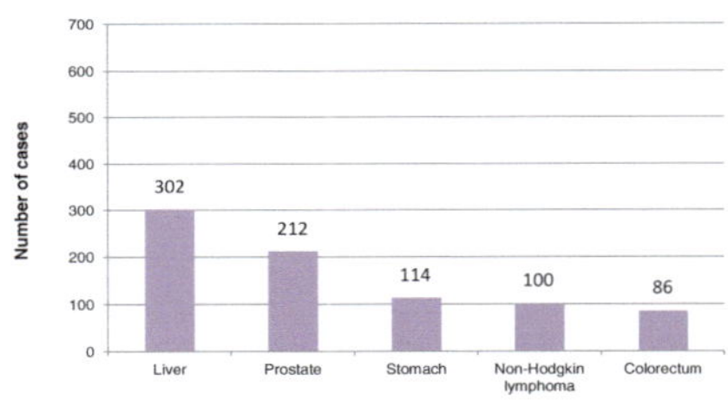

Females

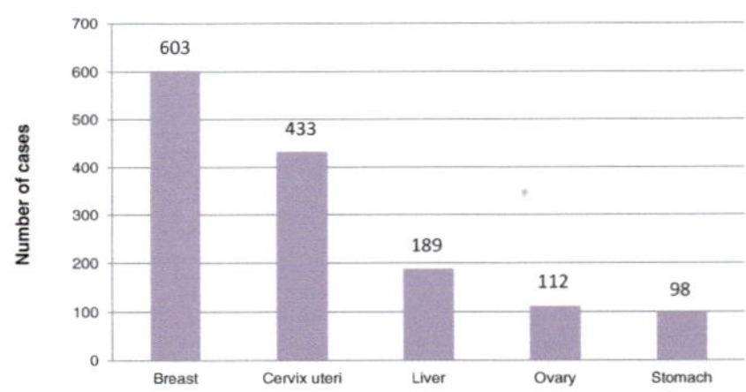

Adult Risk Factors

	Males	Females	Total
Current tobacco smoking (2011)	13.9%	2.3%	8%
Total alcohol per capita consumption, in litres of pure alcohol (2010)	3.8	0.9	2.3
Physical inactivity (2010)	7.6%	9.8%	8.7%
Obesity (2014)	2.6%	10.1%	6.4%
Household solid fuel use (2012)	-	-	95.0%

World Health Organization - Cancer Country Profiles, 2014.

Cancer Plans, Monitoring and Surveillance

Has an operational cancer policy/strategy/action plan	Yes
Has a cancer registry	Yes
Scope	Hospital-based
Coverage	National and Subnational
Last year of data	2012

Cancer Primary Prevention Policies

Tobacco control

Has an operational policy, strategy or action plan to reduce the burden of tobacco use	Yes
Smoke-free legislation	Three to five public places completely smoke-free
Tobacco dependence treatment	NRT and/or some cessation services (neither cost-covered)
Warning labels	Medium size warnings missing some appropriate characteristics OR large warnings missing many appropriate characteristics
Bans on advertising, promotion and sponsorship	Ban on all forms of direct and indirect advertising**
Tobacco taxes	≤25% of retail price is tax

Overweight and obesity prevention and control

Has an operational policy, strategy or action plan for reducing overweight/obesity	Yes

Physical inactivity prevention and control

Has an operational policy, strategy or action plan to reduce physical inactivity and/or promote physical activity	Yes

Harmful use of alcohol prevention and control

Has an operational policy, strategy or action plan to reduce the harmful use of alcohol	Yes

National immunization

Human Papillomavirus vaccination schedule	(starting November 2014, subnational)
Hepatitis B vaccination schedule	...
Hepatitis B vaccination coverage, infants	84%

Cancer Screening and Early Detection

Cervical cancer

Cervical cytology (PAP)	Not generally available at the public primary health care level
Acetic acid visualization (VIA)	Not generally available at the public primary health care level

Breast cancer

Breast palpation / clinical breast exam (CBE)	Not generally available at the public primary health care level
Mammogram	Not generally available at the public primary health care level

Colorectal cancer

Faecal occult blood test or faecal immunological test	Not generally available at the public primary health care level
Bowel cancer screening by exam or colonoscopy	Not generally available at the public primary health care level

Cancer Treatment and Palliative Care

Radiotherapy	Not generally available in the public health system
Total high energy teletherapy units / million inhabitants	...
Number of radiotherapy centres	...
Number of radiation oncologists	...
Chemotherapy (medicines not specified)	Not generally available in the public health system
Oral morphine (formulation not specified)	Not generally available in the public health system
Non-methadone morphine equivalent consumption per cancer death (mg)	...
Community/home care for people with advanced stage cancer and other NCDs	Not generally available

* No mortality data available. Figures are based on national incidence estimates and modelled survival. ... = No data available

** Indicates highest possible level of achievement

World Health Organization - Cancer Country Profiles, 2014.

Ukraine

Total population: 45,530,000
Income group: Lower middle

Total deaths: 686,000
Life expectancy at birth: Total:71 Males:66 Females:76

Cancer Mortality Profile

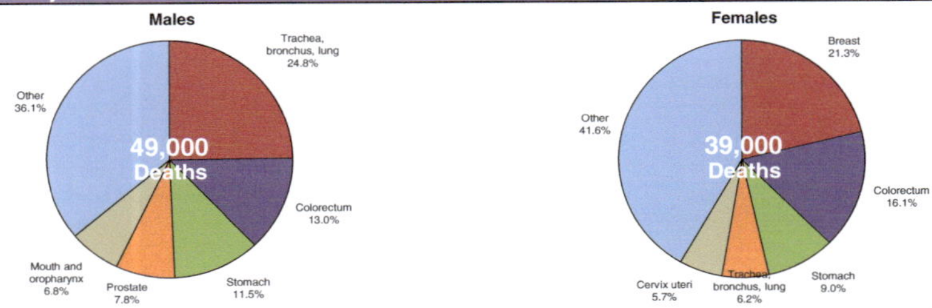

Age-Standardized Cancer Mortality Trends

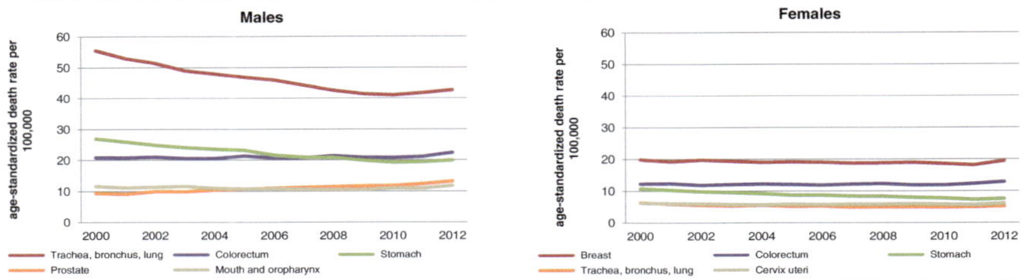

Cancer Incidence

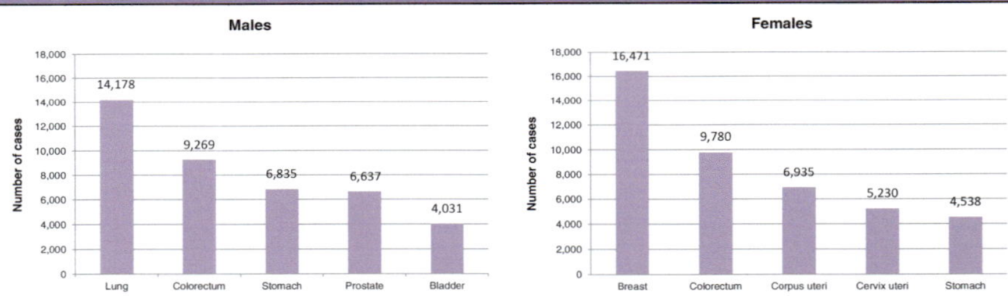

Adult Risk Factors

	Males	Females	Total
Current tobacco smoking (2011)	49.2%	14%	29.9%
Total alcohol per capita consumption, in litres of pure alcohol (2010)	22.0	7.2	13.9
Physical inactivity (2010)	12.2%	16.2%	14.4%
Obesity (2014)	17.9%	24.9%	21.7%
Household solid fuel use (2012)	-	-	3.0%

World Health Organization - Cancer Country Profiles, 2014.

Cancer Plans, Monitoring and Surveillance

Has an operational cancer policy/strategy/action plan	No
Has a cancer registry	Yes
Scope	Population-based
Coverage	National
Last year of data	2011

Cancer Primary Prevention Policies

Tobacco control

Has an operational policy, strategy or action plan to reduce the burden of tobacco use	No
Smoke-free legislation	Six to seven public places completely smoke-free
Tobacco dependence treatment	NRT and/or some cessation services (neither cost-covered)
Warning labels	Large warnings with all appropriate characteristics*
Bans on advertising, promotion and sponsorship	Ban on national television, radio and print media as well as on some but not all other forms of direct and/or indirect advertising
Tobacco taxes	51–75% of retail price is tax

Overweight and obesity prevention and control

Has an operational policy, strategy or action plan for reducing overweight/obesity	No

Physical inactivity prevention and control

Has an operational policy, strategy or action plan to reduce physical inactivity and/or promote physical activity	No

Harmful use of alcohol prevention and control

Has an operational policy, strategy or action plan to reduce the harmful use of alcohol	No

National immunization

Human Papillomavirus vaccination schedule	...
Hepatitis B vaccination schedule	Birth, +1 month, +6 months
Hepatitis B vaccination coverage, infants	46%

Cancer Screening and Early Detection

Cervical cancer

Cervical cytology (PAP)	Not generally available at the public primary health care level
Acetic acid visualization (VIA)	Not generally available at the public primary health care level

Breast cancer

Breast palpation / clinical breast exam (CBE)	Generally available at the public primary health care level
Mammogram	Not generally available at the public primary health care level

Colorectal cancer

Faecal occult blood test or faecal immunological test	Not generally available at the public primary health care level
Bowel cancer screening by exam or colonoscopy	Not generally available at the public primary health care level

Cancer Treatment and Palliative Care

Radiotherapy	Not generally available in the public health system
Total high energy teletherapy units / million inhabitants	2.4
Number of radiotherapy centres	56
Number of radiation oncologists	449
Chemotherapy (medicines not specified)	Not generally available in the public health system
Oral morphine (formulation not specified)	DK
Non-methadone morphine equivalent consumption per cancer death (mg)	...
Community/home care for people with advanced stage cancer and other NCDs	Not generally available

* Indicates highest possible level of achievement

... = No data available
DK = Country responded "don't know"

World Health Organization - Cancer Country Profiles, 2014.

Uzbekistan

Total population: 28,541,000
Income group: Lower middle

Total deaths: 184,000
Life expectancy at birth: Total:69 Males:67 Females:72

Cancer Mortality Profile

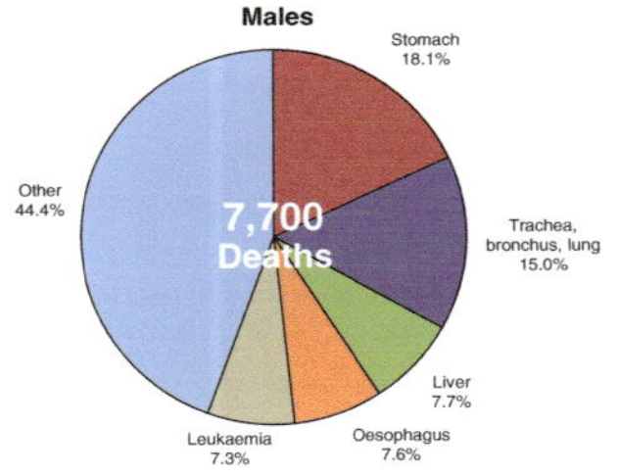

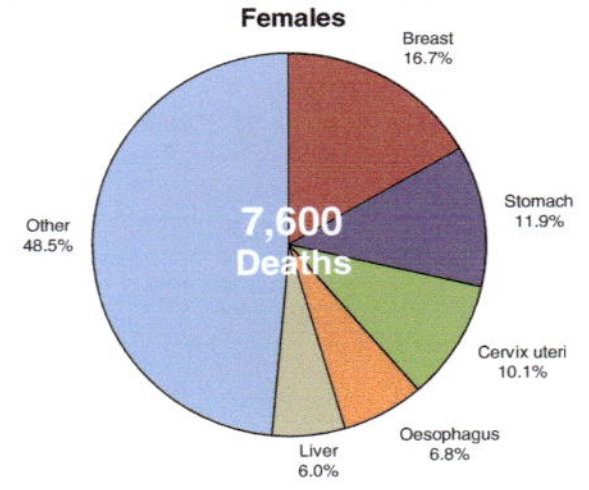

Age-Standardized Cancer Mortality Trends

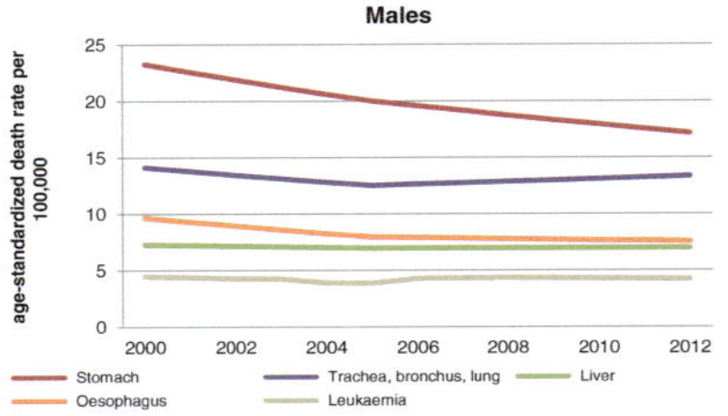

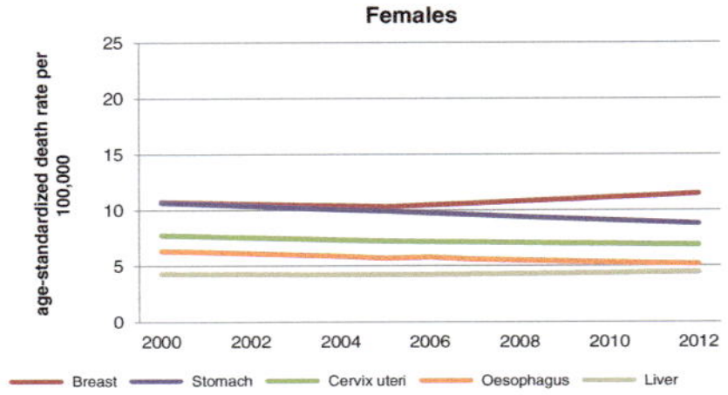

Cancer Incidence*

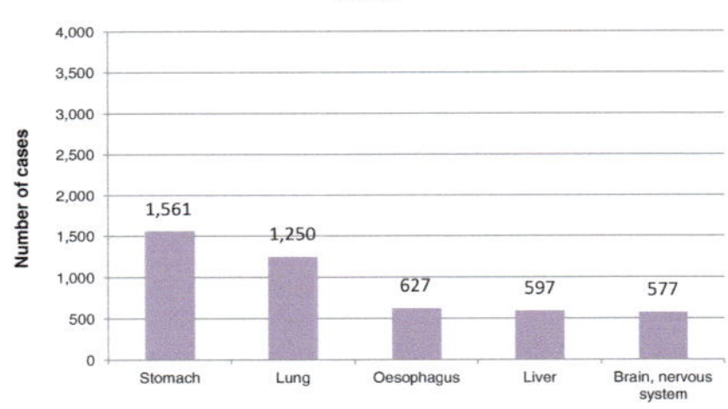

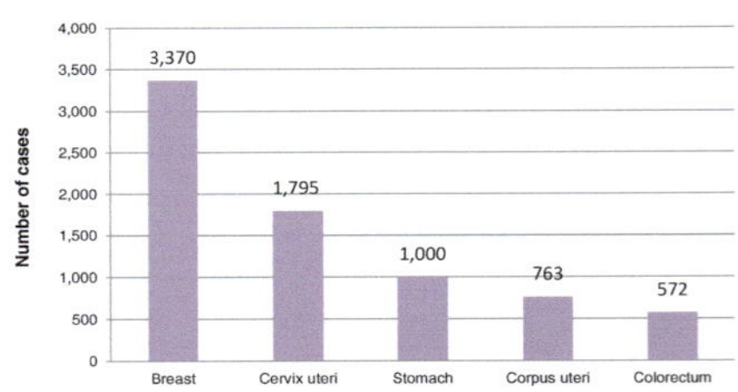

Adult Risk Factors

	Males	Females	Total
Current tobacco smoking (2011)	22.3%	3.5%	12.9%
Total alcohol per capita consumption, in litres of pure alcohol (2010)	7.9	1.3	4.6
Physical inactivity (2010)	11.8%	24.1%	18.1%
Obesity (2014)	11.2%	17.4%	14.3%
Household solid fuel use (2012)	-	-	11.0%

World Health Organization - Cancer Country Profiles, 2014.

Cancer Plans, Monitoring and Surveillance

Has an operational cancer policy/strategy/action plan	Yes
Has a cancer registry	No
Scope	
Coverage	
Last year of data	

Cancer Primary Prevention Policies

Tobacco control

Has an operational policy, strategy or action plan to reduce the burden of tobacco use	No
Smoke-free legislation	Up to two public places completely smoke-free
Tobacco dependence treatment	NRT and/or some cessation services (neither cost-covered)
Warning labels	Medium size warnings missing some appropriate characteristics OR large warnings missing many appropriate characteristics
Bans on advertising, promotion and sponsorship	Ban on national television, radio and print media as well as on some but not all other forms of direct and/or indirect advertising
Tobacco taxes	26–50% of retail price is tax

Overweight and obesity prevention and control

Has an operational policy, strategy or action plan for reducing overweight/obesity	No

Physical inactivity prevention and control

Has an operational policy, strategy or action plan to reduce physical inactivity and/or promote physical activity	No

Harmful use of alcohol prevention and control

Has an operational policy, strategy or action plan to reduce the harmful use of alcohol	No

National immunization

Human Papillomavirus vaccination schedule	(starting January 2015)
Hepatitis B vaccination schedule	Birth
Hepatitis B vaccination coverage, infants	99%

Cancer Screening and Early Detection

Cervical cancer

Cervical cytology (PAP)	Not generally available at the public primary health care level
Acetic acid visualization (VIA)	Not generally available at the public primary health care level

Breast cancer

Breast palpation / clinical breast exam (CBE)	Generally available at the public primary health care level
Mammogram	Not generally available at the public primary health care level

Colorectal cancer

Faecal occult blood test or faecal immunological test	Not generally available at the public primary health care level
Bowel cancer screening by exam or colonoscopy	Not generally available at the public primary health care level

Cancer Treatment and Palliative Care

Radiotherapy	Not generally available in the public health system
Total high energy teletherapy units / million inhabitants	0.6
Number of radiotherapy centres	13
Number of radiation oncologists	...
Chemotherapy (medicines not specified)	Generally available in the public health system
Oral morphine (formulation not specified)	DK
Non-methadone morphine equivalent consumption per cancer death (mg)	...
Community/home care for people with advanced stage cancer and other NCDs	Generally available

* No incidence data available. Figures are based on national mortality estimates and modelled survival.

... = No data available
DK = Country responded "don't know"

World Health Organization - Cancer Country Profiles, 2014.

South Africa

Total population: 52,386,000
Income group: Upper middle

Total deaths: 608,000
Life expectancy at birth: Total:59 Males:56 Females:62

Cancer Mortality Profile

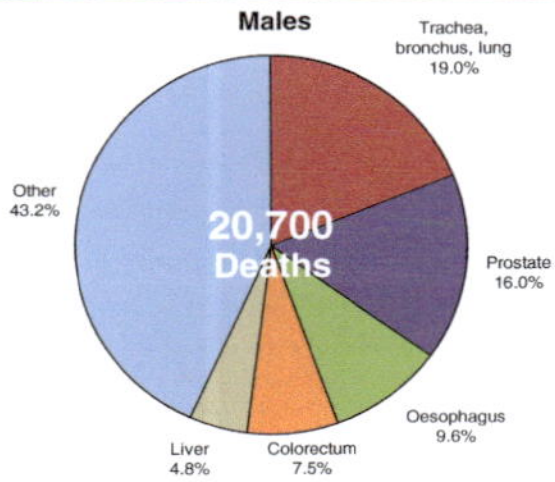

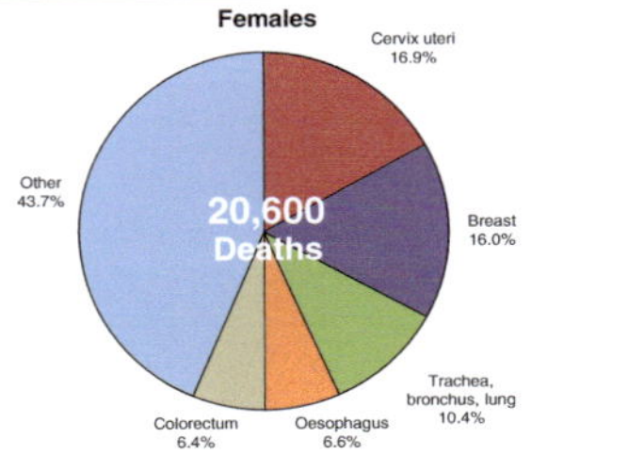

Age-Standardized Cancer Mortality Trends

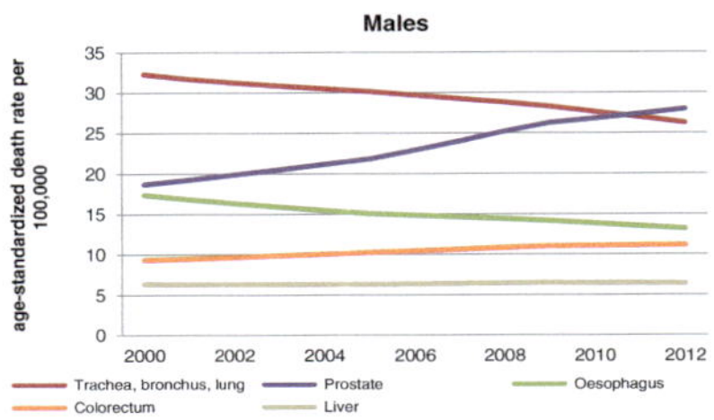

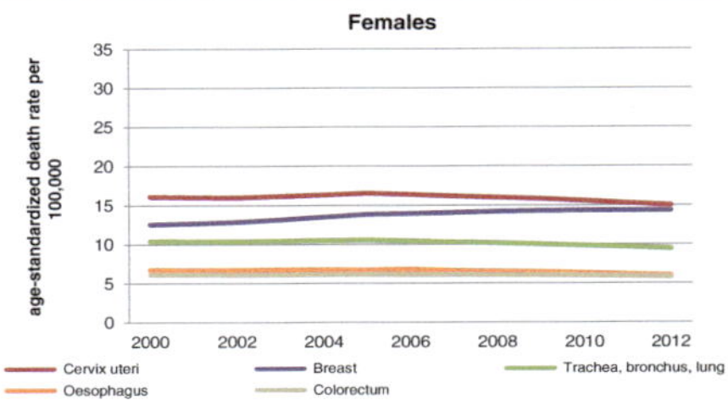

Cancer Incidence

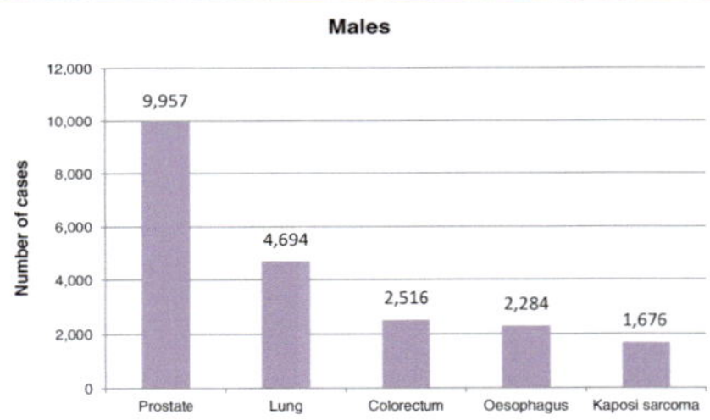

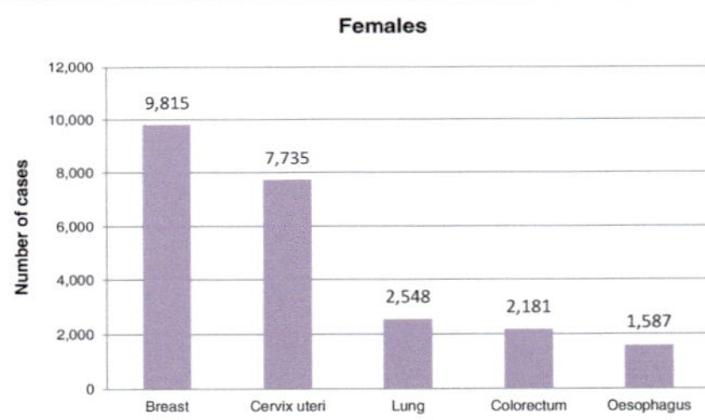

Adult Risk Factors

	Males	Females	Total
Current tobacco smoking (2011)	27.7%	7.7%	17.6%
Total alcohol per capita consumption, in litres of pure alcohol (2010)	18.4	4.2	11.0
Physical inactivity (2010)	40.5%	53.1%	47.1%
Obesity (2014)	14.6%	36.0%	25.6%
Household solid fuel use (2012)	-	-	13.0%

World Health Organization - Cancer Country Profiles, 2014.

Cancer Plans, Monitoring and Surveillance

Has an operational cancer policy/strategy/action plan	ND
Has a cancer registry	ND
Scope	ND
Coverage	ND
Last year of data	ND

Cancer Primary Prevention Policies

Tobacco control

Has an operational policy, strategy or action plan to reduce the burden of tobacco use	ND
Smoke-free legislation	Up to two public places completely smoke-free
Tobacco dependence treatment	NRT and/or some cessation services (neither cost-covered)
Warning labels	No warnings or small warnings
Bans on advertising, promotion and sponsorship	Ban on national television, radio and print media as well as on some but not all other forms of direct and/or indirect advertising
Tobacco taxes	26–50% of retail price is tax

Overweight and obesity prevention and control

Has an operational policy, strategy or action plan for reducing overweight/obesity	ND

Physical inactivity prevention and control

Has an operational policy, strategy or action plan to reduce physical inactivity and/or promote physical activity	ND

Harmful use of alcohol prevention and control

Has an operational policy, strategy or action plan to reduce the harmful use of alcohol	ND

National immunization

Human Papillomavirus vaccination schedule	...
Hepatitis B vaccination schedule	6 weeks, +10 weeks, +14 weeks
Hepatitis B vaccination coverage, infants	65%

Cancer Screening and Early Detection

Cervical cancer

Cervical cytology (PAP)	ND
Acetic acid visualization (VIA)	ND

Breast cancer

Breast palpation / clinical breast exam (CBE)	ND
Mammogram	ND

Colorectal cancer

Faecal occult blood test or faecal immunological test	ND
Bowel cancer screening by exam or colonoscopy	ND

Cancer Treatment and Palliative Care

Radiotherapy	ND
Total high energy teletherapy units / million inhabitants	0.6
Number of radiotherapy centres	39
Number of radiation oncologists	145
Chemotherapy (medicines not specified)	ND
Oral morphine (formulation not specified)	ND
Non-methadone morphine equivalent consumption per cancer death (mg)	...
Community/home care for people with advanced stage cancer and other NCDs	ND

... = No data available
ND = Country did not respond to country capacity survey

World Health Organization - Cancer Country Profiles, 2014.

Zimbabwe

Total population: 13,724,000
Income group: Low

Total deaths: 138,000
Life expectancy at birth: Total:58 Males:56 Females:60

Cancer Mortality Profile*

Males

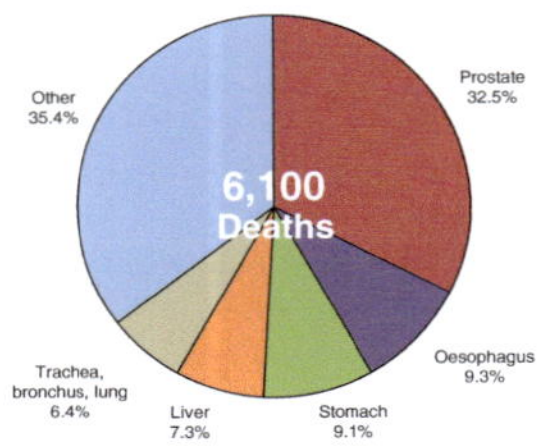

Females

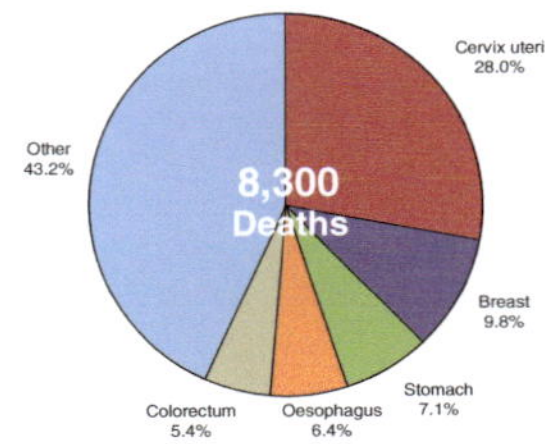

Age-Standardized Cancer Mortality Trends*

Males

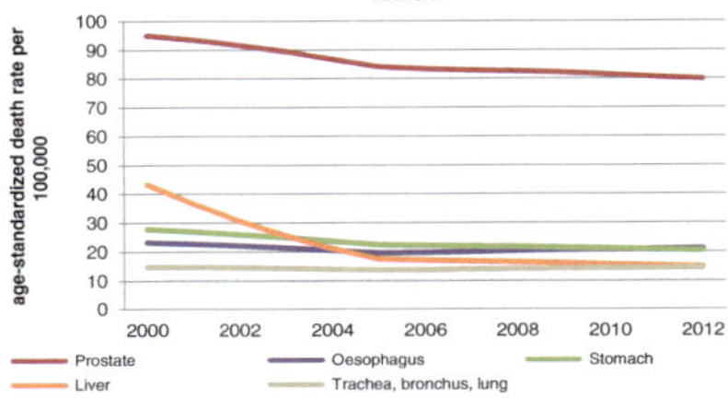

Females

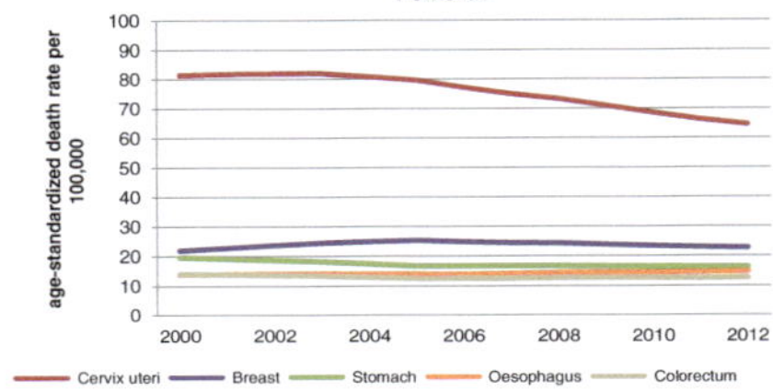

Cancer Incidence

Males

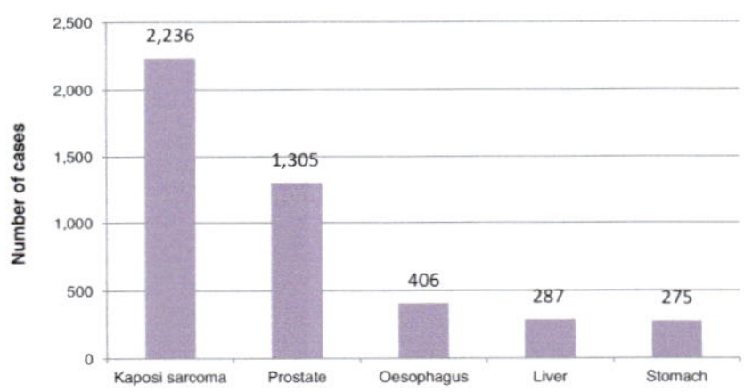

Females

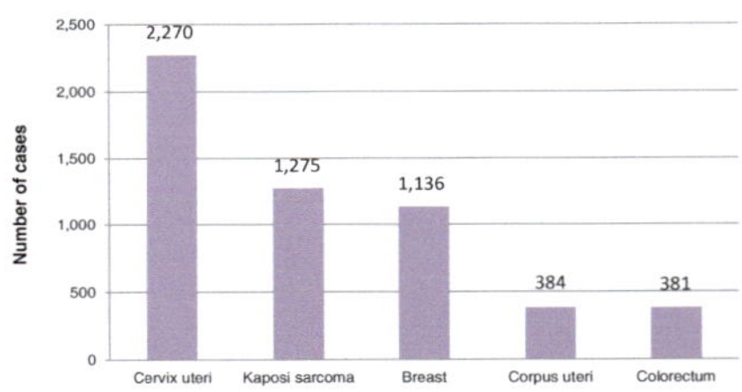

Adult Risk Factors

	Males	Females	Total
Current tobacco smoking (2011)	24.9%	<1%	12.3%
Total alcohol per capita consumption, in litres of pure alcohol (2010)	10.8	0.8	5.7
Physical inactivity (2010)	15.3%	23.8%	19.7%
Obesity (2014)	1.9%	14.8%	8.4%
Household solid fuel use (2012)	-	-	70.0%

World Health Organization - Cancer Country Profiles, 2014.

Cancer Plans, Monitoring and Surveillance

Has an operational cancer policy/strategy/action plan	No
Has a cancer registry	Yes
Scope	Population-based
Coverage	Subnational
Last year of data	2010

Cancer Primary Prevention Policies

Tobacco control

Has an operational policy, strategy or action plan to reduce the burden of tobacco use	No
Smoke-free legislation	Three to five public places completely smoke-free
Tobacco dependence treatment	NRT and/or some cessation services (neither cost-covered)
Warning labels	No warnings or small warnings
Bans on advertising, promotion and sponsorship	Complete absence of ban, or ban that does not cover national television, radio and print media
Tobacco taxes	51–75% of retail price is tax

Overweight and obesity prevention and control

Has an operational policy, strategy or action plan for reducing overweight/obesity	No

Physical inactivity prevention and control

Has an operational policy, strategy or action plan to reduce physical inactivity and/or promote physical activity	No

Harmful use of alcohol prevention and control

Has an operational policy, strategy or action plan to reduce the harmful use of alcohol	No

National immunization

Human Papillomavirus vaccination schedule	10 years, +1 month, +6 months (subnational)
Hepatitis B vaccination schedule	...
Hepatitis B vaccination coverage, infants	95%

Cancer Screening and Early Detection

Cervical cancer

Cervical cytology (PAP)	Not generally available at the public primary health care level
Acetic acid visualization (VIA)	Not generally available at the public primary health care level

Breast cancer

Breast palpation / clinical breast exam (CBE)	Generally available at the public primary health care level
Mammogram	Not generally available at the public primary health care level

Colorectal cancer

Faecal occult blood test or faecal immunological test	Not generally available at the public primary health care level
Bowel cancer screening by exam or colonoscopy	Generally available at the public primary health care level

Cancer Treatment and Palliative Care

Radiotherapy	Generally available in the public health system
Total high energy teletherapy units / million inhabitants	0.4
Number of radiotherapy centres	2
Number of radiation oncologists	6
Chemotherapy (medicines not specified)	Generally available in the public health system
Oral morphine (formulation not specified)	Generally available in the public health system
Non-methadone morphine equivalent consumption per cancer death (mg)	...
Community/home care for people with advanced stage cancer and other NCDs	Generally available

* No mortality data available. Figures are based on national incidence estimates and modelled survival. ... = No data available

World Health Organization - Cancer Country Profiles, 2014.

5.5 Gross Domestic Product - World

List of countries by GDP per capita

From Wikipedia, the free encyclopedia

This is a **list of countries of the world sorted by their gross domestic product (GDP) per capita**. GDP is the worth of all goods and services made in a country in a year.

International Monetary Fund (2010-11)[1]				World Bank (2005–10)[2]				CIA World Factbook (1993–2011)[3]			
Rank	**Country**	Intl. $	**Year**	**Rank**	**Country**	Intl. $	**Year**	**Rank**	**Country**	Intl. $	**Year**
1	Qatar	102,943	2011	1	Luxembourg	86,124	2010	1	Liechtenstein	141,100	2008 est.
2	Luxembourg	80,119	2011	2	Qatar	80,944	2009	2	Qatar	102,700	2011 est.
3	Singapore	59,711	2011	—	*Macau*	63,681	2010	3	Luxembourg	84,700	2011 est.
4	Norway	53,471	2011	3	Singapore	57,932	2010	—	*Bermuda*	69,900	2004 est.
5	Brunei	49,384	2011	4	Norway	57,231	2010	4	Monaco	63,400	2009 est.
—	*Hong Kong*	49,137	2011	5	Kuwait	52,657	2007	5	Singapore	59,900	2011 est.
6	United States	48,387	2011	6	Brunei	49,935	2009	—	*Jersey*	57,000	2005 est.
7	United Arab Emirates	48,158	2011	7	United Arab Emirates	47,213	2010	—	*Falkland Islands*	55,400	2002 est.
8	Switzerland	43,370	2011	8	United States	47,153	2010	6	Norway	53,300	2011 est.
9	Netherlands	42,183	2011	—	*Hong Kong*	46,502	2010	7	Brunei	49,400	2011 est.
10	Austria	41,822	2011	9	Switzerland	46,384	2010	—	*Hong Kong*	49,300	2011 est.
11	Kuwait	41,691	2011	10	Netherlands	42,165	2010	8	United Arab Emirates	48,500	2011 est.
12	Canada	40,541	2011	11	Ireland	40,464	2010	9	United States	48,100	2011 est.
13	Sweden	40,394	2011	12	Denmark	40,163	2010	—	*Guernsey*	44,600	2005
14	Australia	40,234	2011	13	Austria	40,006	2010	—	*Cayman Islands*	43,800	2004 est.
15	Ireland	39,639	2011	14	Canada	39,050	2010	10	Switzerland	43,400	2011 est.
16	Iceland	38,061	2011	15	Sweden	39,024	2010	—	*Gibraltar*	43,000	2006 est.
17	Germany	37,897	2011	16	Australia	38,160	2010	11	Netherlands	42,300	2011 est.
18	Belgium	37,737	2011	17	Belgium	37,631	2010	12	Austria	41,700	2011 est.
19	Taiwan	37,720	2011	18	Germany	37,402	2010	13	Australia	40,800	2011 est.
20	Denmark	37,152	2011	19	Finland	36,473	2010	14	Kuwait	40,700	2011 est.
21	Finland	36,236	2011	20	United Kingdom	35,686	2010	15	Sweden	40,600	2011 est.
22	United Kingdom	36,090	2011	21	Iceland	35,642	2010	16	Canada	40,300	2011 est.
23	France	35,156	2011	22	Equatorial Guinea	34,753	2010	17	Denmark	40,200	2011 est.
24	Japan	34,740	2011	23	France	34,123	2010	18	Ireland	39,500	2011 est.
25	Korea, South	31,714	2011	24	Japan	33,733	2010	—	*Virgin Islands, British*	38,500	2004 est.
—	*European Union*	31,607	2011	25	Spain	32,230	2010	19	Finland	38,300	2011 est.
26	Israel	30,975	2011	26	Italy	31,954	2010	20	Iceland	38,000	2011 est.
27	Bahamas, The	30,959	2011	27	Bahamas, The	31,746	2010	21	Germany	37,900	2011 est.
28	Spain	30,626	2011	—	*European Union*	31,745	2010	22	Taiwan	37,900	2011 est.
29	Italy	30,464	2011	28	Cyprus	31,092	2010	23	Belgium	37,600	2011 est.
30	Cyprus	29,074	2011	29	New Zealand	29,535	2010	—	*Greenland*	37,400	2008 est.
31	Slovenia	28,642	2011	30	Korea, South	29,101	2010	24	Andorra	37,200	2011 est.
32	New Zealand	27,668	2011	31	Israel	28,573	2010	25	San Marino	36,200	2009
33	Bahrain	27,556	2011	32	Greece	28,408	2010	26	United Kingdom	35,900	2011 est.
34	Czech Republic	27,062	2011	33	Slovenia	26,925	2010	27	France	35,000	2011 est.
35	Oman	26,519	2011	34	Oman	26,791	2009	—	*Isle of Man*	35,000	2005 est.
36	Greece	26,294	2011	35	Malta	26,445	2010	28	Japan	34,300	2011 est.
37	Malta	25,428	2011	36	Bahrain	25,799	2008	—	*European Union*	34,000	2011 est.
38	Seychelles	24,726	2011	37	Trinidad and Tobago	25,739	2010	—	*Macau*	33,000	2009
39	Saudi Arabia	24,237	2011	38	Portugal	25,416	2010	29	Korea, South	31,700	2011 est.
40	Barbados	23,417	2011	39	Czech Republic	24,518	2010	30	Israel	31,000	2011 est.
41	Portugal	23,361	2011	40	Slovakia	23,303	2010	31	Bahamas, The	30,900	2011 est.
42	Slovakia	23,304	2011	41	Seychelles	23,115	2010	32	Spain	30,600	2011 est.

International Monetary Fund (2010-11)[1]				World Bank (2005–10)[2]				CIA World Factbook (1993–2011)[3]			
Rank	Country	Intl. $	Year	Rank	Country	Intl. $	Year	Rank	Country	Intl. $	Year
43	Estonia	20,380	2011	42	Saudi Arabia	22,713	2010	—	*Faroe Islands*	30,500	2008 est.
44	Poland	20,334	2011	43	Antigua and Barbuda	20,954	2010	33	Italy	30,100	2011 est.
45	Trinidad and Tobago	20,053	2011	44	Estonia	20,663	2010	34	Cyprus	29,100	2011 est.
46	Hungary	19,591	2011	45	Hungary	20,545	2010	35	Slovenia	29,100	2011 est.
47	Equatorial Guinea[4]	19,356	2011	46	Russia	19,891	2010	36	New Zealand	27,900	2011 est.
48	Lithuania	18,856	2011	47	Poland	19,885	2010	37	Greece	27,600	2011 est.
49	Croatia	18,192	2011	48	Croatia	19,543	2010	38	Bahrain	27,300	2011 est.
50	Antigua and Barbuda	17,981	2011	49	Barbados	19,423	2009	39	Oman	26,200	2011 est.
51	Argentina	17,516	2011	50	Lithuania	18,370	2010	40	Czech Republic	25,900	2011 est.
52	Chile	17,222	2011	51	Libya	16,987	2009	41	Malta	25,700	2011 est.
53	Russia	16,736	2011	52	Saint Kitts and Nevis	16,785	2010	42	Seychelles	24,700	2011 est.
54	Gabon	16,183	2011	53	Latvia	16,340	2010	43	Saudi Arabia	24,000	2011 est.
55	Botswana	16,030	2011	54	Argentina	16,012	2010	44	Barbados	23,600	2011 est.
56	Latvia	15,662	2011	55	Chile	15,779	2010	45	Slovakia	23,400	2011 est.
57	Saint Kitts and Nevis	15,573	2011	56	Turkey	15,687	2010	46	Portugal	23,200	2011 est.
58	Malaysia	15,568	2011	57	Gabon	15,054	2010	47	Antigua and Barbuda	22,100	2011 est.
59	Lebanon	15,523	2011	58	Malaysia	14,731	2010	—	*Aruba*	21,800	2004 est.
60	Uruguay	15,113	2011	59	Mexico	14,564	2010	48	Trinidad and Tobago	20,300	2011 est.
61	Belarus	15,028	2011	60	Romania	14,524	2010	49	Estonia	20,200	2011 est.
62	Mauritius	14,954	2011	61	Uruguay	14,108	2010	50	Poland	20,100	2011 est.
63	Mexico	14,610	2011	62	Lebanon	14,069	2010	51	Hungary	19,600	2011 est.
64	Turkey	14,517	2011	63	Palau	13,976	2010	52	Equatorial Guinea[8]	19,300	2011 est.
65	Panama	14,097	2011	64	Bulgaria	13,931	2010	53	Lithuania	18,700	2011 est.
66	Grenada	13,896	2011	65	Belarus	13,929	2010	54	Croatia	18,300	2011 est.
67	Dominica	13,816	2011	66	Botswana	13,893	2010	—	*French Polynesia*	18,000	2004 est.
68	Bulgaria	13,597	2011	67	Mauritius	13,697	2010	55	Argentina	17,400	2011 est.
69	Iran	13,053	2011	68	Panama	13,608	2010	56	Russia	16,700	2011 est.
70	Kazakhstan	13,001	2011	69	Montenegro	12,861	2010	57	Saint Kitts and Nevis	16,400	2011 est.
71	Saint Lucia	12,607	2011	70	Dominica	12,266	2010	58	Botswana	16,300	2011 est.
72	Venezuela	12,568	2011	71	Venezuela	12,233	2010	—	*Puerto Rico*	16,300	2010 est.
73	Romania	12,476	2011	72	Kazakhstan	12,169	2010	59	Chile	16,100	2011 est.
74	Costa Rica	11,927	2011	73	Iran	11,570	2009	60	Gabon	16,000	2011 est.
75	Brazil	11,769	2011	74	Costa Rica	11,569	2010	61	Lebanon	15,600	2011 est.
76	Montenegro	11,545	2011	75	Serbia	11,349	2010	62	Malaysia	15,600	2011 est.
77	Saint Vincent and the Grenadines	11,491	2011	76	Brazil	11,210	2010	63	Latvia	15,400	2011 est.
—	*World*[5]	11,489	2011	77	Macedonia, Republic of	11,162	2010	—	*Sint Maarten*	15,400	2008 est.
78	South Africa	10,973	2011	—	*World*	11,125	2010	64	Uruguay	15,400	2011 est.
79	Serbia	10,642	2011	78	Saint Vincent and the Grenadines	11,077	2010	65	Mexico	15,100	2011 est.
80	Macedonia, Republic of	10,367	2011	79	Saint Lucia	10,838	2010	—	*Curaçao*	15,000	2004 est.
81	Colombia	10,249	2011	80	South Africa	10,565	2010	—	*Guam*	15,000	2005 est.
82	Azerbaijan	10,202	2011	81	Grenada	10,565	2010	66	Mauritius	15,000	2011 est.
83	Peru	10,062	2011	82	Azerbaijan	9,936	2010	—	*New Caledonia*	15,000	2003 est.
84	Tunisia	9,478	2011	83	Tunisia	9,550	2010	67	Belarus	14,900	2011 est.
85	Suriname	9,475	2011	84	Peru	9,538	2010	68	Turkey	14,600	2011 est.
86	Thailand	9,396	2011	85	Colombia	9,453	2010	—	*Virgin Islands, U.S.*	14,500	2004 est.
87	Dominican Republic	9,287	2011	86	Dominican Republic	9,350	2010	69	Libya	14,100	2010 est.
88	Jamaica	9,029	2011	87	Bosnia and Herzegovina	8,690	2010	70	Dominica	13,600	2011 est.
89	Maldives	8,731	2011	88	Albania	8,592	2010	71	Panama	13,600	2011 est.
90	East Timor	8,701	2011	89	Thailand	8,554	2010	72	Bulgaria	13,500	2011 est.
91	Ecuador	8,492	2011	90	Maldives	8,519	2010	73	Grenada	13,300	2011 est.
92	China	8,382	2011	91	Algeria	8,433	2010	74	Kazakhstan	13,000	2011 est.
93	Belize	8,264	2011	92	Turkmenistan	8,274	2010	75	Saint Lucia	12,900	2011 est.

International Monetary Fund (2010-11)[1]				World Bank (2005–10)[2]				CIA World Factbook (1993–2011)[3]			
Rank	**Country**	**Intl. $**	**Year**	**Rank**	**Country**	**Intl. $**	**Year**	**Rank**	**Country**	**Intl. $**	**Year**
94	Bosnia and Herzegovina	8,133	2011	93	Ecuador	8,028	2010	—	*Northern Mariana Islands*	12,500	2000 est.
95	Turkmenistan	7,846	2011	94	Jamaica	7,673	2010	76	Venezuela	12,400	2011 est.
96	Albania	7,741	2011	95	Suriname	7,664	2009	77	Romania	12,300	2011 est.
97	El Salvador	7,550	2011	96	China	7,599	2010	—	*Anguilla*	12,200	2008 est.
98	Guyana	7,466	2011	97	Ukraine	6,721	2010	78	Iran	12,200	2011 est.
99	Namibia	7,363	2011	98	Belize	6,670	2010	—	*World*	11,800	2011
100	Tonga	7,344	2011	99	El Salvador	6,668	2010	79	Saint Vincent and the Grenadines	11,700	2011 est.
101	Algeria	7,333	2011	100	Namibia	6,475	2010	80	Brazil	11,600	2011 est.
102	Ukraine	7,233	2011	101	Angola	6,186	2010	81	Costa Rica	11,500	2011 est.
103	Kosovo[6]	7,044	2011	102	Egypt	6,180	2010	—	*Turks and Caicos Islands*	11,500	2002 est.
104	Egypt	6,540	2011	103	Swaziland	5,952	2010	82	Montenegro	11,200	2011 est.
105	Bhutan	6,112	2011	104	Jordan	5,749	2010	83	South Africa	11,000	2011 est.
106	Samoa	5,965	2011	105	Armenia	5,463	2010	84	Serbia	10,700	2011 est.
107	Jordan	5,900	2011	106	Bhutan	5,328	2010	85	Macedonia, Republic of	10,400	2011 est.
108	Angola	5,895	2011	107	Syria	5,285	2010	86	Azerbaijan	10,200	2011 est.
109	Libya	5,787	2011	108	Paraguay	5,181	2010	87	Colombia	10,100	2011 est.
110	Kiribati	5,722	2011	109	Sri Lanka	5,078	2010	88	Peru	10,000	2011 est.
111	Sri Lanka	5,674	2011	110	Georgia	5,074	2010	89	Cuba	9,900	2010 est.
112	Georgia	5,491	2011	111	Bolivia	4,849	2010	90	Thailand	9,700	2011 est.
113	Paraguay	5,413	2011	112	Guatemala	4,785	2010	91	Suriname	9,500	2011 est.
114	Armenia	5,384	2011	113	Morocco	4,712	2010	92	Tunisia	9,500	2011 est.
115	Swaziland	5,302	2011	114	Fiji	4,658	2010	93	Dominican Republic	9,300	2011 est.
116	Guatemala	5,070	2011	115	Tonga	4,532	2010	—	*Cook Islands*	9,100	2005 est.
117	Morocco	5,052	2011	116	Vanuatu	4,443	2010	94	Jamaica	9,000	2011 est.
118	Syria	5,041	2010	117	Samoa	4,374	2010	95	China	8,400	2011 est.
119	Vanuatu	4,916	2011	118	Indonesia	4,325	2010	96	Maldives	8,400	2011 est.
120	Bolivia	4,789	2011	119	Congo, Republic of the	4,245	2010	97	Belize	8,300	2011 est.
121	Mongolia	4,744	2011	120	Mongolia	4,036	2010	98	Ecuador	8,300	2011 est.
122	Indonesia	4,666	2011	121	Philippines	3,969	2010	99	Bosnia and Herzegovina	8,200	2011 est.
123	Fiji	4,620	2011	122	Honduras	3,923	2010	100	Palau	8,100	2008 est.
124	Congo, Republic of the	4,589	2011	123	Cape Verde	3,875	2010	—	*American Samoa*	8,000	2007 est.
125	Honduras	4,345	2011	124	Iraq	3,562	2010	101	Albania	7,800	2011 est.
126	Philippines	4,073	2011	125	Guyana	3,432	2010	102	El Salvador	7,600	2011 est.
127	Cape Verde	3,947	2011	126	India	3,425	2010	103	Guyana	7,500	2011 est.
128	Iraq	3,886	2011	127	Micronesia, Federated States of	3,333	2010	104	Tonga	7,500	2011 est.
129	India	3,694	2011	128	Vietnam	3,205	2010	105	Turkmenistan	7,500	2011 est.
130	Tuvalu[6]	3,509	2011	129	Moldova	3,110	2010	106	Namibia	7,300	2011 est.
131	Moldova	3,373	2011	130	Uzbekistan	3,106	2010	107	Algeria	7,200	2011 est.
132	Vietnam	3,359	2011	131	Nicaragua	2,913	2010	108	Ukraine	7,200	2011 est.
133	Uzbekistan	3,302	2011	132	Solomon Islands	2,710	2010	—	*Saint Pierre and Miquelon*	7,000	2001 est.
134	Nicaragua	3,206	2011	133	Pakistan	2,688	2010	109	Egypt	6,500	2011 est.
135	Solomon Islands	3,192	2011	134	Yemen	2,653	2010	110	Kosovo	6,500	2011 est.
136	Ghana	3,083	2011	135	Laos	2,551	2010	111	Kiribati	6,200	2011 est.
137	Pakistan	2,787	2011	136	Papua New Guinea	2,472	2010	112	Bhutan	6,000	2011 est.
138	Sudan & South Sudan[7]	2,726	2011	—	*West Bank and Gaza*	2,465	2005	113	Samoa	6,000	2011 est.
139	Laos	2,659	2011	137	Kiribati	2,457	2010	114	Angola	5,900	2011 est.
140	Djibouti	2,642	2011	138	Mauritania	2,456	2010	115	Jordan	5,900	2011 est.
141	Nigeria	2,578	2011	139	Nigeria	2,399	2010	—	*Niue*	5,800	2003 est.
142	Papua New Guinea	2,532	2011	140	Djibouti	2,308	2009	116	Sri Lanka	5,600	2011 est.
143	Kyrgyzstan	2,372	2011	141	Cameroon	2,294	2010	117	Paraguay	5,500	2011 est.
144	Yemen	2,307	2011	142	Sudan & South Sudan	2,256	2010	118	Armenia	5,400	2011 est.
145	Cameroon	2,257	2011	143	Kyrgyzstan	2,239	2010	119	Georgia	5,400	2011 est.
146	São Tomé and Príncipe	2,252	2011	144	Cambodia	2,194	2010	120	Swaziland	5,200	2011 est.
147	Cambodia	2,216	2011	145	Tajikistan	2,163	2010	121	Morocco	5,100	2011 est.

International Monetary Fund (2010-11)[1]				World Bank (2005–10)[2]				CIA World Factbook (1993–2011)[3]			
Rank	Country	Intl. $	Year	Rank	Country	Intl. $	Year	Rank	Country	Intl. $	Year
148	Mauritania	2,179	2011	146	Burma	1,950	2010	122	Syria	5,100	2011 est.
149	Tajikistan	2,067	2011	147	Senegal	1,935	2010	123	Guatemala	5,000	2011 est.
150	Lesotho	1,960	2011	148	Côte d'Ivoire	1,899	2010	124	Nauru	5,000	2005 est.
151	Gambia, The	1,943	2011	149	São Tomé and Príncipe	1,899	2010	125	Vanuatu	4,900	2011 est.
152	Senegal	1,871	2011	150	Bangladesh	1,659	2010	126	Bolivia	4,800	2011 est.
153	Chad	1,865	2011	151	Kenya	1,651	2010	127	Indonesia	4,700	2011 est.
154	Kenya	1,746	2011	152	Ghana	1,644	2010	128	Congo, Republic of the	4,600	2011 est.
155	Bangladesh	1,693	2011	153	Lesotho	1,601	2010	129	Fiji	4,600	2011 est.
156	Zambia	1,611	2011	154	Benin	1,587	2010	130	Mongolia	4,500	2011 est.
157	Côte d'Ivoire	1,590	2011	155	Zambia	1,562	2010	131	Honduras	4,300	2011 est.
158	Tanzania	1,515	2011	156	Tanzania	1,434	2010	132	Philippines	4,100	2011 est.
159	Benin	1,481	2011	157	Gambia, The	1,410	2010	133	Cape Verde	4,000	2011 est.
160	Burkina Faso	1,466	2011	158	Chad	1,370	2010	134	Iraq	3,900	2011 est.
161	Rwanda	1,341	2011	159	Uganda	1,272	2010	—	*Wallis and Futuna*	3,800	2004 est.
162	Nepal	1,328	2011	160	Burkina Faso	1,256	2010	135	India	3,700	2011 est.
163	Burma	1,325	2011	161	Afghanistan	1,207	2010	136	Moldova	3,400	2011 est.
164	Uganda	1,317	2011	162	Nepal	1,199	2010	—	*Montserrat*	3,400	2002 est.
165	Haiti	1,235	2011	163	Guinea-Bissau	1,186	2010	137	Tuvalu	3,400	2010 est.
166	Comoros	1,232	2011	164	Rwanda	1,163	2010	138	Solomon Islands	3,300	2011 est.
167	Guinea-Bissau	1,144	2011	165	Haiti	1,111	2010	139	Uzbekistan	3,300	2011 est.
168	Mali	1,128	2011	166	Comoros	1,096	2010	140	Vietnam	3,300	2011 est.
169	Ethiopia	1,093	2011	167	Guinea	1,091	2010	141	Nicaragua	3,200	2011 est.
170	Mozambique	1,085	2011	168	Mali	1,065	2010	142	Ghana	3,100	2011 est.
171	Guinea	1,083	2011	169	Ethiopia	1,041	2010	143	East Timor	3,100	2011 est.
172	Afghanistan	956	2011	170	Togo	998	2010	144	Sudan & South Sudan	3,000	2011 est.
173	Madagascar	934	2011	171	Madagascar	969	2010	—	*West Bank and Gaza*	2,900	2008 est.
174	Togo	899	2011	172	Mozambique	942	2010	145	Pakistan	2,800	2011 est.
175	Malawi	860	2011	173	East Timor	928	2010	146	Laos	2,700	2011 est.
176	Sierra Leone	849	2011	174	Malawi	882	2010	147	Djibouti	2,600	2011 est.
177	Niger	771	2011	175	Sierra Leone	827	2010	148	Nigeria	2,600	2011 est.
178	Central African Republic	768	2011	176	Central African Republic	789	2010	149	Marshall Islands	2,500	2008 est.
179	Eritrea	735	2011	177	Niger	728	2010	150	Papua New Guinea	2,500	2011 est.
180	Burundi	615	2011	178	Eritrea	546	2010	—	*Saint Helena, Ascension and Tristan da Cunha*	2,500	1998 est.
181	Zimbabwe	487	2011	179	Liberia	419	2010	—	*Western Sahara*	2,500	2007 est.
182	Liberia	456	2011	180	Burundi	409	2010	151	Yemen	2,500	2011 est.
183	Congo, Democratic Republic of the	348	2011	181	Congo, Democratic Republic of the	347	2010	152	Kyrgyzstan	2,400	2011 est.
								153	Cambodia	2,300	2011 est.
								154	Cameroon	2,300	2011 est.
								155	Mauritania	2,200	2011 est.
								156	Micronesia, Federated States of	2,200	2008 est.
								157	Gambia, The	2,100	2011 est.
								158	São Tomé and Príncipe	2,000	2011 est.
								159	Tajikistan	2,000	2011 est.
								160	Chad	1,900	2011 est.
								161	Senegal	1,900	2011 est.
								162	Korea, North	1,800	2011 est.
								163	Bangladesh	1,700	2011 est.
								164	Kenya	1,700	2011 est.
								165	Côte d'Ivoire	1,600	2011 est.
								166	Zambia	1,600	2011 est.
								167	Benin	1,500	2011 est.
								168	Burkina Faso	1,500	2011 est.
								169	Tanzania	1,500	2011 est.
								170	Lesotho	1,400	2011 est.
								171	Burma	1,300	2011 est.
								172	Mali	1,300	2011 est.
								173	Nepal	1,300	2011 est.

International Monetary Fund (2010-11)[1]				World Bank (2005–10)[2]				CIA World Factbook (1993–2011)[3]			
Rank	Country	Intl. $	Year	Rank	Country	Intl. $	Year	Rank	Country	Intl. $	Year
								174	Rwanda	1,300	2011 est.
								175	Uganda	1,300	2011 est.
								176	Comoros	1,200	2011 est.
								177	Haiti	1,200	2011 est.
								178	Ethiopia	1,100	2011 est.
								179	Guinea-Bissau	1,100	2011 est.
								180	Guinea	1,100	2011 est.
								181	Mozambique	1,100	2011 est.
								182	Afghanistan	1,000	2011 est.
								—	*Tokelau*	1,000	1993 est.
								183	Madagascar	900	2011 est.
								184	Malawi	900	2011 est.
								185	Togo	900	2011 est.
								186	Central African Republic	800	2011 est.
								187	Niger	800	2011 est.
								188	Sierra Leone	800	2011 est.
								189	Eritrea	700	2011 est.
								190	Somalia	600	2010 est.
								191	Zimbabwe	500	2011 est.
								192	Burundi	400	2011 est.
								193	Liberia	400	2011 est.
								194	Congo, Democratic Republic of the	300	2011 est.

* GDP per capita is an essential parameter to assess individual country's ability to fight cervical cancer

References[change | change source]

1. ↑ Data refer mostly to the year 2011. World Economic Outlook Database-April 2012, International Monetary Fund. Accessed on 18 April 2012.
2. ↑ Data refer mostly to the year 2010. World Development Indicators database, World Bank. Accessed on 18 April 2012.
3. ↑ GDP - per capita (PPP), The World Factbook, Central Intelligence Agency. Accessed on 18 April 2012. Note: Data for Guam, Monaco and the World obtained from individual country/grouping pages.
4. ↑ The per capita figure was calculated by the IMF using a 2011 population estimate based on a 2001 census whose validity has been called into question. A 2003 U.S. State Department report on Equatorial Guinea stated that "although the 2002 (sic) census estimated the population at 1,015,000, credible estimates put the number at closer to 500,000. The opposition claimed that the Government inflated the census in anticipation of the December presidential election. (...) Opposition leaders charged earlier in the year that census results showing a twofold population increase were flawed and that numbers were inflated to perpetuate election fraud." [1]
5. ↑ Does not include Syria.
6. ↑ [6.0 6.1] Population data from International Data Base, United States Census Bureau. Accessed on 18 April 2012.
7. ↑ Data for South Sudan are excluded after 9 July 2011.
8. ↑ The World Factbook claims to be using a population of "less than 700,000" to estimate the per capita figure, but the PPP GDP data on Equatorial Guinea's page suggest a population close to double that amount was used.

5.6 Study Summary: The Vision

MarkPap Advantage

Cervical cancer screening from global prospective with emphasis on the developing countries

WHAT IS HAPPENING IN THE TWENTY-FIRST CENTURY? Women are still dying from a preventable disease

In spite of all efforts and new approved technologies, the average outreach among women at risk globally for cervical cancer screening is about 10 %. More than 500,000 women get cervical cancer annually and 360,000 women die, mostly in the low-resource areas. The prognosis are that the situation will get worse. For example in India, the outreach is 6 % and further 150 % increase in mortality is expected by the year 2025.

Is it really impossible to repeat the USA success story, even in shorter period of time? What about two billion women at risk?

It is generally accepted that the best strategy to prevent cervical cancer is cytological screening with Pap test, but also it is generally accepted that Pap test could not be introduced for mass cervical cancer screening globally, because of the following:

1. ***Cost*** **– the existing Pap test is not affordable for most low-resource countries**
2. ***Lack of local infrastructure*** **– qualified personnel to evaluate the result**
3. ***Not accessible*** **– rural areas, without doctor's offices/hospitals**
4. ***Non-comfortable test*** **– requires pelvic exam, cultural sensitivity**
5. ***Slow*** **– takes weeks to get the results back**

Is it possible to mitigate these challenges? The official answer was "No" and governmental official statements from many countries in the developing world were that Pap test cannot be implemented for mass cervical cancer screening.

However, the situation is changing. Twenty-first century is an era of digital technology, digital information creating machines, digital information communications, digital programs for industrial production and for telemedicine and mobile health (M-health).

Digital health is the hope for global health to radically transform delivery of healthcare and reduce health disparity between developed and underdeveloped countries.

For example, what about non-accessibility- women in rural areas of developing countries, including China and India, do not have access to medical institutions. Here, the possibility to take the sample at home and mail it to the laboratory/doctor office would be the solution. This will, in the same time, help dealing with cultural sensitivity allowing, at least at the beginning, women to avoid pelvic exam. But how it can be done, when the Pap test relies on morphology, which is damaged in the vaginal fluids and women could hardly be able to take sample from the cervix.

Although there were attempts, the risk is too high to do this far from a place where any emergency could be treated. However, is it possible to use exfoliated cell in the vaginal fluid and with a Q tip-like device to simply take the sample from the introitus of vagina, smear it on the microscopic slide and proceed with cytological screening. Yes, it is possible, but only if the result does not rely on morphology only, but on another biomarker indestructible in the vaginal fluids.

MarkPap® platform technology is one example of biomarker-based biomedical technology (for self collection) which combined with IT technology could mitigate the 5 challenges cited above and to produce a low-cost, simple, accessible, infrastructure independent platform that is currently the only promise for mass cytological cervical cancer screening [195–219]**.**

If home specimen collection is combined with biomarker based cytology and mobile telemedicine with small surgery at points-of-care the worldwide cervical cancer screening will become reality.

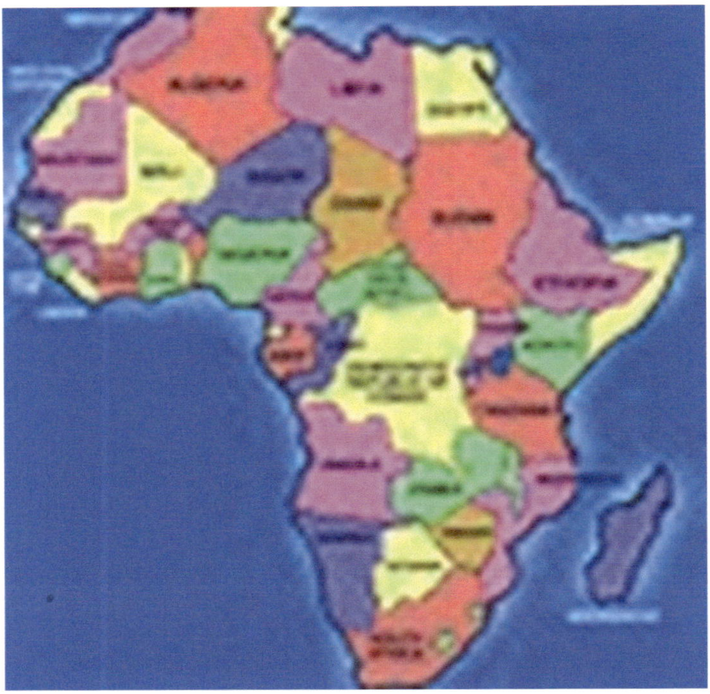

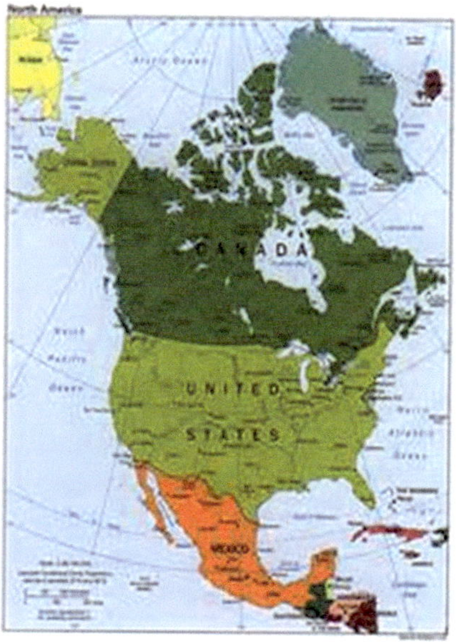

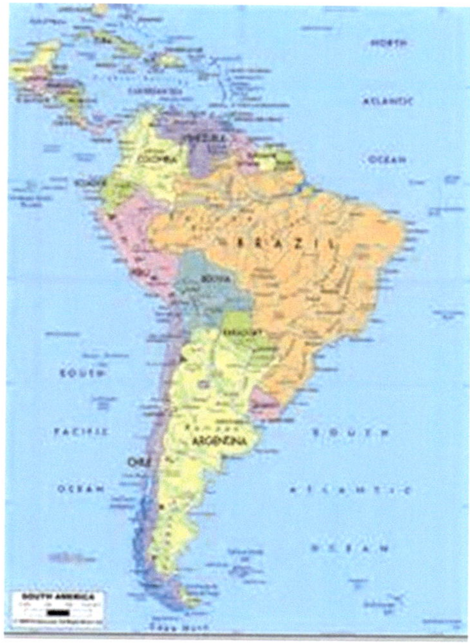

Southern Asia

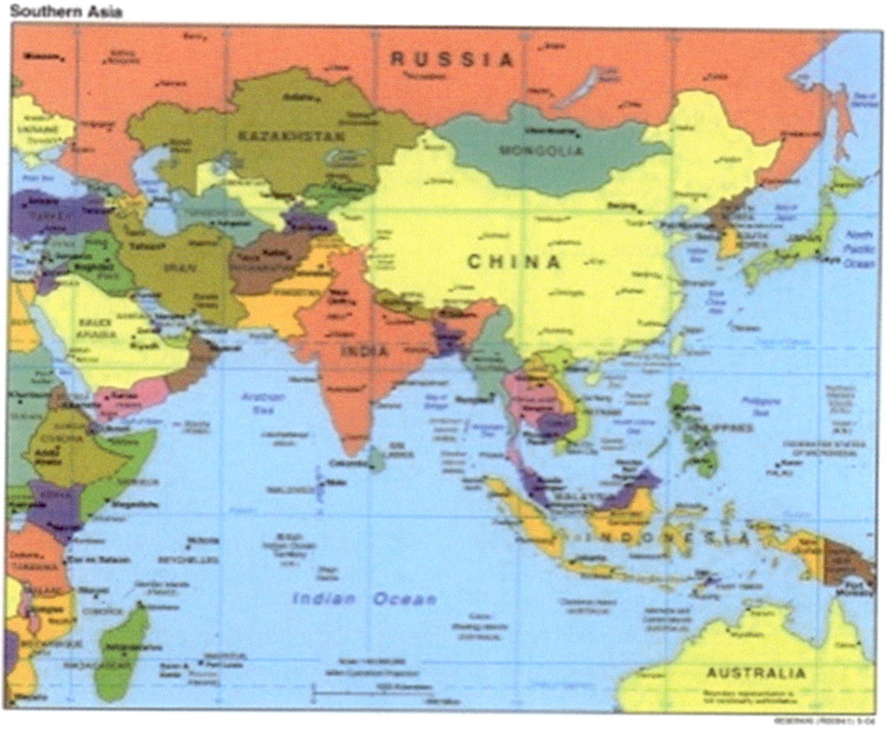

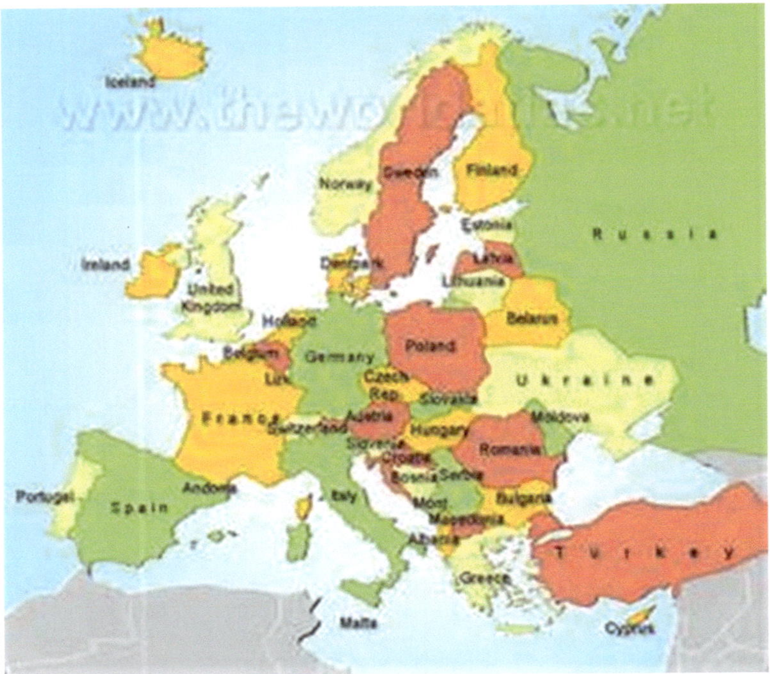

5.7 New Avenues

5.7.1 US-India Symposium on Cervical Cancer

5.7.1.1 Cervical Cancer in India

1. Title of the activity

Strategy for reversing the negative trends of increasing prevalence and mortality of indian women from cervical cancer

2. Proposed venue and dates

The Symposium will be held at the Johns Hopkins University, Montgomery County Campus, where the Global Academy for Women's Health, Inc., the host of this Symposium, is located in Rockville, MD. The Global Academy for Women's Health, Inc. is a non-profit organization with a mission to advance science and education in women's health globally.

The event is planned to be organized during 7 days. Please see the Preliminary Program Agenda below. The event is intended to be held in Fall 2013.

3. **Contact information of US and Indian Principal Investigators**

INDIA
Prof. K. Ganapathy
M Ch (Neurosurgery) FACS FICS FAMS Ph.D
President, Apollo Telemedicine Networking Foundation
Director, Apollo Tele Health Services
Past President, Telemedicine Society of India
President, Indian Society for Stereotactic & Functional Neurosurgery
Former Secretary & Past President Neurological Society of India
Adjunct Professor IIT Madras, Tamil Nadu Dr MGR Medical University & Anna University
Chennai, India
Tel.No.: 91 44 28295447; Fax No. 91 44 28299447
Website: www.telemedicineindia.com, http://www.apollohospitals.com, www.kganapathy.c

UNITED STATES
Olivera Markovic, MD, PhD
Professor and President
Global Academy for Women's Health, Inc.
9601 Medical Center Dr., Suite 111
Johns Hopkins University, Montgomery County Campus
Rockville, MD 20850; Tel/fax: +1 – 301-610-9130
E-mail: info@bioscicon.com, gawh@markpap.com
Web sites: www.bioscicon.com, www.markpap.com

4. **Executive summary**

The Symposium will address the following topics:

1. Global medicine against poverty and disparity
2. Digital Health: The only answer to radically transform delivery of healthcare
3. Low-cost medical devices and digital technology as tools to bridge disparities
4. Cervical cancer in India 2010 mirrors the situation in the US before Pap test
5. How US has transformed the mortality rates and contained cervical cancer?
6. How India can do what US had done?
7. Charting an inclusive strategy to assist India transferring US education and technology assets, which will be focused on special community needs where the largest socio-economic impact could be achieved in India as well in the US.

Problem for Indian Healthcare Providers

India is a country with more than 300 million women at risk for cervical cancer [1]. This disease is completely preventable if detected on time. Unfortunately, in India less than 6 % (18 million) are protected from acquiring and dying from this disease, and about 280 million women at risk do not have proper protection. They get cervical cancer and they die at the unacceptable rate. In 2010 India had 134,420 new cases of invasive cervical cancer and 72,825 deaths. Projections for 2025 are even worse: 203,753 cases and 115, 171 deaths per year [1]. Spending more on diagnosis and therapy than it is necessary (when prevention is not applied) makes India poorer, and the health disparities, between the quality of the same health care services in India and in developed countries, are becoming greater and more visible [2].

However, the main problem, which still has not been addressed properly, is the very low outreach – less than 6 % of Indian women who participate in organized cervical cancer prevention programs. This level is too low for any measure to show its social or socio-economic benefit. The 50 years of US experience is hard evidence to support this contention [3].

How This Problem Was Solved in the US

Before Pap test, US in the first half of Twentieth Century had almost no organized cervical cancer control (screening) and the rates for cervical cancer prevalence and mortality were increasing steadily. In the middle of that Century, the American Cancer Society promoted a comprehensive cervical cancer screening campaign [1] a new cytopathological test recommended by Dr. Papanicolaou (Pap test), [2] following the results of this screening test with diagnostic (colposcopy) and, when indicated, with [3] therapeutic procedures (biopsy/surgery) [3, 4]. This all was done with intention to alter the natural history of cervical cancer in the US and to reverse the negative trends of disease prevalence and mortality. The first results were encouraging to sustain the campaign [2–4].

The tangible social benefit was shown later, when the outreach from <5 % reached 50 %. At this level, both trends reversed, and the disease prevalence and mortality started to move steadily downwards. Currently, in the US, cervical cancer prevalence and mortality rates are below the red line of 10 most frequent diseases and American women who participate in Pap test-based cervical cancer screening (outreach more than 85 %) are assured of being protected and their attention is now turning on reduction of risk factors (education, immunization). There is always a room for further improvement, but this is an excellent example of the efficacious prevention from this grave disease [2].

Indian Awareness of the Problem

Why then this life-saving test and the follow-up management of women at higher risk (positive test – abnormal specimens) have not been applied in India as in the US? Our records show that it is not that the Indian Government is not aware of the problem or is neglecting it, it is not that Indian healthcare providers do not do their best to help their people, it is not that Indian professional societies do not support prevention as they as they do with curative medicine, it is not that India has not funds or cannot raise funds to help women at risk. We have anticipated that *Indian healthcare providers do not have the best tools and strategy to use these tools for fighting the problem*. The former Ambassador of India, Her Excellency Ambassador Shankar was very perceptive; she organized for us to meet with responsible people in the Indian Embassy in USA, where we were convinced that our assessment of Indian circumstances had been on the right track [5].

Symposium Impact: New Strategy

The guests-speakers from India are our long time collaborators with whom we have addressed those questions and exchanged experiences. We feel that a meeting in person, as this Symposium, would be helpful to update our assessment of the situation, to crystallize our thoughts towards a single goal: How to help Indian health care providers to move faster on the same road their American counterparts have passed years ago and, by using the US and our experience and new technologies, to shorten the suffering of Indian women and to relieve them from fear from getting cervical cancer earlier.

If this Symposium will meet the expectations, a concept for a **"New Strategy for Cervical Cancer Screening in low-resources Areas"** (e.g., some regions in India) will evolve. It will be later proposed to Indian and US authorities for consideration and appropriate exploit in both countries [6].

It is expected that the Symposium will elaborate on the New Strategy and, at the end, after Summary and Conclusions such a strategy, if widely adopted and implemented, will help Indian healthcare providers to reverse negative trends of mortality and cervical cancer prevalence in India before year 2025. This would be the most wanted social impact of this Symposium.

See below about Symposium impact on broadening of future collaborative research, inclusion of early career scientists and students, industry participation and establishment of new connections (Annex).

Our collaboration continues and most recent results will be presented at the 18th International Congress of Cytology in Paris, France this year [14].

New Tools for New Strategy: Information Technology, Digital Health

The only answer to radically transform the delivery of healthcare.

Twenty-first century is an era of digital technology. Digital information creating machines, digital information communication, digital programs for industrial production and now for telemedicine and mobile health (M-health) are enabling something that could have not been even considered before in Global Health: The reduction of health disparities between developed and developing countries [2, 7, 15, 16, 20].

Classic Medicine Must Adjust Old Canons to Allow New Technology to Be Safe and Effective

With the growth of digital technology (wired or wireless) there is also an increase of understanding that the classic or standard medical technologies must change to meet the new technical requirements [2]. Current digital equipment lacks artificial intelligence. The modern machines can detect and identify minute changes, can compute terabytes of information, but they alone cannot understand what is going on. The medical utilization of these machines is still at the level of pre-med students for most of clinical issues. Digital technology needs to develop meaningful filtering systems to approach medical decision-making processes. To become health care providers as users-friendly, digital technology must be simplified and must use terminology with proven medical meaning. On the other side, medicine must adopt digital instruments and adjust them to help in prevention, diagnosis and treatment of patients and diseases. This is a long road to go, but there are shortcuts, like biomarker's discovery [8–10, 15, 20].

Biomarkers Are Bridges Between Classic and Digital Medicine

Recently, the biomarkers seem to be able to bridge the gap and are becoming tools for building artificial intelligence for digital technology applied in medicine. It has already been seen in standard medical education. Using biomarkers to develop filters for constructing meaningful digital information is still unexploited filed of medical science. This is our target.

Increasing use of biomarkers and telemedicine is the next period for both digital technology and medicine [7, 8, 10–13, 21].

Education Is Still the Moving Power

Further, The Global Academy for Women's Health, Inc., with its mission to advance education and science in women's health, is currently sponsoring the development of simple, low-cost, life-saving medical devices affordable and available to women in rural, low-resource areas, contingent to local interest and support. Those tools usually combine in vitro diagnostic methods with digital imaging; web networking and mobile phones-upgraded telemedicine devices and processes [2, 9–12, 16].

5. Background, concept and purpose

Cervical cancer is a malignant disease characterized by slow progression and unstoppable growth, first locally, then affecting regional lymph nodes and finally spreading with metastases elsewhere in the body until death of the host. There are two important points here: Slow Progression, and Unstoppable Growth [17, 18].

Unstoppable growth means that at present, once cancer has reached clinical stage of 1B (tumor size of about 1 cm^3) it is already invasive and no matter what diagnostic or therapeutic measures available are used, the prognosis is always grave. This fact turns the focus of health providers to prevention – slow growth allows for early detection, identification and intervention (usually surgical removal) on early, localized lesions before their invasion and/or spread.

In the first half of the Twentieth Century, everywhere in the world, cervical cancer was diagnosed and treated by medical doctors. They were doing their best upon their knowledge, skills and technical abilities. The result was a permanent increase of the prevalence and mortally of this disease – cervical cancer was considered to be number one killer of women from malignant diseases.

Then, in the middle of twentieth century, Dr. Papanicolaou, published his experience with scrapping cervix with spatula, smearing the collected material on microscopic slides, and changing the staining procedure (Pap smear) [18]. In the next 50 years the Pap test was recognized as the best cancer screening test, adopted by vast majority of American health professionals (outreach of more 80 % of American women at risk) and resulted in a dramatic reduction (over 80 %) of cervical cancer mortality and prevalence [3, 19].

The good news about this American success spread over the world and there was no country that did not want to follow this example. But, only few developed countries were able to copy the American experience and obtained the same results. The rest of the world trailed behind, and the health discrepancy started to rise between developed and developing world together with the anxiety and animosity triggering question, "why our women must die?"

India is one of those developing countries where the situation with cervical cancer is similar to the situation in the US before the Pap Test. Why India does not apply this test and have American success story told by their women? The answer is known: Pap test, as it is now, is not affordable – not because of the cost of the test or testing, but because of the infrastructure requiring doctors to collect material, pathologists to read it and gynecologists to manage women with abnormal specimens – all of them present at the point-of care, frequently in low resource areas.

As alternative, Indian health providers began to use different methods that were more available – VIA (visual inspection with acid and cryoablation), Pap smear (but not to the quality control extent as the original Pap test), Liquid based Pap (favored new Pap technology, but very costly), HPV testing which is now coming as introduction to HPV vaccination, and also, a lot of charity money and medical industry discounts and governmental programs [2, 19, 20, 22, 23].

Unfortunately, in spite of all these efforts, only 6 % of Indian women are included in cervical cancer screening programs and only 18 million out of 300 million Indian women at risk are protected. There is no prospective improvement if something more will not be done in the near future. India reports suggest grim prognosis, almost doubling the mortality and prevalence in the next 15–25 years.

The Global Academy for Women's Health, Inc. was organized in 2008, and it immediately renewed contacts with Indian scientists we knew form before and created new contracts asking the same question: How we can help Indian health care providers to overcome the hurdles and to deliver the quality screening test which can make a difference and save tens thousands women's lives in India? Maybe the answer was found in the joint paper we published with AIIMS [13]. This Symposium is a logical extension to that work.

During the years that followed, we have developed a concept which will be presented at the Symposium as the **New Strategy for Cervical Cancer Screening in India (see Figure**, p. 228). The uniqueness of this Strategy is *combining the theory with new tools* (low-cost medical devices – most of them could be produced locally) *and new processes* (IT telehealth in combination with M-health). We envision developing new mobile and IT telehealth medical diagnostics systems for use in preventive medicine. We certainly believe that the modern technology and the IT revolution would be able to reduce the disparities and lessen the frustrations and animosities among people living in fortunate and less fortunate areas of the world. We certainly believe that this strategy will be accepted at the Symposium [6].

Once the Symposium is approved, the Global Academy will undertake a wide activity connecting relevant scientists and health care providers in India, US and all around the world. The Global Academy for Women's Health, Inc. has already established connections with more than 60 centers. The draft of the new strategy will be circulated and responses recorded, classified and reported at the Symposium. All participants will be invited to use video and teleconferencing/webinar tools and to join the Symposium discussions.

To make this concept to succeed, we may keep limited number of persons physically present, however much larger forum will be involved – its number will be known only before the Welcome Reception.

All Symposium materials will be recorded, transcribed, edited and published appropriately. Summary and conclusions will be included in a special chapter of the next edition of our book, "What Every Women Should Know about Cervical Cancer." In the meantime, different media will be used to incite discussion on the same topic and to making the impact as large as possible.

We hope that the long-term impact of this Symposium will be giving new prospective on an old problem and mobilizing communities and government to take more active participation in health prevention. In particular, because of the increased awareness of the disease, the inability to prevent its occurrence, and the requirement to diagnose and treat women with advanced (incurable) disease will increase financial burden to the country economy.

Saving one woman's life is saving population reproductive power, for economy saving educated and trained work force, and for families is saving the essential supporters of their own existence.

6. Specific need for a bilateral invent

During recent years discussing about cervical cancer in India, we have conceived several ideas which are summarized in the Figure below. We recognized that those ideas, as summarized, could become a core for real improvement of cervical cancer problem in India. However, the ideas did not have tools for realizations as they were conceived, Two years ago, in the era of growing telemedicine, BioSciCon came with three products, which promised to serve the purpose of our strategic concept [9–13]. Several feasibility studies have shown that we are on a right track, and both efforts by GAWH to integrate Indian scientists around the new strategy and Indian medical device industry came together. In the same time US launched policy for developing low-cost diagnostic medical devices for developing countries. **These three elements, science, technology and policies will be intertwined in this Symposium and we hope it will result with the acceptance of the Strategy for India.**

5.7.2 India Press Release 2015

Excerpts from web site: www.bioscicon.com/pressrlease.html

August 2015

BioSciCon, Inc. receives 2015 Best of Business Award for Rockville

Small Business Community Association recently selected BioSciCon, Inc. to receive 2015 Best of Business Award for Rockville, MD in the Small Business category.

July 2015

BioSciCon's MarkPap® [CAP-PAP™] Test in India

We have a long-standing collaboration with Indian scientists where the validity of the MarkPap test (CAP-PAP test) in detection of abnormal cells on cervical smears has been confirmed. Please see Publications Annex.

In the beginning of this year two more scientific papers were published on the subject in India.

1. Prof. Santwani with her team at the Department of Pathology, Shah Medical College, Jamnagar and Punjab Institute of Medical Sciences, published a paper "Study of CAP-PAP versus conventional Pap in suspicious cervical lesions" using MarkPap Kit with Combo Control Slides. The paper appeared in Int J Res Med 2015;4(1)102–108, concluding that the CAP PAP test could be the future of cervical cancer screening.
2. Prof. Nenad Markovic supported a doctoral candidate, Dr. Niranjan J, at the Videhu Institute of Medical Sciences in Bangalore, who performed a clinical trial, according to the design provided, confirming the value of CAP-PAP test and published the results in J Evidence Based Med & Healthcare, 2015; 2(6),714–23, 2015, "Cervical Acid Phosphatase; Evaluation as an adjuvant to papanicolaou smear screening in cervical cancer detection". Click here to see the article

India is a country with 70,000 deaths from cervical cancer per year, and below 10 % outreach for the prevention from this disease. Out of 300,000M women at risk only 20M women are protected with preventive cancer screening. Cervical cancer is preventable and curable disease, IF detected on time. But, new strategy is needed.

On June 11, 2015, Drs Olivera and Nenad Markovic met officially with Minister Counselor for Science and Technology Mr. Tarun Mohandra and Attache Mr. Kumar at the Indian Embassy in Washington, DC. The new Strategy for Fighting Cervical Cancer in India with MarkPap technology tools was presented and discussed. The Strategy has been forwarded to the Indian Ministry of Health.

Our book "What every woman should know about cervical cancer" (Springer, 2008) is popular in India. Recently, two Indian distributors joined the list: Delhi Book Store and Meltek Books.

5.7.3 *Cervical Cancer in China Press Release 2015*

China

Overview

Since 2008, BioSciCon has invested lot of resources to implement MarkPap technology in China. This effort was motivated by the visit of high official delegation from China Ministry of Health, who informed us that the China Government is ready to include cervical cancer screening into the yearly check up for women. They expressed interest whether we can develop a methodology that will cost not more than $5.00 per test. We stated that the new MarkPap technology can achieve this goal.

Indeed, China introduced yearly screening and BioSciCon, following this determination, we enter into Trade Agreement with a reputable company, Anke Biotechnology Group, Hefei, Anhui Province, to conduct the whole procedure starting with clinical trials and SFDA approval process for the implementation of the technology in China. The representative of the company, Director of Research and Development, came in USA at BioSciCon for training. The Company took the obligation to protect the intellectual property rights of BioSciCon. The necessary chemicals (kits) were shipped to China, clinical trials started in 2009 and finished in 2009, however during this time the BioSciCon patent has been pirated by a group from Hefei and the MarkPap test started to be manufactured by a new company Anyon Biopharmaceuticals, Ltd from the same city under the name FSC 811 (www, anyon.com.cn). Later, one more company was incorporated in the same city, Anhui Science and Technology Company (www.ahnmst.com). Who joined the manufacturing and sale of MarkPap products counterfeits under the name New Mark, NMPAP, and selling it in many China provinces. The test is well accepted as "innovative technology for the benefit of humanity". Please see excerpts from BioSciCon Press Release www.bioscicon.com/pressrelease.html.

EXCERPTS FROM www.bioscicon.com/pressrelease.html

June 2015

BioSciCon's MarkPap® Images in China.

Original, copyrighted image of a specimen processed with MarkPap® Test, presented on BioSciCon's Gallery page, are plagiarized and published without permission at the website of the Chinese Anhui Science and Technology Co.

Original image from BioSciCon's website

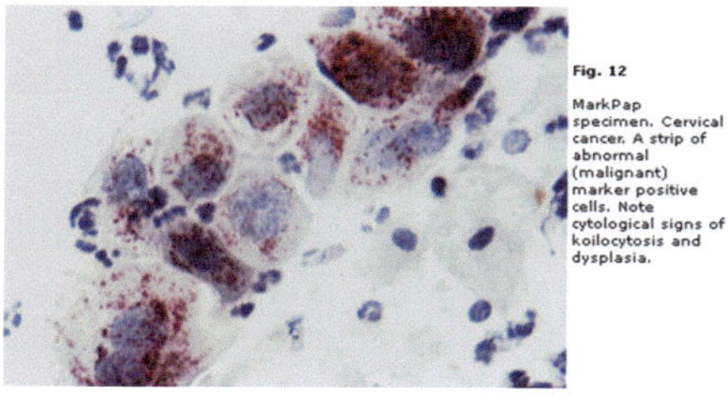

Plagiarized image published at Anhui Science and Technology Co. website

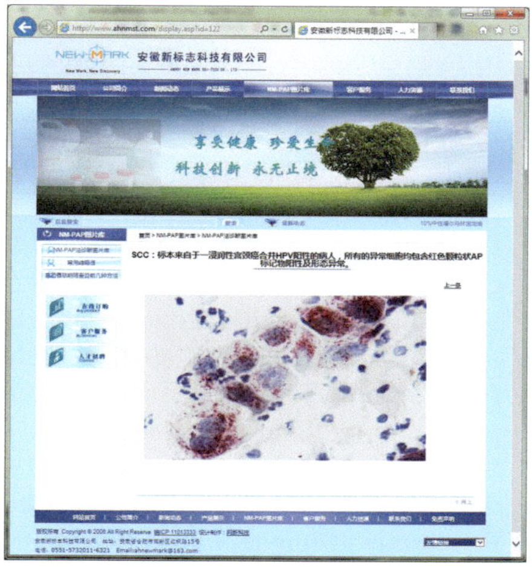
http://www.ahnmst.com/display.asp?id=122
NEW MARK
安徽新标志科技有限公司
科技创新 永无止境
NM-PAP图片库
SCC：标本来自于一浸润性宫颈癌合并HPV阳性的病人，所有的异常细胞均包含红色颗粒状AP标记物阳性及形态异常。

March 2015

MarkPap® in P.R. China

CAP PAP Test, USPTO #6,143,512 (issued in year 2000), MarkPap®, BioSciCon, Inc, USA is gaining popularity in China. It is sold under different names: NewMark-PAP, NM-PAP from Anhui Science and Technology Co., Ltd and FSC-811 from Anyon Biopharmaceuticals, Ltd, both from Hefei, Anhui Province, PR China.

Citation from www.ahnmst.com

(Google translate)

"Abnormal cervical squamous cell early screening kit" to detect chemical and enzyme modified Pap staining of cervical squamous cell early lesions improve the readability of abnormal cells, high sensitivity, shortened reading sheet time, low cost, which is very suitable for large-scale screening of cervical cancer, is suitable for use at all levels of medical institutions. "Innovative technology for the benefit of mankind".

5.7.4 NIH Grant Proposal: Mobile Telecytopathology (Model: Republic of Serbia)

5.7.4.1 Republic of Serbia

Cervical Cancer in Serbia

Klinicko-Bolnicki Centar Zemun – Beograd

Research Strategy

- In response to the call for Technology Transfer assistance from Serbian health care authorities and to help them reduce the incidence and mortality rates in the country, where, recently, those rates were among the highest in Europe (incidence 27.3 and mortality 12.6 per 100,000 women at risk), we have offered a New Strategy for Fighting Cervical Cancer in Serbia. This Exploratory Development (R21) Grant Proposal is to explore if this new Strategy will be effective as expected. If this phase is met, additional funding (e.g., R33, or local sources) will be requested to develop a sustainable service to help women at risk.
- Serbia is a small LMIC country (9.46 million, CIA Book), separated in 1990 from Former Yugoslavia, and has inherited health services infrastructure and policies from the parent country.
- Serbia has established a specialized health care institutions for women and children and from 2011 has a National Cervical Cancer Screening Program based on Pap smear technology with free of charge testing every third year, planning to cover a population of 3.2 millions. In spite of this, the response is insufficient and the outreach is far away from the crucial number of at least one million women participating in regular screening (once every third year).
- Serbian health providers have joined many others worldwide to blame the Pap test for this failure to accomplish better prevention. Thanks to the kindness of Serbian authorities we have studied this situation and we found few crucial elements which can be improved to enable a dramatic improvement of the screening outreach – the speed, accuracy and quality of screening-- for much lower cost and less liability. The keystones for this new approach are (1) Biomarker's improved Pap test, (2) Specimen self-sampling device, and (3) Mobile health using telemedicine network for connecting scattered points-of-care (POC) with expert medical centers, for fast and accurate diagnosis and clinical intervention (if needed) on the same day.
- We will recommend a change the current of Program for Cervical Cancer Screening to the new Strategy for Fighting Cervical Cancer. This Strategy is copying the US experience to stop negative trends of ever increasing cervical cancer prevalence and mortality and to reverse them into positive direction (reduction instead of increase). However, Serbia needs help immediately, and cannot wait 50 years to copy the US experience.

- We have offered a version of this Strategy which may reverse the trends from upward to downward direction within 10–15 years and for cost below $10.00 per test. Applying this new Strategy requires new tools such as: (1) Specimen self-collection devices, (2) MarkPap biomarker based reagents (3) Telemedical exchange of medical image information within a network of hubs scattered in the country, but connected with US specialists for help In difficult cases and for maintenance of the international communications, and (4) Telecytopathology Protocol for reading and interpretation of the Pap slides (with added biomarker signals).
- Naturally, no diagnostic screening test could be successful, if therapy for detected abnormal specimens is not immediately available. However, our partner in this proposal, the Clinical Center Zemun in Belgrade has all these infrastructure and facilities for early removal of suspect lesions and for extended gynecologic surgery, if necessary on the same day.
- In addition, Parallel is an Oracle Expert Team which will be able to make available to this project Oracle Database Server with development tools, Data Warehousing and Business Intelligence tools, Fusion Middleware Infrastructure and Enterprise Content Management Solutions.
- We have received assertions that our partners in Serbia have KSA to meet the R21 requirements and, with our additional help (providing some esoteric instruments and training of the personnel to use them), will be able to conduct feasibility study, to provide data convincing to change the health policy in Serbia, and to build initial infrastructure for moving this Strategy further.
- However, since changing the Governmental program is not an easy task, we have to produce convincing evidence that the new Strategy with the new tools can make the accomplishments which are expected from the Pap test, and which have already been seen and validated in the US.
- There is no better convincing evidence than an NIH study (because of the authority of this institution) and supported by R21 and eventually R33, which will give the power to complete the study as designed and planned for execution.
- Consequently we decided to submit this application for the most appropriate Federal support available at this moment, the Fogarty International Center Grant entitled Mobile Health: Technology and Outcomes in Low and Middle Income Countries.

The Research Study will be conducted as a Randomized Clinical Trial which design is outlined on the Table 5.1, below.

To complete this clinical trial and additional tasks related to the successful completion of the trial, we would need to invest the following:

1. Infrastructure:

   (a) Three workstations (digital microscope with mobile camera, PC with Internet and e-mail, printer and tele/fax connection). Two for Serbia – distant locations, one for an US center.
   (b) One Central Processing Unit with three servers (database, web, administration) for Serbia.

Table 5.1 Clinical trial overview

#	Name	MPT		PAP		Total		Labor
		N	%	N	%	N	%	Budget
1	Recruitment	1000		600		1600	100	
2	Informed C	1000		600		1600		
3	Pelvic exam	1000		600		1600		
4	Self-collect	600		400		1000		
5	MD collect	1000		600		1600		
6	CCRF	1000		600		1600		
7	Slide x 2	1000		600		1600		
8	LCRF	1000		600		1600		
9	Processing	1000		600		1600		
10	Only Pap	600		800		1200		
11	Reading	1600		1200		2800		
12	MPT(+)	140	14	n/a		140		
13	MPT(−)	860	86	n/a		860		
14	PAP(+)	n/a		28	7	28		
15	PAP(−)	n/a		372	93	372		
16	ACT							
17	Statistical analysis	Randomized controlled trial evidence-based decision analysis				3200 units		
18	Colposcopy	28	20	6	20	30		
19	Biopsy	22	80	5	80	27		
20	Histology	22		5		27		
21	Removal	11	50	3		14		
22	Repeat							
23	Database	200	100	1200	100	3200		
24	Conclusion	New strategy is superior to the standard control for more than 50 %						
25	Inference	New strategy to be promoted countrywide						
26	Reporting	Sponsor, SBIR, Local authorities						
27	Publishing	National and international medical journals						
28	Legislative work for promotion of the new strategy							
29	Network	Within Serbia						
30	ITTHC							
31	International	Networking						
32	Reversal of negative trends							

2. Personnel

   (a) Training for three key persons: gynecologist, pathologist and IT operator. Each training will be 15 days in the USA (5 days lecture and 5 days hands on practice.

   (b) Cost of Labor – see in the Budget.

3. Disposables
   (a) Specimen self-collection kits
   (b) Research Reagents Kit
   (c) IT accessories
4. All other facilities, R&D equipment and personnel are available from the participating institutions. BioSciCon's has already assigned appropriate IP for this project. It is incorporated into the proposal as the pre-Grant cost.
5. The cost for Clinical Trial, New Infrastructure, Training of the Personnel, and Disposables is presented in details in the Budget enclosed.

Specific Research Interest of the Participating Institutes and Centers

Mobile health provides a huge opportunity for reducing health care disparity between developed and developing countries. Current strategies and tools are only increasing this gap. Comprehensive mobile ITTHC can bridge the gap and reduce the discrepancy. GAWH is consultant to BioSciCon to sponsor development of a new mHealth to help bridge health disparities between developed and developing countries technology [1, 10].

The new devices and the strategy evolving from the new opportunity is an important new achievement for both, developed and developing countries, because providing better health care is reducing frustrations and promote international collaboration and trade.

Such strategy and models are just occurring in the healthcare practices and on the health care markets; they are still in R&D or Regulatory phase of development, and need additional research (mostly translational) to meet the market requirements (low cost, affordability, accessibility, portability, equitability, energy saving, etc.).

For GAWH, opening a node (hub) in Serbia is another accomplishment in our mission to help all women at risk – 2.4 billion – in the World where only 10 % is protected properly from this fatal, but preventable disease.

For Parallel, becoming a node in an International mHealth network will be qualitative advancement into an area of their long standing business interest. It will also bring financial benefit being connected with many medical institutions in country and abroad and having common long-years health care delivery projects.

For KBC Zemun, it will be an opportunity to confirm its high standing as the opinion leader in Serbia on issues involving Women's Health, Gynecological Health, Gynecological Oncology, and Human Wellbeing and Reproduction. In addition, KBC will renew its connections with local points-of-care providing cancer screening, and it will be able to increase the outreach among the population of women at risk to above 50 %.

Achieving this goal is a big accomplishment for KBC because at this percent of saturation, the negative trends of cervical cancer prevalence and mortality will reverse and will start to decrease – this has not happened so far by efforts of anybody else in Serbia.

Post Grant Maintenance of Infrastructure and Services – Sustain the Social Impact by Self-Sustaining Financial Growth

A future research and development pathway that details the LMIC research capacity will be established at the end of the grant period.

The grant project is designed to test a prototype of mHealth ITTHC (already developed in the US) and to demonstrate on a small scale the full functionality of the system in a small developing country as Serbia. However, the specifics of Serbia are that this country already had a well developed healthcare system which is now in "transition" and suffers from the lack of funding. However, the health professionals are well aware of the benefits their patients have lost, and will not make any barrier to the modern idea of using low-cost medical technology for the same achievements as high-tech systems are producing in the developed world.

With other words, we expect that Serbia health professionals will hailed this project because they know what is good, they have not currently funds for to it, but they will know how to use low-cost technologies, if available. This is exactly the purpose of this grant – to enable educated people to do their job at the same high level of quality, but with new affordable tools.

During the grant period we will assess Serbian capacity to sustain the system with their funds – health insurance, government subsidy, individual payment. Under the System we consider the Strategy, tools (products and services) to enable implementation of the Strategy. This is why the entire mHealth ITTHC is designed to provide the comprehensive service for only $10.00 per service and to be open in membership or insurance formats. At this moment both formats seem sustainable, but the research is needed to confirm this opinion.

We anticipate barriers to entry of the new Strategy, but KBC has sufficient authority to overcome any science or professional barrier. Parallel can do the rest with the technical issues – networking. Their basic system is Oracle, and it is able to scale-up to millions of services per year. A part of our team is a software professor who is creating the network architecture.

Funding remains the major problem for prolonged time of application, but upon our calculations, if widely applied, 1–2 million tests per year, the services can generate sufficient revenue to make the entire system self-sustainable. However, this decision will be made at the end of the grant period as the inference from the conclusions that will come of the research.

Chapter 6
New Strategy and Its Global Application

6.1 Executive Summary

1. **Problem**

   Cervical cancer is a social problem not because it kills about 400,000 women worldwide annually (1 in 6000), but because it is the only cancer which natural history (unstoppable growth until death of the host) can be altered by prevention and disease can be cured, if detected on time.

   Usually, Government legislate a National Program, e.g., Strategy for Fighting Cervical Cancer, provides funding (resources) and delegates it to executive agencies like health care service providers, health insurance, health care industry, and health educators.

   The delegated agencies, within the limitations of their statute, prepare their own Programs and entrust jobs to their executive institutions and/or individuals. These are the real customers who are buying our products and learn our procedures to be able to deliver health services as their job assignments. The end users of services are healthy women at risk for cervical cancer [209].

   However, the chain is much longer. Customers are buying the products and learning the procedures from educators, retailers and distributors, who, on the other hand, are buying from importers/exporters, sellers and wholesalers, who are buying their supply from manufacturers or their direct sales representatives. This is a long chain of intermediaries, and at each step, somebody requires for "customs" to allow products to move forward. The cost is increasing – not the value of the product, but the mercantile cost; an added charge – not added value, which depends upon negotiation. Direct sale could reduce the cost dramatically, but the commercial network of easy earning money through the resale is almost impossible to be avoided. It must be considered very seriously in planning the commercialization strategy.

N. Markovic, O. Markovic, *What Every Woman Should Know about Cervical Cancer*, DOI 10.1007/978-94-017-7560-1_6

This market dictates the selling price of the products and procedures. In low-middle-income countries (LMIC), the average price should be about $10.00 per test including specimen collection, preparation, staining, reading, interpretations, and result reporting back to the originators for decision making what to do with the subject – release her home as healthy and schedule next screening, or continue diagnostic procedure including small surgical intervention for removal of important lesion if required [208, 211, 212, 215, 237] (Annex).

In Twenty-first Century, the entire cycle from specimen preparation through result reporting must be done within hours and if intervention if necessary, the diagnostic procedure and eventual small surgery is expected to be completed within 1 day, or while woman is on the premises. For more complicated diagnostic and/or therapeutic procedures, women should be referred to gynecologists and hospitals. **Such timing is not possible with classic Pap test, and alternatives are sought.**

Among those alternatives, using IT technology, in particular the mobile phone cameras and telemedicine are the most promising. They can reduce both the time and cost of the laboratory service [213, 215–218, 221, 223] (Sects. 7.1 and 7.6).

Using IT technology and automation requires a method with much better accuracy than the classic Pap test and its 20 % inherited false negative rates. The price of $10.00 per test, calculated for one million services per years, includes building the entire infrastructure for this service and a maintenance fee for 1 year. Service will be paid either as fee for service or as membership dues. The selling price is realistic if the markup of each and every intermediary is limited to "up to $0.50." With one million tests sold per year, this markup makes a sizable amount even for the most demanding customers.

The National Consensus Conference on Cervical Cancer Screening was held in Bethesda, Maryland in 1996. The Conference acknowledged Pap smear test as "the best anticancer screening test available," but also admitted that this test has unacceptably high false negative rate. Although much of this rate was blamed to specimen sampling error, it was also recognized that Papanicolaou staining has an inherent false negative rate of 20 %. Indeed, in the years that followed, sampling was improved, but the ability of chemical stain could not be changed and all versions of Pap test performed on smears or on thin-layers (obtained from specimens in solution) stained and examined manually or automatically, continue to have this high false negative rate.

Not emphasized passed the fact that the biggest success of Pap test in the US, the reduction of prevalence and mortality for more than 80 %, was achieved when the outreach rate was raised above 50 % of women at risk in the population. The conclusion was obvious; any social impact could be achieved only if women at risk accept this test and massively participate in voluntary careening.

In 2008, in our first edition, we recommended CAP-PAP test (cervical acid phosphatase- Papanicolaou) as an improvement because CAP emerged as a biomarker for labeling abnormal cervical squamous from normal cells on Pap smears [209, 212, 220].

Nonetheless, instead of improving sensitivity for detection of abnormal specimens with biomarkers, the main stream of cervical cancer screening improvement efforts have been focused on HPV detection (non cytological methods) and on raising the threshold of detection from ASC-US to HSIL or CIN 2/3. Higher detection threshold, by virtue of the technology, had lower false negative rates but false positive have increased exposing healthy women to unnecessary diagnostic procedures. A CIN2/3 threshold is detecting lesions which are almost in cancer symptomatic phase when the early removal could not guarantee the curability rate that was achieved with the lower threshold of the classic Pap test. The ASCUS+ threshold was for an early detection of "abnormality which could develop into cervical cancer" This has been the trademark of classic Pap test.

We believe in biomarkers to improve the sensitivity of detecting cervical cells. It will lower the threshold from ASCUS+ and will detect cases among those currently missed in the category BCC (benign cellular changes) and/or RCC (reactive cellular changes). More slides will be selected for review by pathologists who, in such case, will have the standard Pap test parameters to keep the specificity of detection at the same level, or to improve this specificity with inclusion of HPV markers as disease progress-prognostic factors.

This paragraph and the diagram below conclude our assumptions used for creation of the New Strategy for Fighting Cervical Cancer Worldwide [221, 222].

Conclusion and Inference: Increase the outreach beyond 50 % and obtain reversal of the trends from rising to downsizing.

2. Solution

The new Strategy must be acceptable for the most of the population at risk, must provide easy accessible, affordable, fast, accurate and low cost mass cervical cancer screening with an early intervention while the woman is still on the premises. It must be safeguarded from the role of many intermediaries and the cost for manufacturing and using the products must be below the current market price for the cervical cancer screening in the country. This thoughtfulness, if met, will enable self-sustainability of the procedure until the social goals are reached, and beyond.

Because of these limitations, it is obvious that each and every country should have its own strategy. The role of international health organizations, such as WHO (World Health Organization), is expected to coordinate local and regional programs and to promote the strategy worldwide.

Studying this situation in 28 countries (all continents, more than one third of world population) we came to conclusion that the new Strategy is possible to be implemented, if it is supported with new tools aimed to meet the new requirements.

This new, comprehensive strategy will include the goal to reverse cervical cancer prevalence and mortality within a period of 10–15 years of nationwide implementation by

(a) Increasing the outreach among women at risk to above 50 % (using specimen self collecting devices affordable and accessible to every women),
(b) Reducing the Pap test false negative rates and laboratory's liability by adding specific biomarkers (e.g., cervical acid phosphatase test),
(c) Reducing the procedure turnover time (to few hours instead of days) and the service cost (to less than $10.00 per test) by using digital imaging and tele-cytopathology (to communicate image files between points-of-care and remote expert centers), and by
(d) Using STOMP medical kits for rare gynecological surgery intervention if and when necessary for removal of epithelial lesions.

The diagram below summarizes the complete screening process available for a single woman participating in the cervical cancer prevention program.

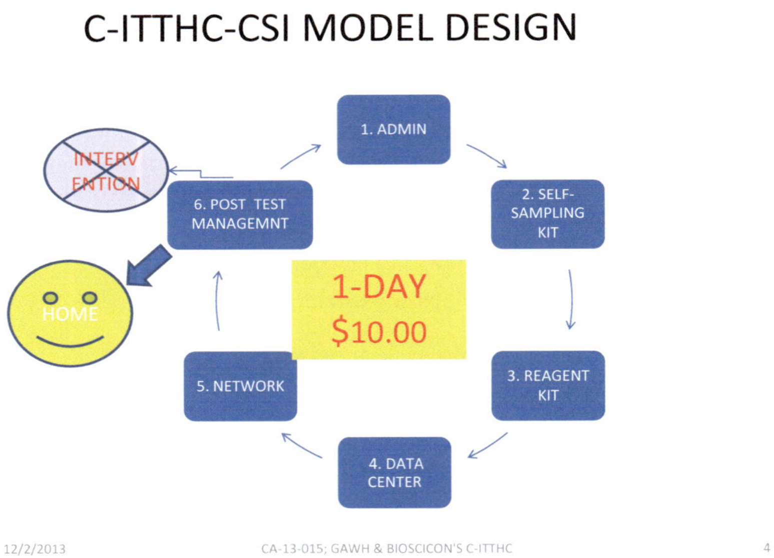

(1) Admin – ITTH team; (2) Self-sampling kit – Specimen collecting device used by women themselves; (3) Reagent kit – MarkPap® Test reagent assembled for laboratory use (300–1000 tests per kit); (4) Data center – a Local CPU connecting image acquisition units at POC with image evaluation units at remote expert centers; (5) Network – a network of ITTHC to cover a region, a country or globally and to enable fast, accurate and low cost exchange of medical information up- and down-stream; (6) Post test management – POC equipped with STOMP Medical kit for small surgical interventions where medical doctors can complete the necessary management of women with positive MarkPap test (intervention). Women with negative test and with successful intervention are considered healthy and will return home the same day (Smile)

Table 6.1 In vitro diagnostic methods are to separate normal (negative) specimens from positive and to grade the abnormality according to the need for clinical action

Threshold	Dysplasia	Pathology	2001-TB	#/year
Th 0	Neg		NLM	
			BCC/RCC	50 M
Th I	Mild	CIN-1	ASC-US	
			ASC-H	3.5 M
Th II	Moderate	CIN-2	LSIL	
	Severe	CIN-3	HSIL	0.6 M
Th III	Carcinoma		CIS	0.08 M
			ICC	0.02 M
Adenoglandular			AGUS	
			AIC	

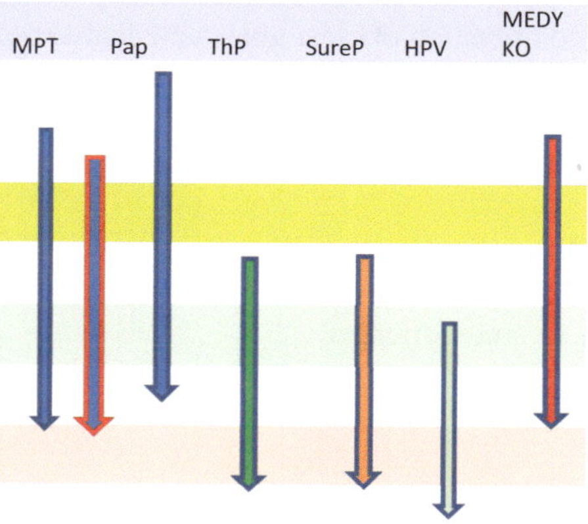

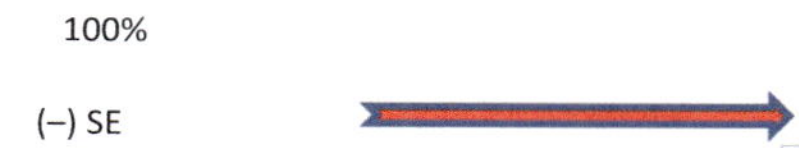

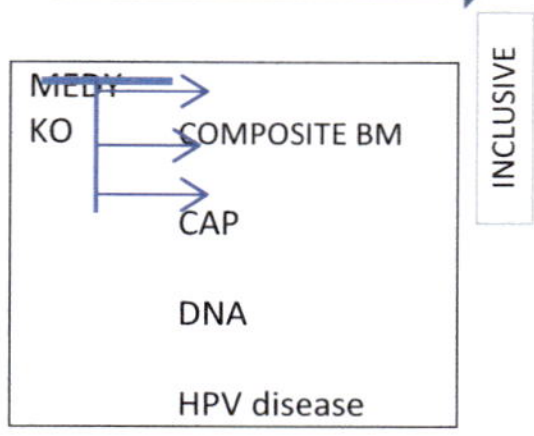

COMMENT

Detection accuracy depends on the threshold of detection.

Th 0	GP specimen	Healthy women – general population
Th I	Dysplasia all degrees	Stratified randomization
Th II	Advanced dysplasia	Stratified randomization

3. **Future Projections**

    BioSciCon, Inc. is already in the latest phases of development of a new, composite biomarker to improve MarkPap®. The trade name of this biomarker will be MEDYKO™ which is an acronym of Metabolic (ME), Dysplasia (DY) and Koilocytes (KO). This composite biomarker is expected to have larger diagnostic specter then any other cervical cancer screening test currently on the market (see Table 6.1) and will keep all other advantages of MarkPap Technology Platform

4. **Instead of Conclusion**

    This Executive Summary is developed by BioSciCon, Inc. from Rockville, Maryland, U.S.A, to test your will to invest into Social Entrepreneurship where the impact is bimodal: health improvement and financial benefits. The testing is important because not very many investors are ready to invest into business when ROI (return on investment) is a long-standing goal. Much larger portion of the investors is looking for fast money (profits) and no other impact. This is why this

Executive Summary could be a good test of what is that you really wish. And, we would be very much interested to share with you the same goal, if it is the social entrepreneurship and the idea to help women with the comprehensive approach, a combination of clear goals and doable programs.

6.2 Global Cervical Cancer Screening

6.2.1 New Strategy for Fighting Cervical Cancer Globally

6.2.1.1 Introduction

Why New Strategy?

Until the middle of Twentieth Century cervical cancer was a ubiquitous disease, the major killer of women from malignant disease, and its prevalence worldwide and mortality was in permanent, unstoppable rise for about 10 % annually as reported from many countries all over the world. The World Health Organization (WHO) was recording statistical data and was trying to influence this trend by issuing guidelines based on the available, at each time, methods and tools for prevention because there was no, then as of now, effective treatment to stop or cure invasive cervical cancer.

In the 2d part of the Twentieth Century the American Cancer Society was credited by introducing, developing and applying the Pap test which became known as "the best anticancer screening test available." As introduced, the Pap test was a composition of several procedures: (1) Recruiting health subjects for screening procedures, (2) Subject examining and specimen sampling for In Vitro Diagnostic evaluation, (3) Specimen collecting, storing and forwarding to cytopathology laboratory. (4) In Lab specimen preparation for staining, (5) Specimen staining for cytopathological microscopic evaluation, (6) Microscope reading and quality control for specimen sampling, preparation and staining, (7) specimen evaluation for pathocytological criteria and interpretation, (8) Result of examination reporting in form of clinical diagnosis found on the specimen, (9) Result reporting as Test (+) or test (−) and degree of positivity (TBS criteria or 2001 BS), (10) Management of women with normal specimens, (11) Management of women with abnormal specimens, and (12) Removal of suspect lesions to cure women.

This entire program requires a special infrastructure (space, equipment, trained personnel, and protocols for service delivery) which were implemented in the US after a massive ACS campaign, support of US Congress and all professional organizations involved in women's health and children development. However, the efforts and the investment had paid off. Over a period 50 years (1950–2000) cervical cancer in the US was placed under control: more than 80 % of women at risk participated in annual cervical cancer screening (once in 3 years), 50 million Pap tests were conducted annually by 10,000 cytotechnologists, 3.5 million women was selected as Pap test positive and subject to further investigation, 0.6 million women were found to be at high risk and 0.04 million women were operated from carcinoma in situ (CIS) and cured. As the result, cervical cancer prevalence and mortality were reduced for 80 % and cervical cancer disappeared from the horizon of 10 most frequent causes of death from malignant disease in the US. It was an unprecedented result, which attracted attention worldwide, and many, including WHO, wanted to copy it in their respected countries.

But, it did not work. Copying American experience became more difficult than anybody had expected. WHO was pressed to declare that although the Pap test is the best test for cervical cancer screening, because of its cost (infrastructure) alternatives are to be sought, and WHO recommended that developed countries create new, low-cost technologies, which may be used in developing world where most of low or immediate income countries and majority of world population belong and most of cervical cancer patients are found.

It did not work again. In 2011, WHO issued new Guidelines and confirmed them in the 2013 publication. This Guidelines have introduced the concept Screen-and-Treat, leaving the Pap test behind, and promoting Visual Inspection with Acid (VIA) in combination with early cryotherapy of visible lesions. In medical terminology, it meant a serious change of strategy from preventive cervical cancer control and screening or surveillance of healthy (asymptomatic) women, to "early diagnosis and treatment" of symptomatic or incidentally found patients. Not surprisingly, this change of guidelines was paralleled by industry and professional organizations, who decreased the sensitivity of the threshold for patient's entry to CIN2+, increased specificity, and left healthy women behind with their fears of cervical cancer , but concentrated to patient care.

As the result, more than 80 % of women at risk for cervical cancer in this countries are not considered in the guidelines, and there is no way the American Success Story to be repeated worldwide. The consequence will be paid by women in developing world and the health discrepancy between developed and developing worlds will only increase.

Which Strategy to Choose for Cervical Cancer Screening?

Options are limited: (1) Screen-and-Treat, (2) HPV and HPV DNA (high risk), (3) CIN2+ (LBP, ThinPrep, SurePath), (4) Pap Test (improved version), or (5) Any other biomarker based test.

If cervical cancer screening is a part of cancer control (surveillance) among healthy women at risk, then option (1) through option (3) should not be considered because (Sect. 4.1.1) Screen and Treat is looking to treat white acid positive or yellowish (lugol/iodine positive) patches of cervical epithelium (which can be positive in other infections, not only in cancer) and the treatment could be either substandard or harmful, HPV tests (HC-2 and HPV DNA) are tests for virus presence, not cancer; their statistical relevance, if used alone w/o cytology, could produce many false positive and false negative results, CIN2+ thresholds will certainly eliminate from consideration as negative many lesions that could have been indeed only false negative.

We have reviewed the excuses published on the issue why classic Pap test cannot be applied in LMIC, and we think, we found that the hurdles could be overcome with introduction of MarkPap biomarker based technology products. How?

<u>Mark Pap Specimen Self-Sampling kit</u> (see below) is designed for women to obtain material in the privacy of their home and to mail it to accredited laboratory for processing.

<u>MarkPap Reagents Kit</u> (see below) is designed (1) to process specimens with a biomarker specific for detection of metabolic changes preceding cancer morphological changes, (2) to identify morphological changes of dysplasia (DNA-nuclear configuration) which is a cytological sign of ongoing malignant alteration, and (3) to present koilocytes (if present) which are cytological sign of HPV disease, a true indicator of worse prognosis.

<u>MarkPap Telecytopathology Service</u> designed to connect points-of-care (POC) with remote expert centers with telemedicine Web-based network to enable fast, accurate, and low cost evaluation of abnormal specimens and to enable health care providers to obtain results the same day when screening is done and to apply any clinical action as recommended – including local surgery if necessary.

New Strategy (Applied for India)

The most important lesson learned from the US experience is that the reversal of negative trends for cervical cancer prevalence and mortality in the US, have happened only when the outreach has reached the 50 % of the populations at risk.

MarkPap technology provides tools to enable application of this principle in each country because this is a biomarker based, telemedicine empowered, low-cost, accurate, accessible and infrastructure independent. For details see Chapter 6.

The following diagram presents an estimate of the utilization of the New Strategy in US, India and China (Fig. 6.1).

How to fund new strategy?

It seems that Hippocrates oath and his Instructions should be applied to make this Strategy available to 2.5 billion women worldwide, The task seems difficult, but award of saving a quarter of million lives annually is too big, that warrant each and any effort to achieve it.

The basic Hippocrates principle that everyone deserve to live healthy life, could resolve the problem of the cost and implementation of the Strategy only if the second principle is accepted, "Rich pay for poor." In this situation, the cost of maintaining regular annual screening could be distributed proportionally to the ability to pay, and the total population at risk may be covered. Indian example confirms these assertions.

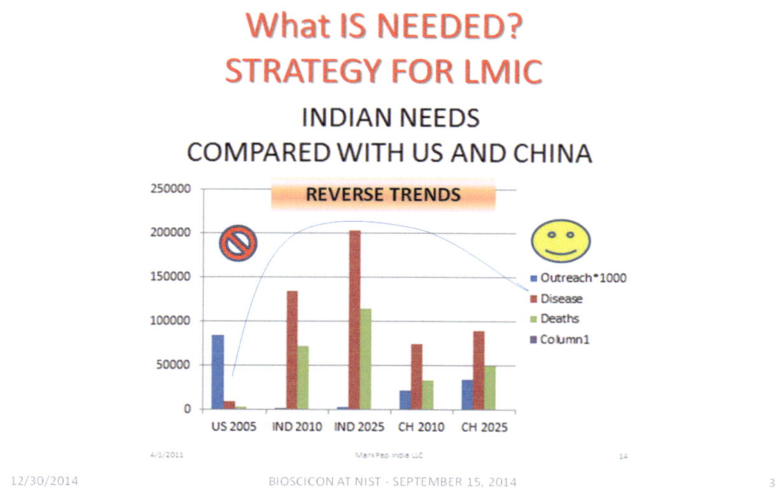

Fig. 6.1 US – Outreach 80 %, Prevalence and mortality under control less than 12 % and respectfully 5 %; India – Outreach less than 6 %, prevalence and mortality without control, constant raising; China: Outreach becoming under control. Prevalence and mortality improving. Outreach in percent, actual numbers of cervical cancer cases, and deaths are compared between USA, India and China during a period of 2005 (actual data) though 2025 (estimates). The *curve* shows how disease and mortality change in relation with the outreach. Note that at the outreach percent of 50 % the curve reverse the trend from upward to downward

Self sustainable cervical cancer screening in India

Population	Pay	Annual tests	Total income
Women at risk	$10.00	100 million	1 billion
Rich	$40.00	10 million	400 million
Moderate	$10.00	20 million	200 million
Poor	$2.00	270 million	540 million
Administration	$0.60	100 million	60 million
Total annual income			1.2 billion
Total annual expenses			1 billion
Total for free distribution			0.2 billion

Instead of Conclusion

We do not pledge the exactness of this estimate, but, even with all uncertainty, it seems that a sustainable program copying a US experience is not impossible to create in India. Naturally, it needs a coordinated action of Indian Government, health care providers, health insurance, health industry and other players interested to improve wellbeing of Indian women and the country human reproduction, social and economic benefits that go with saving women's lives.

Inference to Global Strategy for Fighting Cervical Cancer could be easily outlined from those examples. However, the Global Strategy will need coordination with WHO and all interested governments to initiate changes into direction to achieve a health impact – reverse of cervical cancer prevalence and mortality in the country or in the World – not to stay away of big challenges.

6.3 MarkPap Technology Platform

The name MarkPap® is brand name replacing the previously used trade name Cervical Acid Phosphatase – Papanicolaou Test or CAP-PAP™ test. The new brand name is an acronym of the name of inventors of the new technology and the short name of the basic methodology improved by the invention.

MarkPap technology platform is described as biomarker-based cytopathology, digital imaging, telemedicine web-based networking system for exchange of image files between Points- of-Care and expert centers to improve diagnosis of clinical condition on in vitro diagnostic specimen and enable removal of pathological lesions on time to cure the disease.

The platform is opened for new arrivals and they are coming from the IP and R&D departments of BioSciCon, Inc. (the sponsor of this development), as new patentable inventions, patents, prototypes and products ready for regulatory approval and for sale on world markets.

The following products are considered for market application:

1. **IP on Technology**
2. **MarkPap Reagent Kit**
3. **MarkPap Specimen Self-Collecting Kit**
4. **MarkPap® Digital or Tele-Pap**
5. **MarkPap Workstation: Image Acquisition and Evaluation Unit**
6. **MarkPap IT Telehealth Center**
7. **MarkPap Telecytopathology Service MPPTCPS Global Networking Protocol**
8. **Application of the technology in China**
9. **MarkPap Mobile Health**
10. **MarkPap New Concept: One-Day Service: Screen-Diagnose-Treat**
11. **MarkPap Telemedicine Protocol**

Details are presented in the book in Chap. 7

6.3.1 MarkPap Advantage

Cervical cancer screening from global prospective with emphasis on developing countries

What is happening in the Twenty-first Century?

Women still die from a preventable disease.

In spite of all efforts and new approved technologies, the average outreach among women at risk for cervical cancer screening is about 10 %. More than 500,000 women get cervical cancer annually and 360,000 women die, mostly in the low-resource areas. The prognosis is that the situation will get worse. For example in India, the outreach is 6 % and further 150 % increase in mortality is expected by the year 2025.

Is it really impossible to repeat the USA success story, even in shorter period of time? What about two billion women at risk?

It is generally accepted that the best strategy to prevent cervical cancer is cytological screening with Pap test, but also it is generally accepted that Pap test could not be introduced for mass cervical cancer screening globally, because of the following:

1. ***Cost*** **– the existing Pap test is not affordable for most low-resource countries**
2. ***Lack of local infrastructure*** **– qualified personnel to evaluate the result**
3. ***Not accessible*** **– rural areas, without doctor's offices/hospitals**
4. ***Non-comfortable test*** **– requires pelvic exam, cultural sensitivity**
5. ***Slow*** **– takes weeks to get the results back**

Is it possible to mitigate these challenges? The official answer was "No" and governmental official statements from many countries in the developing world were that Pap test cannot be implemented for mass cervical cancer screening.

MarkPap Technology can mitigate all these pains:

It is low-cost (1), infrastructure independent (2), accessible in rural areas (3) a culture sensitive test (4), results could be obtained in hours (5).

New tools which will provide mass cervical cancer screening.

Currently, we have selected three MarkPap® platform technology products and services MarkPap test kit, MarkPap® Digital Telecytopathology Service and MarkPap-Self Collection Kit.

MarkPap® Test Kit is an assembly of reagents, controls and instructions developed to facilitate the performance of MarkPap® test. This test is a low-cost simple, accurate, affordable and may be performed by low-trained technician at the Point-of

Care (POC). As such, this test will dramatically increase the number of locations where the specimen can be processed. If specialist is available, the diagnosis is made locally. A special MarkPap Reagent Kit is customized for India, MarkPap Kit-India (CPK-50-I) and China. More information about the kits can be found in Sects. 7.1 and 7.2 and Annex www.bioscicon.com/markpapproducts.html

MarkPap® Telemedicine Service for diagnosis at distance (telemedicine- telecytopathology), transmitting microscopic images of biomarker-labeled, red cells (pathologist is not needed at the POC!) digitally or by cell phone to specialists for final diagnosis. This will increase the outreach from rural areas with no infrastructure at the Point-of-Care (Chap. 7 and Annex).

MarkPap® Self-Collection Home Kit for women to take specimen at home and send it to the laboratory for testing. It is only possible with the MarkPap technology, since the biomarker is stable in vaginal fluids. This is to help women who do not have access to doctor's offices or are uncomfortable to visit gynecologist (Chap. 7 and Annex).

In reality, a low trained person processes the specimen with the MarkPap Kit. The same person, put the slide on the microscope and searches for red cells and then transmits those cells digitally or by cell phone camera to pathologist for final diagnosis. Pathologist is not needed at the POC.

This is why MarkPap® technology can be defined as a biomarker-based, telemediciine-empowered, low-cost, simple, affordable, accessible, equitable infrastructure independent platform technology.

When implemented, this technology will be among those which can bring right care at the right place at the right time for lower cost.

These are all highly profitable medical devices which can be immediately implemented by the practicing health providers in the settings of current participants of cervical cancer screening.

Our estimates are that for a population of one million women/screened per year, the use of this strategy could double the number of participants, reduce significantly the cost, increase the revenue, and reduce liability. With other words a better service and more saving for any community (population) that will participate in this program.

These are the advantages of the new technology.

6.4 Social Impact: Alleviating Health Disparities in Low-Middle-Income-Countries (LMIC)

How to provide every woman with *An equal opportunity to fight cervical cancer because it is the most frequent killer of women from malignant diseases worldwide, and the only cancer completely curable if detected and removed on time.*

6.4.1 American Experience

In the beginning of Twentieth Century, cervical cancer was major killer of women from malignant diseases. In the middle of that Century, American Cancer Society started a nationwide campaign to prevent cervical cancer occurrence by screening asymptomatic women for hidden genital (cervical) lesions which could develop into cervical cancer and to remove them on time; consequently, to cure cancer in situ. This campaign was enabled by a new, at that time, in vitro diagnostic test, described by Dr. George Papanicolaou, which included scrapping cervical epithelium (to obtain cells from deeper layers) and using two stain technique with several cleanings to improve clarity of color images for microscopic reading enabling examiners to see more subcellular details than with the standard Hematoxylin/Eosin staining. At the same time, Dr. Papanicolaou (nick name Dr. Pap) started a School on Cytotechnology which has enabled more than 10,000 laboratory technicians to prepare and to read Pap smears before pathologists were to be involved. The screening was designed to select Pap negative specimens (90 %+) from suspect or positive (up to 10 %), which were later reviewed by pathologist for cytopathological diagnosis and grading (from NIL to HSIL, or ICC). The test was completed with the recommendation for management of women who have negative (rescreen after 1 year) and positive results (to confirm diagnosis with a triple – colposcopy, biopsy and surgical removal of the lesion if detected and confirmed), The entire composite procedure (specimen sampling, preparation, staining, reading, interpretation and management) received one short name, the Pap test, and this procedure was widely accepted when applied in the US.

Within the next 60 years, the Pap test was used for annual cervical cancer screening (50 million American women per year) encompassing more than 80 % of populations at risk in 3-year periods. Results are known, the prevalence of cervical cancer disease and the mortality have been reduced for more 80 %, and cervical cancer, from major killer of women from malignant disease, has dropped below the rank of 10 most frequent killers and is of no substantial significance in the US any more. This result was achieved when the outreach has gone above 50 % of women at risk and when the steady increasing trend of the curve showing cervical cancer prevalence and mortality reversed and began a downward trend.

However, the credit for this success cannot be given to Dr. Papanicolaou or to ACS alone, because it is the result of the combined work of the entire team of healthcare providers working strictly in compliance with the prescribed test and the post-test management.

This was the infrastructure necessary for application of the complete Pap test, and the main reason why this test cannot be applied in LMIC where such infrastructure is to be developed and put in service before launching any campaign for mass screening of women at risk.

Unfortunately, the huge success of Pap test created a huge market place of millions of healthy women, which became a target for businesses to enter this space with additions, "improvements" or even replacement of some elements of the Pap test. All this effort, which started in 1996 with the recommendation (the Bethesda System) to accept surrogate endpoints (laboratory results) instead of robust endpoints (clinical outcomes) for measurement of the statistical success of new tests in comparison with standards, and with FDA approvals of studies with surrogate end points has opened doors for many new entries.

As the result, the cost of Pap test has increased, the insurance companies requested prolongation of periods between screening (from annual to once in 3-years) and the downward trend of the curve showing cervical cancer prevalence has leveled and started to rise in 2012–2014.

New ideas are necessary to keep the cervical cancer under control in the US.

6.4.2 Low Medium Income Countries

6.4.2.1 Pains

There are 2.5 billion women worldwide at risk for cervical cancer, more than 600,000 (2.4/100) gets new cervical cancer per year and more than 360,000 (1.4/100) die. These numbers are the same as no preventive measure were used. Indeed, 90 % of women either do not receive any prevention, or receive substandard prevention with alternatives to Pap test or VIA. Only 20 % are protected and even they are not all regular participants in scheduled screenings. The result is as the numbers say – no protection worldwide, and no prospective protection unless the outreach is increased above 50 %.

Obviously, copying American experience is not possible without having the infrastructure to conduct the classic Pap test, and the alternatives have not yet reached the standard as measured by outcomes – although many surrogate endpoints show that the improvements over perform the standard in different ways, but not *quo ad vitam*.

Surrogate end points were made available with liquid-based Pap test (both ThinPrep and SurePath) and the promoters of both techniques claimed to be more sensitive than Pap test, but for detection of C2/C3 specimens because they have more probability to convert into cervical cancer.

Since standard Pap test had inherent 20 % false negative rate, this achievement seemed to be substantial. It was not.

Sensitivity may be increased by moving the threshold up (see Fig. 5.3) introducing new markers which will recruit new positive specimens from earlier categories such as BCC or RCC where the false negatives are hidden, or specificity may be increased by moving the threshold down, trading for the further reduce of the real sensitivity.

Moving cursor up was plausible to introduce HPV testing. However, the HPV general testing method, HC-2 detects many HPV strains and false positives, which would swamp the laboratories and many unnecessary diagnostic tests and/or intervention – some of them even harmful – would have been performed without justification. To avoid it, the threshold went in opposite direction – lower category, LSIL, which has already been described as HPV positive. The higher specificity was obtained, but sensitivity was lost, as well as, the purpose of screening healthy women. With low positioned threshold, the screening procedure recruited women already stratified as Pap positive. The good thing is that the stratified populations are much smaller and cost is proportionally reduced.

All of these manipulations with the threshold and subsequently the control groups used in clinical trials to confirm the advantage of the new test vs. the standard; indeed, have increased the number of substandard Pap test screening in comparison with the classic Pap test.

However, the providers and their financial supporters have proclaimed, even in the US, these substandard technologies as the breakthrough and modern. It was not so long, for them to start requiring the annual standard Pap smear test to be replaced with their modern technologies; this is an ongoing trend right now.

In this galimatias of recommendations, we think, the best advice is to keep with the standard: "Annual Pap smear test for all women age 18 and above." This advice is well supported with 60 years of US experience and data are available for review and comparison at any time.

6.4.3 WHO Guidelines 2013

Only few years ago the World Health Organization hailed Pap test as "the best screening test available," but, since it was not affordable and accessible in developing world, recommended to the health industry in developed countries to "develop low-cost technologies for low-middle-income countries (LMIC)" in order to reduce the fast growing health disparities between people (in this case women) living in these two parts of the world and to calm political tensions built on the health disparity.

Unfortunately, this appeal did not produce the expected effect, and in 2011, WHO issued other guidelines (this time based upon Indian experience with VIA and VILI), and recommended the Visual Inspection with Acid as their alternative for Pap test.

In 2013, WHO went further; in their publication, "Guidelines for screening pre-cancerous lesions for cervical cancer prevention" WHO 2013, (ISBN: 978 924 154869 4), they recommended a new Strategy:" Screen & Treat," requesting an early intervention with cryoablation or LOOP excision, when the cytological diagnosis is CIN2+. As diagnostic methods to reach the target cytological diagnosis, WHO pointed to HPV followed by VIA, HPV alone, VIA alone, Cytology or HPV followed by colposcopy.

The basic problem is here that CIN2+ is cytopathological diagnosis. VIA is a visual assessment of visible lesion, HPV is a test for viral fragments or DNA; neither one without cytology could be confident that CIN2+ was accurately diagnosed. Then, using harmful intervention as cryoablation, or LOOP excision, seems to be somehow "irresponsible" recommendation.

Again, our advice would be to stay with the standard Pap test and to search for options designed to reduce the inherent false negative rate of 20 %. One of these options was CAP-PAP Test (BioSciCon, 2003), but did not attract more attention because it was fast, accurate and low cost method offered in the time when LBP and HPV were on rise. It is time, now, to revisit this option. This book has a chapter MEDYKO discussing the new strategy and new tools to meet this strategy all based on a composite biomarker and cytology followed by standard colposcopy, biopsy and histology, ending with the removal of CIS (carcinoma in situ).

Recommended further readings from the same authors:

STRATEGY FOR INDIA
STRATEGY FOR OTHER LMIC
TOOLS TO ENABLE IMPLEMENTATION OF THE STRATEGY
EDUCATION OF EDUCATORS AND DECISION MAKERS

6.5 Economic Impact – Cost Benefit

6.5.1 Global Funding the New Strategy

The purpose of cervical cancer screening among healthy – asymptomatic – women is to detect presence of lesions that could be developed into cervical cancer, and to remove them; thus, providing cure from cancer. Ultimately, cervical cancer screening test is saving lives of women in fertile periods.

There are 2.4 billion women at risk for cervical cancer world-wide. Each of them needs anticancer screening at least once in 3 years. Implementation of such policy needs substantial societal investment. Not all societies, and particularly not all governments or private enterprises are ready to invest this money without an adequate return.

On the other side, how many women's lives can be saved with a wide campaign of cervical cancer screening. According to the US data, out of 50,000,000 screened healthy women, 7.5 million was found Pap (+), 600,000 was diagnosed as HSIL, and 40,000 had lesions which were to be removed. At that time, Pap test in the US cost was $15.00 per test, and the GDP-PC was $52,000. A simple calculation could show that the saved money was more than four times the cost for this Pap test. The economic incentives were clear. But, how this calculation can be applied to other countries?

Comparison among countries has revealed big differences of GDP-PC causing the value of woman's life to be estimated in a wide range between less than $1,000 and more than $50,000. As much as this calculation seem speculative, it gives a solid base for assessment whether a preventive test, such as cervical cancer screening, is having economical incentives in addition to the social impact. Upon these calculations, a comprehensive cervical cancer screening including management of women with positive test (approximately $10.00 per test) is saving money to the countries with more than $10,000 GDP-PC. Other countries should seek additional funds to compensate for the cost if they need social benefit for their women. This is the point where World Health Organization, Global Health Initiative, churches and many charitable organizations and other social investors may change the outcome for women lives and the health and economic prospective of many countries with the GDP-PC less than $10.000.

Details are presented in Chap. 5, article Economy of MPT. Data in the table shows that 9/11 African countries, 3/9 American, 9/15 Asian, 2/4 Australian, and 6/17 European contrives will need financial and other help, if MarkPap test is to be fully implemented, and if the New Strategy is to deliver the expected results. However, the bright sight is the MarkPap test in this calculation is used as a comprehensive test with post-test management of women free of additional charges. The accuracy of MarkPap test could allow the health care providers to waive the cost of diagnosis and treatment of "missed" cases. This fact changes the financial balance significantly in favor of the comprehensive test combined with management of women after test (Chaps. 6, 7, Annex and Media).

6.5.2 Global Benefit

	A	B	C	D	E	F	G	H	I	J	K	L	M	N	O
1		impact													
2															
3															
4						**MarkPap Test in Global Application**									
5															
6						ECCONOMIC IMPACT ON STATES									
7				MPT will save		COST/BENFIT ESTIMATE FOR 2015									
8															
9															
10					1	0.08 women lives from those screened									
11					2	saving is three lives (woman and two children at average)									
12					3	1 woman also means 1 full per capita bdp									
13							0.5 women, 1/4 each child								
14															
15															
16					Example India										
17														B/C	
18								*2,480 bdp = 4.216*10 e10						Saving	
19										US				Y>or <N	
20								X*10E6	$	Removal		GDP	per capita		
21			region	state		popul		mpt	X*10E6	0.0008		X*10E6			
22	1		1	1		ALG	40	7	70	5,600		5360	30	<1:2.3	1
23	2		Africa	2		SUDAN	38	5	50	4000		2000		<1:3	2
24	3			3		BE	10.3	1.7	17	1360		804	1	<1:17	3
25	4			4		EG	82	14	140	11200		3314	37	<1:3.7	4
26	5			5		ET	96	17	170	13,600		505	7	<1:2.5	5
27	6			6		KE	44	8	80	6400		1245	7.9	<1: 10	6
28	7			7		NG		30	300	24000		3000	720	>2.4 : 1`	7
29	8			8		SA	53	8.5	85	6800		6617	45	<1: 1.9	8
30	9			9		SRILANKA	21	4	40	3200		3300	10.5	<1:4	9
31	10			10		TA	50	8.5	85	6800		695	4.7	<1:18	10
32	11			11		UG	38	6	60	4800		572	2.74	< 1: 3	11
33	TOTAL						472.3	109.7	1097	87,760		27412	865.84		

34				consideration only										
35				c1		Somalia		c6	Rwuanda					
36				c2		Central Africnl R								
37				c3		Libya								
38				c4		Zimbabve								
39				c5		Togo								
40														
41														
42	12		2	1		AR	42	8	80	6400		14500	79	>1,6:1	1
43	13		America	2		BR	202	34	340	27,200		12,500	340	>1:1	2
44	14			3		CA	35.2	6	60	4800		52,200	250	>4: 1	3
45	15			4		CHI	18	3.5	35	2800		12500	35	>1:1	4
46	16			5		CO	48	8.5	85	6800		7830	53.2	<1:1.6	5
47	17			6		GU	16	2.7	27	21600		3375	7.3	<1:4	6
48	18			7		MX	123	21	210	16,800		1,380	23.183	< 1:9	7
49	19			8		VEN	30	6	60	4800		24600	118	>2:1	8
50	20			9		USA	325	55	550	44000		52,000	22,880	>> 4:1	9
51	TOTAL						839.2	144.7	1447	135200		180,885	23,786		
52				Consideration only											
53					c1	Cuba									
54					c2	Dominican Republic									
55					c3	Panama									
56					c4	Uruguay									
57															
58	21		3	1		AFG	31	5.2	52	4160		674	2.8	< 1: 18	1
59			Asia	16		AZ	9.6	1.5	15	1200		7911	9.5	<1:1.5	16
60	22			2		MAM	56	10	100	800		1000	0.8	<1:11	2
61	23			3		CN	1,374	230	2300	184,000		8000	1,472	< 1:1.5	3
62	24			4		IN	1,280	215	2150	172,000		1480	255	< 1:8	4
63	25			5		INDCN*	105	18	180	14400		3000	43.2	>1:4	5
64	26			6		IR	80	14	140	11200		6600	73.9	<1:1.9	6
65	27			7		JP	127	22	220	17600		47000	827	>3.76 : 1	7
66	28			8		KZ	17	3	30	2400		13700	32.8	>1:209	8
67	29			9		KO-S	51	9	90	7200		26000	187	>2:1	9
68	30			10		KU	4	0.7	7	560		52200	34.8	>5:1	10
69	31			11		MO	3	0.6	6	480		5900	2.8	<1:2	11

70	32			12		RUS	143.5	25	250	20000		14511	290.2	>1.6:1	12
71	33			13		PA	190	32	320	25600		1250	32	<1:10	13
72	34			14		TAI	23.5	5	50	4000		32000	128	>2.5:1	14
73	35			15		THAI	66	12	120	9600		5900	56.6	<1:2	15
74	TOTAL						3560.6	603	6030	475200		227126	3448.4		
75				Consideration only											
76					c1	Uzbekistant									
77															16
78	36		4	1		AU	23	4	40	3200		43,000	137.5	>3.4:1	1
79	37		Australia	2		NZ	4.4	1	10	800		31500	25.2	>2.5 :1	2
80	38			3		INDO	250	42	420	33600		3500	117.6	<1:3.5	3
81	39			4		PHIL	103	12	120	9600		4500	43.2	<1 : 2.7	4
82	TOTAL						380.4	59	590	47200		82,500	323.5		
83															
84	40		5	1		DK	6	1.5	15	1200		58,000	69.6	> 4.6:1	1
85	41		Europe	2		FR	66	11.5	115	9200		41000	377	>3.28:1	2
86	42			3		GER	81	14	140	1120		42000	47	> 3.36: 1	3
87	43			4		GR	11	1.9	19	152		31000	4.7	<1:4	4
88	44			5		HU	10	1.7	17	1360		13500	18.36	<1:10.8	5
89	45			6		IT	51	21	210	16800		38000	638.4	> 3:1	6
90	46			7		MK	2.1	0.36	3.6	288		5000	1.4	<1:2.5	7
91	47			8		NOR	5	0.9	9	720		100000	72	>10:1	8
92	48			9		NED	17	6.5	65	5200		51000	265.2	>4:1	9
93	49			10		PO	39	7	70	5600		135007	75.6	>1:1.08	10
94	50			11		PORT	11	1.9	19	1520		23000	34.9	>1.8:1	11
95	51			12		RO	22	3.6	36	2880		13000	37.4	>1:1	12
96	52			13		SRB	9.5	1.6	16	1280		4500	5.7	<1:2.8	13
97	53			14		SP	48	8.5	85	6560		33000	216.5	>2.5:1	14

98	54			15		SW	10	1.7	17	1360		59000	80	>4.7:1	15
99	55			16		TU	76	12.7	127	10160		8900	90.4	<1:1.4	16
100	56			17		UK	64	11	110	8,800		45,000	396	>> 3.6:1	17
101	TOTAL				Actual		528.6	107.36	1073.6	74,200		700,907	2430.16		
102							population	mpt	cost	removal		gdp	capita		
103							`10e6	`10e6	`10e6	`10e3		`10e6	`10e3		
104			WORLD	56			5,581	1,024	10,240	819,560		5,249,327			
105				194	100% UN		7,300	811	8,110			78,000,000	1,068		
106								126%							
107			%	30	%		76.45%	31.50%							
108															
109				Consideration only											
110					c1	Swithzerland									
111					c2	Ukraine									
112															
113															
114															
115			Survey	57	Countries										
116			Consideration												
117				12	Countries										
118			Total	69											
119				36%	UN members										
120															
121			popul	6	of 7.33	or 79% world									

6.5.3 Socio-economic Advantage of the New Strategy

Achieving the main goal of the new strategy, to reverse negative trends of cervical cancer prevalence and mortality in one country, need tools making the application of this strategy accessible, affordable, accurate, independent, low-cost and simple for use needing no or little additional education.

The best solution is robotics or full automation, which is at this time only desirable goal for the future. Currently, alternatives using IT technology, telecytopathology, biomarker -based abnormal image detection, low trained personnel at the POC, laboratory technicians at field laboratories and telepathology networking for exchange of medical image information, will be used instead of unavailable robotics.

Cervical cancer screening is socio-medical program intended for the application to millions of women at risk (age 16–66) majority of whom belong to underserviced and underserved population who cannot afford paying the full price , and are prone to close less expensive –although less efficacious screening modalities, or usually avoid screening.

Consequently, money-sensitivity is becoming a very large issue for any screening of healthy people in low and middle income countries (LMIC).

Because our strategy is to reverse cervical cancer trends, a task achievable only if the outreach of the population at risk is above 51 %, we have to design such strategy and tools which can be affordable to poor population. Specimen self-sampling kit enables women to collect specimen in the privacy of their homes and to avoid going to POC for specimen collection. MarkPap test enable laboratories to easy and accurately detect biomarker-positive specimens, eliminating 90 % of negative specimens for further processing and saving on the cost for processing negative subjects; telecytopathology allows for high quality consultations with experts in big medical centers, thus keeping the quality of diagnosis for those who need it most, and 1–3 h test turnaround is giving the opportunity to women with a positive test to have medical intervention the same day, or while being present at the premises.

All of these advantages could be achieved only because of the biomarker. For details see Chap. 7 and Annex.

On a large scale, the social and financial gains of the new technology are even more visible.

Since the goal of cervical cancer screening is to save women's lives, it is of utmost importance to see whether saving these lives is economically plausible in comparison with the cost of screening millions of healthy women. The first question to answer is what is the value of a woman's life? This is a very sensitive question completely different in different societies, cultures or religions. We simplified the answer using International Monetary Fond measurement of the Gross Domestic Product per Capita (GDP-C). It is already available for each country (see Sect. 5.3). However, if the men's contribution to this product is indexed one, how much is the contribution of one woman. We calculated that woman's contribution to GSDP is one half of a men, but a woman at average deliver two kids who may contribute with one quarter of a men's contribution. It means that both men and woman could be used as calculation units of same value. This how we calculated the cost/benefit of saving women's lives will add at average $20,000 to the community wealth.

The screening cost is easy to calculate and also the cost of other medical interventions, if needed, could be easy to add. The Table shows how this calculation works for 57 most populous countries in the world or for two thirds of world population.

6.6 Policy Change (India)

To:

EMBASSY OF THE REPUBLIC OF INDIA IN THE UNITED STATES OF AMERICA

Washington, DC 20008
2107 Massachusetts Ave. NW
Attention: Embassy of India, Science & Technology
Counselor Tarun Mohindra
From: Drs. Olivera & Nenad Markovic
BioSciCon, Inc. Rockville, MD
Date: Monday, June 15, 2015
Subject:

Proposal for resolution of the problem of Cervical Cancer in India based upon the experience from US (1945–1995) where the concept for cancer screening of healthy women was developed and from the former SFR Yugoslavia where this concept was first applied in a LMIC country (1978–1990).

I. Background

A. US Experience

In the beginning of Twentieth Century, cervical cancer was "the major killer of women from malignant disease" in the U.S.A. In the beginning of Twenty-first Century, cervical cancer is below the horizon of 10 most important malignant disease in the same country. Cervical cancer prevalence and mortality have dropped for more than 80 %. For the first time in history, the natural course for cervical cancer has been changed by medical intervention.

This result was credited to the nationwide application of Pap test, an In Vitro Diagnostic Test for early detection of lesions that could become cervical cancer and their removal. At average, out of 50 million Pap tests, 3.5 million (7 %) suspect specimens could be found, among which 600,000 with advanced lesions that would be subject to further diagnosis, and 40,000 of them would be operated on time to cure.

In the beginning of Twenty-first Century (2010), about 10,000 women developed new cervical cancer and only 4000 died per year. Retrospectively, half was missed by sampling error (inappropriate sample), one half were missed as false negative (interpretation error).

This tremendous achievement was accomplished by a synchronous action of American Cancer Society, (concept, standards and criteria) National Congress (Laws and regulations), and Federal Government (Organizational layout and financial regulations) and their agencies supported by Health Insurance companies (subsidizing the test from specimen collection, preparation, reading and interpretation) and Health Industry (producing new tools to meet the strategy of mass cervical cancer screening with Pap test and alternatives).

This comprehensive approach may be made available to Indian women for much less money and for shorter time than in it was necessary to develop the System in the US.

B. Yugoslavia Experience

Before 1990 SFR Yugoslavia was a Federation of six states, united by the same national government, national policy, and same money, military and judicial system. Otherwise it was a country with a specific socialistic political system, multi-national, multi-cultural, multi-religious, three official languages, and multiple layers of local (state, regions, and municipalities) development.

When in the second part of the Twentieth Century malignant diseases became serious social, economic and individual problem of the citizens, the professional societies united at the Congress of Yugoslav Oncologists, 1982, adopted a Declaration for unique policy for fight against this danger.

The Policy was later presented by the author of this proposal, at the Federal Assembly and resulted in the Declaration on the Fight Against Malignant Diseases in Yugoslavia.

This became the major legal instrument outlining the Federal and States' policies for years before the disintegration of SFRY, and now is still cited in policies of the new countries separated from the Federation.

C. India Experience

India is a fast growing country both by population (demography growth 1.2 % per year) and by GDP (economy). Even faster, the middle class is growing and is demanding better wellbeing including better health care services and protection from grave diseases, including cancer.

India has 300 million women at risk for cervical cancer. Only 18 million women participate in cervical cancer screening programs.

According to the Indian health statics data, cervical cancer is serious problem for the entire country where prevalence and mortality are much higher than in the US, and are increasing with a rate of 10 % annually. This is considered unacceptable, but there is no way to stop this trend because the outreach (percent of women participating in regular cancer control) was only 6 % (data from 2010). With this outreach of 6 % in 2010, 72, 825 women unnecessarily die each year. It is expected that mortality will further increase for 150 % by the year 2025.

Obviously, increasing the outreach must the main target of the new Strategy. But, how to do this in a country where only 20 million women participate and 280 million are left behind. Our calculations show that the proposed Strategy can make a dramatic change here.

II. Bioscicon's Proposal

1. Objectives

(a) To help the Government of the Republic of India to DECLARE that the FIGHT AGAINST CERVICAL CANCER is a part of the STATE POLICY TO PROMOTE HEALTH WELLBEING AND FOR REVENTION OF DISEASES, AS STATED IN THE Chapter CHRONIC DISEASES AND CANCER.
(b) To describe THE FIGHT AGAINST CERVICAL CANCER AS a Compendium of Legislative, Executive, Judicial and Law Enforceable measures imposed to achieve, as the ultimate goal, to REVERSE the increase of cervical cancer into a downward direction.
(c) To measure the effect of the success achieving these goals by reaching the endpoints of (1) outreach among women at risk of at least 51 %, (2) formation of Indian own infrastructure for manufacturing tools necessary for the increase of the outreach, (3) to organize Indian health care providers, health insurance and health industry (pharma, medical devices) into a System for delivery nationwide affordable cervical cancer screening, (4) to set cups on the cost of the services, and (5) to set up the measures for enforcement of the Policy against the non-compliance.

2. Fight Against Cervical Cancer in India

A. Goals

1. To reverse cervical cancer trends of prevalence and mortality within 10–15 years from the implementation of this new strategy and to achieve US accomplishments in curbing this grave disease much faster and for less money.
2. To create the infrastructure (facilities, equipment, trained personnel, tools, medical and technical protocols) to carry on the strategy and to maintain the services as to guarantee the control of cervical cancer for additional 10–15 years.
3. To educate public, educators, politicians, health care professionals and health care workers and to accept and to promote the Strategy and to maintain high outreach (above 51 % of women at risk) as to keep the downsizing the cervical cancer danger.
4. To provide initial investment into the strategy, but to plan ROI which will reimburse for this investment from the revenue obtained for delivery of services under this Strategy.

B. Objectives

To reverse the prevalence and the mortality of cervical cancer in India within 10–15 years of this Strategy application, by:

1. increasing the outreach of cervical cancer screening to above 51 % among 300 million of Indian women at risk
2. educating Indian health care providers to use the new biomarker based technology combined with IT networking
3. supplying Indian market with tools to meet requirements of the Strategy (local manufacturing and co-manufacturing with international suppliers), and by
4. establishing nationwide support and control over compliance with the Strategy.

C. Tools

In addition to already available tools for cervical cancer screening in India, BioSciCon is offering tools specifically designed to be used in the proposed Strategy. These tools are:

1. Specimen self-sampling kit (Home Test) to be used by women individually and at home to collect specimens and send to laboratories for examination
2. MarkPap® reagents kit, an assembly of reagents and instruction to facilitate laboratories performing 300–1000 individual tests
3. Specimen examining work station, a combination of microscope, digital camera or cell phone camera, PC and flat computer monitor, with connection to the Internet, E-mail, and WiFi
4. Comprehensive Information Technology Telehealth Center for India (C-ITTHC-I), a hub to be connected into Indian national and global network for mass cervical cancer screening.

D. Procedures

1. Medical Protocol for individual and mass cervical cancer screening based upon the membership of scattered Points-of Care with the remote expert C-ITTHC-I
2. Technical Protocol to connect POC and C-ITTHC-I into a national network and to extend the connection with the Global Network for cervical cancer screening.

E. Financing

1. Initial financing to be provided by inventors (Government, private, banks, insurance, health industry)
2. Service to be maintained by insurance membership dues, by reimbursement for services rendered to members and others
3. Investment into further improvements to be paid from the profits collected of the revenue obtaining from products and services sold
4. Charities and non-profit investments are welcome. To complete budget requirements.

III. Implementation of the Proposed National Strategy

The new strategy can be implanted by a synchronous action of all of the following elements:

1. LEGISLATIVE (NATIONAL AND STATES' POLICY)
2. EXECUTIVE (ORGANIZATION OF INFRASTRUCTURE AND FINANSING)
3. JUDICIAL (LAW AND REGULATIONS TO PROTECT THE POLICY)
4. PROFESSIONAL (HEALTH STANDARDS AND CRITEORIA TO REACH THEM).

Please also see PPP Visit to I Embassy 2015-Annex, Media, video and Brochure.

Chapter 7
New Tools

7.1 MarkPap® Illustrated

MarkPap Illustrated is a summary of procedures and tools designed and developed to facilitate performing the mass cervical cancer screening under the auspices of the New Strategy.

7.1.1 MarkPap® Test

MarkPap® test is a trademark for CAP-PAP Test [114]. CAP is an acronym for **C**ervical **A**cid **P**hosphatase and PAP indicating dual staining with Papanicolaou stains, as a counterstain. This is to preserve all the advantages of Pap test, which was proclaimed "the best cancer screening test" for decades.

CAP is an isoenzyme, a distinct molecular form of the family of acid phosphatase, present in cervical cells. This isoenzyme typically changes its protein structure (isoenzyme architecture) and its activity along cellular differentiation and tissue maturation. The enzyme is active in basal cells, but gradually reduces its activity from basal to peripheral layers.

Similar pattern of "biochemical maturation" was earlier seen by the same author in megacaryocytes. Megakaryocytic Acid Phosphatase (acid phosphatase present in megakaryocytic lineage) is changing its isoenzyme architecture along the maturation of the cell line from megakaryoblasts to mature megakaryocytes producing platelets. The same isoenzyme, present in mature megakaryocytes was found in trombocytes. This discovery helped differentiate platelet- forming megakaryocytes in different thrombocytopenias [194].

Similarly, CAP is always inactive/negative in normal squamous epithelial cells, while present/positive in basal cells (Fig. 7.1). Only abnormal, less differentiated cells contain this isoenzyme. Precancerous/dysplastic cells and cancerous cells are

N. Markovic, O. Markovic, *What Every Woman Should Know about Cervical Cancer*, DOI 10.1007/978-94-017-7560-1_7

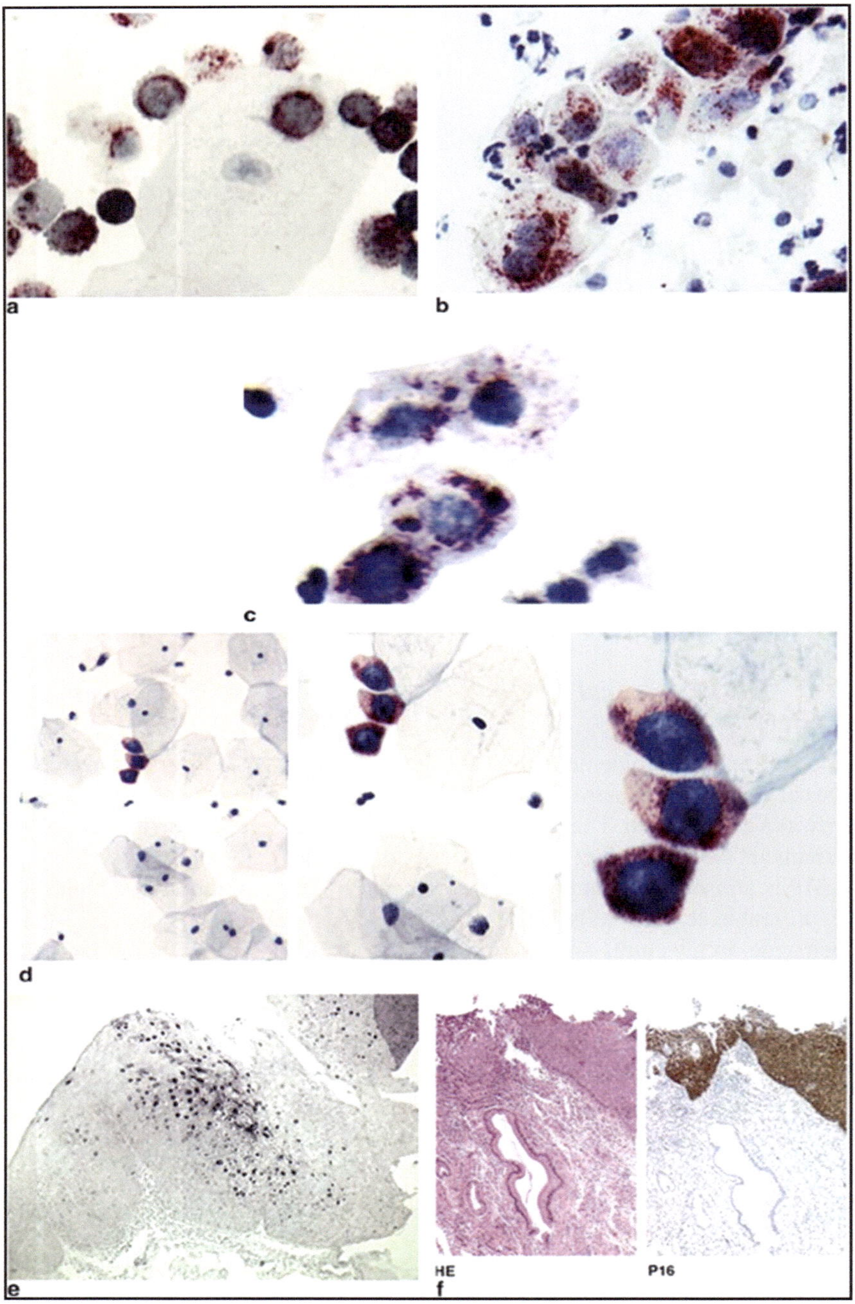

Fig. 7.1 Biomarkers and MPT. (**a**) MarkPap control slides: Cervical acid phosphatase (CAP) marker is the red, granular deposit inside cells counterstained bluish). Control slides are composed of HeLa cell-line cells and buccal cells. HeLa cell line was derived from a human cervical cancer

positive. The red marker is so clearly visible on the bluish Pap counterstaining that can hardly be missed (Fig. 7.1d).

MarkPap® test is the manual version of MarkPap® platform technology and the first product in the MarkPap products pipeline. To visualize the presence of CAP the MarkPap® test has utilized nanotechnology-like reaction producing insoluble deposit of red pigment on the enzyme sites in the cell [21]. Morphological structures are presented with modified Papanicolaou staining procedure.

The red-colored CAP is easily visible and serves to alert the cytoscreener to stop at the "red signal" and more carefully examine the morphology of this cell based on Pap staining (Fig. 7.1b–d).

Therefore, on the normal (healthy) Pap test specimen the squamous epithelial cells are biomarker negative ("no red signal"), only bluish counterstaining visualizing morphological details. However, if abnormal cells are present on the specimen, or lower layer cells have reached the periphery (what would be another sign of dysplasia), those cells will be highlighted with a red biomarker to serve as a "stop light" to alert cytotechnologist to stop and more carefully examine the labeled cell [116–118] (Fig. 7.1b–d). Since Papanicolaou staining is present on the same slide (double staining procedure) cytotechnologist is using morphologic (Pap criteria) to evaluate the cell (Fig. 7.1b–d) [210].

Monocytes are the only other cell type on the slide that are Positive, and serve as an internal quality control. If monocytes are negative, the test should be repeated. For external quality control, we have prepared Combo Control Slides (included in the MarkPap® Reagent Kit), which are cytospin's preparation of normal buccal cells (CAP negative) and HeLa cervical cancer cell line cells always CAP positive (Fig. 7.1a).

The red granular pigment is the image of CAP activity visualized by formation of a color precipitating deposit [114]. It can be used alone (for digital analysis), or in combination with different counterstaining (in this case Pap staining) to visualize the cellular background (for cytology).

The specimen could be obtained by direct smearing (Pap smear) or by transferring suspended cells from specimen collecting solution onto microscopic slides

Fig. 7.1 (continued) is known to be HPV 18 infected and full of cervical acid phosphatase. Buccal cells are negative for CAP activity. (**b**) MarkPap positive cervical cancer (squamous): A strip of abnormal cervical cells (irregular size and shape of cells and their nuclei, but with larger irregular nuclei and darker chromatic, cytoplasmic vacuolization) surrounded with inflammatory cells. (**c**) CAP positive koilocytes: Four abnormal squamous cells with signs typical for dysplasia and HPV infection (irregular nuclei and cavities in cytoplasm). Specimen taken from a patient with high-risk HPV types found on HC 2 test. (**d**) MarkPap biomarker: Three CAP positive abnormal cells surrounded with normal superficial squamous cells and few neutrophils (to compare sizes). Microscope magnification × 20, × 40 and × 100. (**e**) Biomarker for HPV 31 and HPV 32 (With permission from IARC-Histopathology of the uterine cervix – Digital atlas, 2004) Immunohybridization technique (HIS). Thin section of cervical tissue. Several biomarker positive cells identifying presence of HPV virus. (**f**) Biomarker for p16. HE – Hematoxylin/eosin only. P16 – HIS. Cytoplasm and nuclei contain p16 biomarker. (With permission from IARC-Histopathology of the uterine cervix – Digital atlas, 2004)

[84]. Both collection techniques are applicable for MarkPap test. Cytopeservative Solution for specimen collection is supplied together with the Kit, when requested (Fig. 7.4). For developing countries testing in rural areas, and self-collection of specimens, we recommend Pap smears to be used.

This is the most simplified description of MarkPap® test. Otherwise, in the scientific literature, it is described as "*cytoplasmic expression of genetic changes inside nuclei of cervical cells in transformation from normal to dysplastic and malignant, detected by digital imaging after a nano-molecular signal was amplified by chemical catalysis of a substrate in a micro-cellular array system on microscopic slides.*"

In preclinical studies, the analytical sensitivity (positive test when marker is present) of this test was found to be 99.98 %, while the analytical specificity (negative test when marker is not present) 99.99 % [117, 118].

In clinical trials, the diagnostic accuracy (sensitivity/specificity) of correct diagnosis (MarkPap positive/negative) was 88 % or much better than the control Pap smears (51 %) [116, 196, 209, 211, 220]. In addition, it was shown that the biomarker is positive in cells scrapped or shaded from warts (HPV disease which is not cervical cancer). Consequently, CAP biomarker, if present, could serve as a cytological prescreening alert for selection of women probably infected with high risk HPV and suggests further viral testing for HPV presence [165].

7.1.2 MarkPap® Reagent Kit with Accessories

The MarkPap® Kit was created in 2001 with the goal to simplify and standardize the staining procedure. This is a set of reagents necessary for biomarker visualization and Papanicolaou stains for morphological staining. Reagents are ready-made for use. Only the fixative solution should be prepared. The Kit also contains a citrate buffer for the fixative preparation and Combo Control Slides.

Combo Control slides are cytospin preparations of a combination of biomarker positive He-La cultured cells and normal squamous epithelial buccal cells which are

CLINICAL TRIALS RESULTS

2,000 s/s	NEW	CTR-1 Pap	CTR-2 LBP	Advantage
Ancillary	CAP	Pap	ThP	CAP+PAP
MarkPap	CAP+PAP	Pap	ThP	D-Ac, Se, FN
Diagnostic Accuracy*	0.93	0.51	0.82	1.8:1:1.6
Sensitivity	0.88	0.51	0.8	1.7:1:1.5
False negative	4	18	17	1:5:4

July 18, 2015 Business Overview 2007 8

Fig. 7.2 NIH phase III clinical trial (2002–2005): NEW: *CAP* cervical acid phosphatase, *PAP* Papanicolaou staining, *ThP* ThinPrep Pap test. J. Clin. Oncology 2005:23, 165: 1021

biomarker negative. One fully processed Combo slide is provided for the person who is staining specimens at the POC to see the features of a well—processed MarkPap slide. Other slides are Combo specimen slides which are fixed, but left unstained to serve as quality control slides to be processed together with the actual staining of test samples.

He-La small round cells (abnormal cervical cells) must be biomarker positive with red granular deposit in the cytoplasm; big, flat epithelial buccal cells (simulating cervical squamous epithelial cells) must be entirely negative, without any granule of red biomarker presence [210]. If the pattern is any different the specimen should be discarded and new specimen prepared. We ask the person from POC to transmit the images of the microscopic field to BioSciCon for external Quality Control during training. We also recommend control slides to be sent to the pathologist who is performing the telecytopathology service.

The MarkPap Kit is a simple, customer-friendly, easy to use, fast procedure that can be performed by a low-trained technician with 1 day education. We have trained many persons performing MarkPap test on site, and on-line. It was a very successful process. Combo Control Slides secure the success.

The Technical Insert from the MarkPap Kit with detailed information about the reagents, controls, step-by-step technical procedure for processing the biomarker and cytological staining, and precautions is supplied with each Kit. Illustrations with images of MarkPap positive and MarkPap negative cells are also provided together with Evaluation Criteria for reading MarkPap slides (Figs. 7.3 and 7.4).

The specimen could be obtained by direct smearing of the sample on the microscopic slide (Pap smear), or by transferring suspended cells from specimen collected in solution on slides (liquid-based specimens) [84, 115, 226]. Both collection techniques are applicable for MarkPap test. However, the collection fluid must not contain components which will inhibit CAP.

Several papers were published and presented during the last 20 years confirming the utility and the advantages of the MarkPap test increasing the sensitivity of the

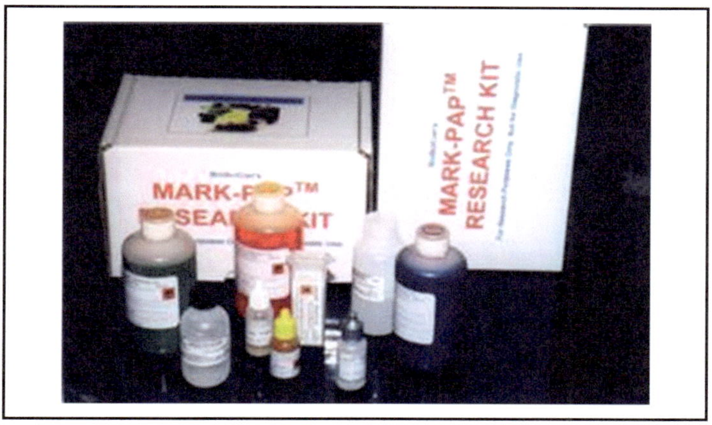

Fig. 7.3 MarkPap Reagent Kit

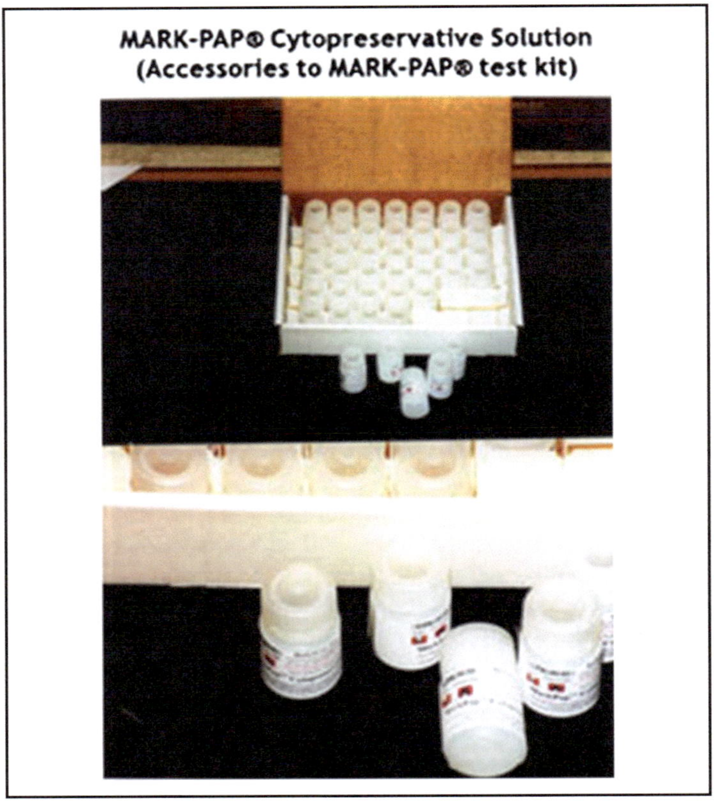

Fig. 7.4 MarkPap cytopreservative solution

test and decreasing the rate of false-negatives to less than 5 %. The specificity is equal to the Pap test [114–122, 194–197, 202, 206–222].

Further advantages were confirmed in the options for specimen self collection MarkPap Self and Telecytopathology Service – diagnosis at distance, see further [20–22, 114–122, 195–197].

The validity of MarkPap test was confirmed outside the US, too.

7.1.2.1 India Study

We had a long standing collaboration with AIIMS, All India Institute of Medical Sciences in New Delhi. The group from Department of Pathology and Department of Obstetrics and Gynecology performed an independent study with MarkPap test Kit and published their results in Indian Journal of Cytology [198]. In 2014, more recent joint results with emphasis on cytological screening in low-resource countries were presented on the International Congress of Cytology in Paris [199].

Both trials were successful and confirmed the validity of CAP-PAP test in detection of abnormal cells.

Prof. Santwani from the Department of Pathology at the MP Shah Medical College, Jamnagar and her assistant at the Punjab Institute of Medical Sciences, Jalandhar, Gujarat, India, performed a clinical trial with MarkPap® Research Kit, and published their results in 2015 concluding that CAP-PAP test could be the future of cervical cancer screening [200].

Prof. Nenad Markovic mentored a doctoral candidate at the Videhi Institute of Medical Sciences in Bangalore, who performed a successful clinical trial confirming the value of CAP-PAP test and published the results in 2015 [201].

7.1.2.2 CAP – PAP in China

In 2008, we started a joint project under Trade Agreement for clinical trials in China, with Anhui Biotechnology Group from Hefei, Anhui Province [205].

Unfortunately, MarkPap technology was stolen from a neighbor company Anyon Biopharmaceuticals [204]. Regardless of published papers and US Patent in the year 2000, the first edition of this book, more than 100 references on the Internet, this firm got Chinese patents in year 2010 and they are selling our Kit under the name FCS-811.

Anyon continues to copy other products from the MarkPap® pipeline, e.g. MarkPap Self [www.anyon.com.cn; 204].

Later, another company, Anhui Science and Technology Co. was incorporated in the same city for the same intention to sell the counterfeit product. This Company is aggressively marketing and selling our Kit under their name New MarkPap and NM-PAP [www.whnmst.com; 203].

7.1.3 MarkPap® Specimen Self-Collection™ Kit

In spite of several attempts, the Pap test could have never been adapted to use exfoliated cells from the vaginal fluids. This is because the morphology of exfoliated cells is changed in vaginal fluids and do not allow proper diagnosis. However, in case of MarkPap test, the red biomarker is not destructible in the vaginal fluids, and it is clearly visible in morphologically damaged cells, even in a part of cell.

The first self-collecting small kit was designed and US Patent is pending (Fig. 7.5).

A woman is supposed to collect specimens at home and send it to the laboratory for further processing and evaluation [21, 121, 122].

The Kit contains two microscopic slides in a slide holder, two sterile Q tips-like applicators, serviette – cleansing wipe, Laboratory Request Form, address label where to send the specimen, with instructions and illustration how to collect the material.

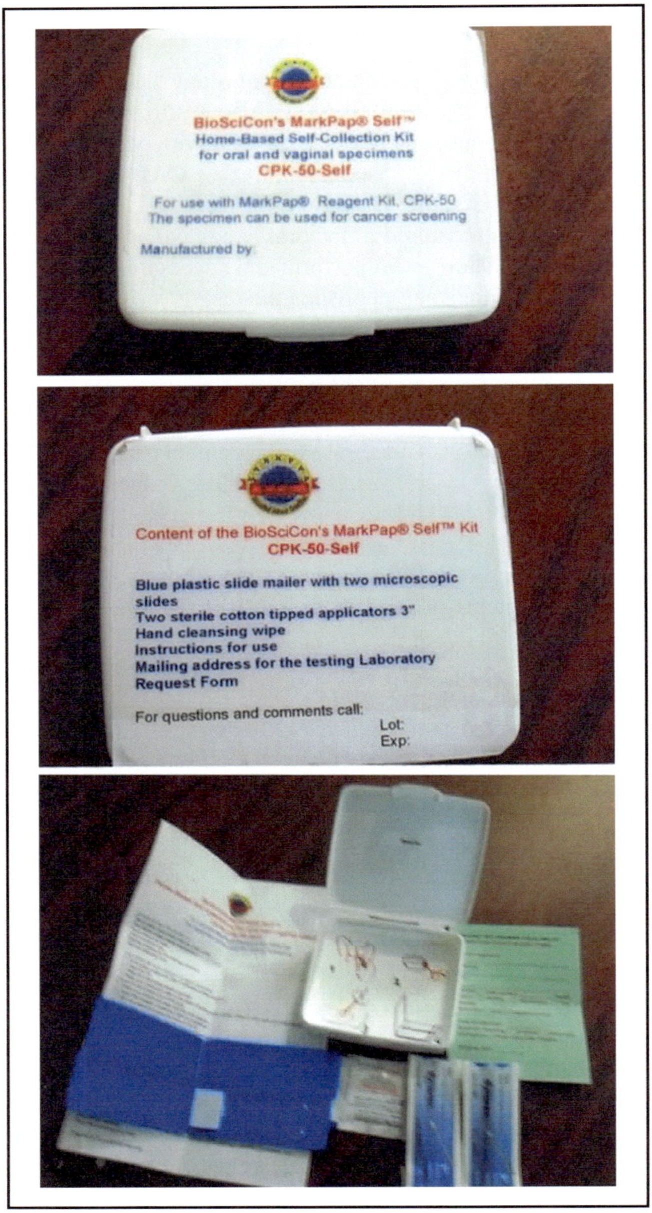

Fig. 7.5 This is home-based self collection kit for oral and vaginal specimen collection, MarkPap® Self-Collection ™ Kit, CPK-50 self. The first two figures are showing the external view, front and back (upper and medium). The interior/content of home kit is shown on the lower part of the figure

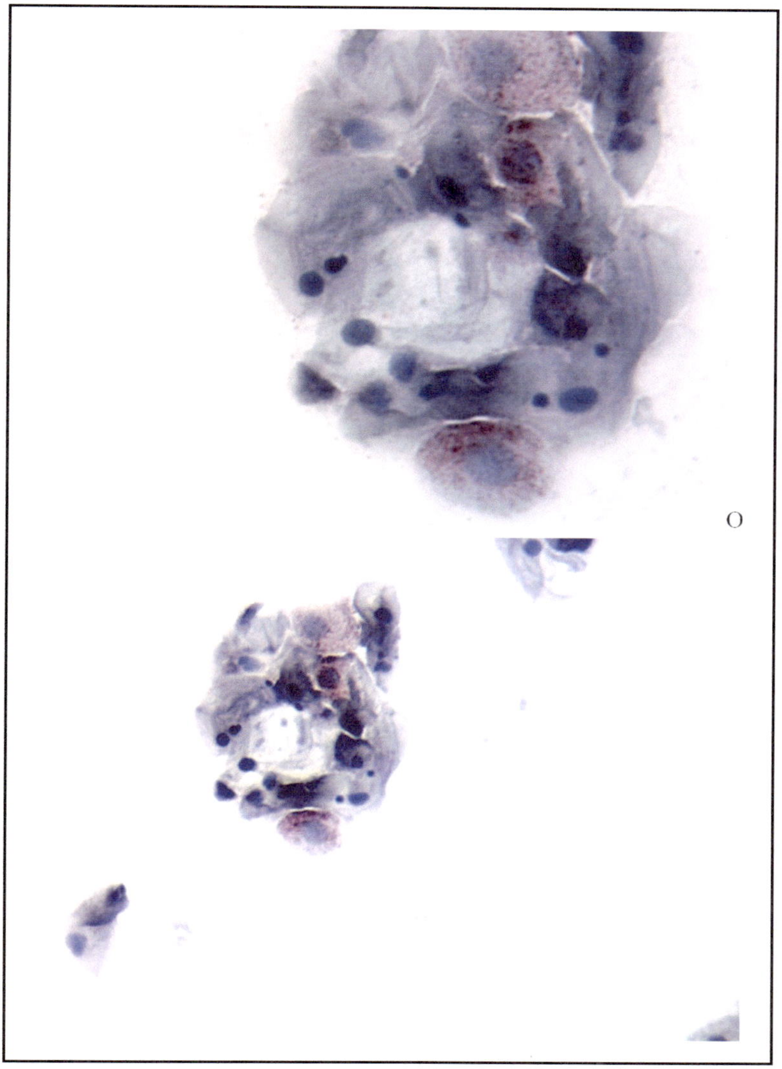

Fig. 7.6 MarkPap test performed on self-collected cervical specimen (two magnifications). Regardless that the cellular morphology is damaged, the non-destructible biomarker is clearly visible

Please see more information and illustration about self-collection test and Kit in Annex of the book. This Kit can also be used for oral specimen collection (Figs. 7.6 and 7.7).

Although the cell morphology is damaged in the vaginal fluids, the cell could usually be identified; however the attention is focused on the MarkPap red biomarker, which is unchanged. Even in much damaged cells, in particles of cytoplasm the marker is clearly visible. The presence of the marker signals suspicious abnor-

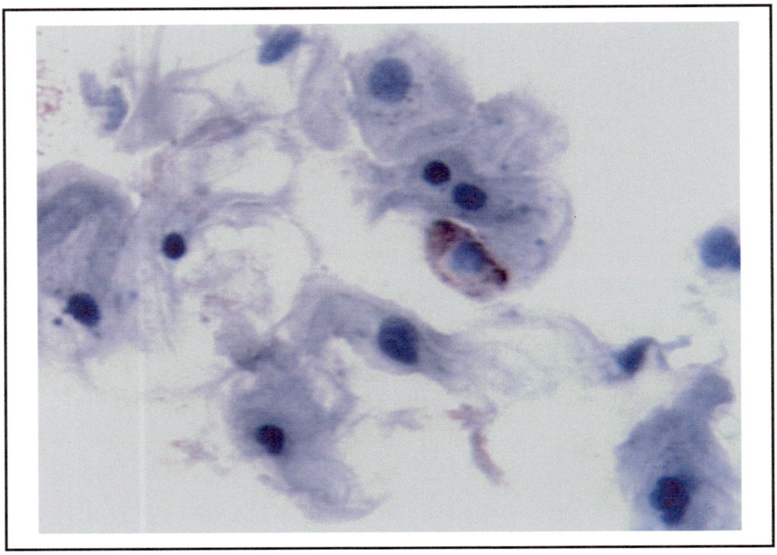

Fig. 7.7 MarkPap positive specimen. Note the biomarker labeled cell

mality, which should be confirmed with the specimen taken from the cervix. First two specimens contain biomarker-positive cells. The last sample is MarkPap negative; there is no red biomarker positive cell.

Having a suspicious or abnormal Home test a woman is now much more motivated to see gynecologist, than without having any symptoms what is frequently seen in the beginning of the disease.

Taking specimens is completely harmless, so women can check the status frequently and have "pre-screening" for cervical cancer (Fig. 7.8).

Please visit www.bioscicon.com/galleries.html, where you can see a gallery of self-collected specimen processed with MarkPap test [210].

MarkPap Self test can be evaluated on site, or the slide can be sent to a distant place for evaluation.

The Fig. 7.9 below presents a scheme for distant reading of slides.

This is a short description on MarkPap Self [21, 103, 121, 122]. The evaluation of slides can be done on site if there is a trained person present, or can be a subject for diagnosis at distance (telecytopathology).

With the introduction of the Self Specimen Collection Test, two of the barriers for not having screening (un-accessibility and cultural sensitivity) could be alleviated, leading to tremendously increased outreach.

7.1.4 *MarkPap Telecytopathology Services*

Mark Pap Telecytopathology Services can be performing with digital transmission of images (MarkPap Digital) and with mobile transmission of images (MarkPap Mobile).

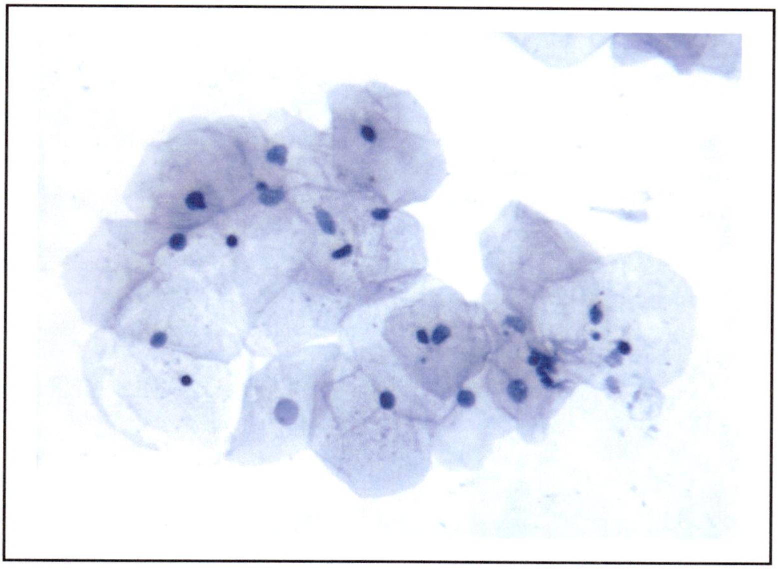

Fig. 7.8 MarkPap negative specimen

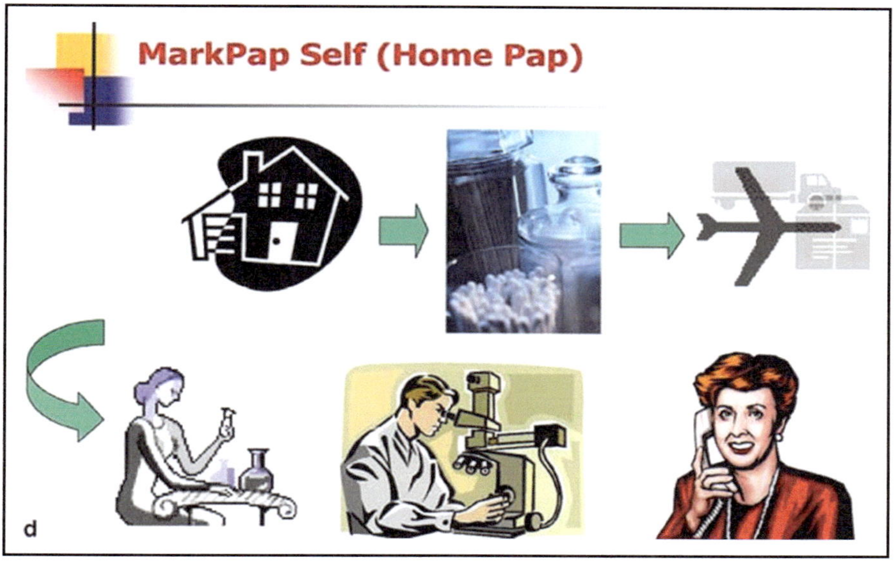

Fig. 7.9 MarkPap self evaluated at distance

7.1.5 MarkPap® Digital – TelePap

MarkPap Digital or Tele-Pap denotes MarkPap test with digital transmission and evaluation at distance, and the service provided is MarkPap Telecytopathology Service.

The visual characteristics of the biomarker make digital imaging easily applicable, an advantage that has been put in development under the name MarkPap® Digital (TelePap) since 2005 [202, 207–212].

The authors of this book frequently emphasize that, not the price, but lack of infrastructure at the POC is the most important barrier to implement mass cervical cancer screening and to fight cervical cancer worldwide. Building infrastructure (including trained cytotechnologists and pathologists) at the POC is most difficult to achieve – needs decades to develop.

However, the MarkPap platform offers a solution to this problem by its Telecytopathology Service, which makes MarkPap test infrastructure independent. At the same time, the cost of the test is being decreased, what again is making the test affordable for greater number of women.

Telecytopathology service is one of the three components of the armamentarium recommended to fight cervical cancer in India (Annex and Media).

The specimen processing is being done at the POC, but evaluation is performed on digitally transmitted images to the specialist at a distant place. When talking about specimen evaluation at distance—telecytopathological diagnosis at distance (either digital or mobile) there is one problem that should always be recognized. In standard telecytopathology (without biomarker), there is still a necessity to have trained person at the POC who will recognize suspicious cells and choose to transmit only those cells to specialist for distant diagnosis. The person at the POC cannot transmit hundreds randomly chosen images for distance diagnosis – it is too expensive. This fact was limiting telecytopathology to occasional consultation or educational purposes only, not for everyday routine practice (See Media).

Here, MarkPap technology is of essential help—abnormal cells are already highlighted with red color with the biomarker, and a low-trained person at the POC can choose to transmit only 8–10 images of the microscopic fields with those marked, pre-selected cells (Fig. 7.10).

VIDEO (see Media).

This fact makes MarkPap Telecytopathology Service possible to use in everyday practice, and MarkPap technology infrastructure independent.

We made a template with data (barcoded) for the patient with all necessary information for the pathologist, space to insert images and space for the response from pathologist. Please see the Template further in this Chapter (Sect. 7.4). We have tested the template between different locations and the POC within the US, and between US India, China and Serbia.

What is the hardware necessary for the telecytopathology service? It depends of the anticipated number of patients and the complexity of the design for functioning.

Generally, it includes three units:

1. Image Acquisition Unit at the POC to acquire images
2. Images Processing Unit to collect the images and forward them to different destinations for evaluation, and collect them back and send reports to the originating POC

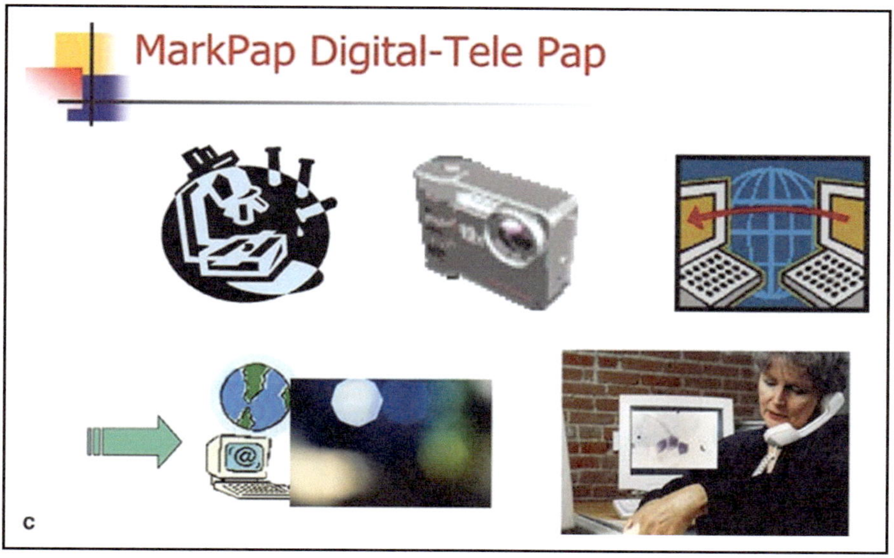

Fig. 7.10 Transfer of images from the microscope equipped with camera through the Image Processing Unit to the Image Evaluation Unit with instant telephone reporting of the result

3. Image Evaluation Units at the hospital or doctor's office where the specimen evaluation is performed and cytopathological results are generated.

It may vary from a simple workstation at the POC and a doctor's office with direct communication between them, to the IT Telehealth Center – ITTHC (local, province, state centers) with multiple Image Acquisition Units and the Image Processing Units, aimed for millions of tests per year (See further Sect. 7.2).

The simplest organization is a Workstation consisting of an Image Acquisition Unit equipped with a microscope with video camera at the POC, as presented on Fig. 7.11, and Image Evaluation Unit at a distant place (doctor's office with a PC or hospital). The communication with the POC is direct, without Image Processing Unit.

Depending on the number of cases, there may be many Image Acquisition Unit workstations.

More cases will require also the addition of the Image Processing Unit to sort and forward images to the Image Evaluation Unit/Units, to collect and to return them to the originator, the Image Acquisition Unit/Units. The Image Processing Unit consists of Database, Web and Administrative Servers.

All three units are becoming structures integrated in the IT Telehealth Centers (ITTHC). See the next Section on ITTHC (Sect. 7.2).

The blue print of the ITTHC is presented on Fig. 7.12 below.

The ITTHC are hierarchically organized in local, province, state centers. The Local IT Telehealth Center is designed for an architecture (application software and hardware) of a local center implemented by a proprietary communication network

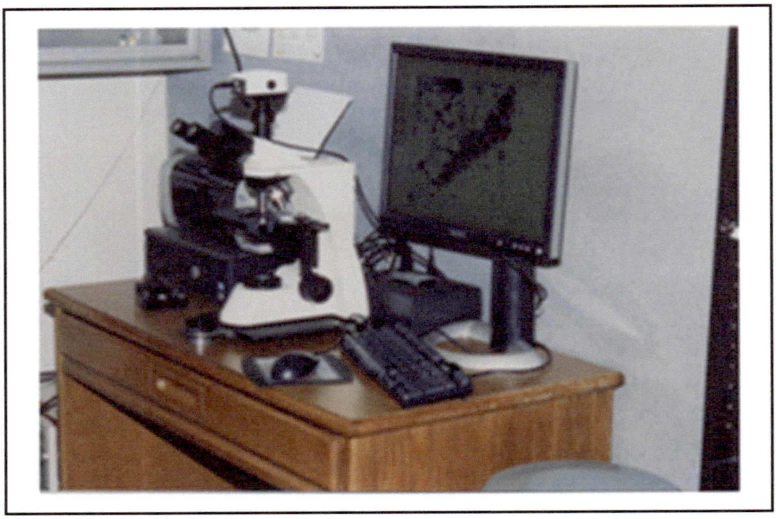

Fig. 7.11 A digital telecytopathology workstation consisting of a microscope, digital camera and computer capture, store and forward image files

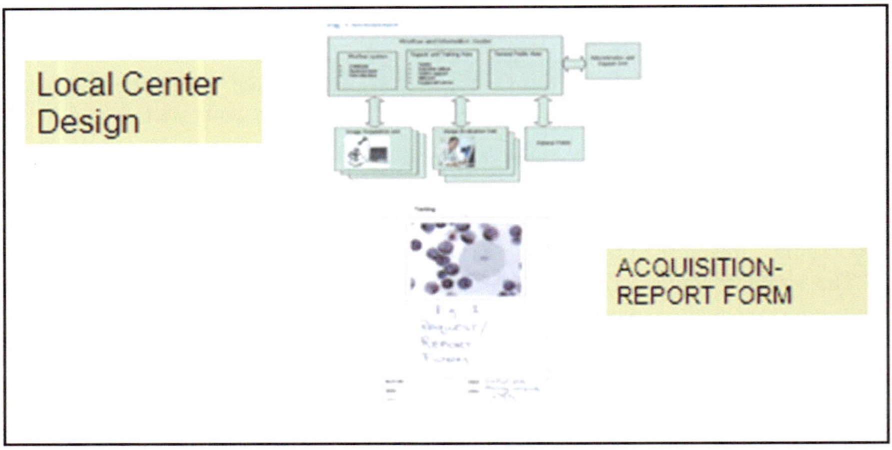

Fig. 7.12 IT Telehealth Center: Architecture (www.bioscicon.com/productsindev.html)

to a global networking system, connected by a unique medical diagnostic protocol to enable automatic exchange of high resolution, still image metadata files between humans on both sides of the networking system (POC and medical centers) (See further ITTHC Sect. 7.2).

The automation makes this Center a low-cost device for cervical cancer screening [206, 207, 209, 213–215].

We have designed and tested MarkPap Telecytopathology Services at different levels within the US and abroad (with India, China, Serbia). The quality of the digital images received in the evaluation units corresponded to the images seen directly in the microscope, and allowed the diagnosis to be made as with (diagnostic images) [225].

7.1.6 *MarkPap® Mobile, Mobile Pap*

7.1.6.1 Transmission of Microscopic Images Using Cell Phone Cameras

Mobile Health (M –Health) denotes delivering healthcare services using mobile wireless communications that have recently emerged as a new viable option for providing healthcare all over the world. According to the United National Foundation, M-Health is high reach, cost-effective method for making healthcare accessible, affordable and effective globally.

Many regions in the world do not have access to the Internet, but 80 % population lives in regions with mobile phone accessibility. This in a huge market for the new M-Health methods, products and services, and a target for Global Health Initiative and its followers.

During the last 15 years, BioSciCon, supported by the Global Academy for Women's Health, Inc., works the application of telemedicine in pathology/telecyto-pathology. During the recent 7 years, our attention was focused on Mobile Telemicroscopy: Capturing and transferring microscopic image files obtained with cell phone cameras from the POC to distant centers for instant diagnosis [207, 208, 209, 214, 215, 217, 218–222].

For this purpose a microscopic adapter to mount the camera on the ocular is a must.

We have developed a proprietary Universal Smartphone – Microscopic Adapter that can be applied on any microscope and any cell phone camera. It simulates human hand movement in 4D and it is unique and distinct from all other commercially available products built for the same purpose. Patent is pending [218].

The next Figure illustrates the Mobile Acquisition Unit, with the Adapter mounted on the microscopic ocular. The Image Acquisition Unit is the same as for Digital Pap Workstation, only instead of Digital camera mounted on the microscope, here, the Universal Adapter is mounted on the ocular holding the cell phone (Samsung). Again, if more cases are to be examined, there may be multiple Image Acquisition Units, connected with the multiple Image Evaluation Unit via the Image Processing Unit in between (Figs. 7.13 and 7.14).

Examples of images of the microscopic fields with cell phone camera using Universal Adapter and images of microscopic fields obtained with digital camera, from the same specimen are presented on Fig. 7.15. The specimen is cervical smear cytological preparation with abnormal cervical cell highlighted by MarkPap biomarker. Images captured with CCD digital microscopic camera (.jpeg format) are in quadrangular frames, images captured with cell phone cameras (AT&T, Samsung, Eternity format) are those in round frames.

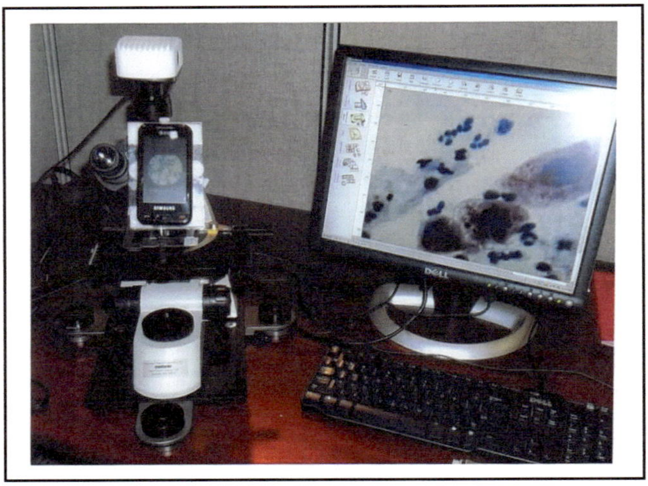

Fig. 7.13 MarkPap mobile image acquisition workstation

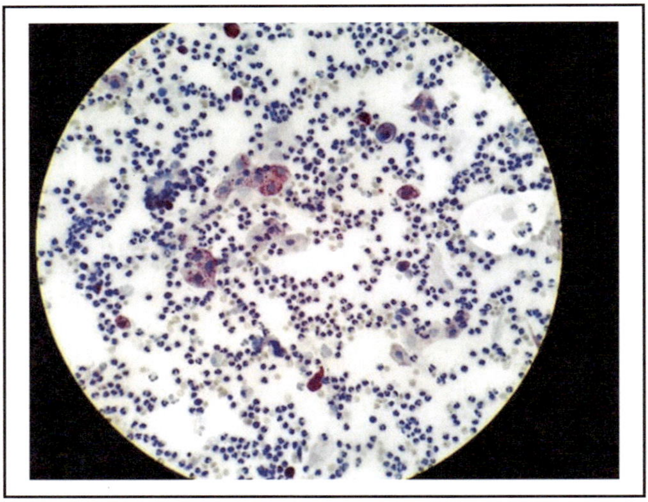

Fig. 7.14 The image from the cell phone screen obtained at the Mobile Workstation Image Acquisition Unit

It is obvious that the images taken by the digital camera and cell phone camera using the Universal Adapter are comparable and the Image analysis or medical diagnosis could be performed interchangeably. Our Universal Adapter that can be used on "any microscope" and "any cell phone camera" is essential to obtain internal consistency and reliability of the measurements, allowing diagnosis of abnormal conditions.

The flowchart for IT Telehealth Center including M-Health is presented on the Fig. 7.16

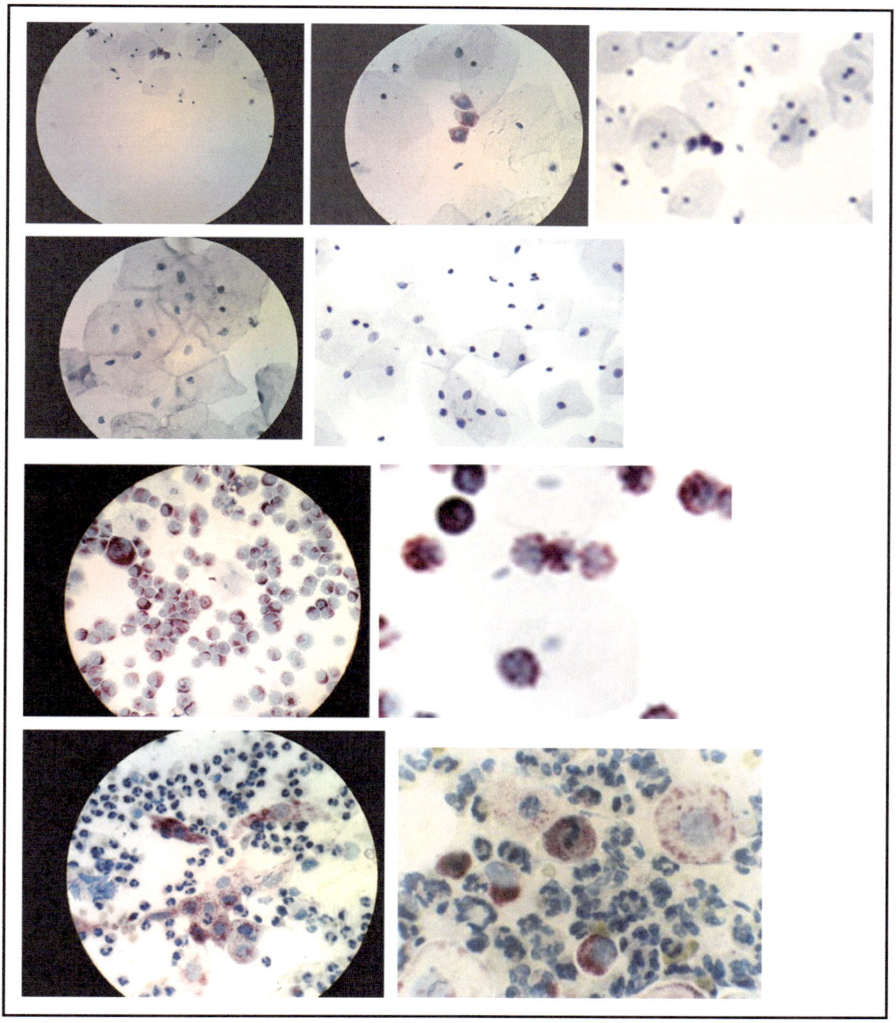

Fig. 7.15 (**1–3**) is different magnification of the same specimen/cells: Three small cells, with dark blue nucleus and red pigment in the cytoplasm, surrounded with big cells which are stained light blue. All images are similar, but the digital camera had the best illumination conditions. (**4–5**). Although in single color (bluish) all morphological features are well preserved to allow cytological diagnosis. Our adapter-model needs more adjustment to provide for better illumination conditions. This adjustment will be done on the prototype (**6–7**) The images captured from a control slide, are made artificially from two types of cells for the purpose of quality control. These are small red cells and big blue cells. Again at different magnifications, but the illumination is better on the cell phone captured image than on the previous slides. (**8–9**) presents images captured with CCD camera and cell phone camera from a cancer specimen. The MarkPap red biomarker (please see BioSciCon' galleries) is present in abundance, both inside cytoplasm of individual cells and in the clusters of positive cells. This diagnosis cannot be missed by either technology

Digital and mobile-acquired images of the same specimens obtained with digital cameras and cell phone cameras

All images captured with digital CCD camera (jpeg format) are in quadrangular frames. All images captured with the cell phone camera are in round frames. Different magnifications are presented. Please contact us for more information

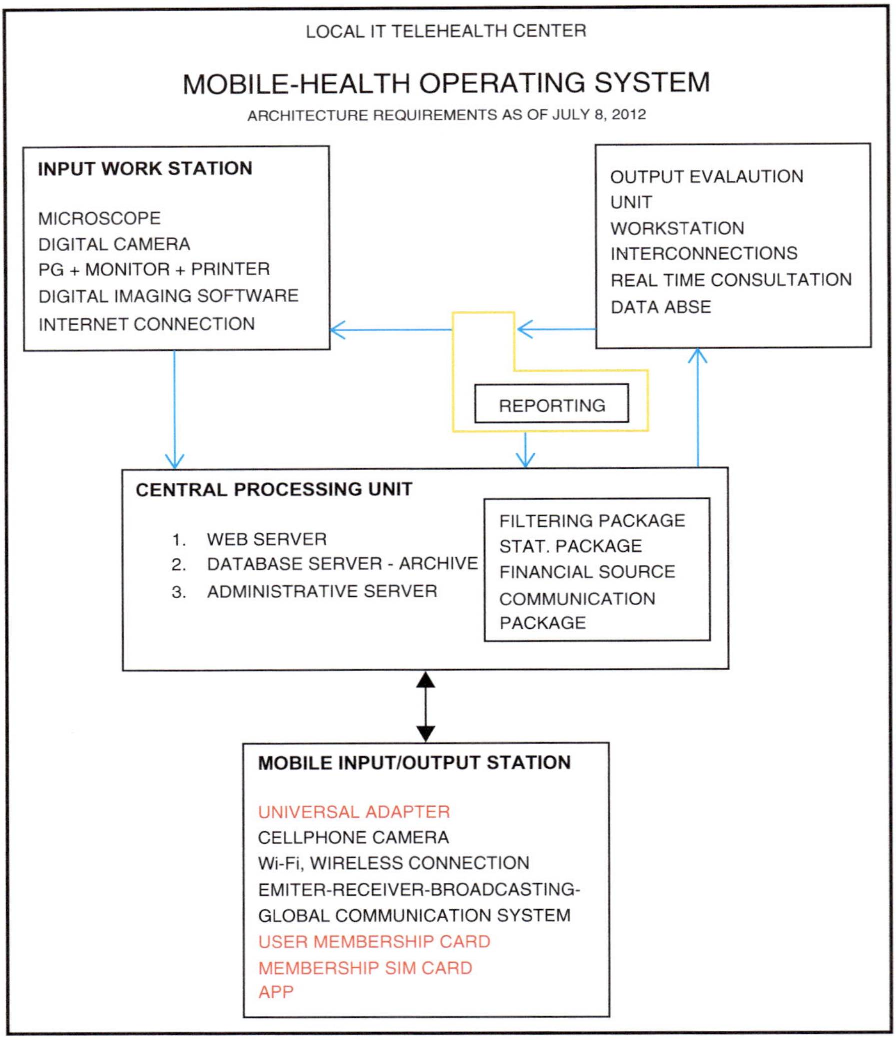

Fig. 7.16 Flowchart for IT Telehealth Center

Practically, it means that the specimen (taken in the medical facility or obtained at home –self sampling) is first processed with MarkPap Reagent Kit by a low-trained technician at the POC. The same person places the specimen on the microscope and looks for "red-labeled" cells. Using a cell phone, attached with adapter on the ocular, or digital camera on the microscope, transmits only those labeled cells to the center for distant diagnosis. It is done as an image file through secure web site using a Template provided for images and other necessary data for the patient with added space for the response-diagnosis. If it is a simple workstation the image file goes directly to the pathologist (Image Evaluation Unit) and it is directly returned to the POC (Image Acquisition Unit).

In 2014 we expanded on the ITTHC, introducing a Comprehensive Information Technology Health Care Center for Cervical Cancer combining it with mobile transmission of images (M-health) and Field medical Intervention Service, with Units for small intervention and colposcopy is performed immediately when necessary. The whole procedure is now called 1-Day Pap Test. The average price per test could be as low as $10.00. See Fig. 7.17 below.

7.1.6.2 More Ideas

The former discussion was focused on Pap smear and liquid-based Pap test specimens. However, cervical cancer screening worldwide is performed with other methods, which all can benefit from addition of biomarker and IT devices and networking. This is the case the Vinegar Test (VIA or VILI), HPV-only and See & Treat. MarkPap testing could be easily attached to these alternative screening procedures. In such "improved" techniques, the nurse taking a specimen and having an instant cytological diagnosis with MarkPap will be more secure and less liable to continue with cryoablation, if appropriate.

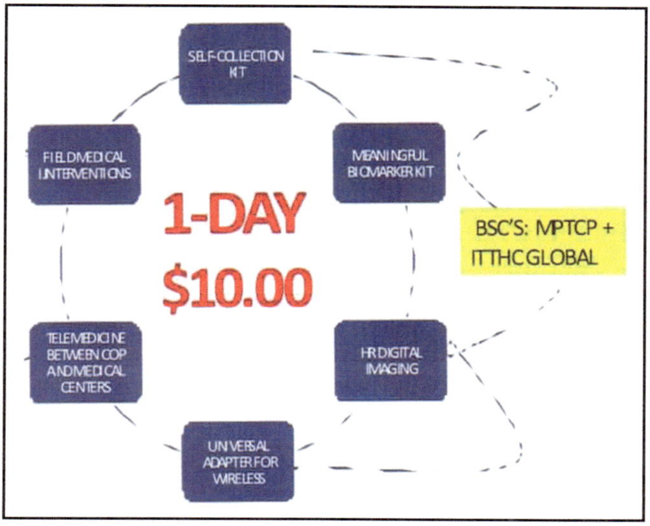

Fig. 7.17 One-day complete service screening-diagnosis-therapy

Instead of naked eye and Vinegar, here is the cytological test and tremendous improvement for VIA tests.

7.1.6.3 Summary of MarkPap Platform Technology: MarkPap Advantage

Based on all its advantage the MarkPap technology can be defined as biomarker-based, telemedicine-enabled, low-cost, simple, affordable, accessible, equitable infrastructure independent platform technology. When implemented, this technology will be among those which can bring right care at the right place at the right time for lower cost. This is currently the only promise for mass cytological cervical cancer screening worldwide.

In Conclusion, for world-wide distribution, we selected and assembled three products and services:

MarkPap(r) Test Kit is an assembly of reagents, controls and instructions developed to facilitate the performance of MarkPap(r) test. This test is a low-cost simple, easy-to-use, accurate, affordable and may be performed by low-trained technician at the Point-of Care (POC). This will dramatically increase the number of locations where specimens can be processed.

MarkPap(r) Telemedicine Service for diagnosis at distance (telemedicine- tele-cytopathology), transmitting microscopic images of biomarker-labeled "red cells" digitally or by cell phone to specialists for final diagnosis. Pathologist is not needed at the POC. This will increase the outreach from rural areas with no infrastructure at POC.

MarkPap(r) Self-Collection Home Kit for women to take specimen at home and send it to the laboratory for testing. It is only possible with the MarkPap® technology, since the biomarker is stable in vaginal fluids. This is to help women who do not have access to doctor's offices or are uncomfortable to visit gynecologist.

In reality, a low trained person processes the specimen with MarkPap Kit. The same person, put the slide on the microscope and searches for biomarker positive cells and then transmit those cells digitally or by cell phone to pathologist for final diagnosis.

This is why MarkPap(r) technology can be defined as a biomarker-based, telemedicine-enabled, low-cost, simple, affordable, accessible, equitable infrastructure independent platform technology. When implemented, this technology will be among those which can bring right care at the right place at the right time for lower cost.

This is currently the only promise for mass cytological cervical cancer screening worldwide.

See also Annex and Media.

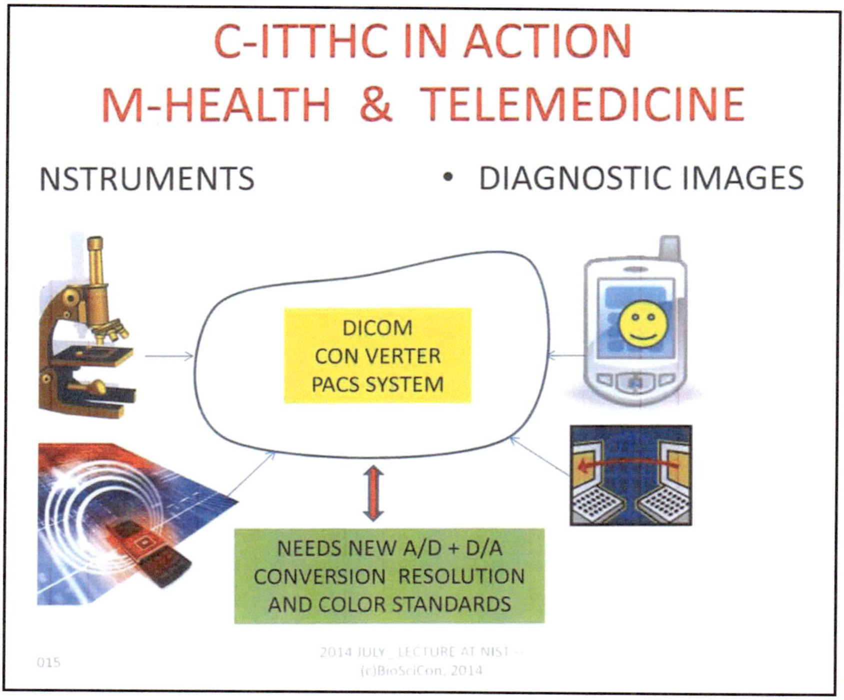

Fig. 7.18 Lecture at NIST, BioSciCon 2014. Analog/Digital connections in mobile telemedicine networking

7.2 Information Technology Telehealth Center (ITTHC)

7.2.1 Introduction

Information Technology Telehealth Centers (ITTHC) is an institutionalized form of a System for mass cervical cancer screening based on a combination of a biomarker-based cytopathology, self-collecting of In Vitro diagnostic specimens, and a network of telemedicine-based hubs connecting distant points-of-care (POC) with remote medical centers (MC) to enable fast, accurate, and low cost cytopathological diagnosis of the specimen and to make the clinical decision on time; thus, enabling same-day clinical intervention, or resolution of the problem while woman is still at the POC (See also Sect. 7.1.5 with the blue print for ITTH) (Fig. 7.19).

7.2.2 Background

While a system is a design, a concept or blue-print, the center is a well-defined institution with identifiable location, mission, vision and affiliations, with paid space occupancy, equipment, personnel, disposables, and with protocols for

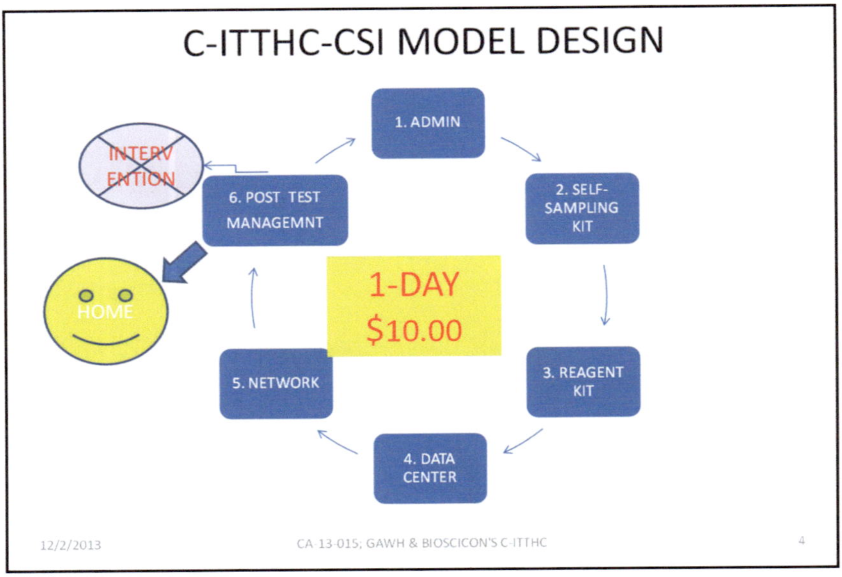

Fig. 7.19 Screen & treat with MarkPap in LMIC
Admin: Headquarters – central unit responsible for organization, funding, functioning and liability of the center; **Self-sampling**: Kit for use by individual women collecting their own sample at home; **Reagent kit**: Assembly of regents, controls and instructions for use by cytopathology laboratories for visualization of specimen cytopathological characteristics; **Data Center**: To manage medical information between POC and MC; **Network**: To maintain 24/7 IT connection between POC and MC; **Post test management**: To provide continuing medical care of participating women including surgical intervention when necessary

technical and medical work, as well as with complete financial construction (income, expenses, ROI and profit) for a sustainable multiyear continuation of jobs towards predetermined goals (See Fig. 7.20).

The System was invented by the American Cancer Society (ACS) in the middle of the Twentieth Century when it was described as, "The Pap test is a method for detection of early signs of lesions that could be developed into cervical cancer, and timely removal of them." This System gained the recognition of the "Best cancer screening method available."

However, this System has shown little, if any efficacy in the developing countries – LMIC (low-middle-income countries).

The ITTHC is an attempt to improve the probability of success of the same System in LMIC. The Center has a defined territory, infrastructure, program of action, objective measures of success/failure, and is easy to implement and to control the compliance. It is designed to serve as a fertilizer for further development of cervical cancer prevention and to enable Indian health care providers to proudly declare that, "Cervical cancer is a fully preventable disease, IF detected on time."

Indian experience with ITTHC could be adjusted for other countries and the network – when automated – could be consider for worldwide application.

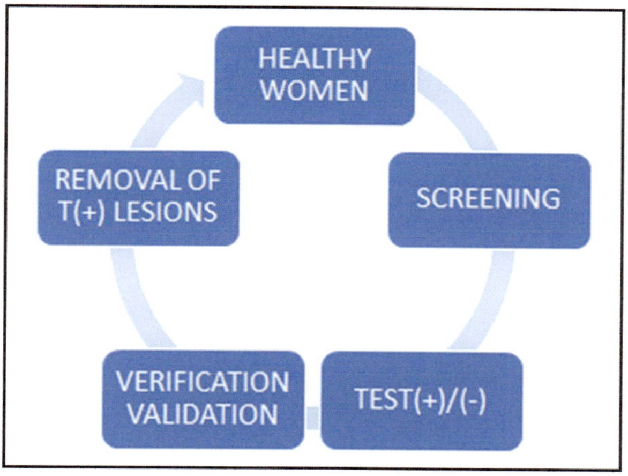

Fig. 7.20 Global cervical cancer control
HW **Healthy women**, *POC* **Points-of-care**, *SDI* **Screening – Diagnosis** (colposcopy-biopsy-histology) – **Intervention**, *SER* **Full service delivery**, *PAY* **reimbursement**, *REV* **Income – (Expenses + ROI + Profit)**, *MPI* **MarkPap India**, *RA* **Regulatory approval,** *IMP* **Importer/export**, *DIS* **Distribution**, *CUS* **Customers** (service providers – service receivers or end users – payers)

This is the vision which feasibility has been tested on the American soil. Is India ready to start moving in this direction even with very small steps? If it is, than the investment into licensing the technology would be warranted.

7.2.3 Purpose

The mission of the ITTHC is to provide long-term sustainable service to a community until the trends of cervical cancer mortality and prevalence are reversed. This goal could be achieved only if the ITTHC is a self-sustainable institution funded from the revenue obtained from services. This is why, institution wise, the center is organized as non-profit social enterprise.

The operational principle of the ITTHC is presented on the following Figure 7.21.

7.2.4 Local ITTHC

The core infrastructure is contained in local ITTHC. There are two types regarding image acquisitions: (1) digital microscope and (2) mobile cell phone camera.

The operating principles of both are presented below as a proposal for China (digital microscope) and India (mobile unit)

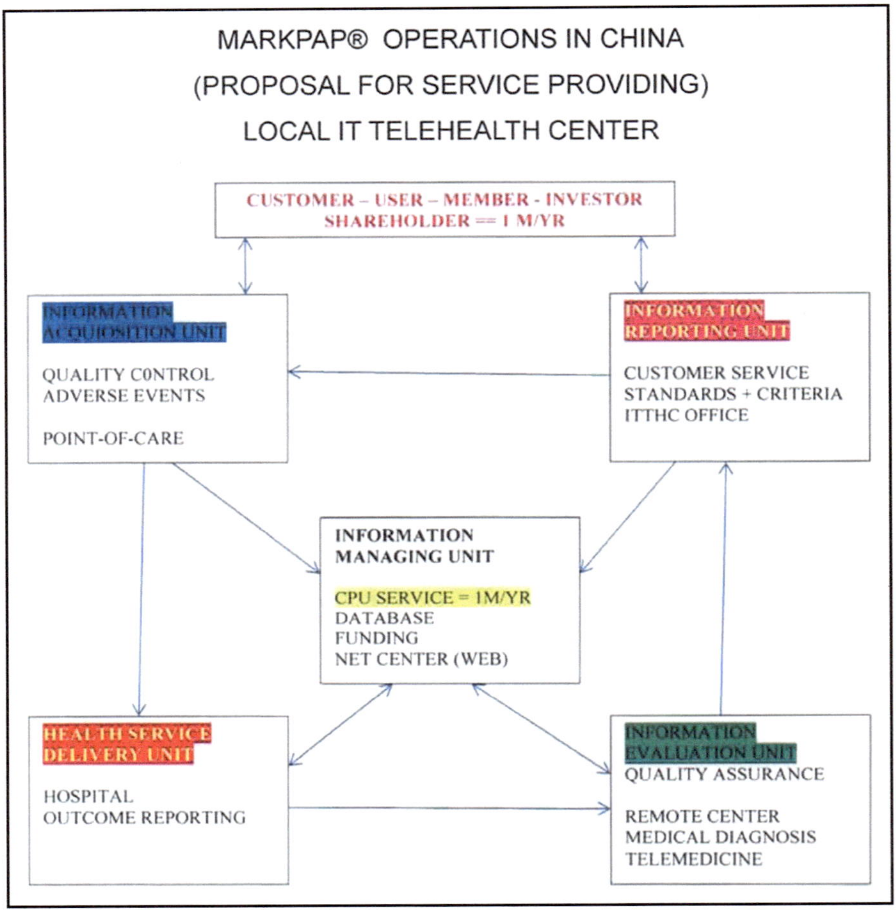

Fig. 7.21 MarkPap™ IT Telehealth Center. Flowchart proposed for a local center in P.R. China (Anhui Province)

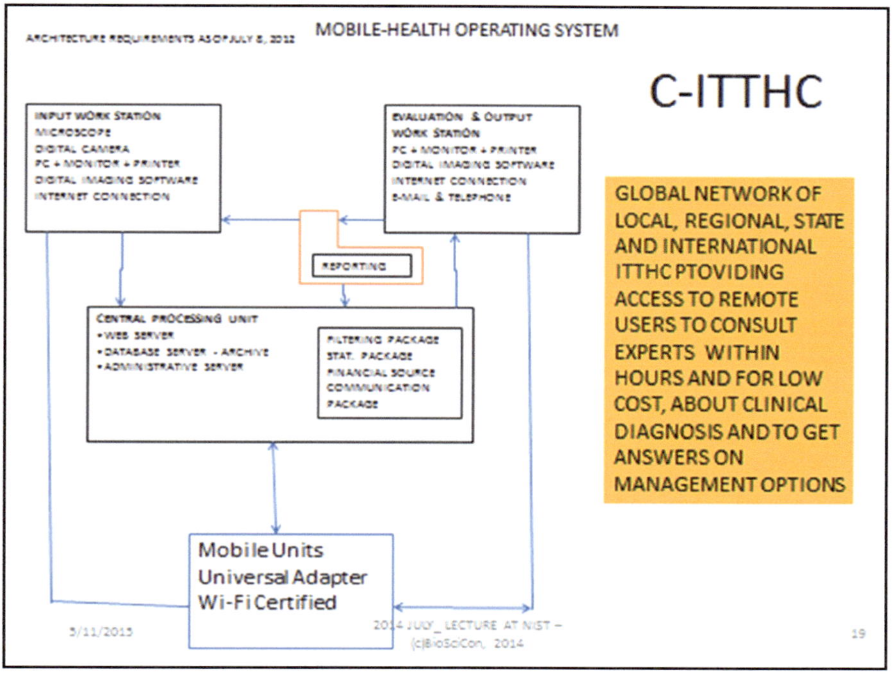

Fig. 7.22 MarkPap™ Health operating system proposed at NIH conference, Jan. 2014. POC Technologies for Cancer

7.2.5 Administrative and Reporting Unit

Administrative and reporting unit is a server in CPU connected directly with the offices at POC and Medical centers, and has open access (Web, e-mail, telephone) for communication with all users. Medical information reports will comply with the US HIPAA regulations. It is also connected with Financial and Analytical departments and with the Statistical Center and serves the Board of Center directors with information on important data for monitoring compliance with old and creation of new policies.

An ITTHC is designed to serve a population with one million services per year. Each center has 28 image acquisition units, one Center Processing Unit (CPU) and 10 Image Evaluation Units. They are connected, (horizontally) to other similar centers in the country they serve, and (vertically) with the regional, state and global ITTHC. A principle of the total network design is presented on the following Figure.

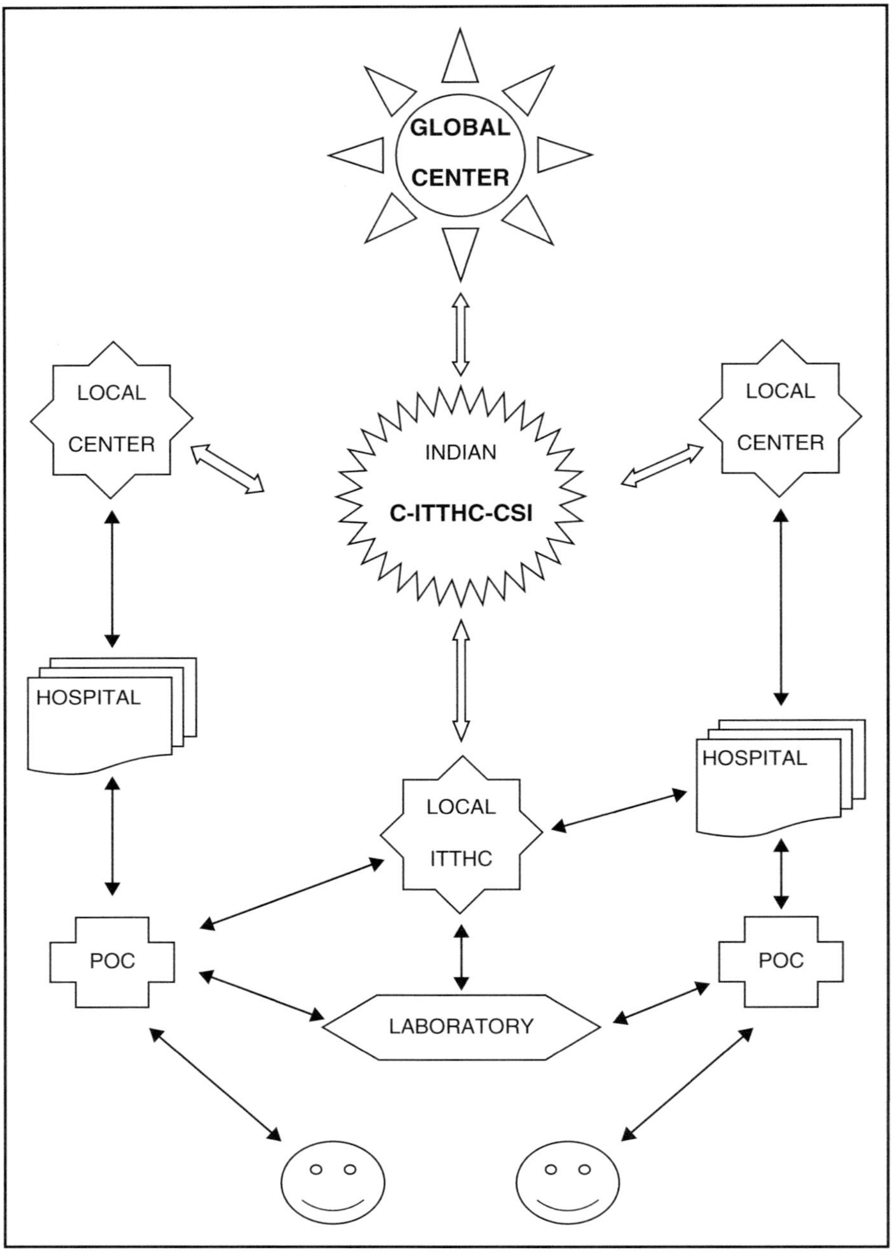

Fig. 7.23

Administrative and Reporting Unit: All units are integrated by the Administrative and the reporting unit. In one Local ITTHC, this unit is a server in CPU connected directly with the offices at POC and Medical centers, and has open access *Web, e-mail, telephone) for communication with all users. It is also connected with

Financial and Analytical departments and with the Statistical Center and serves the Board of Center directors with information on important data for monitoring compliance with old and creation of new policies.

7.2.6 Function – Service Application

The next Figure illustrates how the entire system works.

To make this system more effective and more productive, it is organized under the MarkPap® Telecytopatholgy Protocol, which is described separately.

One of the goals of this organization and the hierarchical functional approach is to reduce the cost and make the entire system much faster (hours instead of days) enabling the screen and treat in the same day. The financial advantage is presented on the next Fig. 7.25.

Finally, just for illustration, our local workstation used as a breadboard for development of the entire system and global network is presented on the picture below. Please note, this unit has double image capturing capability: digital microscope and the cell phone camera attached by a universal adapter (Fig. 7.26).

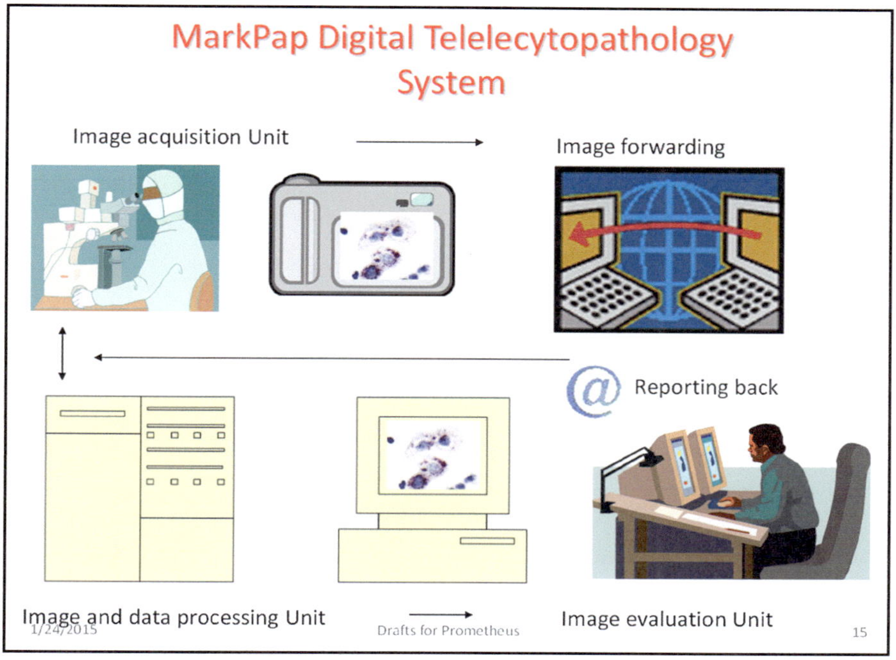

Fig. 7.24

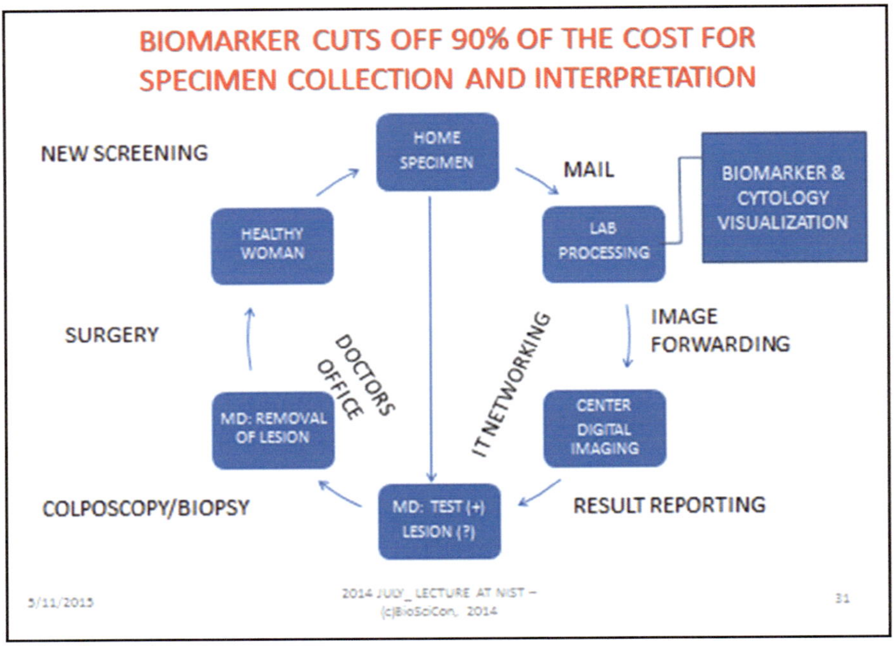

Fig. 7.25 Financial advantage of the ITTH Center

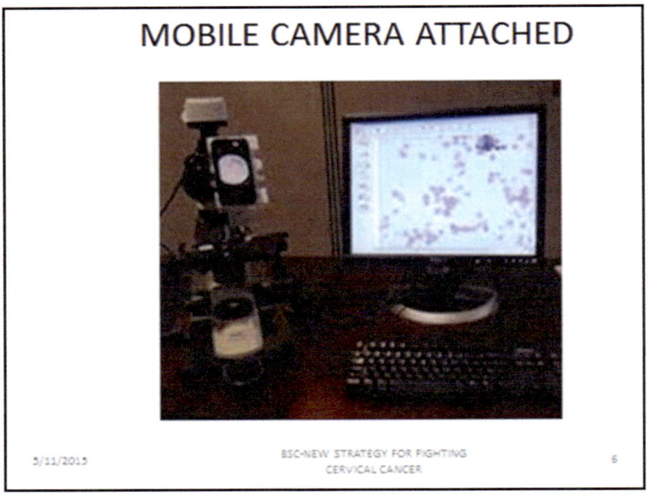

Fig. 7.26 Local Image Acquisition Unit with both digital camera and the mobile camera attached to the microscope

7.3 The New Integrative Complex MEDYKO

7.3.1 MEDYKO 2015

7.3.1.1 Idea and Proof of Concept Via Application in Practice

MEDYKO is a composite biomarker construed of at least two of three markers labeling abnormal condition inside cells; thus, indicating that the cytopathological specimen containing such cells must be classified as "abnormal" and processed for further diagnosis by any standard cytopathology and interpreted in 2001 Bethesda terminology.

MEDYKO is an acronym made of three syllables preceding words metabolism, dysplasia and koilocytes. Each of these words presents an important visual parameter in cytopathology.

ME(tabolism)

Abnormal changes in metabolic pathways precede morphological changes. On specimens stained for visualization of morphology the metabolic identifiers are invisible. They must be visualized with additional staining procedures, usually with chemical reactions activating molecular basis of protein structures (enzyme groups) and producing nanomolecular precipitates of unsolvable stains which form aggregates larger than 1 μm and become visible in addition to the morphology already visualized with standard staining. Presence (+), absence (−), and the degree of this presence (λ), create recognizable pathological conditions and facilitate clinical diagnosis of the impending disease.

DY(splasia)

Nuclear dysplasia – diskaryosis, hyperchromia, segmentation, fragmentation, and other changes of nuclear size, shape and staining, are well known signs of disorder affecting cells and tissues and have been used for more than a century in pathology for diagnosis and classification of diseases. Mild, moderate and severe dysplasia is the first set of categories used to classify clinical condition found on Pap smears. This classification has been replaced with The Bethesda System in 1996, and later with 2001 Bethesda System. This classification does not include biomarkers and their presence/absence must be additionally noted.

KO(ilocyte)

Koilocytes are cells with one large or multiple smaller vacuoles filled with detritus of degraded intracellular material caused by viral infection and phagocytosis. During the cytology staining process this detritus is dissolved and "empty" vacuoles appear intracellular on microscopic preparations. Virus, e.g., HPV is contained inside phagosomes and can be spread after expulsion or cell disruption. These cells represent body's response to infection. In vitro, they are live, can replicate, grow as tumor-like formations (warts) and could behave as benign tumor. They indicate a worse prognosis of the infected tissues.

Combined in a single cell, these markers label the presence of approaching disease (ME), already present disease (DY) and the infection supporting this disease (KO). This is why MEDYKO was named a Meaningful Biomarker.

The illustrations below present the schematic theory described above about the meaningful biomarker, the real image as seen under the microscope with explanation, and the diagram how image analysis can read and interpret those images making automatic screening not only possible, but highly desirable option for mass cervical cancer screening.

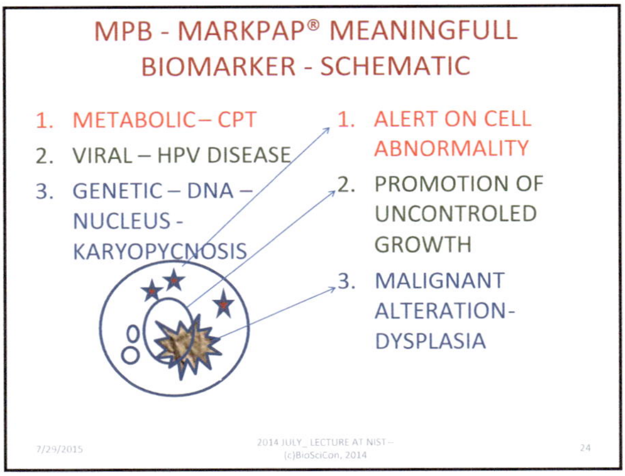

Fig. 7.27

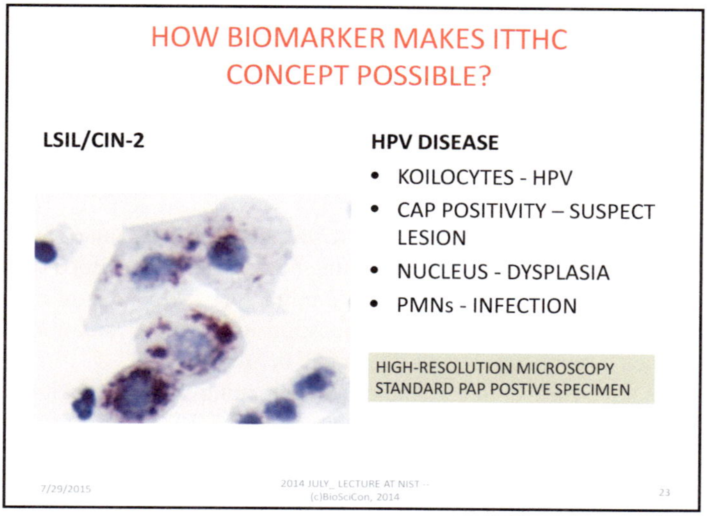

Fig. 7.28

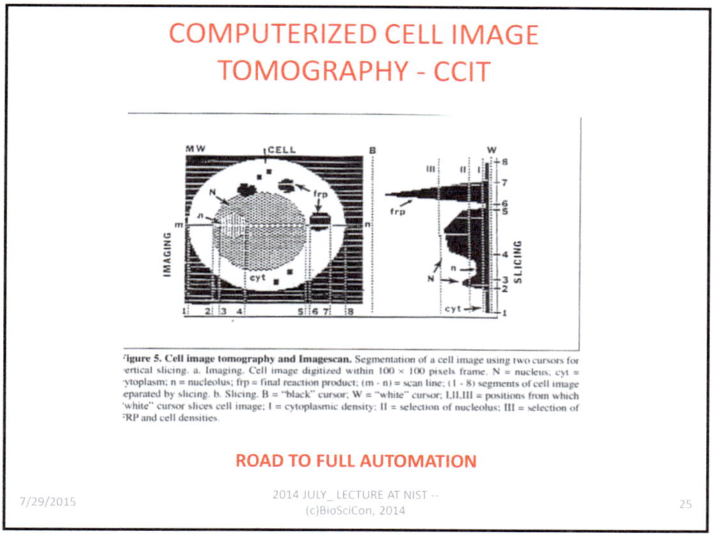

Fig. 7.29

In preliminary studies the principle on which MEDYKO is based was shown extremely productive for application in Low Middle Income Countries (LMIC) and we submitted a Federal Grant Application via NIH. Typically, the complex IT technology design was not clearly understood by our partners in LMIC, and we had to withdraw this application for time when technology for exchange of medical image information will be more affordable – this time is now (2015).

To check the functionality of our design we created a BSC_Template_for Exchange of Image files and have tested it in India, Japan, China, Serbia, Africa, and USA. With no exception, all participating centers have responded on time with expected responses. The transfer time was 2 min for 3–4 MB images, enabling fast a complete exchange of full information (question-image file, evaluation of images-medical diagnosis-reporting) See the Template below.

Finally, we have compared cervical cancer screening with MPT with data available from other modes of screening Pap smear, LBP, HPV testing and have found that Medyko has diagnostic advantage over all other methods because it expands the diagnostic range of both sensitivity and specificity, while other methods can increase either sensitivity or specificity. See Table Comparison.

In Summary, the Global Application of the New Strategy depends upon the will of official and private sector to invest into mass cervical cancer screening and to achieve an outreach rate of 51 % of all women at risk, for over 10–15 years of implementation. This is what the US has done for 50 plus years of Pap test application nationwide and this is what other countries can repeat – less costly and faster – if there is a wish for social entrepreneurships – business model with social and financial impact. In the comprehensive approach, what MarkPap® Technology and Strategy is offering has clear goals and doable programs.

7.3.2 MEDYKO – Introductory Letter

In November 2000, we received a USPTO Patent "CAP-PAP TEST" intended for screening healthy women for early cytological signs of intra-vaginal lesions which, if untreated, could develop into cervical cancer.

Fourteen years later we have accumulated knowledge, skills and experience which helped us, during reexamination of this experience to revise the diagnostic standards and criteria developed when this test was introduced and applied in clinical trials.

During this recent review we observed additional features which, when integrated into a single diagnostic procedure, presented themselves as a new compound endpoint with the same purpose, but more reliable, with less opportunity for false negative and false positive results. This endpoint is the morphological presentation of (1) HPV disease – koilocytosis, (2) of epithelial dysplasia – diskaryosis or nuclear DNA aberrations, and (3), of metabolic aberrations – Cervical acid phosphatase upholding in cytoplasm. Because all these features can be seen instantly – one look – of the affected cells, and since the Pap smear (for cervical cancer screening, has already been categorized as biomarker, we believe that this integrative, unique

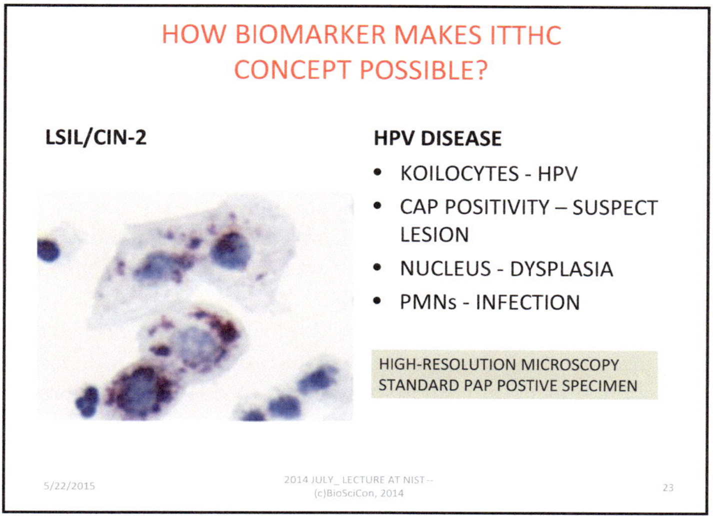

Fig. 7.30

image could be also categorized as a biomarker for early recognition of cytological changes which indicate to a presence of lesions that may develop into cervical cancer.

For better memorizing the long name of this compound biomarker, we are recommending the acronym MEDYKO composed of

ME – metabolic changes (cervical acid phosphatase)
DY – dysplasia, or diskaryosis, DNA changes
KO – Koilocytes, HPV disease – not only HPV infection.

When stained with MarkPap® test, positive (abnormal cells) show blue, white and red features. Dark blue (or maroon) stained is nucleus and light blue is the empty cytoplasm; white are vacuoles (after destruction and elimination of the cellular detritus during alcohol cleaning, and red is cervical acid files an achievable and reliable task, phosphatase aggregates on sites of enzyme activity.

Each of these features has different color and density of color saturation, the characteristics which enable (cell recognition to be) achievable and reliable task, amenable for easy digital image capturing, storing in image database; easy identification, recognition and measuring.

BioSciCon, Inc. is sponsoring development of MarkPap® technology products and services which is a combination of upgraded cytopathology and adjusted digital imaging with wired and wireless telelemedicine integrated to enable global application of mobile-health preventive cancer screening.

MarkPap Pacific LLC was incorporated in 2004 to commercialize these products and services on the markets of the Greater Pacific Area. Since 2004, this company has established a partnership with a Chinese manufacturer to bring MarkPap products to the China cervical cancer markets. Until 2010 this collaboration was successful and MarkPap products became selling in China. In that year, thefts have pirated BioSciCon's patent rights and the cooperation was disrupted. Currently, MarkPap Pacific LLC has invoices for four million dollars and a not resolved trade agreement of 15 million dollars. Because of these debts, LLC went into moratorium in 2013.

However, recently, a known international investment firm offered to BioSciCon to loan (debt-funding) its projects in China up to the total investment necessary to bring the LLC original products to sale in China. The huge potential of this market and the attractiveness of the new IT based technology are the foundation of this offer.

To grant the loan funding, the lender asked for surety bonds instead of other collaterals, and the corresponding insurance company requires a deposit of above $100,000 as a prerequisite for issuing those bonds. A company in moratorium cannot start any such transaction. Therefore, the parent company, BioSciCon, has recommended first to reactivate the LLC, than to offer equity as a collaterals to VC for 100 K–2000 K as a short term loan or investment, to buy those surety bonds, purchase the insurance, and then to get the funding of about 10 millions. As soon as funds will start to arrive, to give back the loan or to return the investment with a certain percent, and to continue with project securely funded until sales, in millions of units, will become sustainable in China and the project self-maintained (revenue from sales).

This is a short overview of the opportunity. If you are interested to invest between 100 K and 200 K on a short term with a substantial profit, please call to continue the discussion. However, the specifics of this opportunity require faster response than your standard 60 days. We would appreciate if you can move faster with this particular project. If we do not hear from you within 4 weeks of this letter, we will consider your company as NOT interested.

I am looking forward to hearing from you soon.

Thank you

Dr. Nenad Markovic
BioSciCon, Inc.
Rockville, MD

7.3.3 *Methods Comparison*

7.3.3.1 MPT Method Comparision with Other cervical cancer Screening Methods

In vitro diagnostic methods are to separate normal (negative) specimens from positive and to grade the abnormality according to the need for clinical action

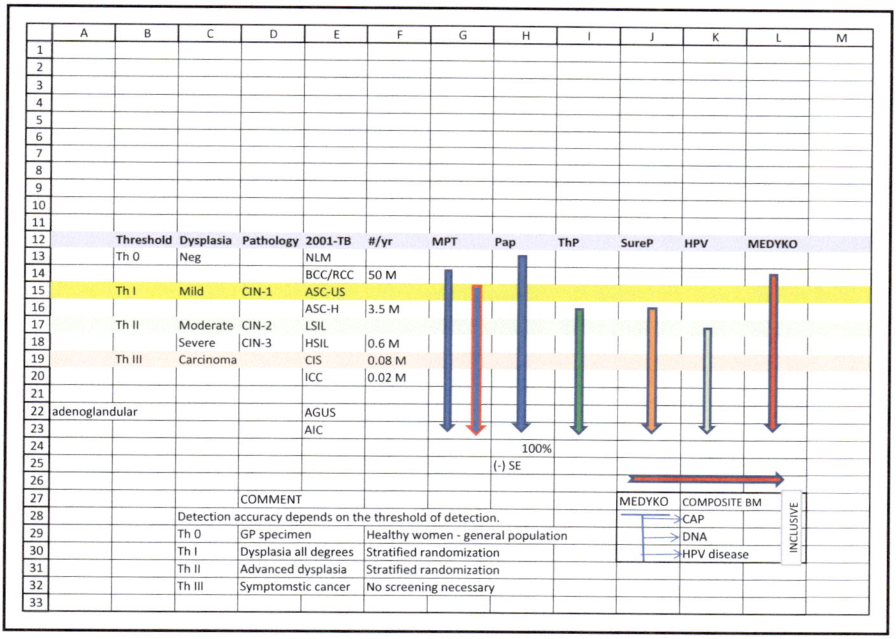

Fig. 7.31

	A	B	C	D	E	F	G	H	I	J	K	L	M
34			Probality for cancer development				ICC in t/y						
35			Th III >>>	Th II >> Th I > Th 0			1:2,500						
36			Control groups: Best - Th 0; Worst Th II.										
37													
38													
39													
40													
41		GUIDELINES											
42	Ref #	Author	Title										
43	194	ACS	American Cancer Society				2012	2002					
44													
45	195	WHO	World Health Organization				2013						
46			WHO Guidelines										
47													
48	196	ASCCP	American Society for Colposcopy and				2013						
49			Cervical Pathology										
50													
51	197	ASCP	American Society for Cytopathlogy				2014						
52													
53	198	CDC	Centers for Disease Control										
54			Cervical Cancer Screening Guidelines				2012						
55													
56	199	CMS	Centers for Medicare Medicaid Services				2014						
57			NCA Trackind Sheet for CC with HPV										
58													
59	200	USPSTF	US Preventive Service Task Force				2012						
60			CC Evidence Based Summary										
61													
62	201	ACOG	American College of Obstetricians and Gynecologists										
63			Guidelines				2009						
64													
65	202	NCI	National Cancer Institute				2014						
66			Cancer statistics										

	A	B	C	D	E	F	G	H	I	J	K	L	M
67													
68	203	ASCT	American Society for Cytotechnology				2012						
69													
70													
71													
72													
73			Major Changes										
74													
75		1	Pap smear remains			20% FN							
76		2	LBP not better than Pap			Se up; SP down							
77		3	HPV - only oncogenic strains										
78		4	Period 1-3 years		3+ limited								
79		5	Surrogate vs. robust end-points										
80		6	IT not yet recommended										
81		7	Incidence and prevalence in US increases after 2010										

Fig. 7.32

7.4 Template for Telecytopathology

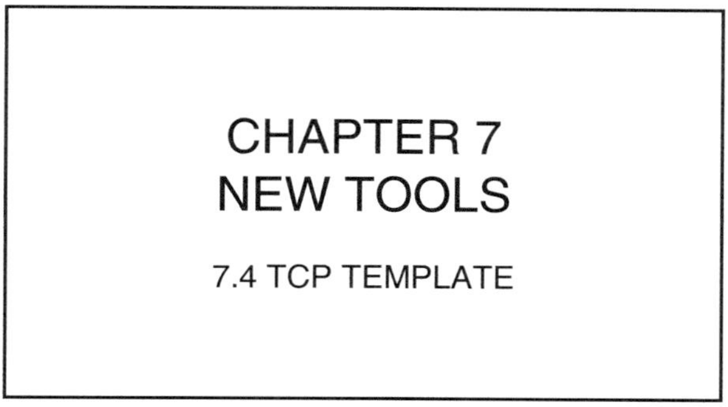

Fig. 7.33 A series of slides from a single template used for exchange of image files between POC and Medical centers – should be connected with additional numbers; e.g. 7.33.1, 7.33.2 etc.

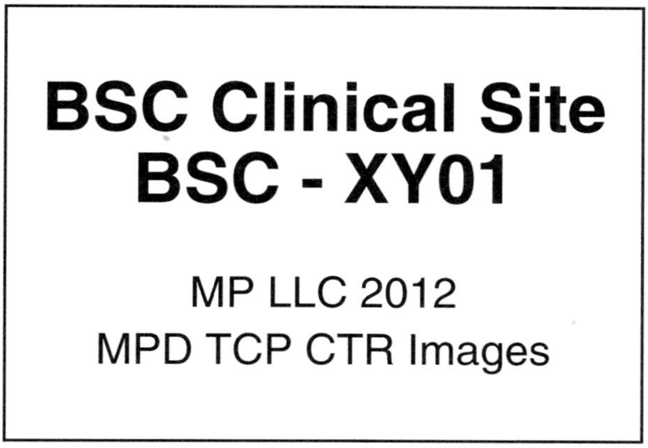

Fig. 7.34 A series of slides from a single template used for exchange of image files between POC and Medical centers – should be connected with additional numbers; e.g. 7.33.1, 7.33.2 etc.

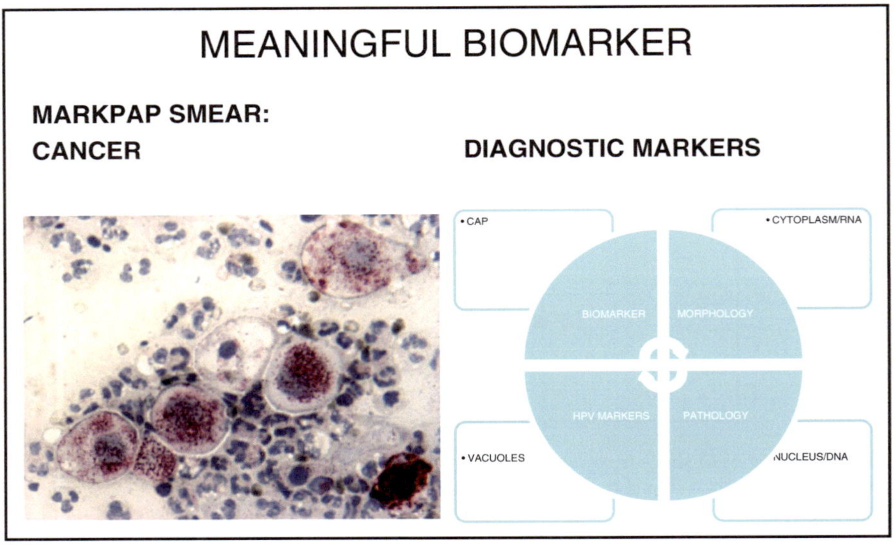

Fig. 7.35 A series of slides from a single template used for exchange of image files between POC and Medical centers – should be connected with additional numbers; e.g. 7.33.1, 7.33.2 etc.

TCP TEMPLATE: Questions

ORIGINATOR

- DATE ________________
- LOCATION____________
- REQUESTER ________
- CASE CODE _________
- SPECIMEN __________
- TEST ________________
- IMAGES # ___________
- TIME WHEN SENT ____

eHEALTH QUESTION

- WHAT IS REQUESTED?
- ADEQUACY OF:
- (1) SAMPLING______
- (2) PROCESSING ____
- GENERAL EVALUATION T(+); T(?); T(-); OTHER
- MEDICAL DIAGNOSIS
- NIL; BCC; ASC-US; ASC-H; LSIL; HSIL; CIS; ICC

Fig. 7.36 A series of slides from a single template used for exchange of image files between POC and Medical centers – should be connected with additional numbers; e.g. 7.33.1, 7.33.2 etc.

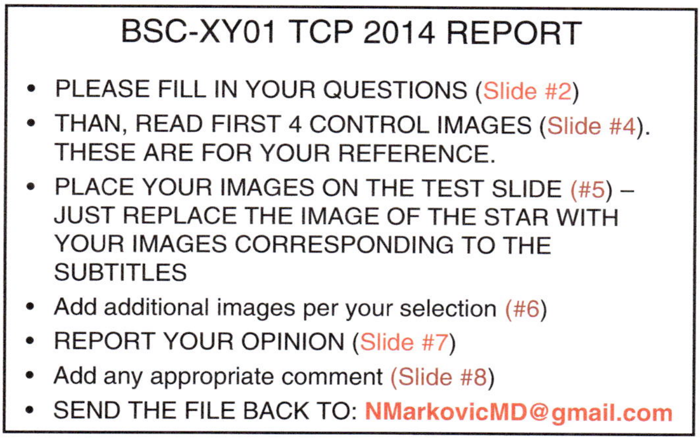

Fig. 7.37 A series of slides from a single template used for exchange of image files between POC and Medical centers – should be connected with additional numbers; e.g. 7.33.1, 7.33.2 etc.

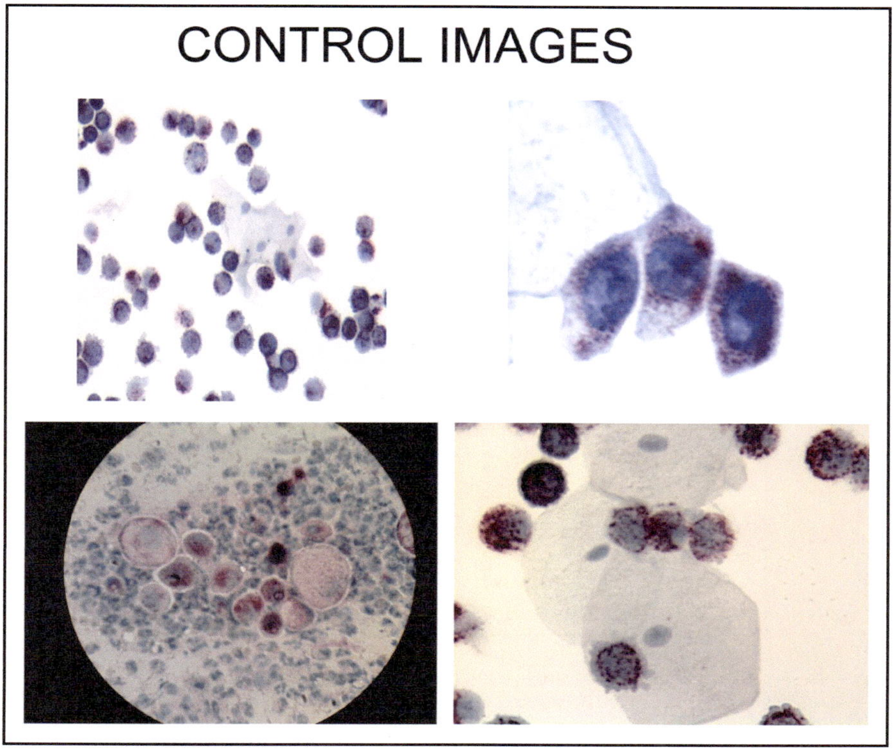

Fig. 7.38 A series of slides from a single template used for exchange of image files between POC and Medical centers – should be connected with additional numbers; e.g. 7.33.1, 7.33.2 etc.

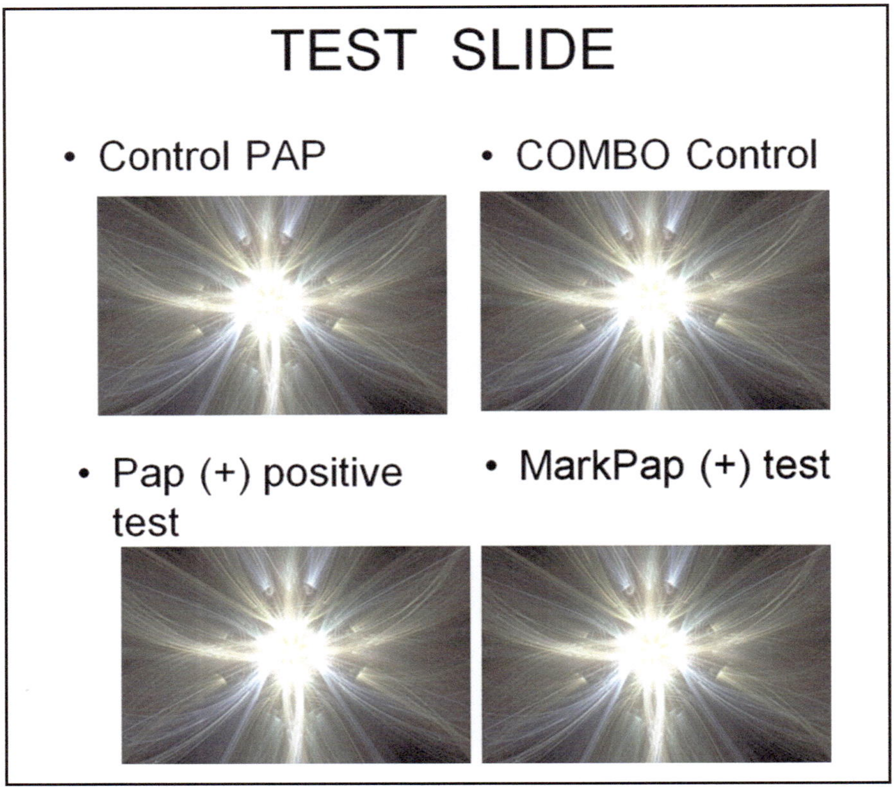

Fig. 7.39 A series of slides from a single template used for exchange of image files between POC and Medical centers – should be connected with additional numbers; e.g. 7.33.1, 7.33.2 etc.

Expert Opinion

- Medical Diagnosis: ____________
  ____
- Comment: ____________________

____

Contact: MN Company, address, t/f, website, e-mail

- Expert: Code, address, contact: ______________

Fig. 7.40 A series of slides from a single template used for exchange of image files between POC and Medical centers – should be connected with additional numbers; e.g. 7.33.1, 7.33.2 etc.

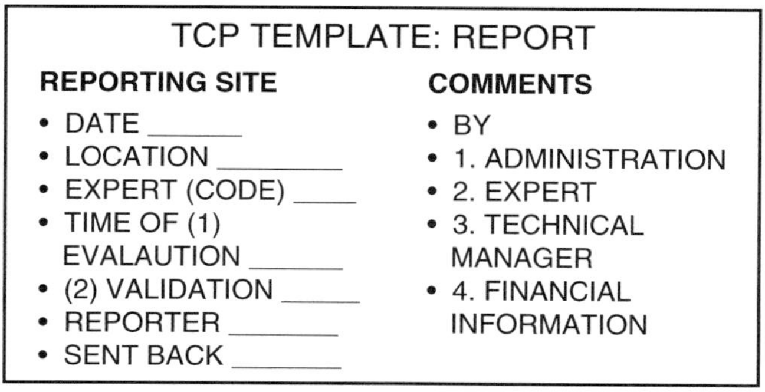

Fig. 7.41 A series of slides from a single template used for exchange of image files between POC and Medical centers – should be connected with additional numbers; e.g. 7.33.1, 7.33.2 etc.

7.5 Screen and Treat with MarkPap® Test

When all strategies including Pap smear, Liquid-Based Pap, HPV testing, Co-testing (HPV & cytology), hrHPV, have failed to reach the majority of population at risk, and the cervical cancer statistics per countries or in the world did not show the expected American data obtained from application of Pap test in the US, the World Health Organization (WHO) has turned to an old idea, for long years rejected as substandard, and upgraded it with addition of cryotherapy (or LEEP) given this strategy new name "Screen and Treat," and hoping this will be solution to recruit more women to participate in cervical cancer control program; thus to save more women lives.

Here are two citations from this newest WHO Strategy:

WHO guidelines for screening and treat.

The expert panel suggests:

- Use a strategy of screen with an HPV test and treat, over a strategy of screen with VIA and treat. In resource-constrained settings, where screening with an HPV test is not feasible, the panel suggests a strategy of screen with VIA and treat.
- Use a strategy of screen with an HPV test and treat, over a strategy of screen with cytology followed by colposcopy (with or without biopsy) and treat. However, in countries where an appropriate/high-quality screening strategy with cytology followed by colposcopy already exists, either an HPV test or cytology followed by colposcopy could be used.
- Use a strategy of screen with VIA and treat, over a strategy of screen with cytology followed by colposcopy (with or without biopsy) and treat. The recommendation for VIA over cytology followed by colposcopy can be applied in countries

that are currently considering either programme or countries that currently have both programmes available.

- Use a strategy of screen with an HPV test and treat, over a strategy of screen with an HPV test followed by colposcopy (with or without biopsy) and treat.
- Use either a strategy of screen with an HPV test followed by VIA and treat, or a strategy of screen with an HPV test and treat.
- Use a strategy of screen with an HPV test followed by VIA and treat, over a strategy of screen with VIA and treat.
- Use a strategy of screen with an HPV test followed by VIA and treat, over a strategy of screen with cytology followed by colposcopy (with or without biopsy) and treat.
- Use a strategy of screen with an HPV test followed by VIA and treat, over a strategy of screen with an HPV test followed by colposcopy (with or without biopsy) and treat.

Annex. Decision-making flowchart for screen-and-treat strategies. This decision-making flowchart or algorithm provides a decision tree to use as a quick reference when choosing a screen-and-treat strategy at the programme level. Programme managers and decision-makers can start at the top and answer the questions accordingly to determine which screen-and-treat option is best in the context where it will be implemented. It highlights choices related to resources, which can include costs, staff and training. However, programme managers will also need to consider other factors, such as the number of women who are lost to follow-up with a strategy that involves more than one screening test.

Screen with an HPV test and treat with cryotherapy, or LEEP when not eligible for cryotherapy When an HPV test is positive, treatment is provided. With this strategy, visual inspection with acetic acid (VIA) is used to determine eligibility for cryotherapy. Negative Determine eligibility for cryotherapy and rule out cervical cancer using visual inspection with acetic acid (VIA) Rescreen after a minimum interval of 5 years Positive Eligible for cryotherapy, treat with cryotherapy Not eligible for cryotherapy, treat with LEEP Suspicious for cancer Post-treatment follow-up at 1 year Refer to appropriate diagnosis and treatment HPV test Note: Refer to the screen-and-treat recommendations provided in Chap. 3 of the guideline for guidance about which strategies are recommended, and for information on the specific factors to consider when deciding on a strategy.

The complete Guidance is presented in the WHO book (Media).

We think that this WHO Guidelines equalizing HPV followed by VIA, HPV alone, VIA alone and Cytology or HPV testing as criteria for treatment (cryotherapy or LEEP) have gone too far from the original Pap test that the original meaning of screening healthy women for silent lesions has been lost.

Consequently, we reviewed what is left, and we found the American guidelines cited in Chap. 4 which are more conservative and closer to the original Pap test screening. Because those other guidelines have their own problems, we have tried to estimate how MarkPap technology may improve the guidelines and make it more acceptable for the LMIC countries where the most of new cervical cases occur each year.

The following Scheme (see below and in the New Strategy) presents Screen & Treat version with MarkPap (example from Federal grant application).

This cycle represents our new strategy for implementation of mass cervical cancer screening in developing world.

Telecytopathology Protocol - Draft:

1. To screen 80 % of eligible women. One woman to be screened once in 3 years minimal requirement. MarkPap technology to be used in 100 % of cases.
2. To collect specimen by women themselves using MarkPap Specimen Self-Collection kit.
3. To use MarkPap Reagents Kit for specimen preparation, biomarker processes and Papanicolaou staining. Technician, who will be controlling the specimen adequacy and quality of staining, will immediately select "abnormal cells" labeled red with the acid phosphatase, and will capture images of microscopic fields containing such cells for further evaluation by pathologists or experts on site or in remote medical centers (using mobile and digital camera systems for image capturing and forwarding.
4. To use MarkPap Telecytopathology membership network for medical information and image exchange and consultations.
5. To report digital image analysis in the point-of-care where colposcopy, biopsy and small surgical intervention (cryotherapy, LEEP, Conization) could be performed the same day using the equipment (e.g.) Medical STOMP provided to POC.
6. To remove all suspect lesions as well as CIS – Approximately up to 2 % of screened women. All other women to return home for the next scheduled control.

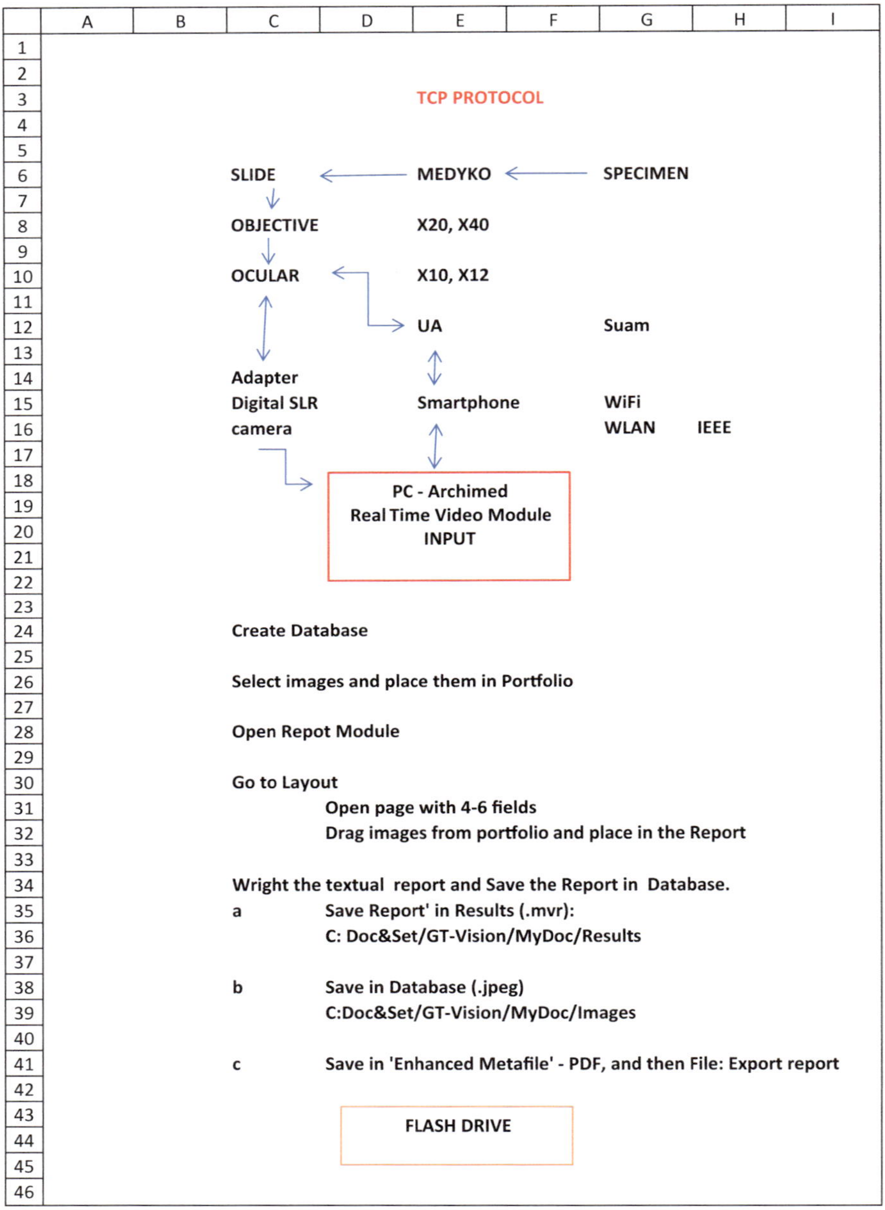
TCP PROTOCOL
SLIDE
MEDYKO
SPECIMEN
OBJECTIVE
X20, X40
OCULAR
X10, X12
UA
Suam
Adapter
Digital SLR
camera
Smartphone
WiFi
WLAN
IEEE
PC - Archimed
Real Time Video Module
INPUT
Create Database
Select images and place them in Portfolio
Open Repot Module
Go to Layout
Open page with 4-6 fields
Drag images from portfolio and place in the Report
Wright the textual report and Save the Report in Database.
a Save Report' in Results (.mvr):
C: Doc&Set/GT-Vision/MyDoc/Results
b Save in Database (.jpeg)
C:Doc&Set/GT-Vision/MyDoc/Images
c Save in 'Enhanced Metafile' - PDF, and then File: Export report
FLASH DRIVE

7.6 Telecytopathology Protocol

	A	B	C	D	E	F	G	H	I
47			TRANSFER						
48			1	EMAIL this folder files					
49			2	COPY this folder to flash drive					
50			3						
51									
52		File image from Video/Microscope etc							
53			Open Archimed						
54				Open Video Module					
55					Start Microscope				
56					Save				
57			My Recent Documents/Desktop/My Documents/Images						
58						*/My Pictures			
59							Create Record Database		
60									
61									
62									
63		Retrieve mage file from one of image databases							
64									
65		Hard disk							
66			My Recent Documents/Desktop/My Documents/Images/My pictures						
67				Open file and Save on a Flash Drive					
68		Software							
69			My Documents/My Pictures/. . .						
70			My Documents/Images/...						
71				Open and Save on Flash Drive					
72			images are saved as individual files in MyPictures and Images						
73			They can also be composed per purpose and saved in additional file folders						
74				with case number names. Both files and folders could be copied					
75				and transferred for emailing, exportin g or publishing.					
76									
77									
78					PC				
79									
80									
81			E-MAILING						
82			1	Open G-MAIL					
83				Open nsmarkovicmd@gmail.com					
84				Open COMPOSE					
85				Compose a new e-mail					
86					To				
87					CC				
88					Bcc				
89					Subject				
90					Text				
91				Add attachment					
92					Browse files from the flash drive				

Fig. 7.42 MarkPap™ telecytopathology protocol flowchart presenting an algorithm for a virtual protocol to test Mobile IT Telehealth centers

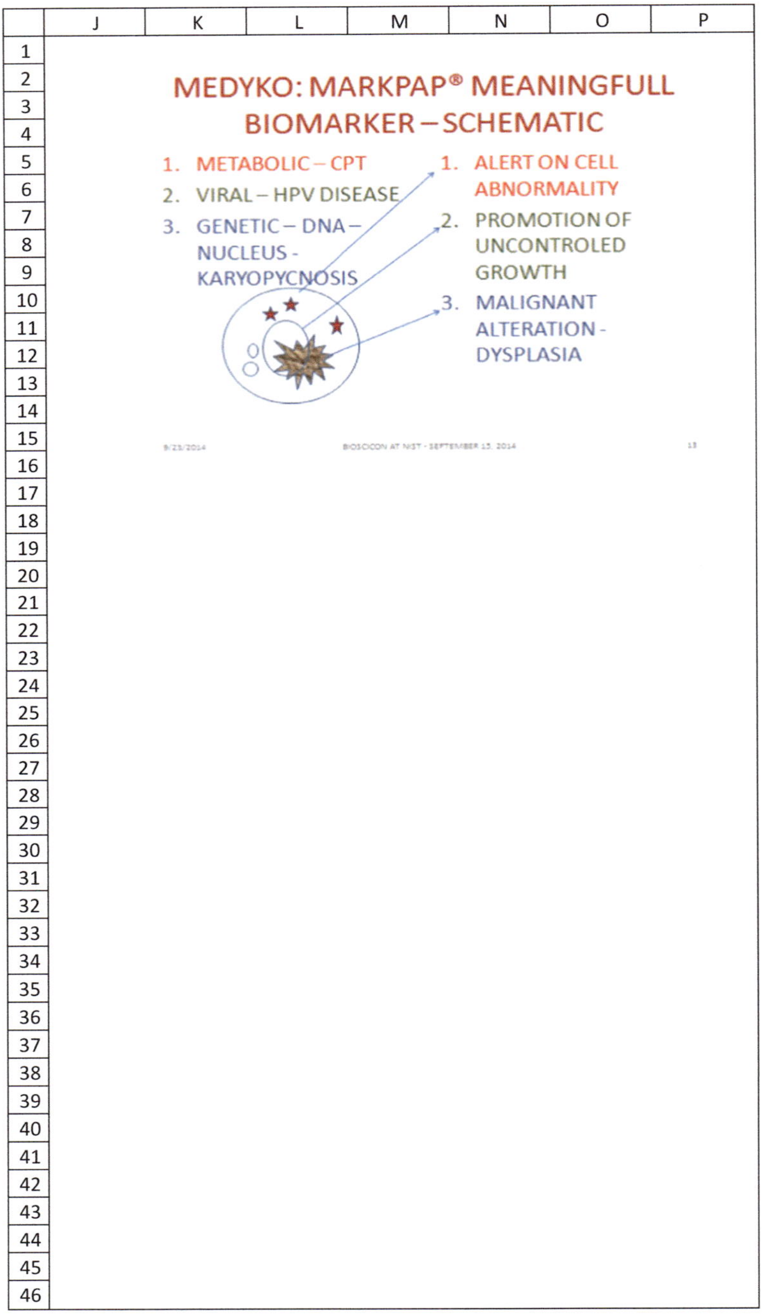

Fig. 7.43 MEDYKO™ Theory behind the discovery of this new composite biomarker

	A	B	C	D	E	F	G	H	I
93					**Find image file and add**				
94				**Save and close, or send**					
95									
96			**2**	**FLASH DRIVE**					
97									
98									
99			**TRANSFERRING**						
100									
101				**E-MAIL**					
102					**POC3**				
103						**SMPT - E-MAIL**			
104						**E-MAIL - MAIL (IMAT)(POC3)**			

Fig. 7.44

Annex: Brochures and PPP Presentations

Contents

N. Markovic, O. Markovic, *What Every Woman Should Know about Cervical Cancer*, DOI 10.1007/978-94-017-7560-1

1 Brochures

1.1 MarkPap India, LLC. Fighting Cervical Cancer. Brochure, 2012

1.1a

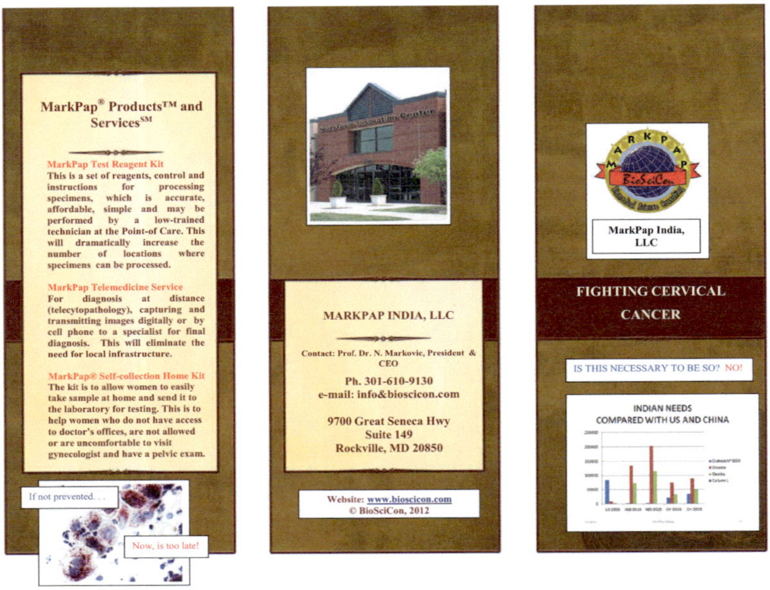

1.1b

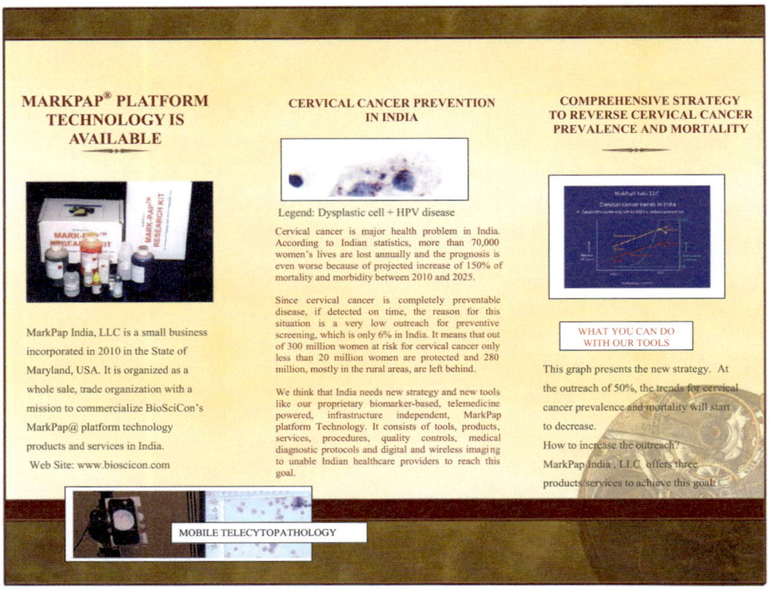

1.2 MarkPap Pacific, LLC. Fighting Cervical Cancer. Brochure, 2012

1.2a

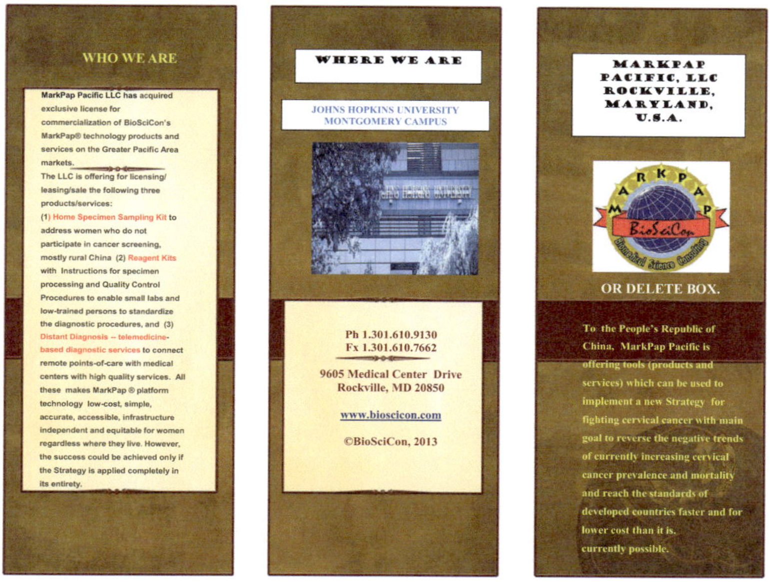

1.2b

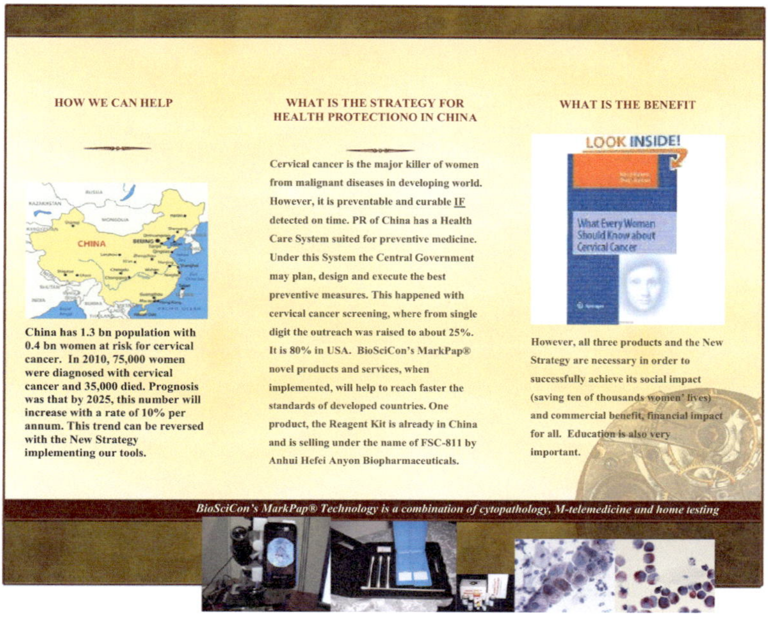

2 Power Point Presentations

2.1 *National Institute for Standards & Technology. (NIST). Lecture on MarkPap® Technology, 2014*

2.1.1

CURRENT STATUS

Tele(cyto)pathology has not yet been utilized in routine healthcare delivery because digital imaging in pathology has not reached diagnostic power of optical imaging. More work from both, medical and IT professionals, is still necessary to adapt both technologies and bridge the gap, synchronize terminology and make medical diagnoses obtained by different technologies interchangeable, more powerful and affordable.

2.1.2

PURPOSE OF THIS LECTURE

TO INCITE YOUR INTEREST ABOUT OUR WORK ON DEVELOPMENT A **STRATEGY**, MANUFACTURING **TOOLS**, DESIGN OF **SERVICES** AND FINALLY TO **DELIVER HELP TO** MILLIONS OF **WOMEN AT RISK** FOR CERVICAL CANCER VIA THE NEW **STANDARDIZATION OF MEDICAL AND IT INFORMATICS** , WHICH WILL ENABLE FASTER, MORE ACCURATE, SAFER AND LESS COSTLY DELIVERY OF **CANCER CONTROL SERVICES** WORLDWIDE.

2.1.3

Epidemic of cervical cancer is not an acceptable occurrence in 21st Century

World

- Total population: 7 bn
- Women at risk: 2.4 bn
- Cervical cancer prevalence: 650 mil; mortality: 280 mil
- Trends: +10%/year
- Outreach: 20% (market restricted)
- Immature market: 280 mil
- **Preventive goals: To reach the US comparable data**

India

- Total population: 1 bn
- Women at risk: 300 mil
- Cervical cancer prevalence: 100 K; mortality: 50 K
- Trends: + 10%/year
- Outreach: 6%
- **Preventive goals: To reverse trends, achievable at outreach of 50%**

2.1.4

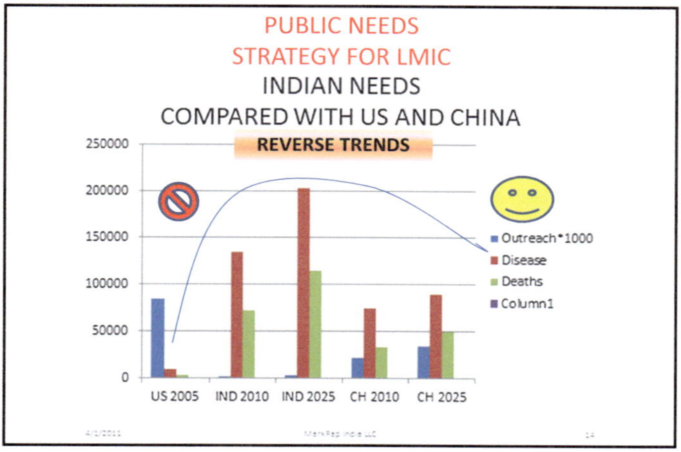

2.1.5

Problems

Technical problems with the standardization of the color of the images, resolution, pattern recognition, the quality and reproducibility of images (quality microscopic adapter needed) has not been fully resolved yet.

The most important problem remains the digital image sampling error : Proper choice of images to be transmitted from the POC for final diagnosis at distance. It implies the necessity to have a trained professional at the POC, what is not usually possible, and why diagnosis at distance is necessary.

It means that both pathological methods designed for optical microscopy should be upgraded for the needs of telecytopathology, and the IT approach for the new requirements .

2.1.6

Solutions

How to mitigate digital image techniques?
In order to avoid the sampling error (which images to choose and send to pathologist at distant place) it is necessary to have a lead for the low-trained person at the POC to decide which images to transmit. For example, a biomarker signaling cervical abnormality that everybody can see. In case of cervical cancer screening, we discovered a cytoplasmic biomarker of cervical dysplasia/cervical cancer that is only present in abnormal cell. The whole platform technology was developed around this biomarker, MarkPap® Technology. When visualized with MarkPap® technology the marker appears as a red colored deposit in abnormal cells only. Normal cells are completely negative.

2.1.7

MarkPap® platform technology illustrated

We have a proprietary technology which is based upon a chemical biomarker positive only in abnormal cells, and always negative in normal cells. This distinction makes the method superior over all competitors.

More....

www.bioscicon.com/gallery.html

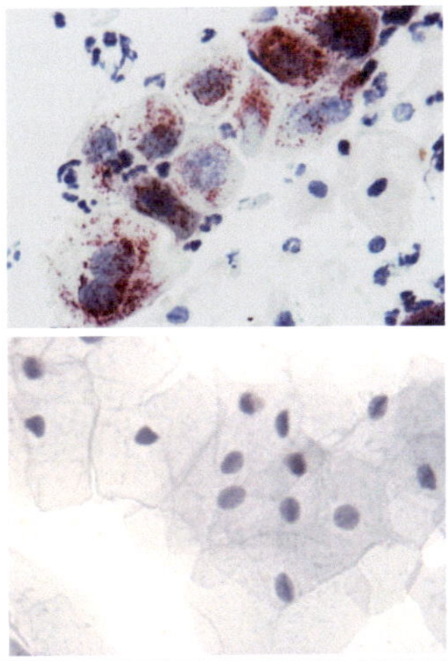

2.1.8

MarkPap® platform technology illustrated.
An ancillary method to Pap test

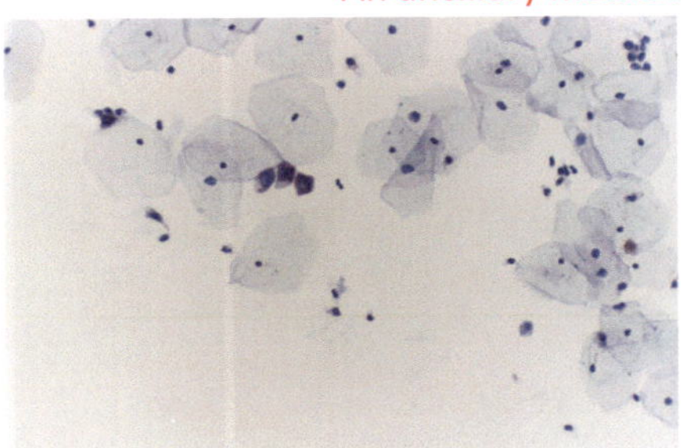

Abnormal specimen, ASC-H.
Three small abnormal (red) cells
among several normal cells.
Screening magnification (left).
Diagnostic magnifications (right).
Abnormal cells cannot be missed!

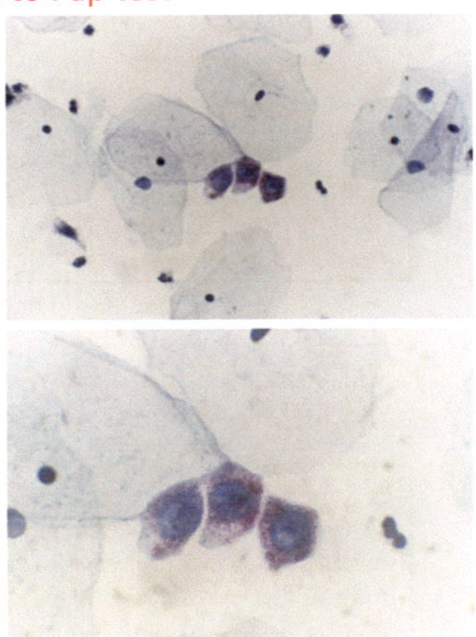

2.1.9

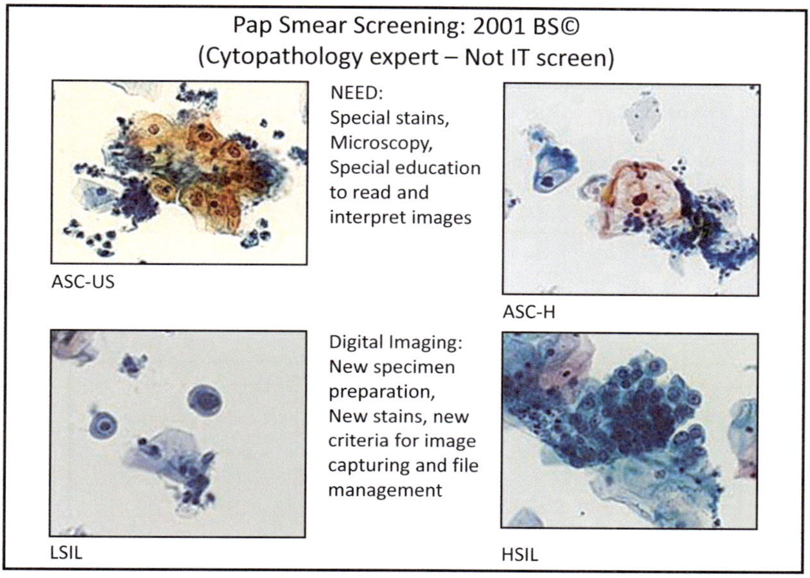
Pap Smear Screening: 2001 BS©
(Cytopathology expert – Not IT screen)
NEED:
Special stains,
Microscopy,
Special education
to read and
interpret images
ASC-US
ASC-H
Digital Imaging:
New specimen
preparation,
New stains, new
criteria for image
capturing and file
management
LSIL
HSIL

2.1.10

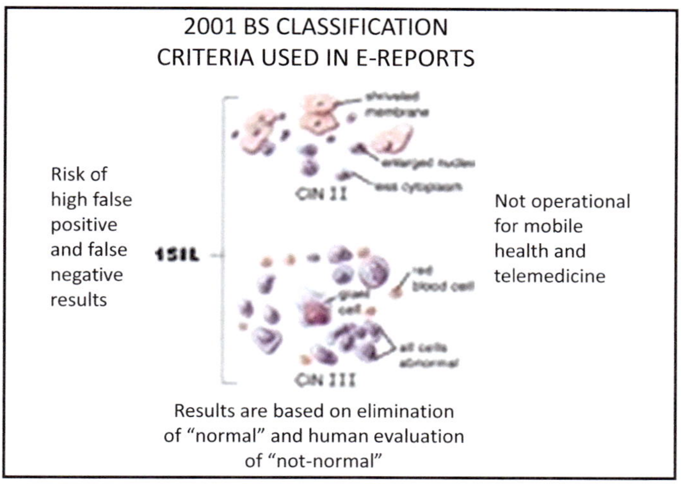
2001 BS CLASSIFICATION
CRITERIA USED IN E-REPORTS
Risk of
high false
positive
and false
negative
results
Not operational
for mobile
health and
telemedicine
Results are based on elimination
of “normal” and human evaluation
of “not-normal”

2.1.11

Further Reading

MarkPap® technology was patented in year 2000: It is biomarker-based, telemedicine empowered, affordable, accessible and infrastructure independent means for mass cervical cancer screening worldwide.
Further readings: www. bioscicon.com
"What every women should know about cervical cancer" "What Every Women Should Know About Cervical cancer (Springer 2008, 2010)
(http://www.springer.com/biomed/cancer/book/978-1-4020-6936-9)

2.1.12

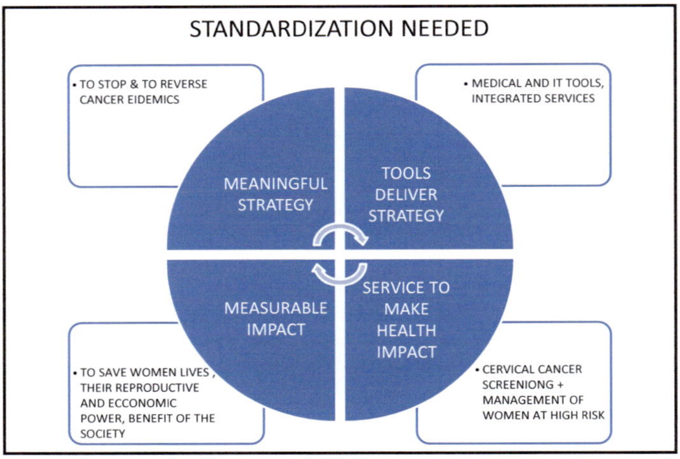

2.1.13

DIFFERENCE A/D

ANALOG IMAGES

- SCANNING SPECIMEN FOR MULTIPLE MEANIGFUL POINTS
- EXAMINE SUCH POINTS WITH DIFFERENT MAGNIFICATION AND FOCUS
- COMPARE OIMAGES WITH MEMORY DATABASE
- MAKE DIAGNOSIS

DIGITAL IMAGES

- COLLECTING MULTIPLE STILL IMAGES FROM THE SPECIMEN
- CAPTURE IMAGES, STORE IN IMAGE FILES, FORWARD TO EXPERTS FOR EVALUATION
- CONSULTATION BEFORE DIAGNOSIS IS ESTIMATED
- REPORT ESTIMATES

2.1.14

How we can help: A meaningful biomarker and WiFi telemedicine

Standard 2014

- Pap smear test
- Liquid-based Pap tests (ThinPrep, SurePath, Papsure)
- HPV related testing (CareHPV, HC-2, Cobas)
- Automation: Image analyzer; PCR,
- Home-based: HPV only

New C-ITTHC

1. Home-based collection
2. MarkPap® biomarker test
3. Digital imaging + Internet or WiFi
4. Telemedicine
5. Post test management
6. Removal of suspect lesions
7. Administration

2.1.15

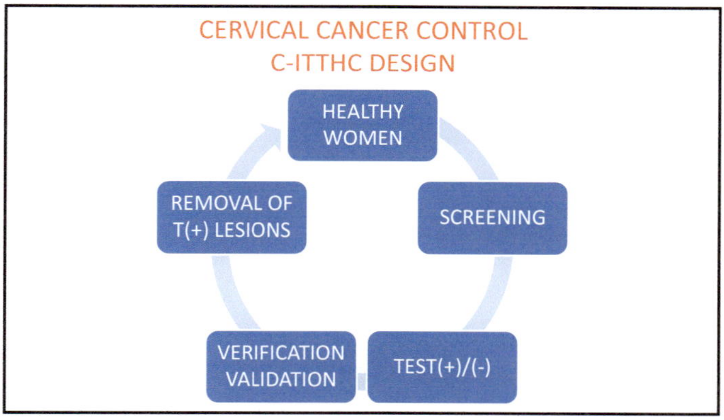

2.1.16

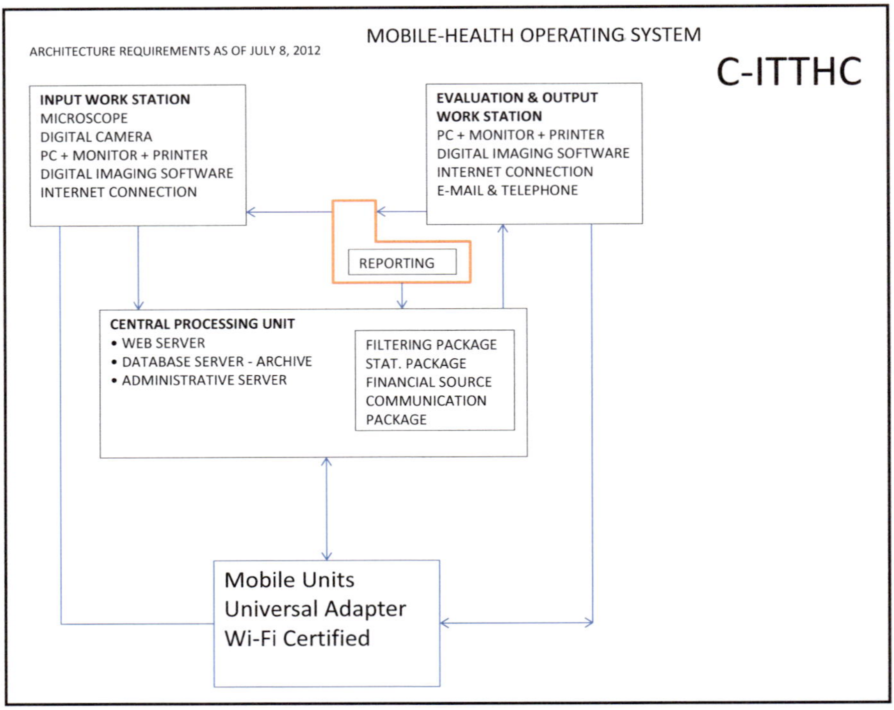

2.1.17

MARKPAP DIGITAL TELECYTOPATHOLOGY SYSTEM

- It is a multi-modular, global medical informatics system encompassing local, regional and global ITTHC with software secured and dedicated to a specific health problem, e.g., cervical cancer control.
- One module is planned to cover population that could need 1 million specific services per year.
- A module provides infrastructure, personnel, mobile and web based networking connections for users around the world, and software for semi-automatic management of the specific job assignments.

2.1.18

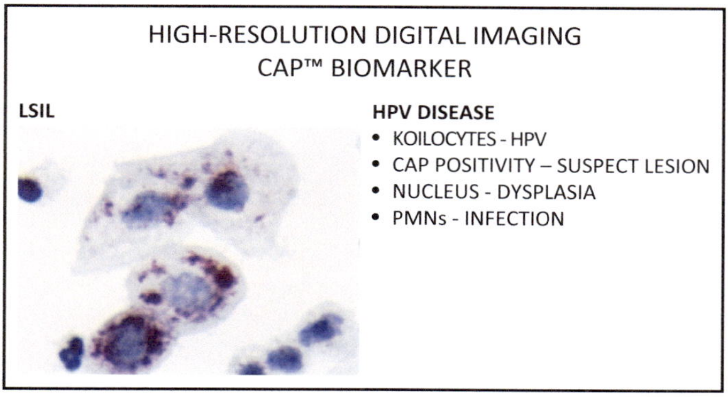

2.1.19

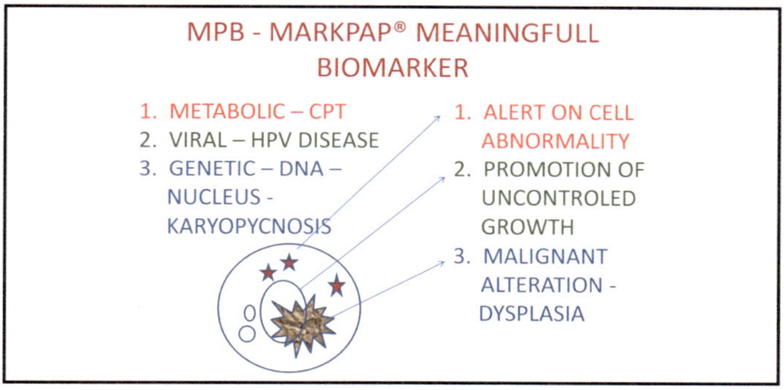

2.1.20

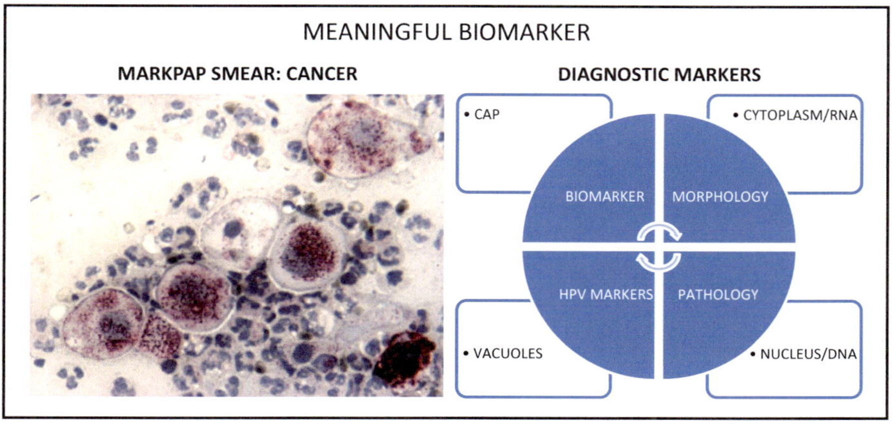

2.1.21

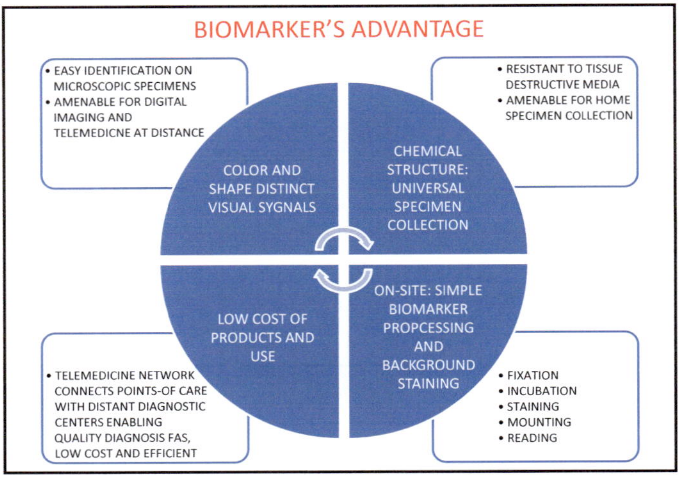
BIOMARKER'S ADVANTAGE
• EASY IDENTIFICATION ON MICROSCOPIC SPECIMENS
• AMENABLE FOR DIGITAL IMAGING AND TELEMEDICNE AT DISTANCE
• RESISTANT TO TISSUE DESTRUCTIVE MEDIA
• AMENABLE FOR HOME SPECIMEN COLLECTION
COLOR AND SHAPE DISTINCT VISUAL SYGNALS
CHEMICAL STRUCTURE: UNIVERSAL SPECIMEN COLLECTION
LOW COST OF PRODUCTS AND USE
ON-SITE: SIMPLE BIOMARKER PROPCESSING AND BACKGROUND STAINING
• TELEMEDICINE NETWORK CONNECTS POINTS-OF CARE WITH DISTANT DIAGNOSTIC CENTERS ENABLING QUALITY DIAGNOSIS FAS, LOW COST AND EFFICIENT
• FIXATION
• INCUBATION
• STAINING
• MOUNTING
• READING

2.1.22

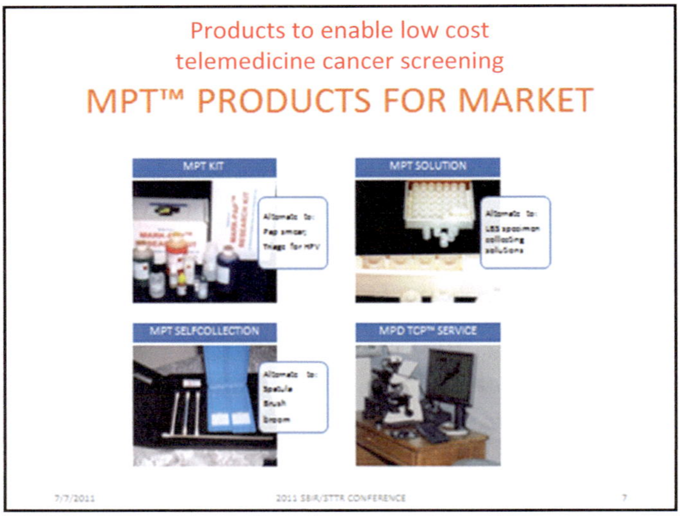
Products to enable low cost telemedicine cancer screening
MPT™ PRODUCTS FOR MARKET
MPT KIT
MPT SOLUTION
MPT SELFCOLLECTION
MPD TCP™ SERVICE
7/7/2011
2011 SBIR/STTR CONFERENCE
7

2.1.23

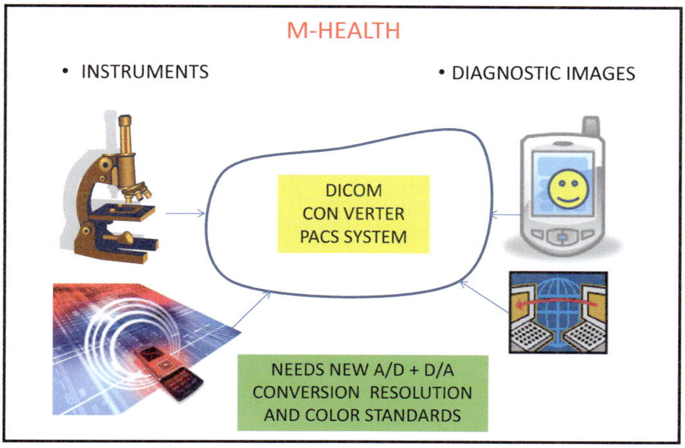
M-HEALTH
• INSTRUMENTS
• DIAGNOSTIC IMAGES
DICOM
CON VERTER
PACS SYSTEM
NEEDS NEW A/D + D/A
CONVERSION RESOLUTION
AND COLOR STANDARDS

2.1.24

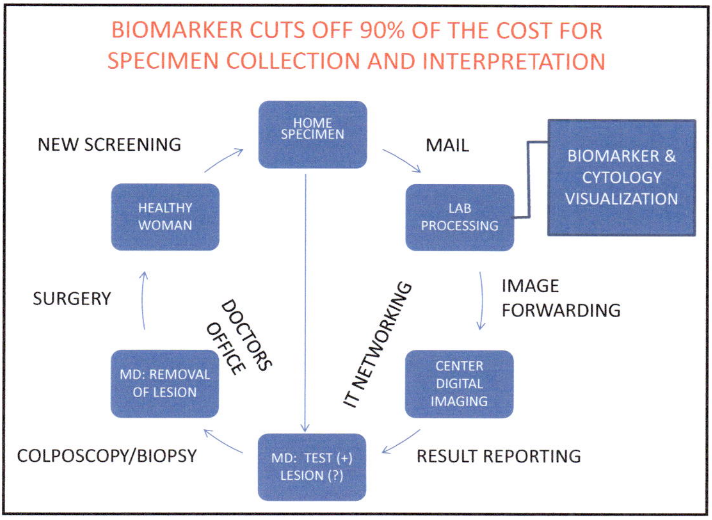
BIOMARKER CUTS OFF 90% OF THE COST FOR
SPECIMEN COLLECTION AND INTERPRETATION
HOME SPECIMEN
NEW SCREENING
MAIL
BIOMARKER & CYTOLOGY VISUALIZATION
HEALTHY WOMAN
LAB PROCESSING
SURGERY
DOCTORS OFFICE
IT NETWORKING
IMAGE FORWARDING
MD: REMOVAL OF LESION
CENTER DIGITAL IMAGING
COLPOSCOPY/BIOPSY
MD: TEST (+) LESION (?)
RESULT REPORTING

2.1.25

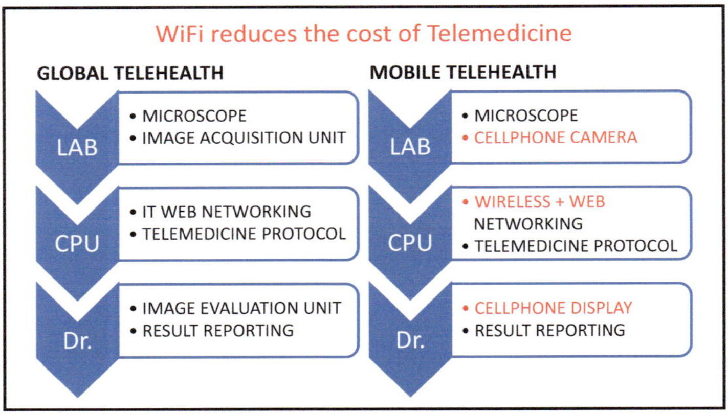

2.1.26

Commercial Demands

Standard testing

- Products to be used in standard procedures – manufacturing, regulatory, marketing, sales
- Standard health delivery services
- Education and training
- Regulatory approvals of standard services

Barriers to newcomers

- 20% of the market is mature and saturated with standard products – it is inaccessible
- 80% of the market is immature, free, but requires education and synchronized actions by industry, health professionals, government and public – this is difficult to achieve

2.1.27

COMMERCIAL STRATEGY

INVESTMENT

- CREATE AN AGENCY IN LMIC TO SERVE AS RESIDENT AGENT
- COMPLETE LOCAL FDA REQUIRMENTS AND OBTAIN REGISTRATION FOR MARKETING AND SALE
- EXPLORE OPTION FOR LOCAL COMPOUND MANUFACTURING
- CONTRACT IMPORTER, DISTRIBUTORS AND CUSTOMERS

MARKETING AND SALE

- SELECT A REGION FOR BETA TESTING
- MARKET GLOBALLY
- EDUCATE POPULATION AND PROFESSIONALS WITH BOOKS AND MEDIA EXPOSURE
- Use Principles, "Rich Pay for Poor," TO ACHIEVE HIGH OUTREACH (ABOVE 50%)
- Sale at the price acceptable to the public and the country.
- Include ROI + Profit in the Revenue

2.1.28

C-ITTHC LOCAL MODUL
Basic Elements for Testing

INPUT DEVICE FOR MOBILE TCP

- Microscope – 20x, 40x, 10x
- Universal adapter
- Mobile wireless camera battery powered
- Recording capability: still image capture, on-screen drawing & texting
- Security: encryption & authentication - SIM
- Designated telelemedicine endpoints for image file sharing – networking plan
- Approval for using as electronic device

OUTPUT TCP EXPERT DIAGNOSIS REPORTING DEVICE

- **MPD TCP Expert**: (1) enables on-screen drawing/ annotations, (2) sharing information quickly and efficiently, (3) long term record keeping (snapshots or video), (4) exporting video to QuickTime formats for portability & encrypting for Windows XP compatible
- **MPD TCP Management Suite**: administrative issues

2.1.29

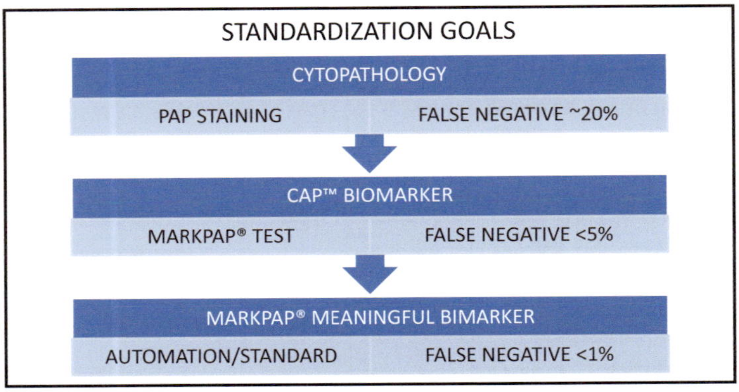

2.1.30

CONTACT

- 1. BIOSCICON, INC. ROCKVILLE, MD
- DR. OLIVERA MARKOVIC, PROFESSOR & DIRECTOR
- 1.301.610.9130
- info@bioscicon.com
- www.bioscicon.com

2.2 *Global Health Challenges: Is worldwide cytological cervical cancer possible? 2015*

2.2.1

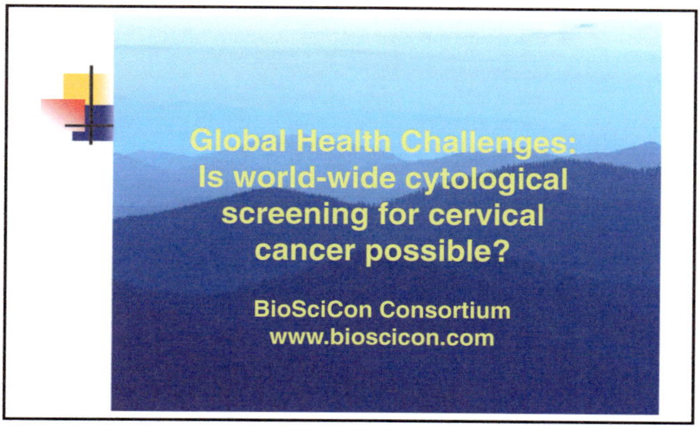

2.2.2

Cervical Cancer is preventable

Cervical cancer is second to the breast cancer cause of women deaths from malignant diseases world-wide. However, cervical cancer is preventable **IF** detected on time. Unfortunately, currently there are 520,000 new cases of cervical cancer each year worldwide and about 260,000 women die from this preventable disease in 21st Century.

Cytological screening (Pap test) remains the best cervical cancer prevention available.

2.2.3

Why women die from cervical cancer?

Because they do not have preventive screening:

- At risk: 1.7 B
- Protected with Pap 110 M or 6.5%
- Developing countries: 20 M Pap tests or 1.2%

2.2.4

Why women do not take a preventive test that makes a difference between health and a grave disease, life and death?

- Because most of women can not afford the expensive Pap test
- Pap test is not available in many countries (lack of infrastructure and qualified personnel)
- Women do not have access to medical institutions
- Can not/do not want to go to gynecologist because of different barriers (cultural, religious)

2.2.5

Is there a solution? YES

- **Can not afford**: Top develop less expensive, affordable Pap test
- **Pap not available**: To develop improved, yet simple Pap test that can be done anywhere in the world and evaluated "at distance" in labs with qualified personnel (telemedicine)
- **No access**: To develop a Pap test with self-collection
- **Cannot/do not want to go to gynecologist**: Self collection and education

2.2.6

The Solution exists: MarkPap® Platform Technology

MarkPap® is a trademark for a line of products, based on the novel biomarker of cellular abnormality, intended to improve the standard of care for cervical cancer prevention.

2.2.7

MarkPap Solution at each step. How?

- **Can not afford**: MarkPap is low cost affordable Pap test.
- **Pap test not available**: Improved (biomarker-based), simple to perform (MarkPap Kit) and can be done anywhere in the world, but amenable for evaluation "at distance" in labs with qualified personnel (telecytopathology).
- **No access**: MarkPap Self (self-collection).
- **Can not/do not want to visit gynecologist**: MarkPap Self and education (

2.2.8

Where , Who?

BioSciCon, Inc.

The Global Academy for Women's Health, Inc.

At Johns Hopkins University, Montgomery County Campus

Rockville, MD, USA

2.2.9

BioSciCon, Inc. develops and manufactures patented biomarker-based MarkPap® platform technology products intended for early detection of cervical cancer and precancerosis. This technology is more accurate, less costly, less invasive than the current Pap test with option for self-sampling and telecytopathology.

2.2.10

MarkPap® Technology: What the biomarker does?

The biomarker is "flagging" dysplastic (precancerous), malignant and HPV induced abnormal cells with a red "flag" increasing their visibility so they cannot be missed even by low-trained professional ("red cells"). Normal cells are entirely negative (blue).

2.2.11

MarkPap® technology: Biomarker is "flagging" abnormal cells

MarkPap biomarker is cytoplasmic expression of genetic changes in cervical cells during transformation from normal to pre-malignant (dysplastic) and malignant, with or w/o HPV infection. When visualized with MarkPap test biomarker appears as a red pigment flagging only abnormal cells.

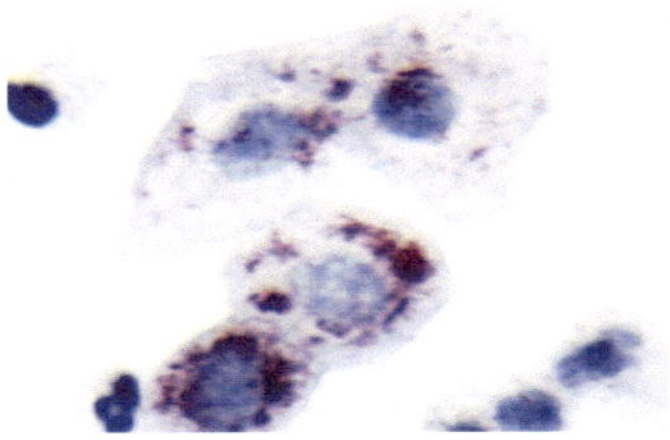

2.2.12

MarkPap® Images

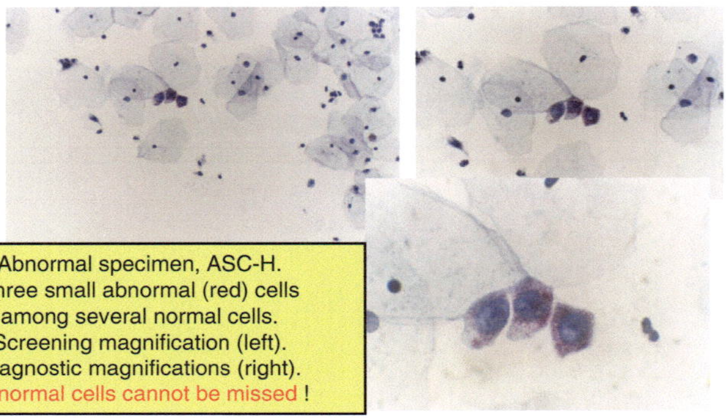

Abnormal specimen, ASC-H.
Three small abnormal (red) cells
among several normal cells.
Screening magnification (left).
Diagnostic magnifications (right).
Abnormal cells cannot be missed !

2.2.13

MarkPap® Images: Biomarker is positive in cancer and HPV induced abnormal cells

MarkPap smear from a patient with invasive cervical carcinoma

Red biomarker is positive in all abnormal cells where micro-vacuolization and dysplastic features are present together

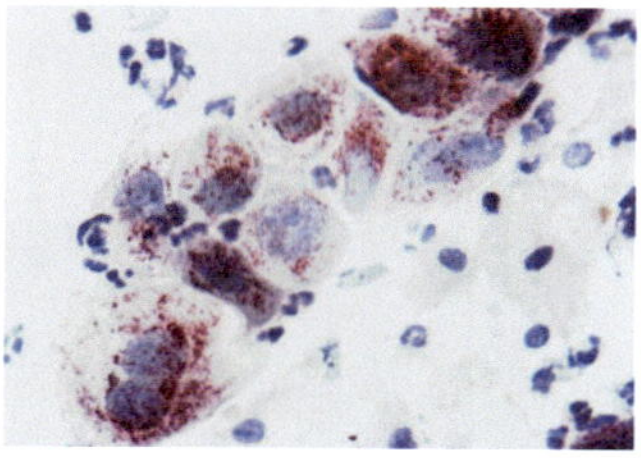

2.2.14

The power of the new biomarker

Because it is based on the new biomarker of cervical abnormality the method is:

- **More accurate**
- **Faster**
- **Simple, customer-friendly kit**
- **Less expensive, affordable**
- **Amenable for telecytopathology (MarkPap Digital)**
- **Self-sampling possible (MarkPap Self)**

The test can be performed in a remote sites, at the point-of-care by a low-trained technician, the same person identifies abnormal cells by the red color and transmit those images in a distant laboratory for diagnosis. The result may be obtained within hours.

2.2.15

MarkPap® Products
(first line of products)

- **MarkPap® Kit** : Assembly of reagents, instructions and controls
- **Kit Accessories**: Cytopreservative solution, COMBO Control slides
- **MarkPapTest**: service, assay for manual and automated staining procedures (**MarkPap Auto**)

2.2.16

MarkPap® Kit

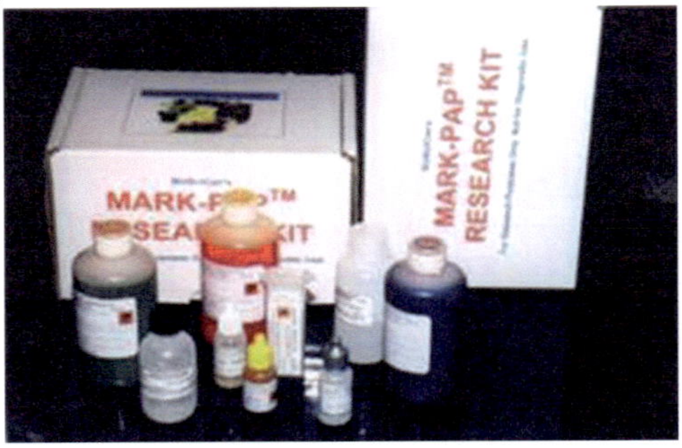

2.2.17

MarkPap® Products
(Second and Third line of products)

- MarkPap® Digital
- MarkPap® Self Kit
- MarkPap® Wireless

All these products are made possible because on the presence of the biomarker. MarkPap® products are available for licensing and sale under local regulations.

2.2.18

MarkPap® Digital Telecytopathology

MarkPap Digital provides opportunity to capture the "red" biomarker positive (abnormal) cells with a digital camera and transmit the images via Internet into laboratories with qualified reviewers for evaluation. The presence of the biomarker, flagging abnormal cells, is critical to allow low-trained person to make selection at the point-of-care which cell images (microscopic fields) to transmit for evaluation The result may be delivered back electronically within hours. This service is available at BioSciCon.

The cost of screening for cervical cancer with MarkPap Digital is affordable for low resource areas.

2.2.19

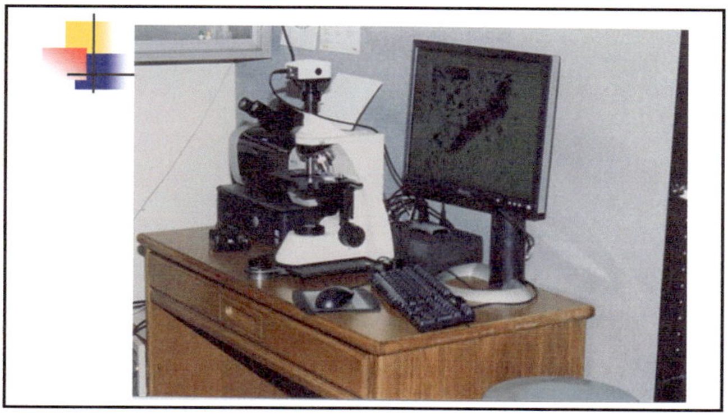

2.2.20

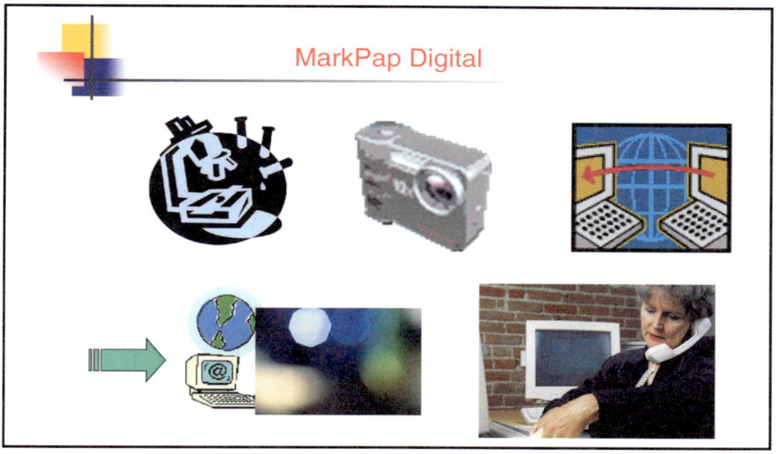

2.2.21

MarkPap Self Test (Kit)

MarkPap elf is an option for women to take the sample in the privacy of their home and to send it in the laboratory. The kit is a simple device for sample collection, that should be available over the counter The Kit is primarily aimed for women who live in remote parts and do not have access to doctors offices..

Since the morphology of cells is damaged in the acidic vaginal fluids, Mark Pap Self is uniquely possible because the biomarker is stable in the vaginal fluids.

MarkPap Self is expected to dramatically increase the number of women who will get preventive testing.

This is third generation product in final phase od development.

2.2.22

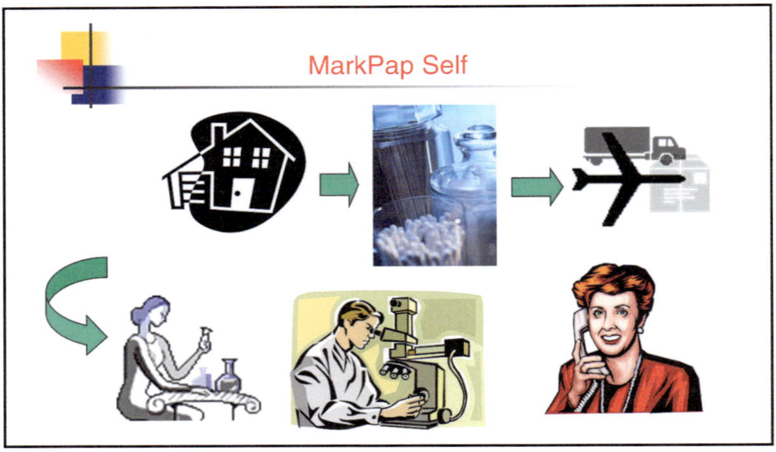

2.2.23

MarkPap® Wireless

Mobile transmission of images with cell phone.
Wireless Telecytopathology

Third generation MarkPap® product still in development.

The cell phone is mounted on the microscopic ocular and images of suspect cells, taken directly from the microscope, are transmitted for distant evaluation.
Since cell phones are widely used, the MarkPap Wireless, e.g., MarkPap® Wireless telecytopathology offers cytological screening (Pap test) anywhere in the world.
Please visit: www.bioscicon.com/publications.html for our progress in this field.

2.2.24

MarkPap®Wireless Telecytopathology

Microscopic image captured directly to the cell phone, (Samsung Eternity). Abnormal specimen with biomarker positive cervical cells.

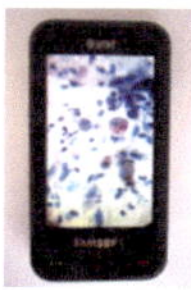

2.2.25

MarkPap® Wireless Telecytopathology

Images of cervical cancer specimen's cells, captured with the same cell phone, transmitted to the for evaluation.
In the expert laboratory images transferred on the computer screen for evaluation.
Biomarker positive cells among many inflammatory cells can be easily differentiated.

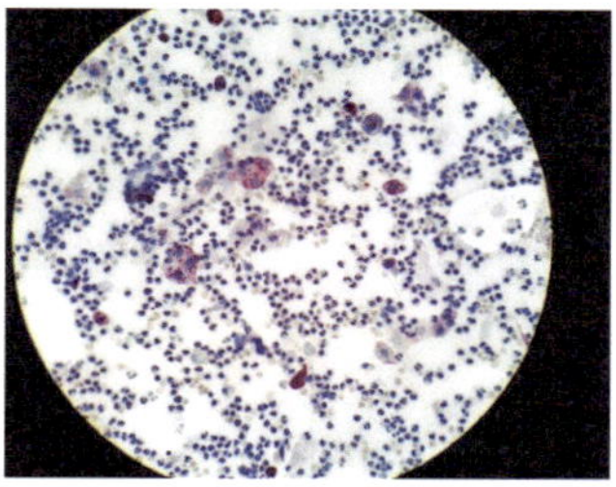

2.2.26

IT Telehealth Center

BioSciCon has designed the Global MarkPap Digital IT Telehealth Center as a modular hierarchal system structure, has built a prototype and successfully tested the feasibility of the concept and the prototype.
One module (Maryland IT Telehealth Center), is designed for 1 million services per year.

2.2.27

BioSciCon Consortium

In order to respond to its mission
BioSciCon developed A Consortium

2.2.28

BioSciCon Consortium

BioSciCon, Inc is biotechnology R&D component of the Consortium with three trade companies MarkPap LLC, MarkPap Pacific LLC and MarkPap India LLC for commercialization of MarkPap® products as they emerge from R&D phase, and an independent non-profit organization, The Global Academy for Women's Health, Inc. with the mission to promote excellence in science and education in women's health.

www.bioscicon.com www.markpap.com

2.2.29

Additional Reading

www.bioscicon.com
www.markpap.com
"What every woman should know about cervical cancer", (Drs. Markovic, edt), Springer, 2008
http://www.springer.com/biomed/cancer/book/978-1-4020-6936-9 **and** www.amazon.com
SBIR and STTR Success Story for BioSciCon, Inc.
http://grants1.nih.gov/grants/funding/sbir_successes/155.htm
SCORE Success Story for BioSciCon. Inc.
www.bioscicon.com/news.html
Virginia Telehealth Network. Video Lecture
http://ehealthvirginia.org/technologywatch2.html

2.2.30

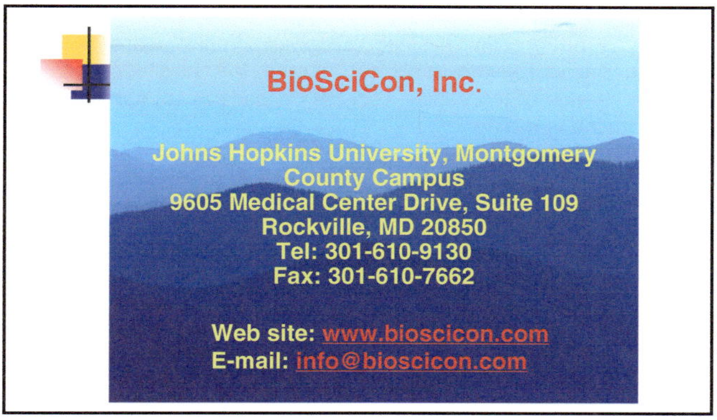
BioSciCon, Inc.
Johns Hopkins University, Montgomery County Campus
9605 Medical Center Drive, Suite 109
Rockville, MD 20850
Tel: 301-610-9130
Fax: 301-610-7662
Web site: www.bioscicon.com
E-mail: info@bioscicon.com

2.3 *MarkPap Pacific Presents: MarkPap® Technology, 2013*

2.3.1

PACIFIC

MarkPap Pacific, LLC

Opportunity in China

2013

2.3.2

MarkPap Pacific LLC

MISSION: To commercialize the BioSciCon's MarkPap® platform technology for prevention of cervical cancer on the markets of Greater Pacific Area – P.R. China in particular.

VISION: To provide Chinese health care providers with tools to reverse the negative trends of increasing cervical cancer prevalence and mortality.

2.3.3

Cervical Cancer is preventable

Cancer of the uterine cervix, cervical cancer is a major cause of women deaths from malignant diseases world-wide. Currently, there are 600,000 new cases of cervical cancer each year, and about 300,000 women die from a disease that is IF detected on time. Unfortunately, only at average 10% of world women population is getting preventive screening. The WHO and all governments are looking for affordable services to overcome this situation. Cytological screening with Pap test is the best solution.

2.3.4

China Needs

- China is the fastest growing cervical cancer market in the world and is still open for new technologies
- There are 440 M women at risk for cervical cancer in China. Every year 75,500 women are diagnosed with cervical cancer and 34,000 die. Prognosis for 2025 are 90,000 new cases and 50,500 deaths
- Current outreach for preventive screening is 17%. Out of 100 women only 17 get prevention. The only way to improve the situation is to increase the outreach
- In the US the outreach is about 80%

2.3.5

Why? What is the problem?

Existing Pap Test Technology

- Costly: Increasing insurance costs in US and prohibitively expensive in developing countries
- Infrastructure: required, with qualified professionals (cytotechnologists/pathologists)
- Insufficient Reliability: (>15% false negatives)
- Slow: Takes weeks to obtain normal results
- Requires visiting a doctor and it is invasive: Not available for women who do not have access to doctor's offices or are not allowed to visit gynecologist

2.3.6

The Solution

MarkPap® Technology is the solution:

- Less costly: Priced lower than Pap test
- Infrastructure: Not required at the POC
- More reliable: <5% false negatives
- Timely: Results within hours (telemedicine service).
- Does not require access to doctor's offices and is less invasive: Self-collection of specimen at home
- Better controlled: QC/QA with control slides and less liability for the laboratory

2.3.7

What is MarkPap® Platform Technology

MarkPap is a trademark for a patented technology that includes instruments, medical devices, reagents (in vitro diagnostics), controls and procedures and instructions which, in different combinations, are intended for early detection of pre-cancerous and cancerous lesions and save women's lives. It is also to improve the quality of life of healthy women relieving them from fear of cervical cancer risk.

2.3.8

Products for Sale in China

Subject to US export and local import regulations

1. MarkPap® Test Kit with accessories

12 individual reagents and control slides with Instruction for the Manual MarkPap® Test

2. MarkPap® Telecytopathology Service (sm)

Instruments and software for distant evaluation

3. MarkPap® Self™ Kit for home specimen collection

2.3.9

What makes MarkPap® Technology unique

MarkPap® technology in a powerful biomarker-based, telemedicine-empowered, simple accurate, fast, accessible, equitable and infrastructure independent technology for early detection of abnormal cells on cervical specimens.

The proprietary biomarker of cellular abnormality is a powerful means to make the test less expensive, more amenable for telecytopathology, does not require pathologist at the Point of Care and opened the possibility for home self-sampling.

More... www.bioscicon.com MarkPap®

2.3.10

MarkPap® platform technology illustrated

We have discovered a proprietary technology which is based upon a molecular biomarker which is positive only in abnormal cells, and always negative in normal cells. The biomarker is visualized as red color deposit. Compare upper, positive specimen (cancer) and lower negative specimen (normal).

This distinction makes the method superior over all competitors. More….

www.bioscicon.com/gallery.html

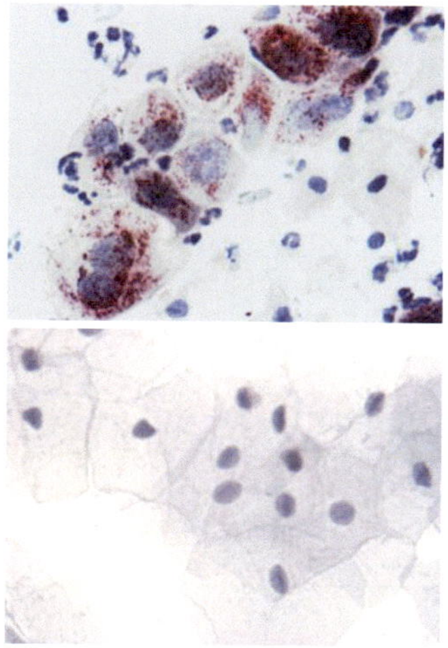

2.3.11

How it works

In practice our products will allow women to take the sample at home (if cannot visit gynecologist) and to mail it to the nearby laboratory. In this laboratory a low-trained technician or a nurse can stain the slide using easy-to-use MarkPap® Kit. The same person examines the slide under the microscope and searches for "red" cells only. The images of those cells are captured with a digital camera or cell phone camera and transmitted for evaluation. The result may be sent back electronically while a women is still on the premises.. More…
www.bioscicon.com/publications.html (40)

2.3.12

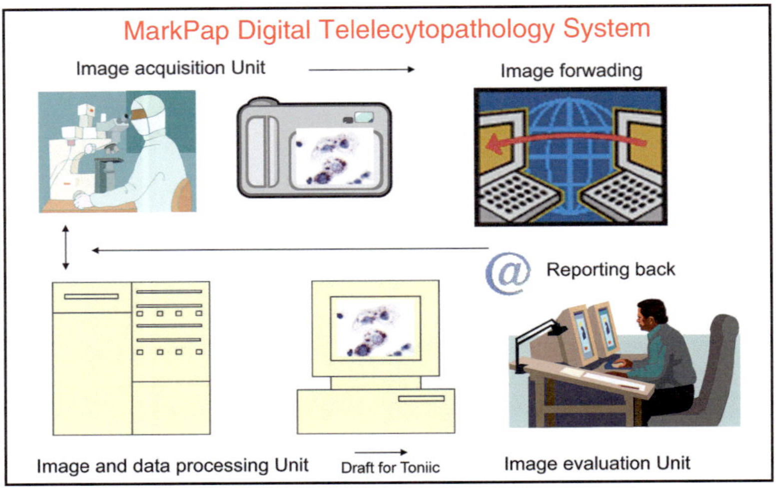

2.3.13

Impact and commercial benefit

- **Mass cervical cancer screening worldwide: Huge societal benefit saving women's lives from preventable cancer, and enormous market with incredible potential for profit (2B women at risk worldwide)**
- MarkPap, Pacific LLC was incorporated to carry this technology in China, to increase outreach, and reduce mortality. When properly applied it is expected to save aproximately100,000 women's lives during 5 years

2.3.14

MarkPap Pacific LLC

MarkPap Pacific is a trade company incorporated by BioSciCon, Inc. in 2007 to commercialize BioSciCon's MarkPap® technology proprietary products and services for preventive cervical cancer screening in China and Greater Pacific Area. BioSciCon has licensed to this company exclusive rights to commercialize selective products and has made available the background history of market research and technology promotion in China

2.3.15

Business Overview

Investment up to date 5M from founders and government grants

MPP estimates to earn $1.00 per MarkPap® product sold, with minimum estimated sales of 1 M products per year, for five years.

Beginning of sales is expecting within 2 years from the investment

- NOTE: When sale phase will start the total value including ROI will be multiplied by equivalent of 10
- See cost /benefit ratio

2.3.16

Investment needed

Investment of up to 1M is needed for:

- Patent protection in China – Legal issues
- Clinical trials in China
- Manufacturing the first delivery package
- Import/export and other licenses
- Insurance
- Operating cost

2.3.17

We need financial and other support from people who are Making Money-Doing Good
ALL DOING WELL

- It is expected an **ENORMOUS** societal impact by saving tens of thousands women's lives, but also a **huge** financial benefit is projected.
- With the beginning of sales the value of the Company will raise significantly, together with the Return on Investment. Consequently, investing into MPP at this time should be considered **WIN—WIN situation**, we think.

2.3.18

Exit Strategy

- As the business model is structured, the Exit is warranted during the pre-sale phase, or when revenue from sales/licensing would began to accrue
- Anytime in the sale phase, because of sales drop or revenue diminishes by otherwise unpredictable and uncorrectable factors, the Company will be offered for sale, first to the founders, then to partners, lastly to others

2.3.19

Education

Education is an essential part of the introduction and implementation of new technologies.

Drs. Nenad and Olivera Markovic authored the book "What every woman should know about cervical cancer" published in 2008 by renown international publisher Springer. The book is available in hard and paperback format, electronic and kindle edition. The book is distributing all over the world and is well accepted.

http://www.springer.com/biomed/cancer/book/978-1-4020-6936-9 and www.amazon.com.

2.3.20

What Every Woman Should Know about Cervical Cancer

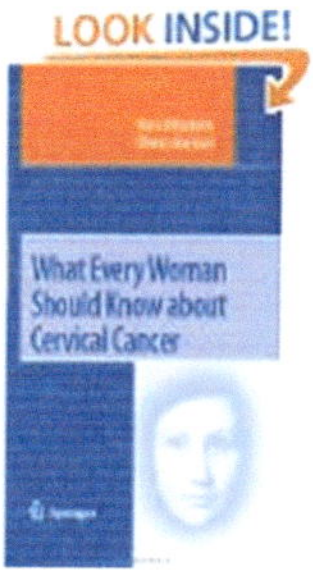

Since the field of cervical cancer is developing fast, Springer invited Drs. Markovic to write the second, extended and updated edition. The work is in progress. See Hopkins News, 2012

http://web1.johnshopkins.edu/~mccblog/?p=1376.

2.3.21

Contact

Prof. Dr. Nenad Markovic
President and CEO MarkPap Pacific, LLC
Johns Hopkins University, Montgomery County Campus
9601 Medical Center Drive, Suite 111
Rockville, MD 20850
www.bioscicon.com
E-Mail: info@bioscicon.com
Tel: 301-610-9130

2.4 *China Deal Overview. MarkPap Pacific, LLC, 2009*

2.4.1

COMPANY

MarkPap Pacific LLC (MPPLLC) is a trade company incorporated in 2007 specially to execute the China Deal – a business contract with Chinese partners for marketing and selling the BioSciCon's MarkPap® platform technology products in China in millions of units.

MPPLLC is located in the Maryland Technology Development Center, 9700 Great Seneca Hwy, Rockville, MD

Contact: Phone: (301) 610-9130; e-mail:
www.bioscicon,com

2.4.2

MarkPap® TECHNOLOGY

Biomarker-based cytology with modified Papanicolaou staining in the background, combined with digital imaging and IT communication for digital transfer of images between remote sites for fast, accurate and low cost evaluation of clinical condition on specimens collected from healthy women or patients.

2.4.3

BIOMARKER

highlighting abnormal **cells with red label**

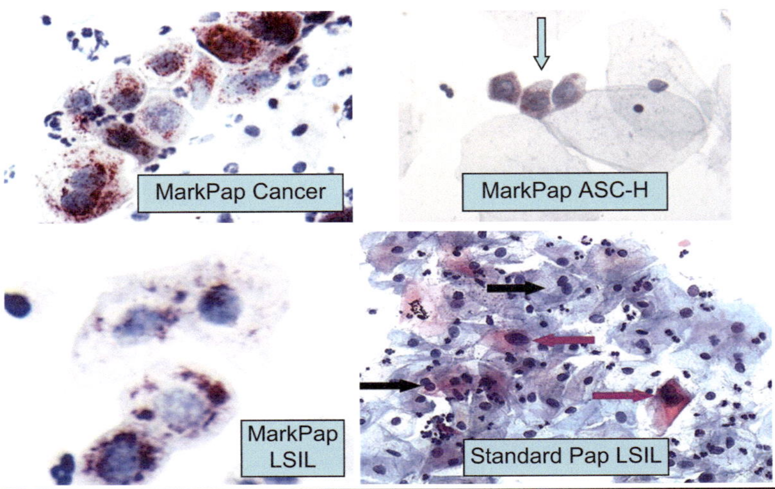

2.4.4

Products for Sale - 1

MarkPap® Kit

- Assembly of reagents, controls and instructions to facilitate performance of 300 MarkPap tests (see image)
- The kit is manufactured by Ricca Chemical Company for BioSciCon, Inc.
- It is available for immediate sale at a price of $900.00 FOB Arlington, TX. Taxes, S&H is additional.

2.4.5

MarkPap® Research Kit

(as available before regulatory approval)

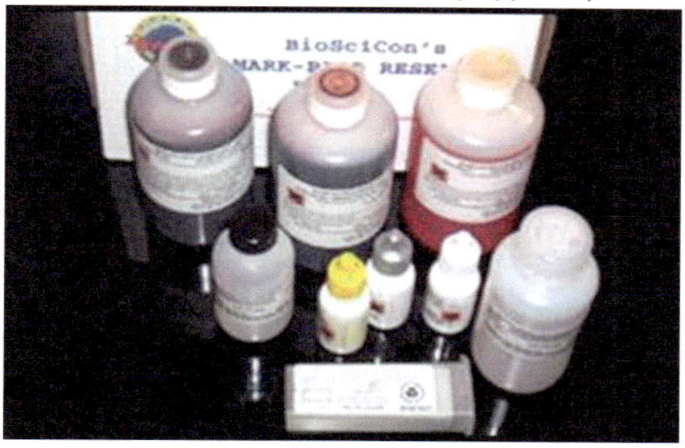

2.4.6

Products for Sale - 2

- MarkPap® Digital™ Telecytopathology Service(sm)
- Connection to the MarkPap Digital Networking Center and using IT communication for medical diagnosis of microscopic images at distance.
- This service is available to customers via a dedicated and secure web site for cost of $2.00 per consultation

2.4.7

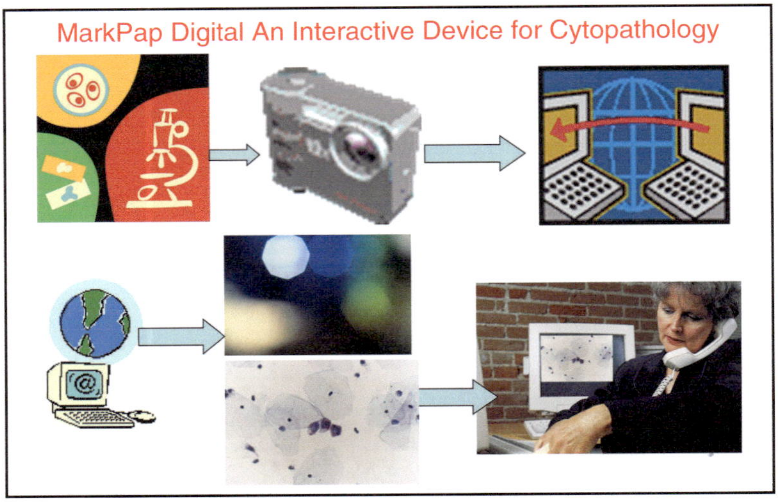

2.4.8

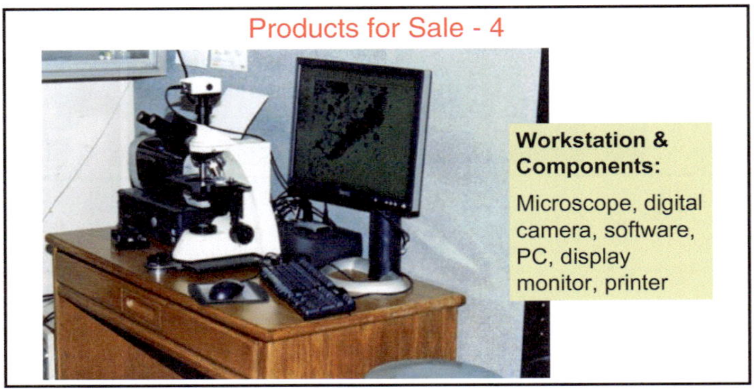
Products for Sale - 4
Workstation & Components:
Microscope, digital camera, software, PC, display monitor, printer

2.4.9

Products for Sale - 3

Accessories

1. MarkPap® Solution Kit™
   Assembly of reagents, controls and instructions for collecting specimens in solution for MarkPap test evaluation
2. MarkPap® Control COMBO slides™
   Individual containers with 1 pre-stained and 4 unstained MarkPap slides for Quality Control and Quality Assurance

2.4.10

MarkPap® Solution™ Kit

MARK-PAP® Cytopreservative Solution
(Accessories to MARK-PAP® test kit)

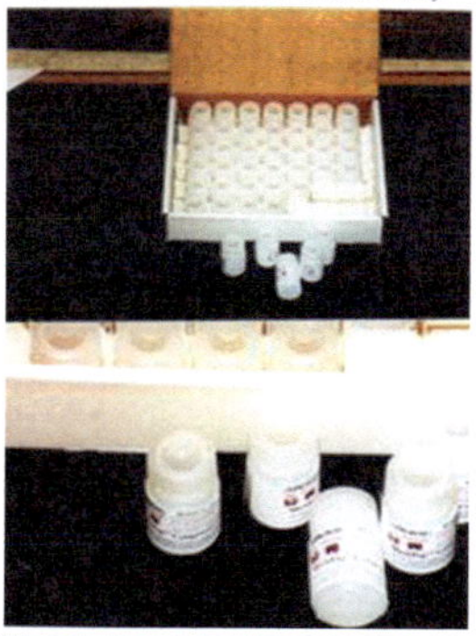

2.4.11

China Deal Outline

- We have signed a Memorandum of Understanding with a Chinese distributor and a contract is in preparation for sale of 1 million tests and up per year for 5 years.
- The same number of services is offered for consideration
- Details are discusses elsewhere

2.4.12

Preface

China is the fastest growing cervical cancer market in the world and is still open for new technologies that could provide, like MarkPap®, fast and accurate diagnostic result for low cost. MarkPap Digital Networking is adding to the testing accuracy via telecytopathology and with bypassing the needs for expensive infrastructure.

2.4.13

China Market

- China Population: 1.3 B
- Women: ½ = 0.65 B
- Women at risk: 2/3 = 0.44 B
- Maximum outreach: 0.80 = 350 M
- Periods: 1/3 = 112 M tests per year
- Penetration: Progressive from 1% up
- Current market (2006): 70 M test per year
- Market growth: 10 M test/year

2.4.14

China Market Needs

- To reduce mortality of cervical cancer which is currently 30/100,000
- Pap test success when implemented: Steady reduction of mortality for 4% per year
- Expected result in China: Approximately 100,000 women lives saved for 5 years of application

2.4.15

US Partners in China Deal

- Owner: BioSciCon, Inc. Rockville, MD
- Seller for China: MarkPap Pacific, LLC
- Reagents and kit manufacturer: Ricca Chemical Company, Arlington, TX
- Digital compound instrument provider: GT-Vision, Hagerstown, MD
- Telemedicine Service provider: MPDN Center in Montgomery County, MD

2.4.16

Chinese partner

Anhui Anke Biotechnology (Group), Ltd.

- Marketing approval (patent protection, clinical trial, import/export licenses)
- Marketing in China
- Distribution and Sale
- Payments

2.4.17

Sources for funding

- 4F
- Grants
- Loans
- Capital investment (A&VC)
- Corporations (co-development)

2.4.18

Value Proposal for Investment Test - Kit

- **According to the MOU, the distributor will buy kits at the sale price $3.00 per test FOB Arlington, TX.**

This sale price includes:

- **Reagents manufacturing with QC and bottling.**
- **Kit packaging and shipping paperwork.**
- **Labeling Insert and labels on the box and reagents.**
- **Free Customer Service for reagents**
- **Markup $0.80 per test**

2.4.19

Value Proposal for Investment
Solution – Control Slides

- MarkPap Solution is another product that is sold in kits containing 30 vials with solution and 30 plastic spatulas for specimen collection
- The estimated price is $5.00 per vial
- Control MarkPap Test Slides are sold in plastic containers with 1 pre-stained and 4 unstained slides for quality control and quality assurance
- Estimates price is $12.00 per container

2.4.20

Value Proposal for Investment MarkPap Digital TCP Service

- MarkPap Digital Telecytopathology Service is the product (service) expected to be provided by the MarkPap Digital Networking Center,which is now in development.
- It is designed to serve customers seeking cytopathology diagnostic services for microscopic specimens from around the world.
- The estimated price is $2.00 per service which includes evaluation of one diagnostic case report (6 digital images)

2.4.21

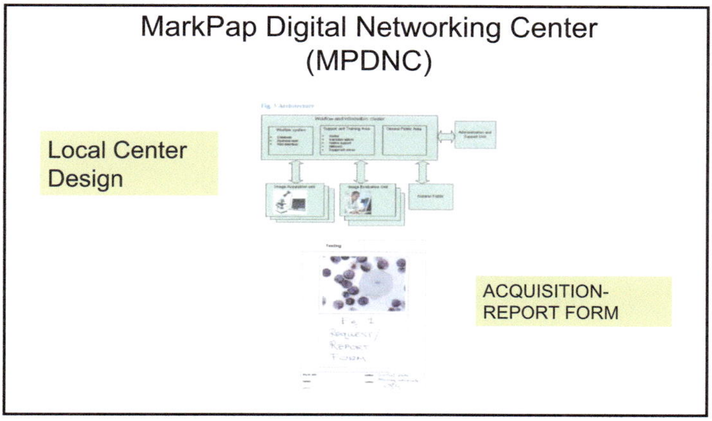

2.4.22

Profit from MPT Sale: $1.00 per test

MP Test Kit sold – Profit in million dollars

2010 -- 70M: 1% = 0.70 M

2011 -- 78M: 2% = 1.56 M

2012 -- 84M: 4% = 3.36 M

2013 -- 88M: 8% = 7.04 M

2014 -- 90M: 9% = 8.10 M

Cumulative profit for 5years = 20.76 ~ 20M

2.4.23

MarkPap Solution Market

MarkPap Solution is needed for HPV and other biomarkers testing. The needs are estimated to be 5% of the total number of tests and to rise for 10% annually. .

70M: 5% = 3.5M + 10%=3.535

78M: 5% = 3.9M + 10%=3.939

84M: 5% = 4.2M + 10%=4.242

88M: 5% = 4.4M + 10%=4.444

90M: 5% = 4.5M + 10%=4.545

Cumulative t for 5y = 20.7M

2.4.24

MPD - Networking System

Local for 1M women
- **Local networking station includes:**
- **20 Input workstations (WS)**
- **1 Local CPU,**
- **6 Image Evaluation Units (IEU)**

Global for 2B women
- **Global system includes:**
- **State CPU**
- **Regional CPU**
- **Local CPU**

Single networking protocol and diagnostic protocol

2.4.25

Business Overview

- Signing the contract should put us in position to plan a multimillion dollar revenue from at least 1 million sold units per year
- We expect approximately 1 million dollar profit each year from the first day of sale
- To come to this point we need cash investment/loan of up to 1 million dollars divided in portions

2.4.26

Investment is needed for:

- Patent protection in China
- Clinical trials in China
- Manufacturing first delivery package
- Import/export and other licenses
- Insurance
- Operating cost
- Overhead

2.4.27

Cost taken by the partner

- Marketing in China
- Distribution from FOB destination to delivery destination in China
- Warehouse service if necessary
- Retail sale: processing orders and pre-payments for both products and services
- Local delivery service
- Local customer service

2.4.28

Cost taken by BioSciCon

- Preparation and printing of labeling special for China
- Design, monitoring and evaluation of RCT in China
- Quality assurance of kits in the US
- Second level Customer Service for Post-marketing troubleshooting

2.4.29

Cost taken by the Manufacturer

- Production of reagents for 300K tests
- Bottling
- Packing 1000 kits
- Internal quality control
- Paperwork for shipping

2.4.30

Cost taken by MarkPap Pacific LLC

- Training of Chinese customers both in the US and China
- Providing logistics for implementation of MarkPap Digital Telecytopathology services) equipment, networking, personnel, funding, legal counseling, office support)
- Business contracts with China and monitoring of the compliance

2.4.31

CONTACT

Dr. Olivera Markovic
Professor and Director
BioSciCon, Inc.
Rockville, MD
Tel: 301-610-9130
Fax:301-6107662
E-mail: info@bioscicon.com
Web site: www.bioscicon.com

2.5 *MarkPap Pacific, LLC. Opportunity in China, 2008*

2.5.1

MarkPap Pacific LLC Presents:
MarkPap® Technology

A new opportunity in PR
of China 2008

2.5.2

The Consortium of Organizations Caring for Women's Health

- BioSciCon, Inc, the parent R&D corporation for a proprietary, platform MarkPap® technology for cervical cancer prevention
- MarkPap LLC, organized for commercialization of the technology (marketing, distribution and sale)
- MarkPap Pacific LLC, incorporated specifically for commercialization in greater Pacific Area
- The Global Academy for Women's Health, Inc, an independent non-profit dedicated to women's health education

2.5.3

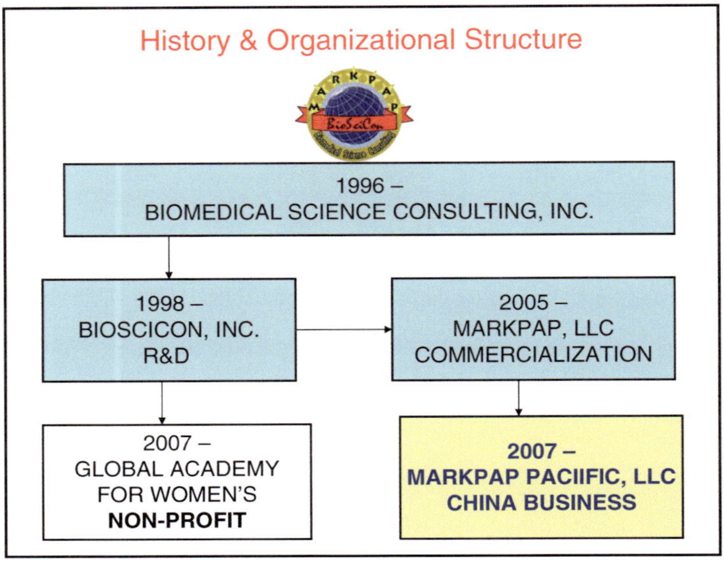
History & Organizational Structure
1996 –
BIOMEDICAL SCIENCE CONSULTING, INC.
1998 –
BIOSCICON, INC.
R&D
2005 –
MARKPAP, LLC
COMMERCIALIZATION
2007 –
GLOBAL ACADEMY
FOR WOMEN'S
NON-PROFIT
2007 –
MARKPAP PACIIFIC, LLC
CHINA BUSINESS

2.5.4

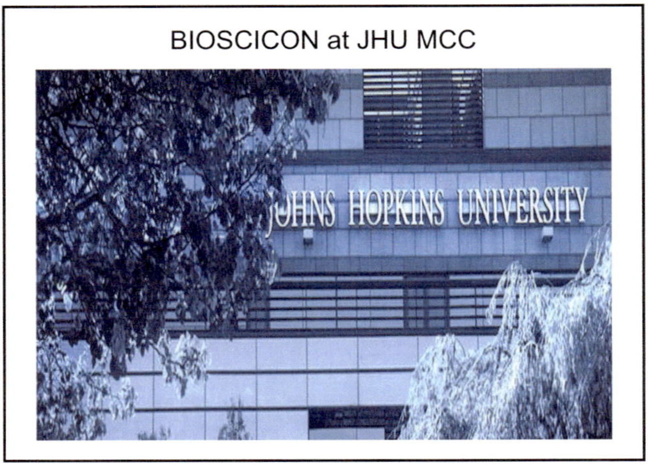
BIOSCICON at JHU MCC
JOHNS HOPKINS UNIVERSITY

2.5.5

Company

- **MarkPap Pacific [MPP] is LLC incorporated as subsidiary to MarkPap LLC which mission is to commercialize the BioSciCon's MarkPap technology worldwide.**
- **MPP is an independent entity but limited to the PR China market.**
- **The initial assets of MPP is 4 million dollars in IP and the operational cost on loan from BioSciCon.**

2.5.6

MARKPAP PACIFIC LLC AT
SHADY GROVE INNOVATION CENTER

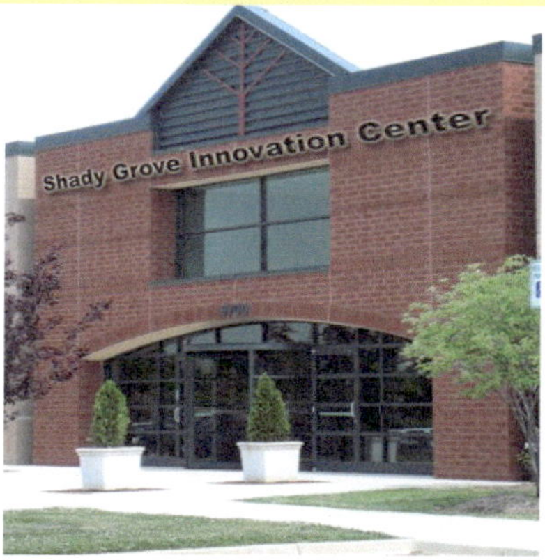

2.5.7

World Needs

Cervical cancer was the major killer of women with malignant disease. This history has changed for countries where Pap test is available. However, because of lack of qualified personnel, only 10% of world women population is protected. The WHO and all governments are looking for affordable services to overcome this shortage. Telehealth offers the best solution

2.5.8

Why China?

Population 2006: 1,300 million

- Female 50% = 630 million
- Female above age 18 (2/3) = 420 million
- Expected participants 80% = 336 million
- 1% penetration = 3.5 million

Fastest growing market:

- Pap test in 2006 = 74 million
- Estimated growth = 10 million per year
- Estimated number of tests in 2009 = 90 million
- 1% = 0.93 million
- 3.5 million = 3.7%
- Target = 4% niche

2.5.9

China's market drivers:Emphasis on screening

- **China Government programs for protection of all women at risk (mostly directed to rural and low income parts of the country)**
- **Fear of cervical cancer and awareness of possible prevention (urban China and new middle class paying for services).**
- **Awareness that HPV vaccine must be combined with cytological screening for maximum effect**.

2.5.10

How we can meet these needs?

- We can provide our test (kits) to any place in the world that has minimal laboratory facilities to process the specimen, and a microscope with Internet connection to send digital images.
- We can remotely connect this clinical site with our IT Telehealth Center for prompt diagnosis of the medical condition on this specimen.

2.5.11

Why we?

- **BioSciCon is the sole owner of a proprietary biomarker-based in vitro diagnostic technology which, due the biomarker characteristics, is amenable for telecytopathology – medical diagnosis on distance.**
- **Our brand products includes: MarkPap®, test, kit, solution, MarkPap Digital workstation, Telehealth networking centers, automatic and robotic devices.**

2.5.12

Technology

- MarkPap is a trademark for a patented technology that includes instruments, medical devices, reagents (in vitro diagnostics), controls and procedures and instructions which, in different combinations, are intended to improve the quality of life of healthy women relieving them from fear of cervical cancer risk.

2.5.13

MarkPap® platform technology

We have a proprietary technology which is based upon a chemical biomarker positive only in abnormal cells, and always negative in normal cells. This distinction makes the method superior over all competitors.

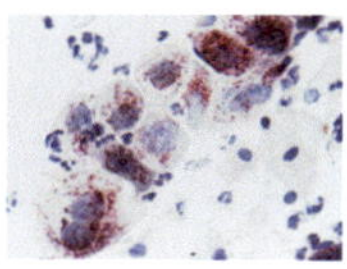

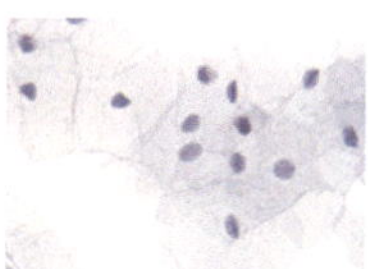

2.5.14

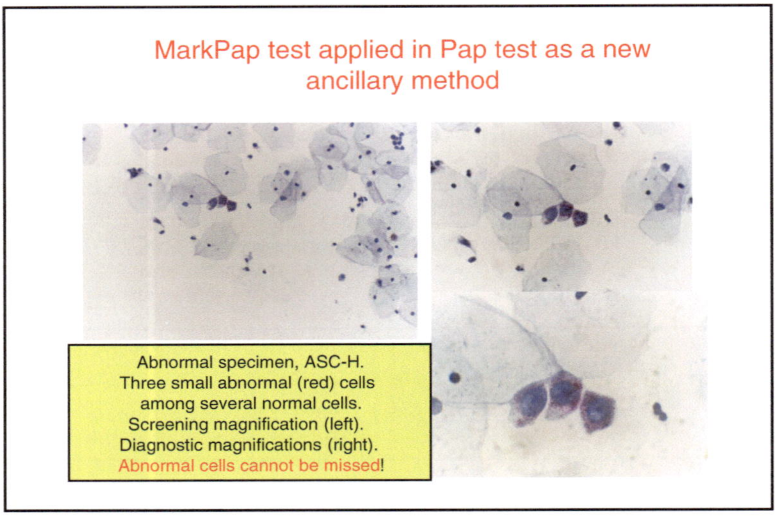
MarkPap test applied in Pap test as a new ancillary method
Abnormal specimen, ASC-H.
Three small abnormal (red) cells
among several normal cells.
Screening magnification (left).
Diagnostic magnifications (right).
Abnormal cells cannot be missed!

2.5.15

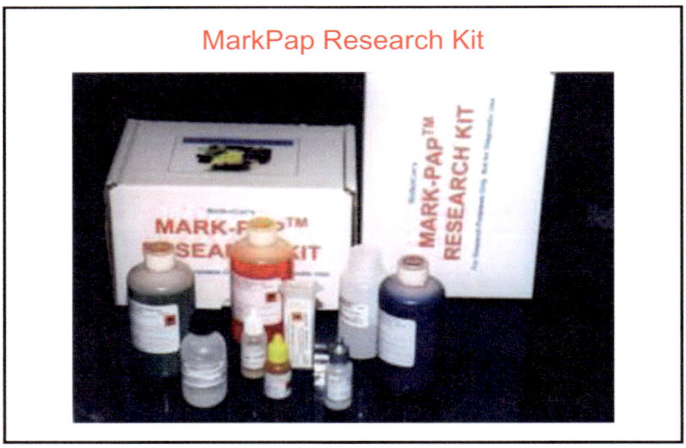
MarkPap Research Kit
MARK-PAP™
RESEARCH KIT

2.5.16

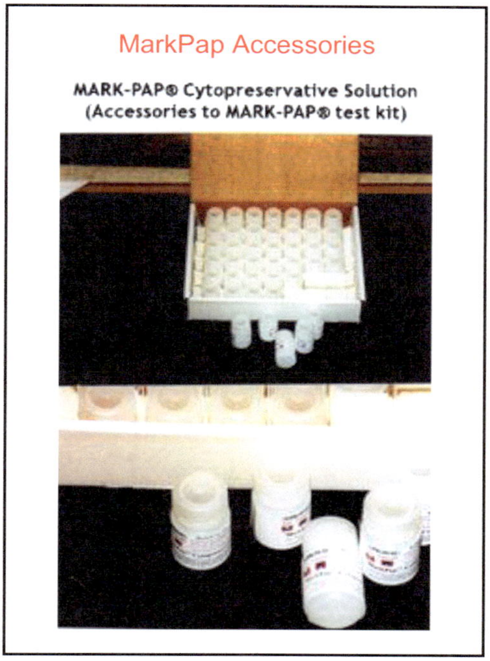
MarkPap Accessories
MARK-PAP® Cytopreservative Solution
(Accessories to MARK-PAP® test kit)

2.5.17

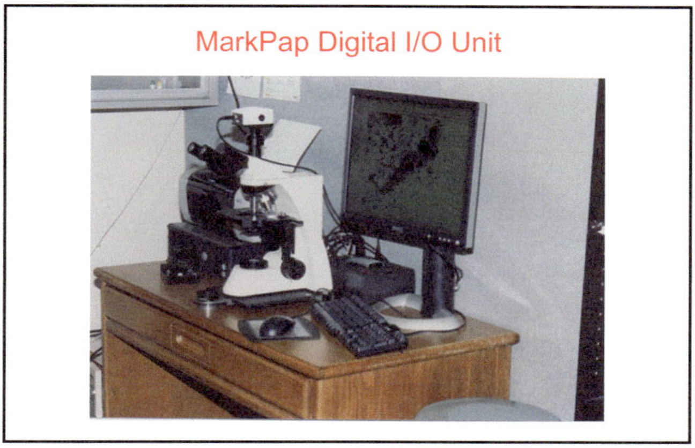
MarkPap Digital I/O Unit

2.5.18

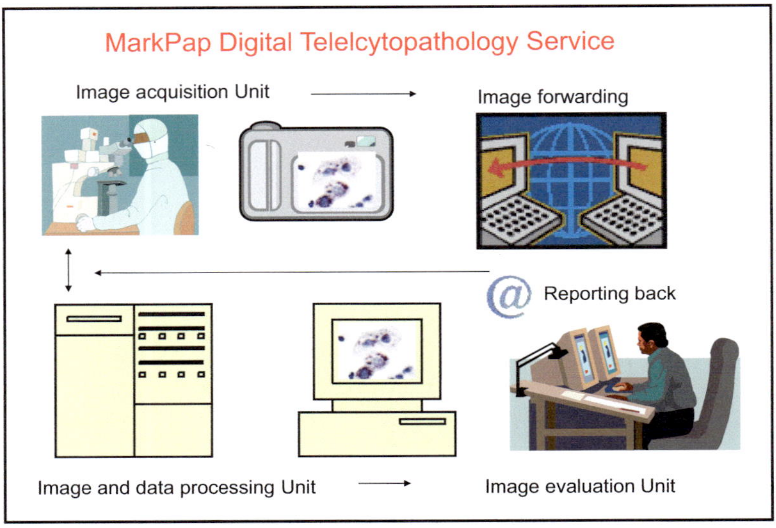
MarkPap Digital Telelcytopathology Service
Image acquisition Unit
Image forwarding
Reporting back
Image and data processing Unit
Image evaluation Unit

2.5.19

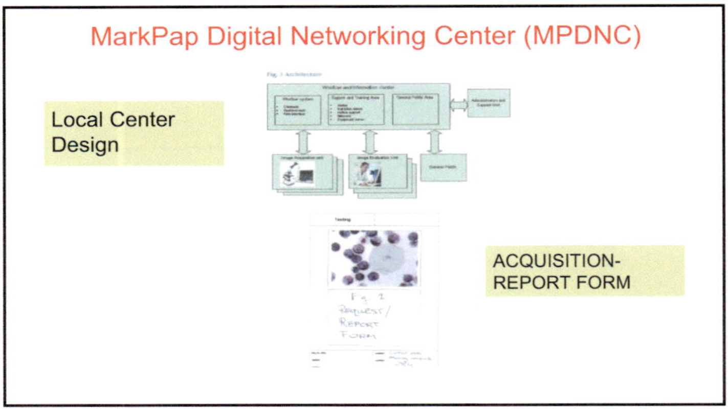
MarkPap Digital Networking Center (MPDNC)
Local Center Design
ACQUISITION-REPORT FORM

2.5.20

- BioSciCon has designed the Global MarkPap Digital Networking Center as a modular hierarchal system structure, has built a prototype and successfully tested the feasibility of the concept and the prototype.
- One module (Maryland IT Telehealth Center), designed for 1 million services per year, was given to MPPLLC for commercialization

2.5.21

MarkPap® Technology Competitive Advantages

The presence of the biomarker makes a difference:

- **MORE ACCURATE, FASTER, LESS EXPENSIVE**
- **TELEMEDICINE: The marker can be seen by less-trained technician, who transmits images of suspect cells in the laboratory for final diagnosis (TelePap: MarkPap® Digital, MarkPap® Wireless)**
- **Future Home Pap (MarkPap® Self)**

Mass cervical cancer screening worldwide: Huge societal benefit saving women's lives from preventable cancer, and enormous market with incredible potential for profit(2B women at risk)

www.bioscicon.com

2.5.22

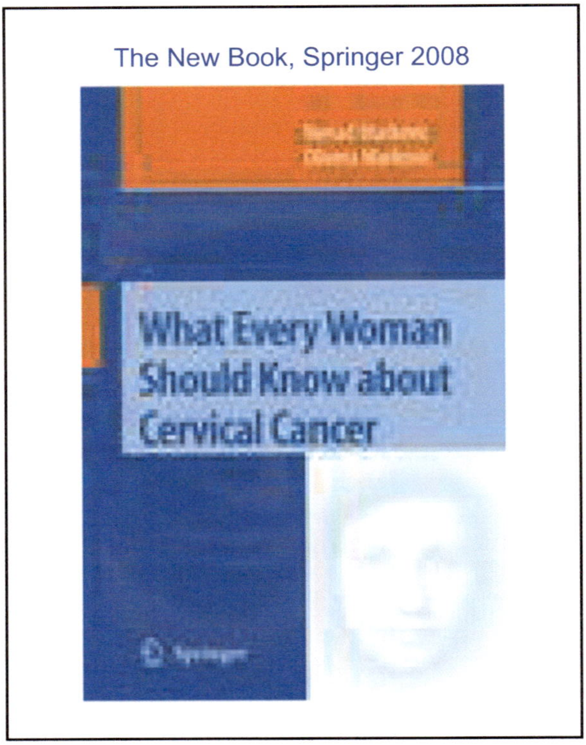

2.5.23

Supporting Organizations

- Maryland Department of Business and Economic Development, Office of International Investment and Trade, Baltimore, MD
- Maryland Center in Shanghai, China
- SCORE, District Office, Washington, DC
- Rockville Economic Development, Inc., Rockville, MD
- National Institutes of Health, Bethesda, MD
- Montgomery County Incubator Network, MD

2.5.24

Our Partner in China

Anhui Anke Biotechnology (Group) Co., Ltd.
Hefei, Anhui, P.R. China
http://www.ankebio.com
Prof. Dr. Song LiHua, President
Dr. Xu ZhenShan, Director of R&D Department

2.5.25

Anke Bio Visit

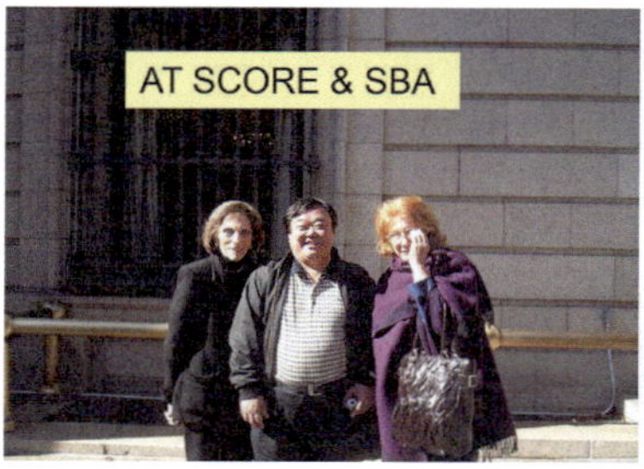

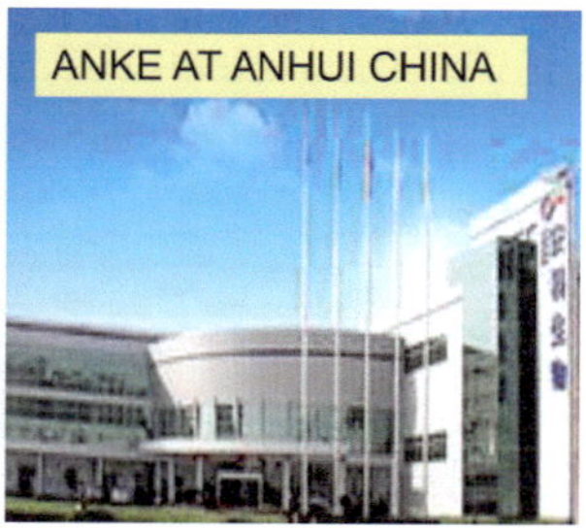

2.5.26

Additional Information

For more information on the technology please visit our web site: http://www.bioscicon.com

For more information on the Company please contact Prof. Dr. Nenad Markovic, President and CEO, MarkPapPacific, LLC at info@bioscicon.com, or Ms. Jane Jing, VP for China Affairs, MarkPap Pacific, LLC at janezzjing@gmail.com T: 202-498-5808

MarkPap Pacific, LLC
9700 Great Seneca Hwy, Suite 149
Rockville, MD 20850

2.6 MarkPap India, LLC. Cervical Cancer in India. How we can help? 2012

2.6.1

BioSciCon Consortium of Companies

- BioSciCon, Inc, the parent R&D corporation for a proprietary, platform MarkPap® technology for cervical cancer prevention.

  More…www.bioscicon.com
- MarkPap LLC, organized for global commercialization of the technology (marketing, distribution and sale)
- MarkPap Pacific LLC, incorporated specifically for commercialization in China and greater Pacific Area
- MarkPap India LLC incorporated specifically for commercialization in India and South East Asia
- The Global Academy for Women's Health, Inc, an independent non-profit dedicated to women's health education

  More.. www.markpap.com/index.html

2.6.2

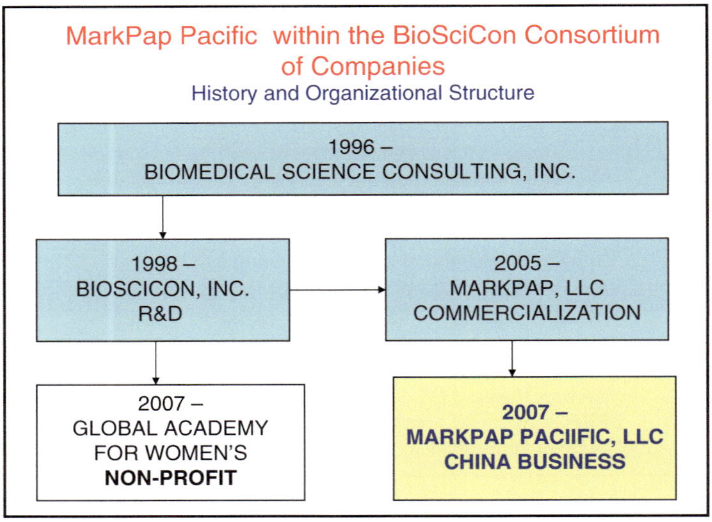

2.6.3

Mission

Introduction of simple, low-cost life-saving medical devices affordable and available globally.

Example: CERVICAL CANCER preventive MarkPap platform technology , which is biomarker-based and telemedicine powered technology.

2.6.4

Cervical Cancer is Preventable

Cervical cancer is second to the breast cancer cause of women deaths from malignant diseases world-wide. Currently, there are 560,000 new cases of cervical cancer each year, and about 250,000 women die from this preventable disease. However, cervical cancer is preventable **IF** detected on time. Cytological screening (Pap test) remains the best cervical cancer prevention. More… www.bioscicon.com/publicinformation.html

2.6.5

WORLD

Problem

- At risk: 2 B
- Protected with Pap 150M or about 10% at average
- The number of tests in the developing world recently increased to 80M Pap tests, but outreach is still only 5%.

Other technologies

- Screen & treat
- VIA
- HPV testing
- Vaccination

2.6.6

Cervical Cancer in India

- 300 million women at risk
- 18 million protected with screening. Outreach 6%.
- 280 million women without any prevention from a preventable cervical cancer
- 134,000 cancer cases and 72,825 deaths per year
- Prognosis that the cancer incidence and mortality will further increase in India for 150% by the year 2025.

Current prevention efforts failed.

2.6.7

The Problem

In spite of the tremendous help provided to women the existing Pap test technology is

- Costly: The test is not affordable for mass screening in low-resource areas
- Infrastructure: Required, with qualified professionals locally (cytotechnologists/pathologists)
- Not accessible: Rural areas without local doctor's offices
- Invasive and non-comfortable test: Requires pelvic exam, that is culture sensitive
- Slow: Takes weeks to obtain normal results

2.6.8

The Solution of the Problem

MarkPap® Technology is the solution:

- Costly: Less expensive and affordable (MarkPap Kit)
- Infrastructure: Not required locally (MarkPap Digital Telemedicine Services).
- Not accessible: Home Self-sampling Kit
- Invasive and non-comfortable test: Home Self-sampling
- Slow: Results within hours

2.6.9

MarkPap® Platform Technology

MarkPap is a trademark for a patented technology that includes instruments, medical devices, reagents (in vitro diagnostics), controls, procedures and instructions in different combinations to improve the quality of life life of women.

In India, we will introduce 3 products:

1. MarkPap Reagent Kit (customer friendly easy to use kit to perform the test)
2. MarkPap Telecytopathology Services (telemedicine, reading the result at distance)
3. MarkPap Self-Collection Kit (home specimen self-collection)

More… www.bioscicon/markpapproducts/html

2.6.10

How MarkPap Test Can Do This?

The proprietary MarkPap biomarker (patented in the Year 2000) is a powerful means to make the test less expensive, more accurate, faster and amenable for telecytopathology (distant reading) and home self-sampling.

More… www.bioscicon.com

2.6.11

Products for Sale: Subject to US export and local import regulations

1. **MPK: Research Kit**
   - 12 individual reagents
   - control slides
2. **MPS: Cell preservative solution**:
3. **Individual reagents from the Kit**
4. **Manual Procedure**

5. **MPD: MarkPap Digital-Telecytopathology**
   - Instruments and software for distant evaluation

5. **MPSCK: Home Pap Kit (Avail. 2011)**
   - 8 individual device

2.6.12

This is How and Why the MarkPap® Technology is the Solution: MarkPap Advantage

- **It is less expensive and affordable (MarkPap Kit)**
- Does not require local infrastructure and pathologist at the point-of-care Because of the biomarker, low-trained person can decide which cells to transmit by telecytopathology for evaluation (MarkPap Digital/Wireless Telemedicine Services)
- **Home self-sampling is only possible with MarkPap technology, because of the presence of the biomarker.**
- **Home self sampling makes the Pap test more accessible for women in remote areas and more comfortable for women, so much more women can have this test**
- **Fast, results within hours**
- Clinical trial showed that the test is more accurate than the conventional Pap test
  More… www,bioscicon.com

2.6.13

MarkPap® Platform Technology Illustrated

Our proprietary technology is based upon a molecular biomarker which is positive only in abnormal cells (upper image) and always negative in normal cells (lower image). The red color of the biomarker signals the cell abnormality (ID for cervical cell abnormality).

The biomarker makes a difference and this distinction makes the method superior over all competitors. More….
www.bioscicon.com/gallery.html

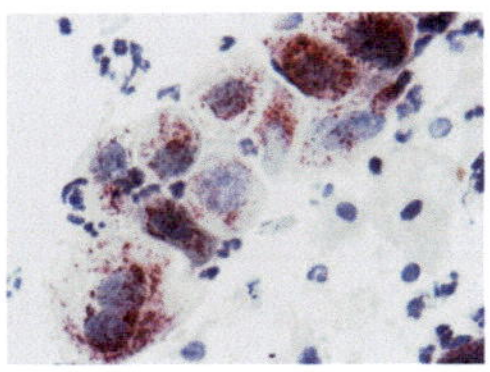

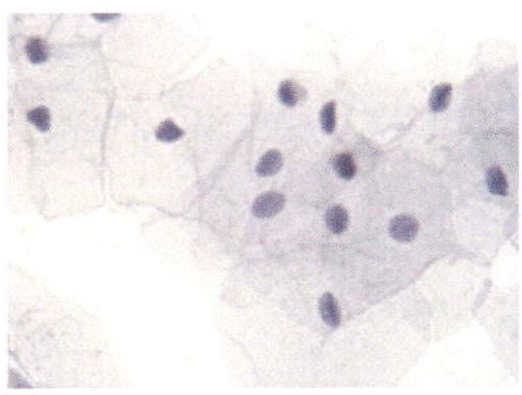

2.6.14

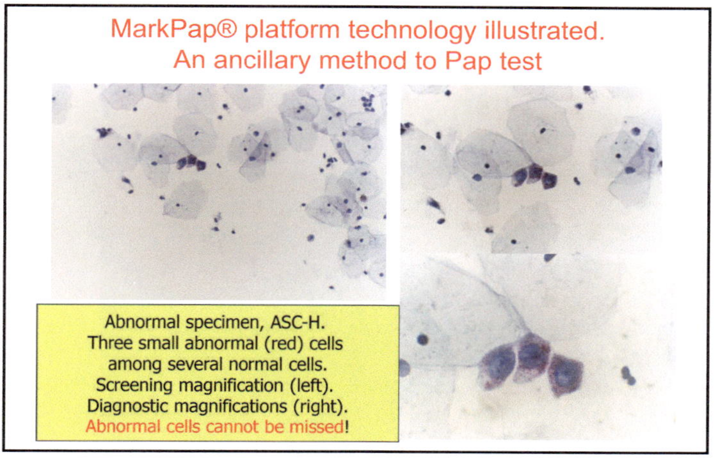
MarkPap® platform technology illustrated.
An ancillary method to Pap test
Abnormal specimen, ASC-H.
Three small abnormal (red) cells
among several normal cells.
Screening magnification (left).
Diagnostic magnifications (right).
Abnormal cells cannot be missed!

2.6.15

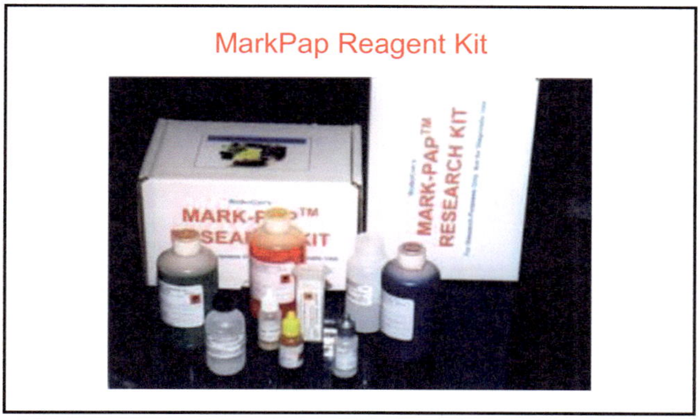
MarkPap Reagent Kit
MARK-PAP™
RESEARCH KIT

2.6.16

A Digital Telecytopathology Workstation consisting of a microscope, digital camera and computer capture, store and forward image files

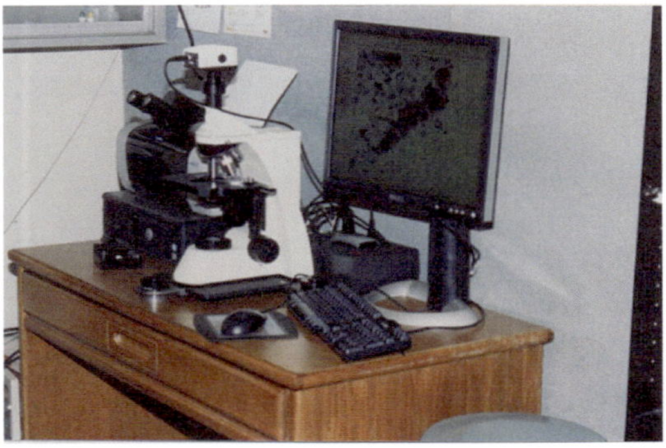

2.6.17

What Happens When the Specimen Arrives in the Laboratory?

In the laboratory, the specimen is stained with the MarkPap Reagent Kit. The kit is customer-friendly, easy-to-use and the test can be performed by a low-trained technician or a nurse. The same person put the slide under the microscope and look for biomarker-positive ("red") cells. Pathologist is not needed there! If there are red cells on the slide he/she transmits the images of those cells/microscopic fields to the specialist for evaluation. Images can be sent via computer or with a cell phone.

2.6.18

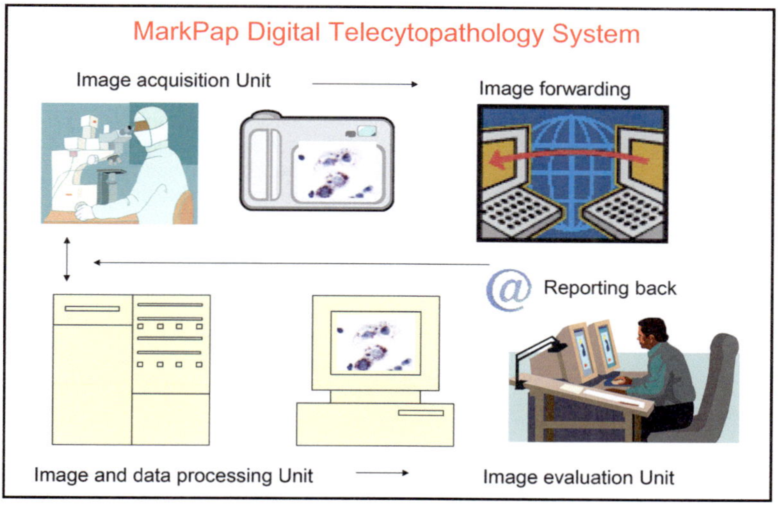
MarkPap Digital Telecytopathology System
Image acquisition Unit
Image forwarding
Reporting back
Image and data processing Unit
Image evaluation Unit

2.6.19

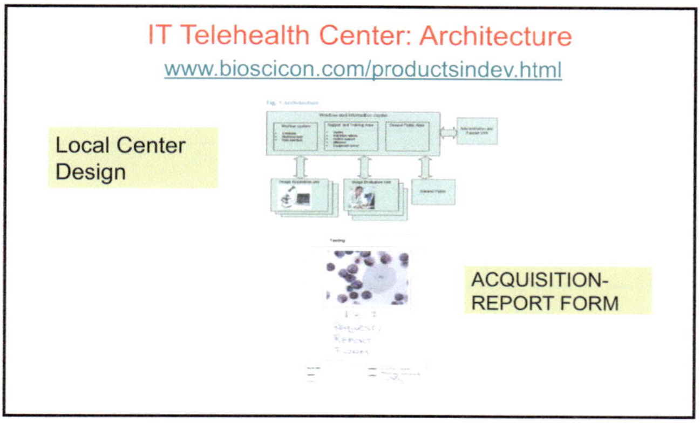
IT Telehealth Center: Architecture
www.bioscicon.com/productsindev.html
Local Center Design
ACQUISITION-REPORT FORM

2.6.20

MarkPap® Wireless Telecytopathology Service

We are currently working on the use of cell phone cameras, instead of digital cameras, for the transmission of images from the remote sites. In many parts of the world where computers are not available or affordable, cell phones could substitute the computers. We are working on the development of an Universal Adapter to connect any cell phone to any microscope. More ...www.bioscicon.com/pressrelease.html

2.6.21

MarkPap® Advantages

- Unique biomarker makes possible an instant and simultaneous detection of cervical dysplasia and HPV disease
- Accurate (diagnostic sensitivity >90%, low FN rates)
- Fast (results within hours of sampling)
- Affordable (low cost of supplies and labor)
- May be used for primary cervical cancer screening and for pre-screening for HPV

2.6.22

Summary of the MarkPap

In practice, MarkPap Self and MarkPap Digital would allow women to take the sample at home and to mail it to the nearby laboratory. In this laboratory a low-trained technician or nurse can stain the slide using easy-to-use MarkPap Kit. The same person examines the slide under the microscope and searches for "red" cells only. The images of those cells are captured with a digital camera or cell phone camera and transmitted for evaluation. The result may be sent back electronically within hours.. More... www.bioscicon.com/publications.html (40)

2.6.23

Education Goes Together With Technology: The book

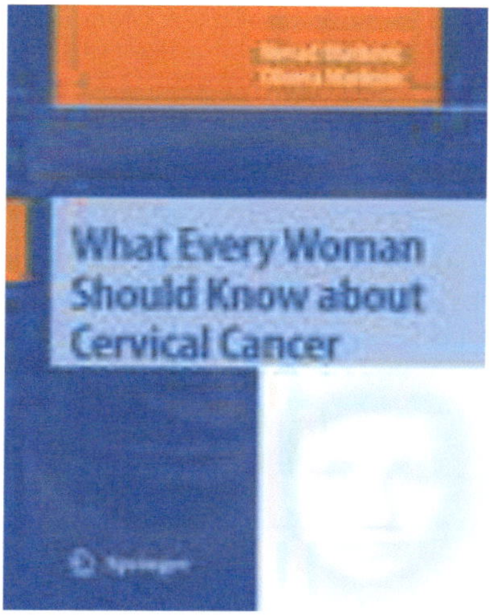

2.6.24

More about The Book

www.bioscicon.com/publications.html
www.amazon.com
www.markpap.com

Education is the essential part in introducing and successful implementation of a new technologies.

2.6.25

CONTRIBUTION

Mass cervical cancer screening worldwide: Huge societal benefit saving women's lives from preventable cancer, and enormous market with incredible potential for profit (2B women at risk)

2.6.26

BioSciCon and MarkPap Pacific Featured

- MarkPap Pacific and BioSciCon efforts to bring the technology to China using telehealth services, appeared in Washington Post on December 2009.
- BioSciCon and its cutting edge MarkPap® platform technology was presented in the US Congress in March 2011 as a success story (US Senator Olympia Snow).
- BioSciCon was proclaimed two consecutive years the best Rockville company in Biotechnology Sector .

2.6.27

Contact

Prof. Dr. Nenad Markovic
President and CEO
BioSciCon, inc.
Johns Hopkins University. Montgomery County Campus
6901 Medical Canter Drive, Bld 9605, Suite 10
Rockville, MD 20850
E-mail: info@bioscicon.com
www.bioscicon.com
T: 301-610-9130
F: 301-610-7662
www.bioscicon.com/contact.html

2.7 BioSciCon, Inc., Special Health Strategies for fighting cervical cancer in India. 2015

2.7.1

YOUR HOSTS

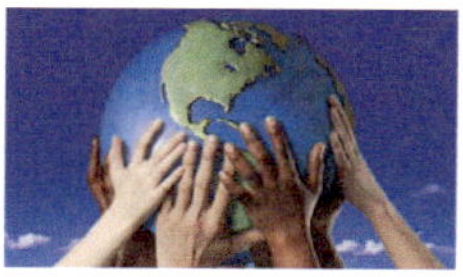

GLOBAL ACADEMY FOR WOMEN'S HEALTH, INC.
IRS code: 501(C)(3)
www.markpap.com

BIOMEDICAL SCIENCE CONSULTING, INC.
www.bioscicon.com

2.7.2

Why cervical cancer

- Cervical cancer is second to the breast cancer cause of women deaths from malignant diseases world-wide. Currently, there are 600,000 new cases of cervical cancer each year, and about 300,000 die, mostly in the developing world. However, cervical cancer is preventable <u>**IF**</u> detected on time.
- Women in developed countries are well protected with regular screening and early removal of suspect lesions.
- Unfortunately, because of lack of qualified personnel, only 10% of world women population is protected with preventive screening.

2.7.3

Cervical cancer in India

- India has 300 million women at risk for cervical cancer. Only 18 million women participate in cervical cancer screening programs.
- With this outreach of 6% in 2010, 72, 825 women unnecessarily die each year. It is expected that mortality will further increase for 150% by the year 2025.

2.7.4

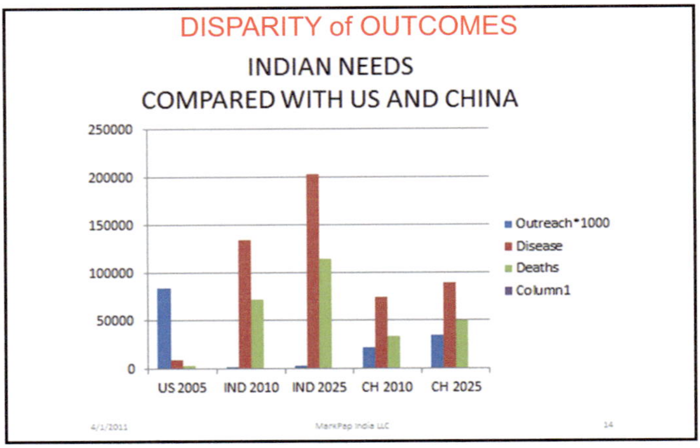
DISPARITY of OUTCOMES
INDIAN NEEDS
COMPARED WITH US AND CHINA
250000
200000
150000
100000
50000
0
US 2005
IND 2010
IND 2025
CH 2010
CH 2025
Outreach*1000
Disease
Deaths
Column1
4/1/2011
MarkPap India LLC
14

2.7.5

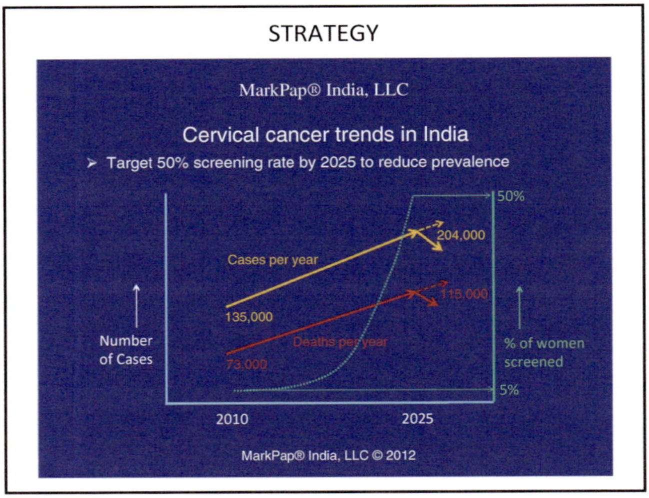
STRATEGY
MarkPap® India, LLC
Cervical cancer trends in India
➢ Target 50% screening rate by 2025 to reduce prevalence
50%
204,000
Cases per year
115,000
135,000
Number
of Cases
Deaths per year
73,000
% of women
screened
5%
2010
2025
MarkPap® India, LLC © 2012

2.7.6

New opportunity for mass screening

- Indian Government has best intentions and is putting a lot of efforts, the Indian population is aware of the danger , the Indian health providers are aware of the advantage of prevention versus treatment of cervical cancer, but apparently they do not have the appropriate tools to do more.
- We believe that we can provide those tools introducing a new biomarker/telemedicine based platform technology, with possibility for specimen self-collecting.

2.7.7

Old Problems

Existing Pap Test Technologyis:

- Costly: Prohibitively expensive in developing countries
- Infrastructure: Required, with qualified professionals (cytotechnologists/pathologists) at the Point–of-Care (POC)
- Accessibility: Women in rural regions do not have access to the POC
- Uncomfortable exam/culture sensitive: Acquiring the sample requires a pelvic exam, that is invasive and women avoid it, or women are not allowed to visit gynecologist
- Slow: Take weeks to obtain normal result

2.7.8

The Solution

MarkPap ® technology is the solution

- Costly: Less expensive test
- Infrastructure: Not required at POC
- Accessibility:Does not require access to doctor's offices.
- Uncomfortable exam/culture sensitive: Does not require visit to a gynecologist and it is less invasive
- Slow: Timely, results within hours (immediate service)
- It is also better standardized and controlled (QC/QA with control slides and less liability for the laboratory

2.7.9

How MarkPap Test can make this happen

The proprietary biomarker is a powerful means to make the test less expensive, more amenable for telecytopathology and to open the possibility for home self-sampling.
More... www.bioscicon.com

2.7.10

MarkPap® Platform Technology

MarkPap is a a trademark for a patented technology that includes instruments, medical devices, reagents (in vitro diagnostics), controls and procedures and instructions which, in different combinations, are intended for early detection of pre-cancerous and cancerous lesions and save women's lives. It is also to improve the quality of life of healthy women relieving them from fear of cervical cancer risk.

2.7.11

MarkPap® platform technology illustrated

We have a proprietary technology which is based upon a chemical biomarker positive only in abnormal cells, and always negative in normal cells. This distinction makes the method superior over all competitors.
More....
www.bioscicon.com/gallery.html

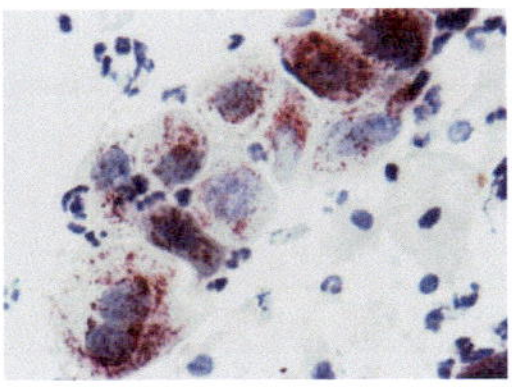

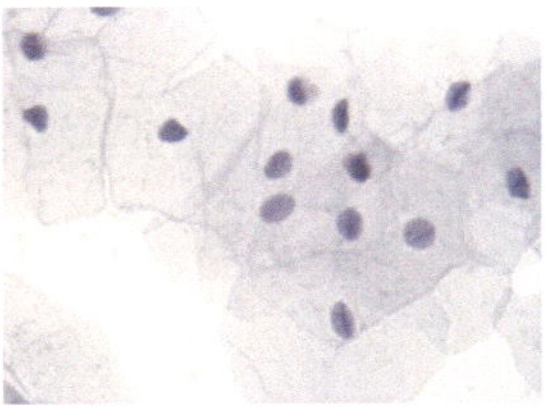

2.7.12

MarkPap® platform technology illustrated. An ancillary method to Pap test

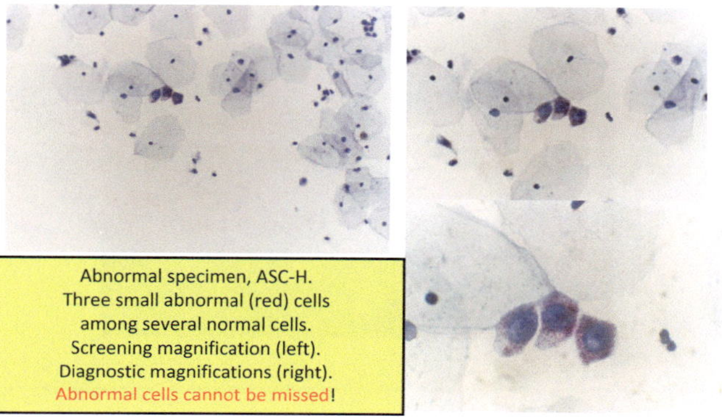

Abnormal specimen, ASC-H.
Three small abnormal (red) cells among several normal cells.
Screening magnification (left).
Diagnostic magnifications (right).
Abnormal cells cannot be missed!

2.7.13

Products for Sale: Subject to US export and local import regulations

1. MarkPap® Test Kit with accessories

12 individual reagents and control slides with Instruction for the Manual MarkPap® Test

2. MarkPap® Telecytopathology Service (sm)

Instruments and software for distant evaluation

3. MarkPap® Self™ Kit

for home specimen collection. Will be available in 2012

2.7.14

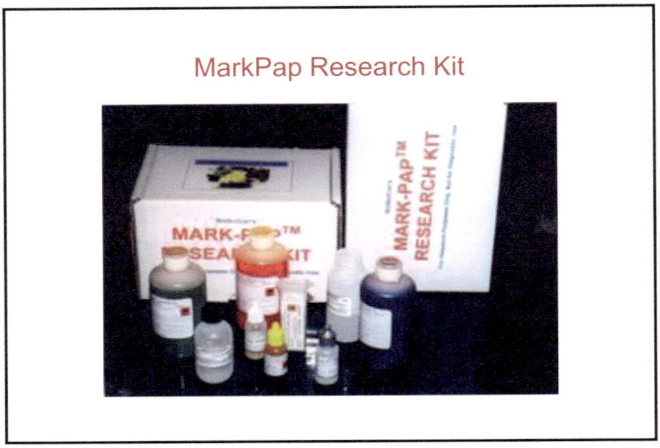
MarkPap Research Kit
MARK-PAP™ RESEARCH KIT

2.7.15

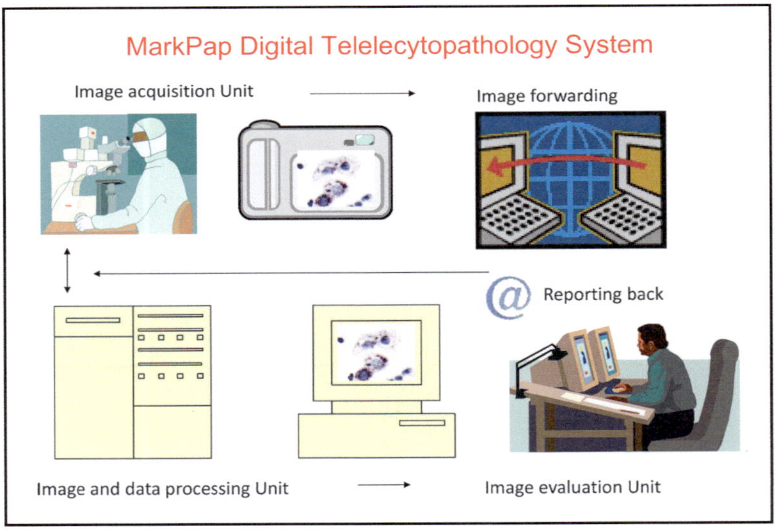
MarkPap Digital Telelecytopathology System
Image acquisition Unit
Image forwarding
Reporting back
Image and data processing Unit
Image evaluation Unit

2.7.16

MarkPap® Wireless: Our recent focus

We are currently working on the use of cell phone cameras in the transmission of images from the remote sites. In many parts of the world where computers are not available or affordable, cell phones could substitute the computers. We are working on the development of an Universal Adapter to connect any cell phone any microscope.

More ... www.bioscicon.com/pressrelease.html

2.7.17

MarkPap® wireless: MOBILE PAP

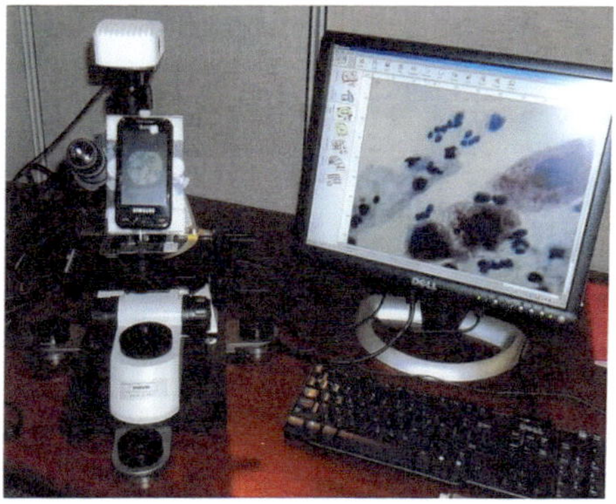

2.7.18 .

Home self-collection of specimens
(MarkPap-Self)

MarkPap-Self is an option for women to take the specimen in the privacy of their home and to send it for processing in a laboratory. MarkPap-Self is aimed for women who live in remote regions and do not have access to a amedical institution, for those who (because of different tradition /religious restrains)are not allowed to visit gynecologist, or women who are not simply comfortable with pelvic exam and prefer to take a sample at home.

We believe that MarkPap-Self will dramatically increase the number of women who get preventing screening.

2.7.19

Anticipated Service

In practice our products will allow women to take the sample at home and to mail it to the nearby laboratory. In this laboratory a low-trained technician or nurse can stain the slide using easy-to-use MarkPap Kit. The same person examines the slide under the microscope and searches for "red" cells only. The images of those cells are captured with a digital camera or cell phone camera and transmitted for evaluation. The result may be sent back electronically within hours..
More... www.bioscicon.com/publications.html (40)

2.7.20

CONTRIBUTION

Mass cervical cancer screening worldwide: Huge societal benefit saving women's lives from preventable cancer, and enormous market with incredible potential for profit (2B women at risk)

2.7.21

New Definition of MarkPap® Platform

MarkPap® platform technology which is biomarker-based, telemedicine-empowered, accurate, simple, low-cost, infrastructure independent, accessible, equitable, culture-sensitive platform that can bring quality cervical cancer prevention in a right time, on the right place for a low cost.

Qualified professionals are not needed at the POC, that makes this technology infrastructure independent.

2.7.22

Unique opportunity

MarkPap ® technology is currently the only promise for mass cervical cancer prevention in the developing world.

Not only in India, but in the whole developing world.

There are 3B women at risk for cervical cancer in the world. Timely prevention may save hundreds of thousands women lives in the years to come.

2.7.23

CONTACTS

Business contacts:
BioSciCon, Inc.
MarkPap India, LLC
E-mail: info@bioscicon.com
www.bioscicon.com
Non-profit:
Global Academy for Women's Health, Inc
gawh@markpap.com
www.markpap.com

For specific questions, please contact
Prof. Dr. Nenad Markovic
President and CEO
MarkPap India, LLC

2.8 *BioSciCon, Inc. Fighting Cervical Cancer in Azerbaijan, 2013*

2.8.1

FIGHTING CERVICAL CANCER IN AZERBAIJAN

OVERVIEW OF BUSINESS OPPORTUNITY
PREPARED BY GLOBAL ACADEMY FOR WOMEN'S HEALTH AND BIOSCICON, INC.
2013

2.8.2

PREAMBLE

- In response to the ElizarovConsulting Group invitation to US Tech Companies to join ICT Trade Mission in Baku, Azerbaijan –presented at the W. Hanna Innovation Center in Shady Grove, MD on October 31, 2013, the Global Academy for Women's Health, Inc., JHU MCC, Rockville, MD, has prepared this Overview of Business Opportunity for consideration of Azerbaijan Ministry of Health and relevant authorities.
- It will be presented in Azerbaijan by the Elizarov Consulting Group, Wheaton, MD, U.S.A.

2.8.3

CONTENTS

1. BUSINESS WITH SOCIAL (HEALTH) AND FINANCIAL IMPACT
2. HEALTH PRIORITY NEEDS IN AZERBAIJAN (GOVERNEMENT ACTION PLAN ON PREVENTION OF CERVICAL CANCER (NATIONAL RH STRATEGY: 2008– 2015)
3. NEW STRATEGY
4. ROAD MAP TO SUCCESS – FIRST STEPS

2.8.4

1. SOCIAL ENTREPRENEURSHIP

HEALTH IMPACT

- TO REVERSE NEGATIVE TRENDS OF CERVICAL CANCER PREVALENCE AND MORTALITY AND TO START POSITIVE TRENDS.
- TO INCREASE THE OUTREACH OF CERVICAL CANCER SCREENIG TO ABOVE 50% OF WOMEN AT RISK (1.5 Million in Azerbaijan)

FINANCIAL IMPACT

- To accept the program only if the Profitability Index (return/[investment + service]) is shown to be above 1.2
- Return is ROI + Profit
- Service is 5-year self-sustainable delivery of health benefits

2.8.5

2. CERVICAL CANCER AS HEALTH PRIORITY

- Azerbaijan (A.) Ministry if Health (MOH) has National RH Strategy for 2008 –2015, including cervical cancer as one of the priorities.
- Currently there are 3 million women at risk, one half of them needs annual screening.
- Only 2% women participate in screening programs; 5 times less than world average
- Women in A. die from cervical cancer ten times more than in the US.

2.8.6

NEW STRATEGY FOCUSED ON FIGHTING CERVICAL CANCER IN AZERBAIJAN

ORGANIZATION

- INSTITUTE OF ONCOLOGY, OBGYN INSTITUTE AND MEDICAL FACULTY ARE ALREADY ASSIGNED BY MOH TO CARYON THE ACTION PLAN
- WE CAN HELP THEM DEVELOP A COMPREHENSIVE PROGRAM FOR CERVICAL CANCER PREVENTION AND TO BUILD AN INSTITUTIONAL CENTER FOR MPLEMENTATION OF THIS PROGRAM

MARKPAP TOOLS

- Biomarker-based cytopathology (Reagents Kit)
- Digital Imaging – Workstation with wired and wireless connections
- Mobile and telemedicine networking between points-of-care and medical centers - ITTHC
- Home-Based Specimen Self-Collecting Kit
- See www.bioscicon.com

2.8.7

ROAD MAP TO SUCCESS FIRST STEPS

- HAVE LEGISLATIVE AND FINANCIAL SUPPORT FOR GOVERNMENNT – DONE
- REVISE THE CURRENT AND DETERMNE THE NEW IMPRPOVED STRATEGY TO FIGTH CERVICAL CANCER - TO BE DONE
- ENGAGE THE ELIZAROV CONSULTUNG GROUP AND THE GLOBAL ACADEMY FOR WOMEN'S HEALTH, INC. TO CONDUCT A FEASIBILITY AND A PROFITABILITY STUDY – NEXT STEP

2.8.8

FINANCIAL ASPECTS

FEASIBILITY STUDY

- COMBINE AVAILABLE RESOURCES (SPACE, EQUIPMENT, PERSONNEL), PROVIDE NEW TOOLS , EDUCATE, TRAIN AND CONDUCT A SMALL EFFICACY STUDY IN AZERBAIJAN WITH CONTROL CENTER IN THE US.
- Total const: ~ 1 million USD

PROFITABILITY INDEX

- CONDUCT MARKET RESEARCH – AZERBAIJAN AND CASPIAN SEA REGION FOR POTENTIAL USERS OF THE SERVICES. IDENTIFY CUSTOMERS AND PRICE RANGE FOR SERVICES.
- CALCULATE THE PROFITABILITY INDEX
- Total cost: ~ 1million USD

2.8.9

GOLD STANDARDS

FEASIBILITY

- Financial calculations are made upon NIH SBIR Phase 1 and Phase 2 studies per product
- Azerbaijan "free health services" included in the Action Plan, are not calculated because they have their cost no matter who pays for it.

PROFITABILITY

- Feasibility will be assessed as the ability to achieve the results equal to those achieved in the US.
- Once the result equivalence will be confirmed as [test – control] ≥ delta ±0.25 control, the cost of the pre-money investment, the space, equipment, supply and service delivery will be compared with the cost of reimbursement for the standard "best" services as the potential "return".

2.8.10

ADDITIONAL READINGS

- Technology:
- www.bioscicon.com
- www.markpap.com
- Markovic O&N. What every woman should know about cervical cancer. Springer 2008.

2.8.11

SUMMARY

- An overview of Azerbaijan's health policy and capabilities together with the assessment of the cervical cancer globally and in the Caspian region, strongly indicates that Azerbaijan has ability, infrastructure, health care providers' quality and technical skills to develop and implement a new strategy for Fight Against Cervical Cancer based on IT technology achievements which could be faster, more accurate and of lower cost than the current standards, and can bring new infrastructure, new jobs, and new income to the State in addition to health benefits to much more women in the country and the neighboring states.

2.8.12

CONTACTS

GAWH

- Prof. Dr. Olivera Markovic
- Global Academy for Women's Health, Inc.
- Johns Hopkins University MCC
- 9601 Medical Center Drive
- Rockville, MD 20850
- T: 1.301.610.9130
- Web: gawh@markpap.com

ECG

- Mr. Yakov Elizarov
- Elizarov Consulting Group
- 11002 Veirs Mill Road, Ste. 735, Wheaton, MD 20902
- T: 1.301.962.3131
- Email: info@ECGDC.com
- Skype: ECGDC@live.com

2.9 *MarkPap, LLC. MarkPap® Technology for Prevention Cervical Cancer in Africa, 2014*

2.9.1

MARKPAP® Technology
for Cervical Cancer Prevention in
Africa 2014

Low-cost, simple tests, empowered
with IT/mobile technologies for
global cancer prevention

2.9.2

NIGERIA IN AFRICA

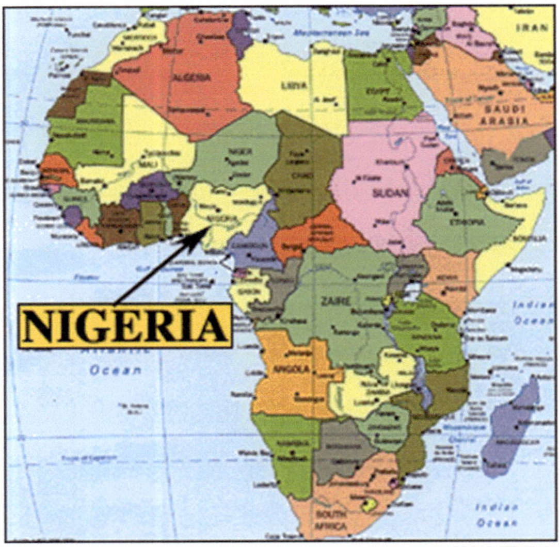

NIGERIA IS SHARING CERVICAL CANCER PROBLEMS WITH ALL AFRICA, BUT BECAUSE OF THE AIDS PREVALENCE THIS PROBLEM IS LESS VISIBLE AND MORE DANGEROUS

2.9.3

CERVICAL CANCER IS PREVENTABLE

Cancer of the cervix of the uterus (cervical cancer) is second to the breast cancer cause of women deaths from malignant diseases world-wide. Currently, there are 600,000 new cases of cervical cancer each year, and about 300,000 die from this disease. However, cervical cancer is preventable **IF** detected on time. Prevention is done by cervical cancer screening. Pap test remains the best cervical cancer prevention. However, existing Pap test, as it is, cannot be implemented in low-resource countries.

2.9.4

WHY NOT Existing Pap Test ?

Because of the

- Cost of the Test
- Lack of Infrastructure - qualified professionals at the Point-of Care required
- Not Accessible for women living in rural areas (visiting doctor' office required)
- Invasive and culture sensitive
- Global Health Disparity

2.9.5

HEALTH DISPARITY

AFRICA

- POPULATION: 1 BN
- WOMEN AT RISK FOR CERVICAL CANCER: 300 M
- OUTREACH: 2-10%
- CERVICAL CANCER TRENDS: INCREASE FOR 10% ANNUALLY

  90,000 deaths per year .
  High AIDS prevalence
- increases the risk.

US

- POPULATION: 0.33 BN
- WOMEN AT RISK FOR CERVICAL CANCER: 110 M
- OUTREACH: 80%
- CERVICAL CANCER TRENDS:
- INITIAL DECREASED OF ABOUT 80% FOLLOWED BY 4% DECREASE ANNUALLY
- 4,000 deaths per year

2.9.6

HOW TO REDUCE DISPARITY

- GOAL: TO REVERSE THE TRENDS FROM CERVICAL CANCER PREVALENCE AND MORTALITY INCREASE INTO DECREASE
- OBJECTIVE: TO ADOPT NEW STRATEGY FOR FIGHT AGAINST CERVICAL CANCER IN OTHER TO INCREASE THE OUTREACH to more than 50% for women at risk
- TO PROVIDE TOOLS, TO TRAIN PERSONNEL, TO EDUCATE WOMEN AND HEALTH PROVIDERS, TO LAUNCH COUNTRYWIDE CAMPAIGN FOR PARTICIPATION IN SCREENING

2.9.7

STRATEGY TO FIGHT CERVICAL CANCER IN AFRICAN COUNTRIES

WE KNOW WHY, BUT QUESTIONS REMAIN:
WHAT? WHEN? WHO? HOW?

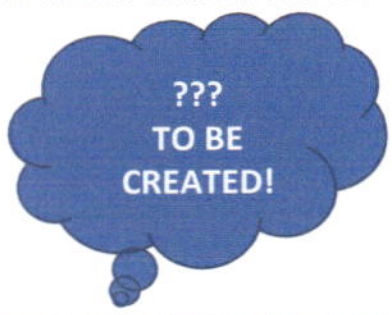

2.9.8

Problems and Solutions

PROBLEMS AT POC

1. Insufficient diagnostic of early pre/cancerous lesions
2. Lack of pathologists to evaluate the specimen
3. Accessibility, cultural sensitivity

SOLITIONS

1. Low-cost, simple test for processing the specimen at POC.
2. Use mobile phones for medical diagnosis at distance. Send microscopic images to a professional.
3. At home, self-specimen collection.

2.9.9

ROLE OF THE GOVERNMENT

GOVERNMENT:

1. TO ADOPT STRATEGY
2. TO PROVIDE TOOLS FOR IMPLEMENTATION
3. TO ORGANIZE HEALTH CARE PROVIDERS AND THE CAMPAIGN
4. TO ESTABLISH MILESTONES AND MONITORING FOR RESULTS
5. TO PROVIDE COMPLIANCE OF ALL PARTICIPANTS

2.9.10

MarkPap® Technology can help

MarkPap® technology is biomarker-based, simple, low-cost, telemedicine-empowered (wired or wireless), accessible, equitable, culture sensitive, infrastructure independent technology that can provide right health care on a right place in a right time. This is an advanced version of Pap test that can be used for mass cervical cancer screening for women worldwide.

2.9.11

MarkPap® Products for Sale in Africa

1. MarkPap Reagent Kit (low-cost, customer-friendly easy-to-use kit, can be performed at the POC in small labs with low-trained personnel)
2. MarkPap Telecytopathology Service (telemedicine, diagnosis at distance)
3. MarkPap Self-Collection kit (home specimen self-collection)

2.9.12

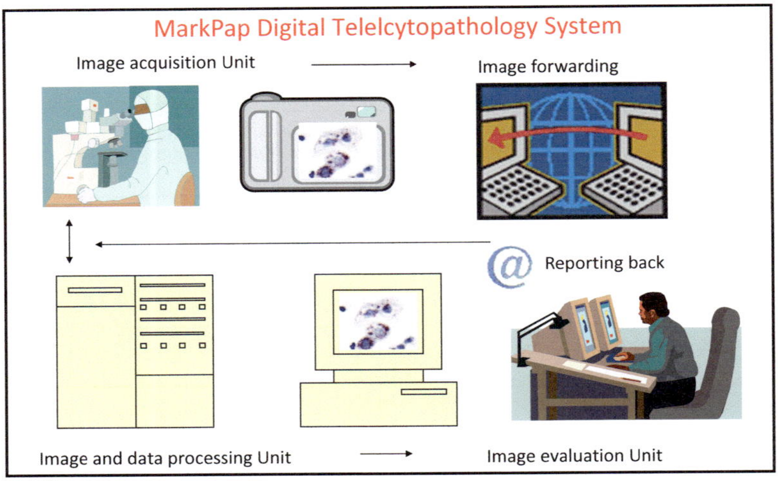

2.9.13

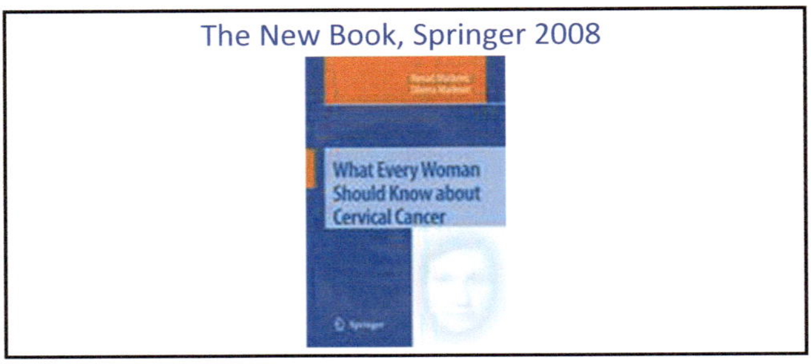

2.9.14

CONTACT

Prof. Dr. Nenad Markovic
MARKPAP LLC
(Wholesaler for MarkPap products worldwide)
9605 Medical Center Drive
Johns Hopkins University, MCC
Rockville, MD 20850
Tel: 1.301.610-9130 (voice)
E-mail info@bioscicon.com
Web Site: www.bioscicon.com

2.10 Global Academy for Women's Health, Inc. Cervical Cancer: Past, Present and Future. Invited Lecture, 2013. Northern Virginia Community College, NOVA, Annandale, VA

2.10.1

CERVICAL CANCER:
PAST, PRESENT AND FUTURE

PROF. DR. OLIVERA MARKOVIC
Lecture 2013 at the Northern VA
Community College,
Annandale, VA

2.10.2

DEFINITION

- Cervical cancer, is a malignant disease affecting cervix of the uteri and DOES NOT discriminate between women
- The disease is an unstoppable growth of malignant cells which destroy tissue around the lesion, spreads to lymph nodes and can metastasize around the body
- If this natural history is not interrupted by preventive or curative measures the outcome is ultimately fatal within few years of the detection of first symptoms

2.10.3

OVERVIEW OF THE DISEASE

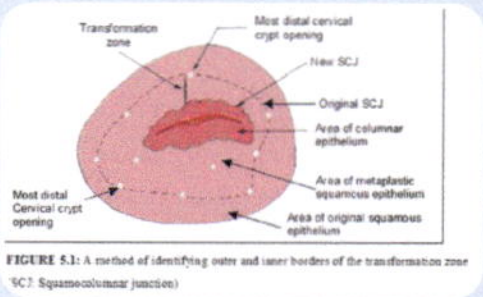

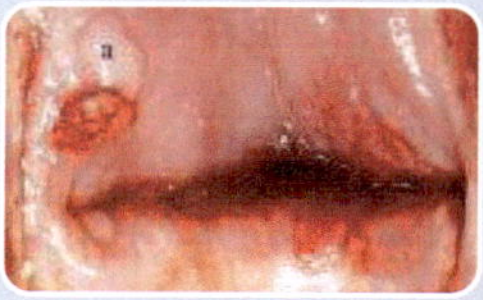

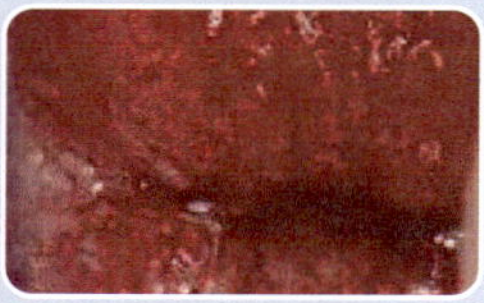

LOCATION
FOR CANCER DEVELOPMENT

LESION
OPERABLE
SCREENING AND REMOVAL FOR CURE

ADVANCED
INOPERABLE
DIAGNOSIS THERAPY INEFFECTIVE

2.10.4

CLINICAL STAGING AND THERAPY

CURE

CIS:
- Conization,
- LOOP,
- Partial cervicotomy

Curable

ICC-- 1A:
- Diagnostic intervention
- Surgery
- Surgery + Local Radiation

All are curable

IMPROVEMENT

ICC--1B & up:
- Local surgery
- Radical surgery,
- Radiation,
- Chemotherapy
- Combination therapy
- Alternative therapy

None is curable

2.10.5

Cervical cancer is preventable

- The disease is preventable and curable **IF** detected on time.
- Women in developed countries are well protected with regular screening and early removal of suspect lesions.
- Cytological screening (Pap test) remains the best cervical cancer prevention.

2.10.6

EPIDEMIOLOGY

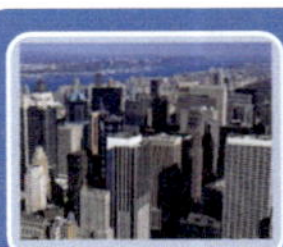

US [STANDARD]: 350 million
- Women at risk: 110 million
- Screening outreach: >80%
- CC (2012) prevalence: 12,000; mortality: 4,000

Per 10e6
P: 11; M:4

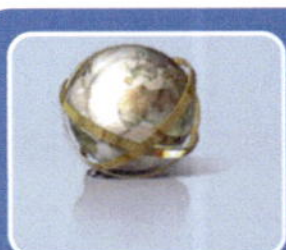

WORLD: 7.3 BN
- Women at risk: 2.5 bn
- Screening outreach: < 20%
- CC(2012) prevalence: 600,000; mortality: 360,000

Per 10e6
P: 2.4; 1.44

Egypt: 84 million
- Women at risk: 28 million
- Screening outreach: ? Diagnosis???
- CC (2010) prevalence: 514; mortality: 299

Per 10e6
P:1.7; 1.06

2.10.7

COMPARISON USA VS. EGYPT

USA

- PRE: PAP TEST (80% red)
- PRESENT: PAP + ADDITIONALS (LBP, HPV, VIA, DNA)
- FUTURE: IMPROVED PAP
- THERAPY: STILL OBSOLETE

EGYPT

PRE PAP SITUATION

- DISEASE ***NOT RECOGNIZED*** AS SERIOUS PENDING PROBLEM

NEEDS:

- BETTER DIAGNOSIS
- BETTER PREVENTION OF RISK FACTORS AND CANCER CONTROL – SCREENING

2.10.8

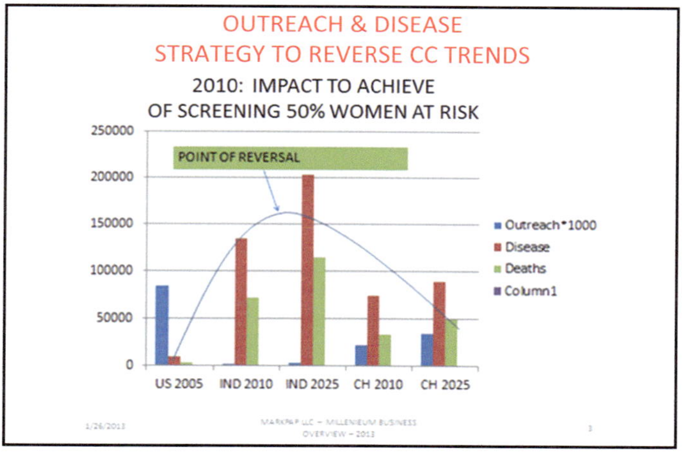

2.10.9

US Example

Before Pap test in the first half of the 20th Century, Us had almost no organized cervical cancer control (screening) and the rates for cervical cancer prevalenece and mortality were increasing steadily. Then, in the middle of that Century the American Cancer Society promoted a cytological screening developed by Dr. Papanicolaou (Pap test). The outreach from about less than 5% was raised to 80% and the prevalence and mortality was decreased for 80%. There are about 50 mil Pap test done each year in this country, and CC cancer prevalence and mortality decreased below the red line of 10 most frequent diseases in the US.

2.10.10

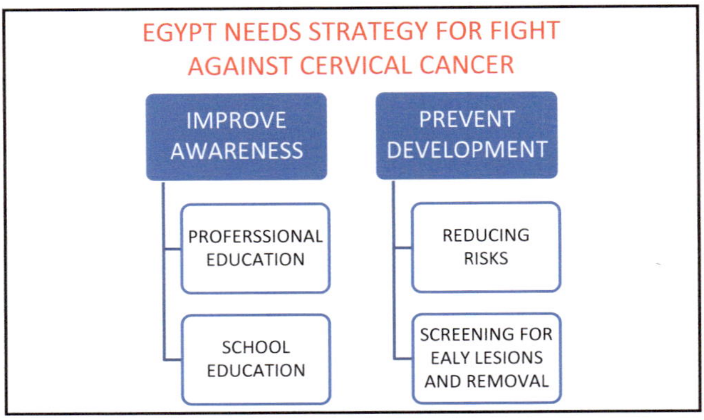
EGYPT NEEDS STRATEGY FOR FIGHT AGAINST CERVICAL CANCER
IMPROVE AWARENESS
PREVENT DEVELOPMENT
PROFERSSIONAL EDUCATION
REDUCING RISKS
SCHOOL EDUCATION
SCREENING FOR EALY LESIONS AND REMOVAL

2.10.11

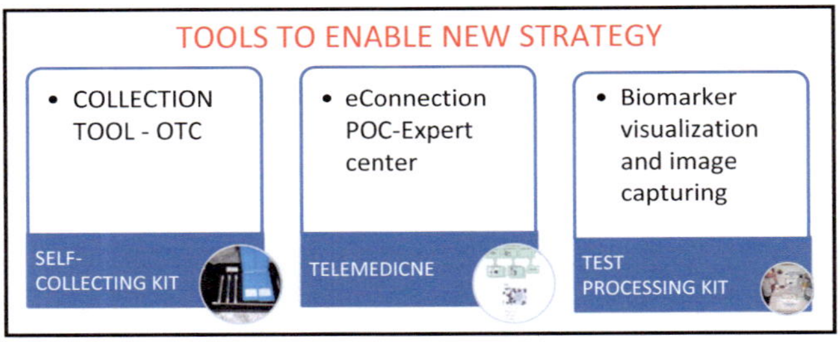

2.10.12

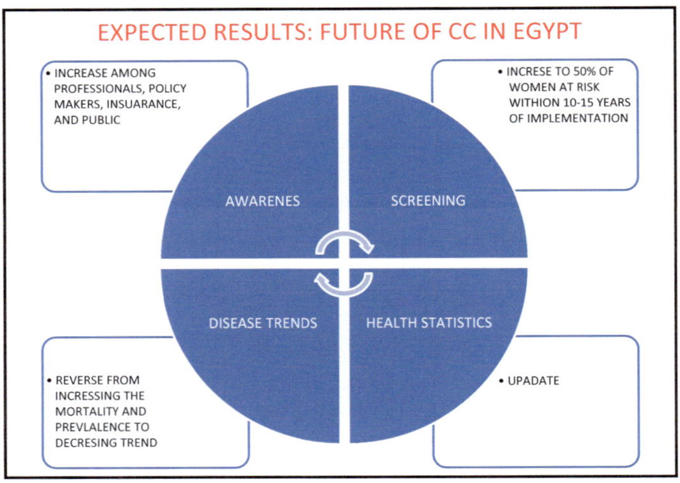

2.10.13

CONTACT

FOR ADDITIONAL INFORMATION PLEASE CONTACT:

GLOBAL ACADEMY FOR WOMEN'S HEALTH, INC.
9601 MEDICAL CENTER DRIVE, RM 111
JOHNS HOPKINS UNVERSITY, MCC
PROF. DR. OLIVERA MARKOVIC
P/F: 1.301.610.9130
Web-site: www.markpap.com

Where to Read More?

Guidelines where and how to look for information covering topics for cervical cancer from essentials to advanced research.

In this chapter you will learn where to seek further help having direct links to excellent resources from American Cancer Society (ACS), National Cancer Institute (NCI), other governmental and public institutions, private founda- tions, support groups and survivors groups.

This is a list of institutions with addresses and telephone numbers where to ask questions and learn more), links to support groups and other useful links where you may find answers on specific questions.

Internet is an enormous resource for health information. In the previous text we were trying to provide referent literature cited on the Internet. You will find most of them in Literature Cited.

However, a woman who is searching Internet by herself, should always read the source of information. Governmental Agencies, e.g., National Cancer Institute (NCI), National Cancer Society (NCS), Food and Drug Administration (FDA) Centers for Disease Control (CDC), International Union Against Cancer (UICC), are excel- lent credible resources. You can find addresses and telephone numbers of these institutions. Women who do not have Internet connection may wish to get in touch by telephone or write a letter. I would suggest calling by phone – it is more interactive and you can immediately ask questions and get answers. Learning the basics from the book will help you to learn what every woman should know about cervical cancer and you will feel more comfort- able to discuss and ask questions.

There are lot of information from different other sources, e.g., non- profit orga-nization, where articles may be written by persons who are not medical doctors, for-profit organizations that might be driven by commercial motives. Discussion groups among patients are useful for many women sharing information with other women who had or are having similar problems. In most cases, these are sincere testimoni- als, but have in mind that these women are patients, not professionals and be critical. Again, if you like to take any action, consult your doctor.

N. Markovic, O. Markovic, *What Every Woman Should Know about Cervical Cancer*, DOI 10.1007/978-94-017-7560-1

Institutions available for support of cancer patients
National Institutes of Health

National Cancer Institute (NCI)
Public Inquires Office, #3036A
6116 Executive Blvd. MSC 8322
Bethesda, MD 20892-8322
Tel.: 301-435-3848
Toll-Free: 1-800-422-8237
1-800-4- CANCER (1-800-422-6237)
www.nci.nih.gov
www.cancer.gov
www.cancernet.nci.gov

American Cancer Society (ACS)
1599 Clifton Rd., NE
Atlanta, GA 30329-4251
Toll-Free: 800-227-2345
1-800-ACS-2345 at any time, 24 h
http://www.cancer.org
www.naric.com
ASC National Information Center http://cancer.org/docroot/ESN/content/ESN_3_1X_ASC_NationalP_Cancer _information....

Other helpful links from ACS
ACS: The Cancer Survivors Network (ACS)
www.acscsn.org/index.html?popup=1

Local chapters of American Cancer Society as a source of sup- port (ASC)
http://www.cancer.org/docroot/ESN/content/ESN_2_3XA_Message of Hope.... (ASC)

By giving your zip code you can find out about local chapters (ASC)
http://www.cancer.org/docroom/COM/COM_0.asp

Finding Support (ASC)
http://www.acssn.org/index.html?popup=1

I Can Cope (ASC)
http://www.cancer.org/docroot/ESN/content/ESN_3_1X_I_Can_Cope,asp

Take a Free Class Now
http://www.cancer.org/docroot/ESN/content/ESN_3_1X_I_Can_Cope_online.asp

The Association of Cancer Online Resources, Inc. (ACOR)
www.acor.org
All About Cancer
http://www.cancer.org/doctoor?CRI/CRI_2x,asp?sitearea=LRN

ASC Support Program and Services
http://www.caner.org/docroot/ESN/_3asp?sitearea=ESN

Reach to Recovery
http://www.cancer.org/docroot/ESN/content/ESN_3_1Xreach_to_Recovery

Cancer Research Institute
681 Fifth Ave
New York, NY 10022-4209
Toll-Free 1-800-992-2623
Fax: 212-832-9376
e-mail: info@cancerresearch.org
http://www.cancerresarach.org

Center for Disease Control
1600 Clifton Rd,
Atlanta, GA 30333, USA
Switchboard: (404) 639-3311
Public Inquiries: (404) 639-3534
Toll-Free: 1-800-311-3435
www.cdc.gov

Cancer Care, Inc.
Tel.: 212-302-2400
Counseling line: 1-800-813-4673
e-mail: www.cancercare.org

National Institute for Mental Health
NIMH public Health Inquires
Tel.: 301-443-4513
Toll-Free: 1-866-615-6464

Substance Abuse and Mental Health Service Administration
Mental Health Information Center
Tel.: 1-800-789-2647
e-mail: www.samhsa.gov

Food and Drug Administration
www.fda.gov

Association of Cancer Online Resources
www.acor.org

Global Academy for Women's Health, Inc.
14905 Forest Landing Circle
Rockville, MD 20850
Tel.: 301-610-9130
e-mail: info@bioscicon.com
www.markpap.com

Health on the Net Foundation
www.hon.ch

Health Summit Working Group
www.hitweb.mitretek.org/hswg

Support Group in the US
National Cervical Cancer Coalition (NCCC)
7247 Hayvenhurst Ave, Suite A-7
Van Nuys, CA 91406
Toll-Free: 1-800-685-5531
Tel.: 818-909-3849 Office
e-mail: info@nccc-online.org
http://www.nccc-online

American Cancer Society
www.cancer.org

Different helpful links
Association for Home Care and Hospice
Tel.: 1-202-547-7424
e-mail: www.nahc.org

National Coalition for Cancer Survivorship
www.cansearch.org

Hospice Net
www.hospicenet.org

Hospice Association of America
www.nahc.org

National Association of Home Care
www.nahc.org

Meals on Wheels Association of America
www.projectmeal.org

Clinical Trials
www.cancertrials.nci.gov
www.centerwactch.com
www.oncolink.upenn.edu/clinical_trials

Alternative and Complementary Medicine
NIH Office of Alternative Medicine
www.altmed.od.nih.gov
NIH Center for Alternative and Complementary Medicine

http://nccam.nih.gov/health/camcancer
University of Texas Center for Alternative Medicine Research
www.sph.uth.tmc.edu/utcam/default.htm

http://www.cancer.org/docroot/ETO/content/ETO_5_1_Introduction. asp (ASC)

International Cancer Resources
International Union Against Cancer (IUCC)
www.iucc.ch
Telescan
www.telescan.nki.ni
Cancer Help UK
www.medweb.bham.ac.uk/cancwerhelp/index.html
Cancer Backup
www.cancerbackup.org.uk
World Health Organization
www.who.ch

ASCCP GUIDELINES 2012: Stewart Massad et al. 2012 updated Consensus Guidelines for the Management of Abnormal Cervical Cancer Screening tests and cancer precursors. American Society for Colposcopy and Cervical Pathology. J of Lower Genital Tract Diseases, Vol 17, Nov 5, 2013, 51–527.

Ethics

Ethics Statements

Conflict of Interest

The authors declare the following:

(a) Authors, as principal investigators and investigators in clinical trials received research grants from NIH (see above) and were salaried for their contribution.
(b) Authors are inventors of the technology (US PTO # 6,143,512 of year 2000) and directed MarkPap® technology development from idea to current products and concepts for application.
(c) If and when the technology will be licensed, the authors will receive royalty.

Funding Source

(a) Invention and R&D for the MarkPap® technology was funded by owners, and in part by family, friends and US Federal Grants via NIH SBIR phase 1 and 2 grants No. 1R43CA086767 (2001), 2R44CA086767 (2002–2005) and 1R43CA094628 (2003).
(b) NIH funding was principally used to support clinical trials necessary to prove the concept and to determine clinical utility of the technology.
(c) Custom manufacturing of products by Ricca Chemical Company was based on "fee for service" principle.
(d) Clinical trials conducted internationally, were funded by BioSciCon as the sponsor (free product and trial design) and the local sources (patient and laboratory management – study conduct) to guarantee the independence of the study.

N. Markovic, O. Markovic, *What Every Woman Should Know about Cervical Cancer*, DOI 10.1007/978-94-017-7560-1

Epilogue

Unfinished Story

The purpose of cancer screening is to postpone the inevitable death once the malignant disease had started and was detected. The cervical cancer screening goes a step beyond: it can cure cancer by removal of local lesion if tumor is detected on time. On time means at any moment during carcinogenesis and tumor-genesis, but before the invasive phase when local therapy is not effective and other means are needed (above clinical stage 1A).

Cervical cancer screening is a part of cancer control measures – surveillance of healthy population to detect early signs of the disease. It is not cancer prevention – management of risk factors, not cancer diagnosis and treatment – management of symptomatic patients.

Human papilloma virus is one of risk factors for development of cervical cancer. As other chronic inflammation, if HPV causes a persistent disease, it can cause spontaneous mutations and carcinogenesis. Once cancer has developed, HPV infection is promoting the tumor growth and underlines the worse prognosis of the cancerous lesions. HPV immunization should be considered for stopping and postponing cancer growth, not only for prevention of cancer genesis where this effect is still dubious.

Unfortunately, as much as cervical cancer screening is effective for individual woman if cancer is detected on time, the screening is ineffective if the outreach among women at risk is below 50 % of population. Only after this crucial percent is reached, the cervical cancer prevalence and mortality in a population at risk can reverse its increasing trends and become to decrease. This is the American experience after 60 years of screening applied on millions of women at risk.

If this outreach is not reached, as in the most of the world population, the cervical cancer will continue to rise (by 10 % annually, while population growths by rate of 1.2–1.4 %) and will stay as the major killer of women from malignant diseases. Hopefully, this social aspect has been recognized, the well known American experi-

N. Markovic, O. Markovic, *What Every Woman Should Know about Cervical Cancer*, DOI 10.1007/978-94-017-7560-1

ence has become an inspiration in other countries and a targeted goal for their health policies.

The new edition of our book, has addressed this social aspect of cervical cancer screening, and we hope, the better understanding of the country, state and community engagement will help health care providers to reach the target and to award the society with the reversal of cervical cancer trends – saving women's lives and their human development, social, economic and cultural contributions.

This book is also addressing another aspect of the same puzzle, the cost/benefit ratio between investment into mass cervical cancer screening (more than 51 % of women at risk), and the economic benefit on return to investment, the countries participating in this global program could gain. With the current prices we have estimated that countries with GDP above $10,000 per capita, could easily take the challenge and in a period of 10–15 years will be rewarded with reversal of the currently increasing trends.

Countries with BDP below this threshold, must ask for additional funds to obtain the same benefit and the global goals.

We predict that the most of LMIC will decide for the benefits of the suggested policy change –the new strategy and tools—and that women at risk will be better protected from cervical cancer in the next 20–30 years, than they are now protected.

Literature Cited

1. ACCP. Cervical cancer prevention. Fact Sheet. 10 key findings and recom-mendations for effective cervical cancer screening and treatment programs. Cited Internet http://www.alliance-cxca.org/. Cited September 25, 2007
2. Agoff SN, Lin P, Morihara J et al (2003) p16^{INK4a} expression correlates with degree of cervical neoplasia: a comparison with Ki-67 expression and detection of high-risk HPV types. Mod Pathol 16(7):665–673
3. AHRQ, Agency for Healthcare Research and Quality. Patient Fact Sheet. 20 tips to help prevent medical errors. http://www.ahrq.gov/consumer/20tips.html on August 1 2007. Cited August 24, 2007
4. American Cancer Society Home. http://www.cancer.org. Cited September 17, 2007
5. American Cancer Society. Prevention & early detection. ACS guidelines for early detection of cancer. http://www.cancer.org/docroot/PED/content. Cited September 15, 2007
6. American Cancer Society Guidelines on nutrition and physical activity in cancer patients. http://caonline.amcancersociety.org. Cited August 17, 2007
7. Anonymous. Hysterectomy. Medical encyclopedia. http://www.answers.com/topic/hysterectomy. Cited June 30, 2007
8. Anonymous. Statistics about cervical cancer. WrongDiagnosis.com http://www.wrongdiagnosis.com/c/cervical_cancer/stats.html. Cited July 12, 2007
9. Anonymous. Chlamydial genital tract infections. Chlamydia as a cofactor in cervical cancer. http://www.chlamydiae.com/restricted/docs/infections/gentrac_cervical_cancer. Cited September 14, 2007
10. Anonymous. University of Florida Shands Cancer Center. Stress and depression frequent among women treated for gynecological cancers. http://www.ufscc.ufl.edu/patient/cancernews.aspx. Cited June 23, 2007
11. Anonymous. New biomarker for cervical cancer. Medical observer, December 1999. http://findarticles.com/articles/mi_m3230/is_12_31/ai. Cited July 4, 2007
12. Arrossi S, Sankaranayanan R, Parkin D. Incidence and mortality of cervical cancer in Latin America. IARC, WHO. http://www.scielosp.org/scielo.php?script=sci. Cited July 15, 2007
13. Arbyn M, Raifu AO, Autier P, et al (2007) Burden of cervical cancer in Europe: estimates for 2004. 2007 European Society for Medical Oncology. Ann Oncol online ISSN 1569–8041
14. ASCCP Practice recommendations. The cervix: histology. http://asccp.org/edu. Cited February 4, 2007
15. Austin R. Marshal. Information for ASC member posted on members list@cytopathology.org and ASCCP Home. http://www.asccp.org/consensus.shtml. Cited September 4, 2007
16. BBC News on April 9, 2007. Staining 'spots cervical cancer' http://news.bbc.co.uk/go/pr/fr/-/2/hi/health/6518685.stm. Cited August 28, 2007

N. Markovic, O. Markovic, *What Every Woman Should Know about Cervical Cancer*, DOI 10.1007/978-94-017-7560-1

17. Beutner KR et al (1997) Human papilloma virus and human disease. Am J Med 102(5a):9–15. www.brown.edu/courses/Bio_160/Projects1999/path.html. Cited April 4, 2006
18. Bioscreening Industry News. November 7, 2005. TriPath Imaging, Inc. (NASDAQ) PRNewswire-First Call. New research study provides further evidence of strong correlation of TriPath Imaging ProEx C Biomarkers with biopsy evidence of high-grade cervical intraepithelial neoplasia (CIN 2+)
19. Bibbo M (1997) Comprehensive cytopathology. W.B. Saunders, Philadelphia
20. BioSciCon's electronic Survey. Web Site link. http://www.surveymk.com/s.aspx?sm=aKALIgzj7AwSthXcp0nI1w_3d_3d. Cited September 25, 2007
21. BioSciCon's web portal: http://www.bioscicon.com
22. BioSciCon' MarkPap Self test. http://bioscicon.com/productsindev.html
23. Biswas R. Rural Indian women face heightened cervical cancer risks. PRB Population Reference Bureau. http://www.prb.org/Articles/2004/RuralIndian. Cited June 8, 2007
24. Bischoff R, van der Greef J, van der Zee AGJ. Project: discovery of new biomarkers for cervical cancer. KNAW-Research Information. http://www.onderzoekinformatie.nl/en/oi/nod/onderzoek. Cited 10 August, 2007
25. Blonna R (2000) Coping with stress in the changing world. McGraw-Hill, Boston
26. Bokemeyer C, Hartmann JT, Kuczyk MA, et al (1996) The role of paclitaxel in chemosensitive urological malignancies: current strategies in bladder cancer and testicular germ-cell tunics. World J Urol 14(6):354–359. Springer, Berlin. ISSN 0724–4983 and (online) 1433–8726
27. Bosch FX, Munoz N, de Sanjose S et al (1992) Risk factors for cervical cancer in Colombia and Spain. Int J Cancer 52(5):750–758
28. Brake T, Connor JP, Petereit D, Lambert PF (2003) Comparative analysis of cervical cancer in women and in a human papillomavirus-transgenic mouse model. Cancer Res 63:8173–8180
29. Brinton LA (1992) Epidemiology of cervical cancer-overview. IARC Sci Publ 119:3–23
30. Campbell NA (1977) Biology. Benjamin/Cummings, Menlo Park
31. Cancer Research UK. Cervical cancer chemotherapy http://cancerhelp.org.uk/help/default.asp?page=2779. Cited September 9, 2007
32. CancerHelp UK (sponsored by NHS Direct Online). Which surgery for cervical cancer, from Internet http://www.cancerhelp.org.uk/help/default/asp?page=9188. Cited January 6, 2007
33. Cancer Centers of America. Complementary & alternative medicines for cervical cancer treatment. http://www.cancercenter.com/cervical-cancer/complementary. Cited July 17, 2007
34. Cancer Research UK. About cervical cancer radiotherapy. http://cancerhelp.org.uk/help. Cited July 7, 2007
35. Cancer Research UK. Cervical cancer chemotherapy. http://cancerhelp.org.uk/help/default.asp/page=2779. Cited September 19, 2007
36. CAP Advocacy Group. Guidelines for the review of Pap tests in the context of litigation or potential litigation. College of American Pathologists Policy Guidelines adopted February 1998, reaffirmed October 2005. http://www.cap.org/cap.portal?. Cited September 29, 2007
37. Cass I, Kaplan BY (2003) Neoplasm of the ovary and fallopian tube. In: Scott JR, Gibbs RS, Kaplan BY, Haney AF (eds) Danforth's obstetrics and gynecology. Lippincott, Williams & Wilkins, Philadelphia, pp 518–603
38. Castellisage X, Diaz M, de Danjose S et al (2006) Worldwide human papillomavirus etiology of cervical adenocarcinoma and its cofactor: implications for screening and prevention. J Natl Cancer Inst 98(5):303–315
39. Centers for Disease Control and Prevention. Genital HPV Infection – CDC Fact Sheet. http://www.cdc.gov/std/HPV/STDFact-HPV.htm on July 31 2007. Cited July 7, 2007
40. Centers for Disease Control and Prevention. STD Surveillance. http://www.cdc.gov/std/stats/tables/table42.htm. Cited July 31, 2007
41. Centers for Disease Control and Prevention. Vaccines and immunization. HPV vaccination. http://www.cdc.gov/vaccines/vpd-vac. Cited July 25, 2007

42. Cervical cancer in Latin America and the Caribbean. PAHO (Pan American Health Organization), Regional Office of WHO (World Health Organization). PAHO, Fact Sheet 2001
43. CDC. DES Home. DES update: consumers. Potential health risks for DES daughters. http://www.cdc.gov/des/consumers. Cited June 27, 2007
44. CDC. MMWR (2007) QuickStats: prevalence of HPV infection among sexually active females aged 14–59 years, by age group. National Health and Nutrition Examination Survey, United States 2003–2004, MMWR weekly report 24 August 24, 2007/56(33):852
45. Cervical Cancer/HPV Community. Daily Newsletter Online. September 16, 2007. Post Conference Reports. Publisher National Cervical Cancer Coalition cervicalcancer@clinica-health.com. Cited September 16, 2007
46. CNN.com. Health library. Diseases and conditions. Cervical cancer from Mayo clinical special to CNN. On June 22 2007. http://www.cnn.com/HEALTH/library/DS/00167.html. Cited July 12, 2007
47. Center for Disease Control and Prevention. AIDS/HIV multitude of pages for review available http://www.cdc/hiv.gov. Cited April 3, 2007
48. CLIA, Clinical Laboratory Improvement Amendments of 1988. See CDC web site http://cdc.gov/. Cited August 1, 2006
49. Clinical Laboratory Improvement Amendments 1988. Title 42 CFR 493 of 1988
50. Cohen BJ, Wood DL (2000) Memmler's human body is health and disease. Lippincot, Williams & Wilkins, Philadelphia
51. Cortez D, Glick G, Ellege SJ (2004) Minichromosome maintenance proteins are direct targets of the ATM and ATP checkpoint kinases. Proc Natl Acad Sci U S A 101(30):10845–10846
52. Curtis P. Cancer fear as fewer women take routine pap smear. http://www.guardian.co.uk/medicine. Cited September 12, 2007
53. Cytyc Corp. The ThinPrep system – how it works? http://www.cytyc.com/85506?prd/prep-work.html. Cited February 26, 2007
54. de Cherney A, Nathan R (2007) Lange medical book. Current obstetrics and gynecology diagnosis and treatment. McGraw-Hill, New York
55. Denny L, Kuhn L, Pollack A et al (2000) Evaluation of alternative methods of cervical cancer screening for resource-poor settings. Cancer 89(4):826–833
56. DeNoon D (2006) Soking boosts cervical cancer risk. According to Gunelli A. Cancer epidemiology, biomarkers & prevention 15:2141–2147. News release, American Association for Cancer Research
57. Digene. Hybrid Capture 2 Technology. http://digene.com/labs. Cited July 19, 2007
58. Diamics. C-map cervical cancer screening system. http://www.diamics.com/mo5.htm. Cited April 30, 2007
59. Donnatelle RJ, Davis LG (1997) Health: the basics. Allyn & Becon, Boston
60. Dunne EF, Unger ER, Stenberg M et al (2007) Prevalence of HPV infection among females in the United States. JAMA 298(8):813–819
61. Edelman CI, Mandel C (1994) Health promotion throughout the lifespan. Mosby, St.Louis
62. Eluf-Neto J, Booth M, Munoz N et al (1994) Human papillomavirus and invasive cervical cancer in Brazil. Br J Cancer 69(1):114–119
63. Eltoum IA, Robeson J. Impact of HPV testing, HPV vaccine development, and changing screening frequency on national Pap test volume (Projections from the National Health Interview Survey). Cancer Cytopathol. Published Online 29 January 2009 in Willey InterScience www.interscience.willey.com. Cited May 4, 2007
64. Epigee Women's Health. Herpes resource. From http://www.epigee.org/guide/stds.html. Cited May 28, 2007
65. Eschenbach DA (2003) Pelvic infections and STD. In: Scott JR, Gibbs RS, Kaplan BY, Haney AF (eds) Danforth's obstetrics and gynecology. Lippincott, Williams & Wilkins, Philadelphia, pp 518–603

66. Evantosh E, Hill EC, Pernoll ML (2007) Benign disorders of the uterine cervix. In: de Cherney A, Nathan R (eds) Lange medical book. Current obstet-rics and gynecology diagnosis and treatment. McGraw-Hill, New York, pp 677–692
67. Eysenck HJ (1994) Synergistic interaction between psychological and physical factors in the causation of lung cancer. In: Lewis C, O'Sulivan C, Baraclough J (eds) The psychoimmunology of cancer. Oxford University Press, Oxford, pp 163–178
68. Fox SI (1999) Human physiology. WCB/McGraw-Hill, Boston
69. Franco EL, Schlecht NF, Saslow D (2003) The epidemiology of cervical cancer. Cancer L 9(5):348–359
70. Garcia-Hernandez E, Gonzales-Sanchez JL, Andrade-Manzano A et al (2006) Regression of papilloma high-grade lesions (CIN 2 and CIN 3) is stimulated by therapeutic vaccination with MVA E2 recombinant vaccine. Cancer Gene Ther 13:592–597
71. Gill G. Personal citation of CLIA*88 paragraph (f). Published on mest@cytopathology.org. Cited May 6, 2007
72. Girdano D, Everly G, Dusek D (1993) Controlling stress and tension. A holistic approach. Prentice Hall, Englewood Cliffs
73. Glaxo SmithKline. Cervarix a GSK's candidate vaccine for cervical cancer, demonstrated sustained efficacy for up to 4.5 years and broader protection against cancer causing HPV types. http://www.gsk.com/ControllerServlet. Cited July 25, 2007
74. Glickman J. Basic facts on HPV. Health science report. http://health-science-report.com/alotek/topics1/article3/ of January 2 2007. Cited January 2, 2007
75. Goddard K (1991) Morita Therapy. A literature review. Transcult Psych Res Rev 28(2):93–115
76. Greenwell P, Dwek M. Biomarkers for HPV and cervical cancer: proteomics and glycomics. University of Westminster. Project design. http://wmin.ac.uk/bioscience/page-530. Cited July 5, 2007
77. Guccione K. Women in government issues new state policy recommendation. Women in government. http://www.judicialwatch.org/printer_6299.shtml. Cited August 5, 2007
78. Guyton AC, Hall JE (2000) Medical physiology. W.B. Saunders, Philadelphia
79. Guyton AC, Hall JE (1997) Human physiology and the mechanism of disease. W.B. Saunders, Philadelphia
80. Gunstream SE (2000) Anatomy and physiology. McGraw-Hill, Boston
81. Hartman LC, Loprinzi CL (2005) Mayo Clinic guide to women's cancers. Mayo Foundation for Medical Education and Research, Rochester
82. Health & Medical News. A PAP test replacement? http://www.abc.net.au/science on April 20 2001. Cited December 8, 2006
83. Hildesheim A, Herrero R, Castle PE et al (2001) HPV co-factors related to the development of cervical cancer: results from a population-based study in Costa Rica. Br J Cancer 84(9):1219–1226
84. Histopathology Atlas. Histopathology of the uterine cervix – digital atlas. Frappart L, Fontaniere B, Lucas E, Sankaranaranayan R. IARC Screening Group. ISBN 92 832 2424 8. http://screenijng.iarc.fr/atlashisto. Cited September 29, 2007
85. Hubard RA. Human papillomavirus testing methods. Archives of pathology and laboratory medicine, August 1, 2003. From LookSmart on Internet http://findarticles.com/p/articles. Cited June 30, 2007
86. Hughes EF, Jacobs BD, Berman BM (2007) Complementary and alternative medicine. In: McFee ST, Papadakis MA, Tierney L (eds) Lange 2007 current medical diagnosis and treatment. McGraw-Hill Medical, New York, pp 1743–1773
87. Human Anatomy on line. Female reproductive system. http://www.inner-body.com/image. Cited September 21, 2007
88. IARC Screening Group. Colposcopy and treatment of cervical intraepithe-lial neoplasia. Chapter 2. An introduction to cervical intraepithelial neoplasia (CIN). http://screening.iarc.fr/colpochap.php. Cited June 23, 2007

89. IARC Screening Group. The Bethesda system http://screening.iarc.fr/atlas-classifbethesda.php. Cited January 5, 2007
90. International Union Against Cancer (UICC). TNM classification of malignant tumors http://www.uicc.org/index2.php?option=com. Cited April 2, 2007
91. IARC Handbooks on Cancer Prevention (2005) Vol 10. Cervix cancer screening. ISBN 92 832 3010 8
92. IARC Screening Group Home Page. Cervical cancer. http://screening.iarc.fr/. Cited June 15, 2007
93. Idman PD. Treatment of cervical dysplasia. Advanced gynecology solutions http://www.gyn-alternatives.com/cervical_dysplasia_treatment.html. Cited August 2, 2007
94. Incidence (epidemiology) from Wikipedia. http://en.wikipedia.org/wiki/Incidence_(epidemiology). Cited September 14, 2007
95. Internet Health Library. Cervical cancer research. Diet & lifestyle. http://www.internethealthlibrary.com/Health_problems/Cervical%20Cancer%%20. Cited June 22, 2007
96. Judicial Watch. Judicial Watch uncovers three deaths relating to HPV vac-cine (Gardasil) and 1637 adverse reactions. http://judicialwatch.org/printer_6299.shtml. Cited September 2, 2007
97. Kodner CM, Nastraty S (2004) Management of genital warts. Am Fam Physician 70:2335–2346. http://www.aafp.org/afp/20041215/2335.htoml. Cited September 2, 2007
98. Kjaer SK (1998) Risk factors for cervical neoplasia in Denmark. APMIS Suppl 80:1–41
99. Kendall-Tackett KA (2005) Handbook of woman stress and trauma. Routledge/Taylor & Francis, New York
100. Kautsky LA (2007) Quadrivalent vaccine against human papilloma virus to prevent high-grade cervical lesions. NEJM 356(19):1915–1927
101. Kolonel LH, Hankin JH et al (1981) Nutrient intakes in relation to cancer in Hawaii. Br J Cancer 44:332
102. Koss LG (1992) The Papanicolaou stain. Diagnostic cytology and its histopathology basis, 4th edn. Lippincott, Philadelphia
103. Kumar S. Nanolithography. In vivo optical detection of intracellular cancer biomarkers using gold nanoparticles. Spie Digital Library. http://spiedl.aip.org/getabs.servlet. Cited August 30, 2007
104. Lang LH. UNC researcher study new biomarker to improve screening for cervical cancer. University North Carolina News Services, October 1, 1999, No 584. http://www.unc.ed/archives/oct99. Cited September 3, 2007
105. Li HQ, Jin SQ, Xu HX, Thomas D (2000) The decline in the mortality rates of cervical cancer and a plausible explanation in Shandong, China. Int J Epidemiol 29:398–404
106. List of causes of death by rate. From Wikipedia. http://en.wikipedia.org/wiki/List_of_causes_of_death_by_rate. Cited September 14, 2007
107. Liton SC et al (2005) Mayo clinical family health book, 3rd edn. Genetic Testing, HarperCollins, ISBN-10: 0-06-0002590-6
108. Ludwig JA, Weinstein JN (2005) Biomarkers in cancer staging, prognosis and treatment selection. Nature reviews/cancer. Nature Publishing Group 5:845–856, and http://www.nature/reviews/cancer. Cited September 14, 2007
109. Maslow AH (1968) Toward a psychology of being. Van Nostrand, Princeton
110. McFee ST, Papadakis MA, Tierney L (2007) Lange 2007 current medical diagnosis and treatment. McGraw-Hill Medical, New York
111. Mac Kay HT (2007) Gynecology. In: McFee ST, Papadakis MA, Tierney L (eds) Lange 2007 current medical diagnosis and treatment. McGraw-Hill Medical, New York, pp 747–781
112. Malinowski DP (2007) Multiple biomarkers in molecular oncology. I. Molecular diagnostics application in cervical cancer detection. Expert Rev Med Diagn 7(2):117–131
113. Marcial-Toledo S, Cortez-Guzman J, Chavez L et al (2006) Screen-and treat colposcopy as public health strategy fore cervical cancer early detection in high risk population: the experience of the Centro de Estudios y Prevencion del Cancer (CEPREC) in indigenous population

of Southern Mexico. J Clin Oncol, 2006 ASCO Annual meeting proceedings Part 1, Vol. 24, No. 18S (June 20 Supplement), 5012. http://www.gardasil.com. Cited January 2, 2007
114. Markovic N, Markovic O (2000) CAP-PAP test. US Patent 6,143,512, 20 Nov 2000
115. Markovic O, Markovic N (2003/2004) Cervical acid phosphatase: a biomarker of cervical dysplasia and a potential surrogate endpoint for colposcopy. Dis Markers 19:279–286
116. Markovic N, Markovic O, Sundeen J (2004). BioSciCon Cervical Cancer Study Group. Pap test and a new biomarker-based technology for enhancing the visibility of abnormal cells. 2004 ASCO annual meeting, New Orleans, J Clin Oncol Suppl 22(1):9561. Slide presentation available on http://www.asco.org/portal/site/ASCO/menuitem. Cited September 19, 2007
117. Markovic N, Markovic O, Henderson E et al (2005) MarkPap test for cervical cancer screening. 2005 ASCO annual meeting. J Clin Oncol Suppl 23(1):1021 Slide presentation available on the Internet www.asco.org/portal/site/ASCO/menuitem. Cited September 25, 2007
118. Markovic N, Markovic O (2006) The power of the biomarker for cervical cancer control. 2006 ASCO annual meeting. J Clin Oncol Suppl 24:11001(18S). http://www.asco.org/portal/site/. Cited July 7, 2007
119. Markovic N, Markovic O, Henderson E (2006) MarkPap digital, a new prospective for biomarker-based gynecological cytology. Ann meeting of the AACR, April 2006, Washington, DC
120. Markovic N, Markovic O (2007). MarkPap test and HPV vaccination. BIO international convention. 2006, innovative corridor, Boston http://72.14.209.104.../Poster/Listing.aspx. www.bioscicon/publications.html. Cited August 1, 2007
121. Markovic O, Markovic N (2007) Will home Pap test be soon available. Experimental biology 2007 annual meeting, Washington, DC. The FASEB J 21(6):708.10
122. Markovic N, Markovic O (2003–2007). publications are available on the Internet at the BioSciCon web site http://www.bioscicon.com/publications.html
123. Maugh T, Chong J (2007) The highly tooted treatment to prevent cervical cancer may be less effective than previously thought. Article in Los Angeles Times on May 10, 2007
124. Merck & Co., Inc. Products. Gardasil [Quadrivalent HPV vaccine]. Risk for HPV. Information. From Internet http://meck.com and http://www.gardasil.com. Cited September 29, 2007
125. Metcalf CV, Felible R (1992) Lighten-up: survival skills for people under pressure. Addison Wesley, Reading
126. Mikolaj AA (2005) Stress management for emergency care providers. Pearson/Prentice, Upper Saddle River
127. Miller K, Blumenthal P, Blanchard K (2004) Oral contraceptives and cervical cancer: critique of a recent review. Contraception 69:347–351
128. Minkin MJ, Wright CV (2003) The Yale guide to women's reproductive health. Yale University Press, New Haven
129. Mutch D (2003) Uterine cancer. In: Scott IR, Gibbs RS, Kaplan BY, Haney AF (eds) Danforth's obstetrics and gynecology. Lippincott, Willliams & Wilkinis, Philadelphia, pp 951–964
130. National Cancer Institute Fact Sheets. Cancer advances in focus. Cervical cancer (posted October 30 2006). Retrieved from Internet http://www.cancer.gov/aboutnci/cancer-advances-in-focus/cervical. Cited May 31, 2007
131. National Cancer Institute Home. http://www.nci.nih.gov
132. National Cancer Institute. Antioxidants and cancer prevention. Fact Sheet. http://www.cancer.gov/cancertopics/factsheet/antioxidantsprevention. Cited June 28, 2007
133. National Cancer Institute. Notice for contract solicitations. NOT-CA-02-011. Defining and validating biomarkers of risk for progressive cervical cancer. http://grants.nih.gov/guide/notice-files/NOT-CA-02-011.html. Cited September 2, 2007
134. National Cancer Institute. Med News. Screening statement for health professionals (Data last modified 2-20-2007). Screening for cervical cancer. http://www.meb.uni-bonn.de/cancer.gov. Cited September 16, 2007

135. National Cancer Institute. Surveilance Epidemiology and End Results (SEER), cervical cancer, http://seer.cancer.gov/statfacts/html/cervix.htm. Cited September 12, 2007
136. NIH, NCI, FactSheet. Oral contraceptives and cancer risk: Q&A. http://www.cancer.gov/cancertopics/faxtsheer/Risk/oral-contraceptives. Cited June 23, 2007
137. NIH Center for Alternative and Complementary Therapy. http://nccam.nih.gov/health. Cited September 12, 2007
138. NIH Consensus Conference on Cervical Cancer (1966) NIH consensus statement online 1–3: 43(1):1–38
139. NIH, NCI, FactSheet. Antioxidants and cancer prevention: Fact Sheet. http://cancer.gov?cancertopics/factsheet/antioxidantsprevention, of June 22 2007. Cited September 12, 2007
140. NIH Consensus Statement No. 102. Cervical cancer. NIH Consent/Statement 1996 April 1–3; 14(10):1–38
141. Nisl J. Colposcopy and cervical biopsy. WebMD. Cancer Health Center. F http://www.webmd.com/cancer/Colposcopy-and-Cervical-Biopsy. Cited September 12, 2007
142. Northrup C (1998) Women's bodies, women's wisdom. Bantam Books, New York
143. Obermair A, Bancher-Todesca D, Bilgi S et al (1997) Correlation of vascular endothelial growth factor expression and microvessel density in cervical intraepithelial neoplasia. J Natl Cancer Inst 89:1212–1217
144. Oberman E, Went F, Zimpfer A et al (2005) Expression of minichromosome maintenance protein 2 as a marker for proliferation and prognosis in diffuse large B-cell lymphoma; a tissue microarray and clinico-pathological analysis. BMC Cancer 5:162–172
145. Orr JW Jr, Wilson K, Bodiford C et al (1985) Corpus and cervix cancer: a nutritional comparison. Am J Obstet Gynecol 153(7):775–779
146. PATH:Alliance for Cervical Cancer Prevention. Low-resource approaches to a high-stakes health problems. http://www.path.org/projects/accp.php. Cited August 8, 2007
147. Peck MS (1987) The road less traveled. Simon & Schuster, New York
148. Public Law US 102–139, Title 1, Section 101, 105 Statute 742 (1991)
149. Quotations. My Quotation Book from ThinkExist. http://thinkexist.com/quotes/top. Cited September 29, 2007
150. Reynolds D (1984) Playing ball on running water. Williams Morrow, New York
151. Reynolds D (1992) The teacher student relationship in Japanese culture and Morita therapy. Int Bull Morita Ther 5(1):18–21
152. Reesink-Peters N, Wisman GBA, Jeronimo C et al (2004) Detecting cervical by quantitative promoter hypermethylation assay on cervical scrapings: a feasibility study. Mol Cancer Res 2:289–295
153. Ruffin MT, Ogaily MS, Johnston CM et al (1995) Surrogate endpoint biomarkers for cervical cancer chemoprevention. J Cell Biochem Suppl 23:113–124
154. Sankaranarayanan R et al (2005) A cluster randomized controlled trial of visual, cytology and human papilloma virus screening for cancer of the cervix in rural India. Int J Cancer 116(4):617–623
155. Sankaranarayanan R et al (2007) Effect of visual screening on cervical cancer incidence and mortality in Tamil Nadu, India: a cluster-randomized trial. Lancet 370:398–406
156. Scanlan RA. Nitrosamines and cancer. The Linus Pauling Institute. Oregon University. http://lpi.oregonstate.edu/f-w00/nitrosamine.html. Cited September 6, 2007
157. Schmale AH, Iker H (1971) Hopelessness as a prediction of cervical cancer. Soc Sci Med 5:99–100
158. Seely RR, Stephens TD, Tate P (2003) Anatomy and physiology. McGrawHill, Boston
159. Selye H (1973) The evolution of stress concept. Am Sci 61:692
160. Shields TS, Brinton LA, Wang SS et al (2004) A case-control study of risk factors got invasive cervical cancer among U.S. women exposed to oncogenic types of human papilloma virus. Cancer Epidemiol Biomark Prev 3(10):1574–1582

161. Smith JS, Lindsay L, Hoots B et al (2007) Human papilloma virus type distribution in invasive cervical cancer and high-grade cervical lesions. A metaanalysis update. Int J Cancer 121:621–632
162. Solomon D, Davey D, Kurman R et al (2002) The 2001 Bethesda system. Terminology for reporting results of cervical cytology. JAMA 287(16):2114–2119
163. Solomon D, Schiffman M (2001) Comparison of three management strategies for patients with atypical squamous cells of undetermined significance: baseline results from a randomized trial (ALTS). J Natl Cancer Inst 93(12):293–299, and Response in J Natl Cancer Inst 93(12):251–252
164. Suba EJ, Donnelly AD, Furia L et al (2007) Cervical cancer prevention for all the world's women: genuine promise resides in skilled quality management rather than novel screening approaches. Diagn Cytopathol 35(3):187–191
165. Tang YW, Stratton CW. Advanced techniques in Diagnostic Microbiology. Amazon. http://www.amazon.com/exec/obidos/. Cited September 4, 2007
166. Takahashi Shoji. Diagnosis and treatment of cervical cancer. Office of Technology Development. GTU, Washington, DC. http://otl.georgetown.edu/industry/inventions. Cited September 24, 2007
167. Temoshok L, Dreher H (1992) Type C behavior and cancer. Random House, New York
168. Thomas DB, Ray RM, Koetsawang A et al (2001) Human papillomaviruses and cervical cancer in Bangkok. I. Risk factors for invasive cervical carcinomas with human papillomavirus types 16 and 18 DNA. Am J Epidemiol 153(8):723–731
169. Thomson FE, Patterson BH, Weinstein SJ et al (2002) Serum selenium and the risk of cervical cancer among women in the United States. Cancer Cause Control 13(6):517–526
170. ThermoShandon. Thermo scientific. Anatomic pathology. Products. http://www.thermo.com. Cited September 29, 2007
171. TNM Classification of Malignant Tumors. From Wikipedia on Internet, http://en.wikipedia.org/wiki/TNM
172. TriPath Imaging Home. http://www.tripathimaging.com
173. http://www.abc.net.au/science on April 20 2001
174. Velema JP, Ferrera A, Figueroa M et al (2002) Burning wood in the kitchen increases the risk of cervical neoplasia in HPV-infected women in Honduras. Int J Cancer 97(4):536–541
175. World Health Organization (1947) Constitution of the WHO. Chronicles of the WHO, Geneva
176. WHO HIV/AIDS Guidelines. http://who.int/hiv/pub/guideline/en. Cited on September 29, 2007
177. WHO Department of Vaccine Research and Biologicals. Human HPV and HPV vaccines: technical information for policy makers and health professionals. WHO Press 2007. Cited on September 6, 2007
178. Women in US Government. Challenge to eliminate cervical cancer. Policy Recommendation. http://www.womeningovernment.org/prevention. Cited on September 29, 2007
179. Wikipedia, the free encyclopedia. Epidemiology. http://en.wikipedia/wiki/Epidemiology. Cited August 27, 2007
180. Wikipedia. Histology http://en.wikipedia.org/wiki/Histology. Cited September 12, 2007
181. Wikipedia, the free encyclopedia. Radiation therapy. http://en.wikipedia.org/wiki/Raiationtherapy. Cited September 7, 2007
182. Wright VC (1984) Carbon dioxide laser surgery for cervical intraepithelial neoplasia. Laser Surg Med 4(2):145–152
183. Wright T et al (2002) ASCCP 2001 consensus guidelines for the management of women with cervical cytological abnormalities. JAMA 287(16):2120–2129
184. www.nccn.org NCCN clinical practice guidelines in oncology. Cervical cancer screening, V1.2008. Cited September 8, 2007
185. www.brown.edu/courses/Bio_/Products1999/path/html

186. Yoon SK, Lim NK, Ha SA, et al (2004) The human cervical cancer oncogene protein is a biomarker for human hepato-cellular carcinoma. Cancer Res 64:5434–5441. http://cancerres.aacrjournals.org/cgi/content/abstract/64/15/5434. Cited July 5, 2007
187. Youngerman-Cole S et al Pelvic examination. WebMD. Women's health http://women.webmd.com/Women-MedicalReference/Pelvic-Examination. Cited June 28, 2007
188. Zalopa AR, Katz MH (2007) HIV infection. In: McFee ST, Papadakis MA, Tierney L (eds) Lange 2007 current medical diagnosis and treatment. McGraw-Hill Medical, New York/Chicago, pp 1346–1377
189. Zenillman JM (2001) Chlamydia and cervical cancer: a real association? JAMA 285:81–83
190. de Zelmanowicz A, Hildesheim A (2004) Family history of cancer as a risk factor for cervical carcinoma: a review of the literature. Papillomavirus Rep 15(3):113–120
191. Ziegler RG (1986) Epidemiologic studies of vitamins and cancer of the lung, esophagus, and cervix. Adv Exp Med Biol 206, ISSN 0065–2598 Journal Code:2LU
192. Ziegler RG, Jones AC, Rosenthal JF, et al (1991) Diet and the risk of in situ cervical cancer among white women in the United States. Cancer Cause Control 2(1):17–29, ISSN 0957–5243
193. Zuna RE, Allen RA, Moore WE, et al (2004). Comparison of human papilloma virus genotypes in high-grade squamous intraepithelial lesions and invasive cervical carcinoma: evidence for differences in biologic potential of precursor lesions. Mod Pathol 17:1314–1322 (presented at the 92nd annual meeting of the US and Canadian Academy of Pathology, Washington, DC, March 2003)
194. Markovic O, Shulman NR (1977) Megakaryocyte maturation indicated by methanol inhibition of an acid phospahatase shared by megakariyocytes and platelets. Blood 50:905
195. Markovic N. BioSciCon presents the MarkPap technology. Larta-CAP Venture Forum 2007, San Francisco, May 2007. http://www.theventureforum.com/PresentingCompaniesList.asp
196. Markovic N, Markovic O. Biomarker plus. 55th annual meeting of the American Society of Cytopathology, Nov 2007, Houston. Cancer cytopathology Suppl. 11/5,385,2007. Click here to download the abstract. (PDF format)
197. Markovic N, Markovic O. Ask for women' s opinion first. Teaching and computer session. FASEB experimental biology, 2008. Today's research: tomorrow's health. San Diego California, April 5–9, 2008. Click here to download the abstract
198. Prabal D, Wenkateswaran Y, Bhatla N, Markovic O, Verma K (2008) Cervical acid Phosphatase detection: a guide to abnormal cells in cytology smear screening for cervical cancer. J Cytol 25(1):1–5. Click here to view the article
199. Iyer VK, Mathur SR, Bhatla N, Markovic O. Evaluation of cytology screening strategies for cervical cancer in resource poor settings. 18th International Congress of Cytology, Paris, May 2013. Click here to view the abstract
200. Neha B, Agrawal PM, Santwani M (2015) Staudy of CAPPAP versus conventional papa in suspicious cervical lesions. Int J Res Med 4(1):102–108
201. Niranjan J, Prakash CJ (2015) Cervical acid Phosphatase: evaluation as a an adjuvant to Papanicolaou smears screening in cervical cancer detection. J Evid Based Med Healthc 2(6):714–732
202. Markovic O, Markovic N. MarkPap technology: a prospective for global cervical cancer control. FASEB annual meeting, experimental biology 2006, San Francisco
203. Anhui Science Technology Company. www.ahnmst.com. Assessed June 2015
204. Anyon Biopharmaceuticals in Anhui, China. www.anyon.com.cn. Assessed July 2016
205. Anhui Anke Biotechnology Group Co, Ltd ankebio@mail.hf/ah.cn. Accessd July 2015
206. Markovic O, Markovic N (2007) Will home Pap test be soon available? Experimental biology 2007. The FASEB J 2007 21(6), A 754, 708.10. Click here to view the article
207. Markovic O, Markovic N (2012) Is mass cytological cancer screening possible worldwide? The FASEB J 26, 657.1. Click here to view the abstract

208. Markovic O, Markovic N. Meeting the recommendations for cervical cancer screening in developing counties. 2014 national conference on cancer detection, diagnosis and treatment for global health. NIH, Bethesda, January 2014. Click here to view
209. Markovic N, Markovic O (2008/2010) What every women should know about cervical cancer. Springer, Dordrecht. http://www.springer.com/biomed/cancer/book/978-1-4020-6936-9
210. www.bioscicon.com/gallery.htlm. Accessed June 2015
211. www.bioscicon.com/pressrelease.html. Accessed June 2015
212. www.bioscicon.com
213. Markovic O, Markovic N (2013) IT telehealth center for telecytopathology. The FASEB J 27:874.20. Click here to view the abstract
214. Markovic N, Markovic O, Panashchenko O, McJonathan S. A tool for integration of cytology, HPV screening and telecytopathology. BIO 2008 international convention. San Diego, June 2008. Click here to download the abstract
215. Markovic O, Markovic N. IT enables same-day Pap test. Experimental Biology 2009, FASEB, April 2009. Click here to read the abstract
216. Markovic O, Markovic N. Cell phones as a new m-Health opportunity for mass cervical cancer screening. Experimental Biology 2010, FASEB, April 2010. Click here to read the abstract
217. BioSciCon's most recent advances in wireless telecytopathology. Click here to view the document
218. Markovic O, Markovic N. Further studies on the application of wireless cytopathology for detection of cervical cancer and initial screening for oral cancer. FASEB national meeting, Experimental Biology 2011, Washington, DC, April 2011. Click here to download the abstract
219. Markovic O, Markovic N (2012) Universal adapter for telecytopathology. The FASEB J 26, 1b476. Click here to view the abstract
220. www.bioscicon.com/publications html. Accessed June 2015
221. MarkPap India, LLC. Fighting cervical cancer in India. Brochure that can be retrieved by clicking on the link.Ch9/1
222. MarkPap Pacific, LLC. Cervical cancer in China. Brochure. Annex. China_13_brochure, F_2.pdf.Ch.9/2
223. Prof. K. Ganapathy. eHealth – The Enterprise of Healthcare ehealth.eletsonline.com/2011/04/tele-health-is-being. Personal Communication 2006–2015
224. Markovic N, Markovic O. MarkPap® test and human papilloma virus infected cells. ASCP annual meeting, 2005
225. Personal communications 2006–2015
226. Markovic N, Markovic O, Sundeen J (2004) Cervical acid phosphatase and Preservecyt®. Inv Med 52(Supp 2):80. See also reference 220, #10
227. Markovic N, Markovic O. Low-cost medical devices combined with telemedicine reduce reduce health disparities between developed and underdeveloped countries. National NIH conference on cancer detection and diagnostic technologies for global health, Bethesda 2011. Book of abstracts, p.138. www.bioscicon.com/publications.htlm #47. Retrieved August 2015
228. Athena HPV Trial. Roche diagnostic medical release. www.thealthenatrial.com. Retrieved August 2015
229. Cobas 600 Analyzer. Roche diagnostics. http://usdiagnostics.roche.com. Retrieved July 2015
230. Who Statistical Information System. www.who.int. Retrieved June 2015
231. List of counties by GOP per capita. https://en.wikipedia.org. Retrieved June 2015
232. Lantinal Cancer Institute. Surveilance Epidemiology and Results (SEER) Cervical cancer. http://seer.cancder.gov. Retrieved June 2015
233. Markovic N, Markovic O. Cervical Acid Phosphatase-Papanicolaou (CAP-PAP Test). Kit, method and accessories. Processes for producing and using the same. CAP-PAP test kit (short title). Published patent application #10/339.760. PCT. MarkPap system (Method, kit, solution and accessories). FP/W02004/063710

234. ACOG Guidelines. Screening for cervical cancer, topic page. March 2012. U.S. Preventive Services Task Force. http://www.uspreventiveservicestaskforce.org/uspstf/uspsc. Updated 2014. Retrieved May 2014
235. Saslow D, Solomon D, Lawson H, Killackey M, Kulasingam S et al (2012) American Cancer Society, American Society for Colposcopy and Cervical Pathology, and American Society for Clinical Pathology screening guidelines for the prevention and early detection of cervical cancer. J Low Genit Tract Dis 16(3):175–204 (ASCCP,ASC,ASCP)
236. New screening guidelines for cervical cancer, ACS (2012) www.cancer.org. Retrieved May 2014
237. WHO Guidelines (2013) Guidelines for screening and treatments of precancerous lesions for cervical cancer prevention. http://www.who.int
238. MarkPap India, LLC. See www.bioscicon.com

Index

N. Markovic, O. Markovic, *What Every Woman Should Know about Cervical Cancer*, DOI 10.1007/978-94-017-7560-1

MIX
Papier aus verantwortungsvollen Quellen
Paper from responsible sources
FSC® C105338

If you have any concerns about our products,
you can contact us on
ProductSafety@springernature.com

In case Publisher is established outside the EU,
the EU authorized representative is:
Springer Nature Customer Service Center GmbH
Europaplatz 3, 69115 Heidelberg, Germany

Printed by Libri Plureos GmbH
in Hamburg, Germany